The Environmental Threat to the Skin

Preparation of this book has been supported with a grant from Schering AG, Germany

The Environmental Threat to the Skin

Edited by

Ronald Marks
Professor of Dermatology
University of Wales College of Medicine
Cardiff, UK
and
Gerd Plewig
Professor of Dermatology
University of Düsseldorf
Düsseldorf, Germany

MARTIN DUNITZ

© Martin Dunitz 1992

First published in the United Kingdom in 1992
by Martin Dunitz Ltd, The Livery House, 7–9 Pratt Street
London NW1 0AE

All rights reserved. No part of this publication may be reproduced, stored in a retrieval system, or transmitted, in any form or by any means, without the prior permission of the publisher.

A CIP catalogue record of this book is available from the British Library.

ISBN 1-85317-057-7 (Martin Dunitz edition)
ISBN 1-85317-097-6 (Schering edition)

Composition by TecSet Ltd, Wallington, Surrey
Printed and bound in Great Britain by
The University Press, Cambridge.

Contents

Contributors   xi
Introduction   xix

Part I: Solar radiation and other climactic influences

1 Human exposure to ultraviolet radiation   3
   B. L. Diffey

2 Ozone depletion: historical review and prospects for the 21st century   11
   R. Russell Jones

3 The epidemiology of malignant melanoma   15
   R. M. MacKie

4 The epidemiology of non-melanocytic skin cancer in Australia   19
   Robin Marks

5 Sun exposure and solar damage in a Welsh population   23
   S. D. Shalom, R. Marks and I. Harvey

6 Photodysplasia: significance and measurement   27
   R. Marks, A. D. Pearse, P. Laidler and A. G. Knight

7 The effects of ultraviolet-B irradiation on proto-oncogene expression in normal human epidermis   33
   S. Takahashi, A. D. Pearse and R. Marks

8 From Slip! Slop! Slap! to SunSmart: the public health approach to skin cancer control in Australia in the 1990s   39
   Robin Marks

9 What do children know about the effects of sun on their skin?   43
   S. Blackford and D. Roberts

10 Ultraviolet radiation and the immune system   47
   W. L. Morison

11 Photoallergens and photosensitivity: current problems   51
    I. R. White

12 Drug and chemical photosensitization   57
    B. E. Johnson

13 Ultraviolet radiation and the photosensitivity disorders   67
    J. L. M. Hawk

14 Ultraviolet irradiation and thiazides: in vitro effects   73
    E. Selvaag, Th. Bergner and B. Przybilla

15 Mechanisms of photoaging   77
    K. Scharffetter-Kochanek, M. Wlaschek, K. Bolsen, G. Herrmann, P. Lehmann, G. Goerz, C. Mauch and G. Plewig

16 Assessment of actinic elastosis by means of high-frequency sonography   83
    K. Hoffmann, T. Dirschka, S. el-Gammal, and P. Altmeyer

17 Pigmented facial macules: a sign of photoaging?   91
    L. R. Lever and R. Marks

18 Differences between basal cell carcinoma arising in light-exposed and non-light-exposed skin   97
    R. J. Motley and R. Marks

19 Objective assessment of intra- and interindividual skin colour variability: an analysis of human skin reaction to sun and UVB   99
    S. el-Gammal, K. Hoffmann, P. Steiert, J. Gaβmüller, T. Dirschka and P. Altmeyer

20 Ultraviolet radiation induced erythema: a proposal for a computerized quantification   117
    G. C. Fuga, C. Spina, A. Di Palma, F. Acierno, G. F. Cirillo and W. Marmo

21 Microcirculatory damage in subjects exposed to the risk of ionizing radiation: image analysis and statistics of a 5-year observation   121
    G. C. Fuga, C. Cavallotti, A. Di Palma, F. Leonetti and W. Marmo

22 Mast cell degranulation results in endothelial activation after acute exposure of human skin to ultraviolet irradiation   125
    R. M. Lavker, M. S. Kaminer and G. F. Murphy

23 Advances in sunscreen protection and evaluation   131
    N. J. Lowe

24 Microfine titanium dioxide: a new route to dermatological sun protection   137
    E. Galley, D. Roberts and J. Ferguson

25 Visual display units and facial rashes: fact or fiction?   143
    A. J. Carmichael and D. L. Roberts

26 Skin complaints and visual display unit work: a psychophysiological approach   147
    M. Berg, B. Arnetz, S. Lidén, P. Eneroth and A. Kallner

27 A small solid state meter for measuring melanin pigmentation   149
    C. Edwards and R. Heggie

28 Subacute cutaneous lupus erythematosus probably caused by occupationally acquired chronic ultraviolet radiation   155
    M. Buslau

29 Seasonal influences on the occurrence of dry flaking facial skin   159
    M. D. Cooper, H. Jardine and J. Ferguson

Part II: Chemical Hazards in the Environment

30 Xenobiotic metabolism in the skin   167
    D. R. Bickers and H. H. Mukhtar

31 Cutaneous hazards associated with the use of cosmetics   173
    A. C. de Groot

32 Occupational plant dermatitis   177
    R. J. G. Rycroft

33 Xenobiotic experimentation: predicting percutaneous penetration   179
    J. Hadgraft and K. R. Brain

34 Chemical irradiation and predisposing environmental stress (cold wind and hard water)   185
    W. E. Parish

35 Immunotoxicity of heavy metal compounds   195
    H-C. Schuppe, P. Kind, C. Stringer and E. Gleichmann

36 Human skin response to irritants: the effect of UVA and UVB radiation on the skin barrier   203
    P. Lehmann, E. Hölzle, B. Melnik and G. Plewig

37 Sodium lauryl sulphate penetration through human skin   211
    B. Forslind, A. Emilson and M. Lindberg

38 Do transition metals in household and personal products play a role in allergic contact dermatitis?   215
    D. A. Basketter, E. G. Barnes and C. F. Allenby

39 The effect of area of application on the intensity of response to a cutaneous irritant   219
    P. J. Dykes, S. Hill and R. Marks

40 Contact dermatitis to paraphenylenediamine in hairdressers   225
    B. Santucci, G. C. Fuga, C. Cannistraci, W. Marmo, A. Cristaudo and M. Picardo

41 Euxyl K 400: a new allergen in cosmetic products   231
    A. Tosti, L. Guerra and F. Bardazzi

42 The skin equivalent as a genotoxicity model   233
    M. J. Edwards, P. J. Dykes, V. R. Merrett and R. Marks

43 Some new and alternative approaches to skin irritation testing   239
    D. Jirová, Z. Nikolová, S. Fiker and H. Janči

44 Cutaneous manifestations of tetrachlorodibenzo-*p*-dioxin in children and adolescents   247
    R. Caputo

45 Systemic toxicity in man secondary to percutaneous absorption   249
    S. Freeman and H. I. Maibach

46 Ivy shield: a new barrier cream for the prevention of poison ivy dermatitis   265
    D. F. Murrell and E. A. Olsen

47 Can health hazard associated with chemical contamination of the skin be predicted from simple in vitro experiments?   269
    C. Surber, K-P. Wilhelm, H. I. Maibach and R. H. Guy

48 Skin surface pH after short exposure to model solutions   277
    C. Surber, P. Itin and Th Rufli

49 Surfactant damaged skin: which treatment?   283
    E. Berardesca, G. P. Vignoli, G. Borroni, C. Oresajo and G. Rabbiosi

50 Three cases of urticaria caused by chronic exposure to pentachlorophenol   287
    J. Lambert, L. Matthieu, Ph. Jorens, P. Schepens and P. Dockx

51 Non-melanoma skin cancer and therapeutic agents   291
    J. H. Epstein

52 Skin tumour promotion and the wound response: two sides of a coin   297
    F. Marks, G. Fürstenberger and M. Gschwendt

53 The role of protein kinase C in epidermal differentiation and neoplasia   309
    A. A. Dlugosz, J. E. Strickland, G. R. Pettit and S. H. Yuspa

54 Effects of short-term surfactant exposure on stratum corneum capacitance and skin surface water loss   313
    K-P. Wilhelm, A. B. Cua and H. I. Maibach

55 The influence of hyaluronic acid on wound healing controlled by a standardized model for humans   319
    K. Winkler, K. Hoffmann, S. el-Gammal, B. Karmann and P. Altmeyer

56 Influence of short daily exposure to thermal water on the hydration state of the skin   333
    P. Clarys, C. Eeckhout, J. Taeymans, P. Gross and A. O. Barel

57 Experimental modelling of percussive mechanical trauma to the skin and its monitoring in the workplace   339
    C. Graves, C. Edwards and R. Marks

Part III: The Microbial Threat

58 The effects of global warming on skin infections and infestations   351
    D. Taplin, A. M. Allen, T. L. Meinking and S. L. Porcelain

59 The effects of arthropods on the skin   359
    D. A. Burns

60 Mediterranean sea and swimming pool dermatoses   **363**
J-P. Ortonne, M. Weiler, P. el Baze and A. Genollier-Weiler

61 The role of animals in the spread of fungal skin infections in humans   **377**
C. M. Philpot

62 Dermatophytes and human frequentation: a mycological environmental study   **381**
R. Mercantini, G. C. Fuga, D. Moretto and W. Marmo

63 The role of the cutaneous microflora in host defence and its response to the environment   **385**
J. H. Cove, E. A. Eady, J. L. Tipper and W. J. Cunliffe

64 The host's immunological contribution to the ecological battle on the skin surface   **391**
W. G. Gebhart and A. Kersten

65 The aetiology and treatment of fungal nail infection   **395**
D. T. Roberts

66 Microbiological, environmental and industrial challenge to an industrially orientated hydrocolloid dressing   **399**
P. G. Bowler and H. Delargy

Index   **407**

Contributors

F. Acierno	Istituto Dermatologica, Ospedale S. Maria and S. Gallicano, 00153 Rome, Italy
A. M. Allen	Pierce County Public Health Department, Tacoma, WA, USA
C. F. Allenby	Lister Hospital, Stevenage, Herts, UK
P. Altmeyer	Dermatologische Klinik der Ruhr-Universität, D – 4630 Bochum, Germany
B. Arnetz	National Institute for Psychosocial Factors and Health, Stockholm, Sweden
F. Bardazzi	Istituto di Clinica Dermatologica dell'Universita, via Massarenti 1, 40138 Bologna, Italy
A. O. Barel	Vrije Universteit Brussel, Pleinlaan 2, 1050 Brussels, Belgium
E. G. Barnes	Environmental Safety Laboratory, Unilever Research, Sharnbrook, MK44 1LQ, UK
D. A. Basketter	Environmental Safety Laboratory, Unilever Research, Sharnbrook MK44 1LQ, UK
E. Berardesca	Department of Dermatology, University of Pavia, IRCCS Policlinico S. Matteo, 27100 Pavia, Italy
M. Berg	Department of Dermatology, Karolinska Hospital, Stockholm, Sweden
Th. Bergner	Department of Dermatology, University of Munich, Munich, Germany
D. R. Bickers	Skin Diseases Research Center, Department of Dermatology, Case Western Reserve University, Cleveland, Ohio, USA
S. Blackford	Department of Dermatology, Singleton Hospital, Sketty Lane, Swansea SA2 8QA, West Glamorgan, UK
K. Bolsen	Department of Dermatology, University of Düsseldorf, Germany
G. Borroni	Department of Dermatology, University of Pavia, IRCCS Policlinico S. Matteo, 27100 Pavia, Italy
P. G. Bowler	ConvaTec, Newtec Square, Deeside Industrial Park, Deeside, Clwyd CH5 2NU, UK
K. R. Brain	The Welsh School of Pharmacy, University of Wales, Cardiff CF1 3XF, UK

D. A. Burns	Department of Dermatology, Leicester Royal Infirmary, Leicester LE1 5WW, UK
M. Buslau	Zentrum der Dermatologie und Venerologie, Abt. I, J. W. Goethe-Universität, Frankfurt am Main, Germany
C. Cannistraci	Istituto Dermatologica, Ospedale S. Maria and S. Gallicano, 00153 Rome, Italy
R. Caputo	1st Department of Dermatology, University of Milan, 20122 Milan, Italy
A. J. Carmichael	Department of Dermatology, University Hospital of Wales, Cardiff CF4 4XN, UK
C. Cavallotti	Istituto Dermatologica, Ospedale S. Maria and S. Gallicano, 00153 Rome, Italy
G. F. Cirillo	Istituto Dermatologica, Ospedale S. Maria and S. Gallicano, 00153 Rome, Italy
P. Clarys	Vrije Universteit Brussel, Pleinlaan 2, 1050 Brussels, Belgium
M. D. Cooper	Consumer Products Development, Boots Pharmaceuticals, 1 Thane Road, Nottingham NG2 3AA, UK
J. H. Cove	Department of Microbiology, University of Leeds, Leeds LS2 9JT, UK
A. Cristaudo	Istituto Dermatologica, Ospedale S. Maria and S. Gallicano, 00153 Rome, Italy
A. B. Cua	Dermatology Department, University of California Hospital, San Francisco CA 94143–0989, USA
W. J. Cunliffe	Departments of Dermatology and Microbiology, Leeds Foundation for Dermatological Research, Leeds General Infirmary, Leeds, LS1 3EX, UK
A. C. de Groot	Department of Dermatology, Carolus Hospital, 5200 BD 's-Hertogenbosch, The Netherlands
H. Delargy	ConvaTec, Newtec Square, Deeside Industrial Park, Deeside, Clwyd CH5 2NU, UK
B. L. Diffey	Regional Medical Physics Department, Dryburn Hospital, Durham DH1 5TW, UK
A. Di Palma	Istituto Dermatologica, Ospedale S. Maria and S. Gallicano, 00153 Rome, Italy
T. Dirschka	Dermatologische Klinik der Ruhr-Universität, D – 4630 Bochum, Germany
A. A. Dlugosz	Laboratory of Cellular Carcinogenesis and Tumor Promotion, National Cancer Institute, Bethesda MD 20892, USA
P. Dockx	Department of Dermatology, University of Antwerp, Universiteitsplein 1, B – 2610 Antwerp (Wilrijk), Belgium
P. J. Dykes	Department of Dermatology, University of Wales College of Medicine, Heath Park, Cardiff CF4 4XN, UK
E. A. Eady	Departments of Dermatology and Microbiology, Leeds Foundation for Dermatological Research, Leeds General Infirmary, Leeds, LS1 3EX, UK
C. Edwards	Department of Dermatology, University of Wales College of Medicine, Heath Park, Cardiff CF4 4XN, UK
M. J. Edwards	Department of Dermatology, University of Wales College of Medicine, Heath Park, Cardiff CF4 4XN, UK
C. Eeckhout	Vrije Universteit Brussel, Pleinlaan 2, 1050 Brussels, Belgium

P. el Baze	Laboratoire de Bactériologie, Hôpital Pasteur, Nice, France
S. el-Gammal	Dermatologische Klinik der Ruhr-Universität, D – 4630 Bochum, Germany
A. Emilson	Department of Medical Biophysics, Karolinska Institute, S – 104 01, Stockholm, Sweden
P. Eneroth	Research and Developmental Laboratory, Huddinge Hospital, Stockholm, Sweden
J. H. Epstein	Department of Dermatology, University of California, San Francisco CA 94143, USA
J. Ferguson	Consumer Products Development, Boots Pharmaceuticals, 1 Thane Road, Nottingham NG2 3AA, UK
S. Fiker	Institute of Hygiene and Epidemiology, Department of Environmental Health, Srobarova 48, 100 42 Prague 10, Czechoslovakia
B. Forslind	Department of Medical Biophysics, Karolinska Institute, S – 104 01, Stockholm, Sweden
G. C. Fuga	Istituto Dermatologica, Ospedale S. Maria and S. Gallicano, 00153 Rome, Italy
G. Fürstenberger	Institute of Biochemistry, German Cancer Research Center, Im Neuenheimer Feld 280, D – 6900 Heidelberg, Germany
J. Gaßmüller	Schering AG, D – 1000 Berlin, Germany
E. Galley	Boots Pharmaceuticals, Crooke's Healthcare, 1 Thane Road, Nottingham NG2 3AA, UK
W. G. Gebhart	Department of Dermatology II, University of Vienna, Alserstrasse 4, A – 1090 Vienna, Austria
A. Genollier-Weiler	Service de Dermatologie, Hôpital Pasteur, B.P. 69–06002 Nice cedex, France
E. Gleichmann	Medical Institute of Environmental Hygiene, Düsseldorf, Germany
G. Goerz	Department of Dermatology, University of Düsseldorf, Germany
C. Graves	Department of Dermatology, University of Wales College of Medicine, Heath Park, Cardiff CF4 4XN, UK
P. Gross	Kurzentrum, Lenk, Switzerland
M. Gschwendt	German Cancer Research Center, Institute of Biochemistry, D-6900 Heidelberg, Germany
L. Guerra	Istituto di Clinica Dermatologica dell'Universita, via Massarenti 1, 40138 Bologna, Italy
R. H. Guy	School of Medicine and School of Pharmacy, Departments of Dermatology, Pharmacy and Pharmaceutical Chemistry, University of California, San Francisco, USA
J. Hadgraft	The Welsh School of Pharmacy, University of Wales, Cardiff CF1 3XF, UK
I. Harvey	Centre for Applied Public Health Medicine, University of Wales College of Medicine, Heath Park, Cardiff CF4 4XN, UK
J. L. M. Hawk	Photobiology Unit, St Thomas' Hospital, London SE1 7EH, UK
R. Heggie	Department of Dermatology, University of Wales College of Medicine, Heath Park, Cardiff CF4 4XN, UK

P. C. Heinrich	Department of Biochemistry, RWTH Aachen, Germany
G. Hermann	Department of Dermatology, University of Düsseldorf, Germany
S. Hill	Department of Dermatology, University of Wales College of Medicine, Heath Park, Cardiff CF4 4XN, UK
K. Hoffmann	Dermatologische Klinik der Ruhr-Universität, D – 4630 Bochum, Germany
E. Hölzle	Department of Dermatology, Heinrich-Heine-University, Düsseldorf, Germany
P. Itin	University of Basel, Department of Dermatology, CH – 4031 Basel, Switzerland
H. Jančí	Institute of Hygiene and Epidemiology, Department of Environmental Health, Šrobárova 48, 100 42 Prague 10, Czechoslovakia
H. Jardine	Consumer Products Development, Boots Pharmaceuticals, 1 Thane Road, Nottingham NG2 3AA, UK
D. Jírová	Institute of Hygiene and Epidemiology, Department of Environmental Health, Šrobárova 48, 100 42 Prague 10, Czechoslovakia
B. E. Johnson	Department of Dermatology, University of Dundee, Dundee, UK
Ph. Jorens	Department of Toxicology, University of Antwerp, B-2610 Antwerp (Wilrijk), Belgium
K. Kaidbey	Department of Dermatology, University of Pennsylvania, Philadelphia PA 19104 – 6142, USA
A. Kallner	Department of Clinical Chemistry, Karolinska Hospital, Stockholm, Sweden
M. S. Kaminer	Department of Dermatology, University of Pennsylvania School of Medicine, Philadelphia PA, USA
B. Karmann	Dermatology Department, University of Bochum, Gudrunstrasse 56, 4630 Bochum, Germany
A. Kersten	Department of Dermatology II, University of Vienna, Alserstrasse 4, A-1090, Vienna, Austria
P. Kind	Department of Dermatology, Heinrich-Heine-University, Düsseldorf, Germany
A. G. Knight	Department of Dermatology, University Hospital of Wales, Cardiff CF4 4XN, UK
P. Laidler	Department of Pathology, University of Wales College of Medicine, Cardiff CF4 4XN, UK
J. Lambert	Department of Dermatology, University of Antwerp, Universiteitsplein 1, B – 2610 Antwerp (Wilrijk), Belgium
R. M. Lavker	Department of Dermatology, University of Pennsylvania, Philadelphia PA 19104 – 6142, USA
P. Lehmann	Department of Dermatology, Heinrich-Heine-University, Düsseldorf, Germany
F. Leonetti	Istituto Dermatologica, Ospedale S. Maria and S. Gallicano, 00153 Rome, Italy
L. R. Lever	Department of Dermatology, University of Wales College of Medicine, Heath Park, Cardiff CF4 4XN, UK
S. Lidén	Department of Dermatology, Karolinska Hospital, Stockholm, Sweden

M. Lindberg	Department of Occupational Dermatology, University Hospital, Uppsala, Sweden
N. J. Lowe	Skin Research Foundation of California, UCLA School of Medicine, 2001 Santa Monica Boulevard, Santa Monica CA 90404–2115, USA
R. MacKie	Department of Dermatology, University of Glasgow, Glasgow G11 6NU, Scotland, UK
H. I. Maibach	Dermatology Department, University of California Hospital, San Francisco CA 94143–0989, USA
F. Marks	Institute of Biochemistry, German Cancer Research Center, Im Neuenheimer Feld 280, D–6900 Heidelberg, Germany
R. Marks	Department of Dermatology, University of Wales College of Medicine, Heath Park, Cardiff CF4 4XN, UK
Robin Marks	Anti-Cancer Council of Victoria, 1 Rathdowne Street, Carlton South 3053, Australia
W. Marmo	Istituto Dermatologica, Ospedale S. Maria and S. Gallicano, 00153 Rome, Italy
L. Matthieu	Department of Dermatology, University of Antwerp, Universiteitsplein 1, B–2610 Antwerp (Wilrijk), Belgium
C. Mauch	Department of Dermatology, University of Cologne, Germany
T. L. Meinking	Department of Dermatology and Cutaneous Surgery, University of Miami School of Medicine, Miami FL, USA
B. Melnik	Department of Dermatology, Heinrich-Heine University, Düsseldorf, Germany
R. Mercantini	Istituto Dermatologica, Ospedale S. Maria and S. Gallicano, 00153 Rome, Italy
V. R. Merrett	Department of Dermatology, University of Wales College of Medicine, Heath Park, Cardiff CF4 4XN, UK
D. Moretto	Istituto Dermatologica, Ospedale S. Maria and S. Gallicano, 00153 Rome, Italy
W. L. Morison	Department of Dermatology, The Johns Hopkins Medical Institutions, 600 N. Wolfe Street, Baltimore, MA 21205, USA
R. J. Motley	Department of Dermatology, University of Wales College of Medicine, Heath Park, Cardiff CF4 4XN, UK
H. H. Mukhtar	Skin Diseases Research Center, Department of Dermatology, Case Western Reserve University, Cleveland, Ohio, USA
G. F. Murphy	Department of Dermatology, University of Pennsylvania, Philadelphia PA 19104–6142, USA
D. F. Murrell	Department of Dermatology, North Carolina Memorial Hospital, Chapel Hill, NC 27514, USA
Ž. Nikolová	Institute of Hygiene and Epidemiology, Department of Environmental Health, Šrobárova 48, 100 42 Prague 10, Czechoslovakia
E. A. Olsen	Division of Dermatology, Duke University Medical Center, Durham NC 27710, USA
C. Oresajo	Elizabeth Arden Biosciences, Trumbull CT, USA
J. P. Ortonne	Service de Dermatologie, Hôpital Pasteur, B.P. No. 69–06002 Nice cedex, France

W. E. Parish	Unilever Research, Colworth House, Sharnbrook, Bedford MK44 1LQ, UK
A. D. Pearse	Department of Dermatology, University of Wales College of Medicine, Heath Park, Cardiff CF4 4XN, UK
G. R. Pettit	Arizona State University, Tempe AZ 85287, USA
C. M. Philpot	Department of Medical Microbiology, University Hospital of Wales, Heath Park, Cardiff CF4 4XN, UK
M. Picardo	Istituto Dermatologica, Ospedale S. Maria and S. Gallicano, 00153 Rome, Italy
G. Plewig	Department of Dermatology, Heinrich-Heine-University, Düsseldorf, Germany
S. L. Porcelain	Departments of Dermatology and Cutaneous Surgery, and Epidemiology and Public Health, University of Miami School of Medicine, Miami FL, USA
B. Przybilla	Department of Dermatology, University of Munich, Munich, Germany
G. Rabbiosi	Department of Dermatology, University of Pavia, IRCCS Policlinico S. Matteo, 27100 Pavia, Italy
D. Roberts	Boots Pharmaceuticals Consumer Products Development, D98, 1 Thane Road, Nottingham NG2 3AA, UK
D. T. Roberts	Department of Dermatology, Southern General Hospital, Glasgow, G51 4TF, UK
D. L. Roberts	Department of Dermatology, Singleton Hospital, Sketty Lane, Swansea SA2 8QA, West Glamorgan, UK
Th Rufti	University of Basel, Department of Dermatology, CH – 4031 Basel, Switzerland
R. Russell Jones	St John's Dermatology Centre, St Thomas' Hospital, London SE1 7EH, UK
R. J. G. Rycroft	St John's Dermatology Centre, St Thomas' Hospital, London SE1 7EH, UK
B. Santucci	Istituto Dermatologica, Ospedale S. Maria and S. Gallicano, 00153 Rome, Italy
K. Scharfetter-Kochanek	Department of Dermatology, University of Düsseldorf, Germany
P. Schepens	Department of Toxicology, University of Antwerp, Universiteitsplein 1, B – 2610 Antwerp (Wilrijk), Belgium
H.-C. Schuppe	Department of Dermatology, Heinrich-Heine-University, Düsseldorf, Germany
E. Selvaag	Department of Dermatology, University of Munich, Munich, Germany
S. D. Shalom	Department of Dermatology, University of Wales College of Medicine, Heath Park, Cardiff CF4 4XN, UK
C. Spina	Istituto Dermatologica, Ospedale S. Maria and S. Gallicano, 00153 Rome, Italy
P. Steiert	Dermatologische Klinik der Ruhr-Universität, D – 4630 Bochum, Germany
J. E. Strickland	Laboratory of Cellular Carcinogenesis and Tumor Promotion, National Cancer Institute, Bethesda, MD 20892, USA
C. Stringer	Division of Immunology, Medical Institute of Environmental Hygiene, Heinrich-Heine-University, Düsseldorf, Germany
C. Surber	University of Basel, Department of Dermatology, CH – 4031 Basel, Switzerland, and University of California, San Francisco, USA

J. Taeymans	Kurzentrum, Lenk, Switzerland
S. Takahashi	Department of Dermatology, University of Wales College of Medicine, Heath Park, Cardiff CF4 4XN, UK
D. Taplin	Departments of Dermatology and Cutaneous Surgery, and Epidemiology and Public Health, University of Miami, Miami, Florida 33101, USA
J. L. Tipper	Department of Microbiology, University of Leeds, Leeds LS2 9JT, UK
A. Tosti	Istituto di Clinica Dermatologica dell'Universita, via Massarenti 1, 40138 Bologna, Italy
G. P. Vignoli	Department of Dermatology, University of Pavia, IRCCS Policlinico S. Matteo, 27100 Pavia, Italy
L. J. Walsh	Department of Dermatology, University of Pennsylvania, Philadelphia PA 19104–6142, USA
M. Weiler	Service de Dermatologie, Hôpital Pasteur, B.P. No. 69–06002 Nice cedex, France
I. R. White	St John's Dermatology Centre, St Thomas' Hospital, London SE1 7EH, UK
K.-P. Wilhelm	Department of Dermatology, Medical University of Lübeck, Germany, and University of California, San Francisco, California, USA
F. Wilmroth	Department of Biochemistry, RWTH Aachen, Germany
K. Winkler	Dermatologische Klinik der Ruhr-Universität, D – 4630 Bochum, Germany
M. Wlaschek	Department of Dermatology, University of Düsseldorf, Germany
S. H. Yuspa	Laboratory of Cellular Carcinogenesis and Tumor Promotion, National Cancer Institute, Bethesda MD 20892, USA
H. W. L. Ziegler-Heitbrock	Department of Immunology, University of Munich (LMU), Germany

Introduction

It has long been recognized that the skin's role as a barrier between a homeostatically maintained constant internal environment and the potentially hostile world outside is vital to life. Despite this recognition by all involved in some aspect of human biology, there seem to have been few attempts to gather together available information on the various environmental hazards between the covers of one book. Perhaps this has not been undertaken until now because of the logistical difficulty inherent in the cross disciplinary nature of the subject. Apart from dermatologists, some of the other major professional groups involved are toxicologists, internists, environmental scientists, pharmacologists, oncologists and microbiologists.

The other major stimulus to the study of environmental effects has been the dramatic rise in incidence in disorders resulting from interaction between the environment and the skin. Skin cancer, various forms of dermatitis and exotic infections are forcing their attention on physicians, and this has generated a general concern in the community. Clearly alterations in the earth's atmosphere and in the range and nature of chemical substances and microbes that contact human skin are to blame. But these alterations are mostly man made as well as being due to changed social patterns. It seems that the answer is in our hands and we hope that the work of the numerous scientists in different countries represented here will help persuade legislators and stimulate general awareness of the problems.

For the most part the contents are based on a conference held in Cardiff in April 1991, and we are extremely grateful to the large number of industrial concerns who generously gave their support for this symposium. We are particularly appreciative of an educational grant by Schering AG, Germany making possible the production of this book.

R. MARKS
G. PLEWIG

Part I: Solar radiation and other climatic influences

1
Human exposure to ultraviolet radiation

B. L. Diffey
Regional Medical Physics Department, Dryburn Hospital, Durham, UK

The radiant energy from the sun has been responsible for the development and continued existence of life on Earth. Approximately 5% of solar terrestrial radiation is ultraviolet radiation (UVR) and is the major source of human exposure. Prior to the beginning of the century, the sun was the only source of UVR but, with the advent of artificial sources, the opportunity for additional exposure has increased. Exposure may be intentional, e.g. cosmetic tanning from sun or solaria, or unintentional, often a consequence of occupational exposure. Within UVR, the biological effects can vary enormously with wavelength, and for this reason UVR is further subdivided into three regions: UVC, UVB and UVA.

UVC (280–100 nm) rays do not pass through the Earth's atmosphere. Nevertheless, UVC is produced by many artificial sources and can be particularly damaging to the eyes.

UVB (315–280 nm) rays are primarily responsible for nearly all biological effects following exposure to sunlight, namely sunburn, suntan and, after many years, premature aging of skin and skin cancer. Exposure of the eyes can produce photokeratitis and conjunctivitis. The only well-established benefit of exposure of normal skin is the production of vitamin D.

UVA (400–315 nm) rays are closest to the visible spectrum, pass through window glass and are least harmful on a dose-for-dose basis. They can produce erythema, tanning, skin aging, and cancer, but at doses about 1000 times greater than for UVB.

Sunlight

The spectrum of terrestrial sunlight extends from about 290 nm in the UV region up to about 2500 nm in the infra-red region. At noon during the summer in northern Europe, the irradiance on an unshaded horizontal surface is approximately 40 W/m^2 in the UVA spectrum and less than 3 W/m^2 in the UVB.

There are six principal factors that modify terrestrial UVR flux: time of day, season, geographical latitude, cloud cover, surface reflection and altitude.

Time of day: about 20–30% of total daily UVR is received from 11 am to 1 pm in summer, with 75% between 9 am and 3 pm.

Season: in temperate regions, seasons play an important role with regard to the UVR, especially UVB intensity at the Earth's surface. Seasonal variation is much less nearer the equator.

Geographical latitude: annual UVR flux decreases with increasing distance from the equator. Roughly, the annual number of minimal erythema doses (MEDs) on an unshaded, horizontal surface at midlatitudes (20–60°) can be estimated as annual MEDs = $2 \times 10^4 \exp(-\text{latitude}/20)$.

Cloud cover: clouds reduce UV intensity, although UVR changes are not so great as those of total intensity because water in clouds attenuates sunlight infra-red much more than UVR. The risk of over-exposure is thereby increased because the warning sensation of heat is diminished.

Even with heavy cloud cover, the scattered UVB

component of sunlight (often called skylight) is seldom less than 10% of that under clear sky; light clouds scattered over blue sky make little difference to sunburning effectiveness, unless directly covering the sun. Complete light cloud cover gives about 50% of the UVB energy, relative to clear sky, reaching the surface of the Earth. However, very heavy cloud cover can virtually eliminate UVB even in summer time.

Surface reflection: reflection of sunlight from the ground is normally unimportant as far as personal exposure is concerned. A grass lawn scatters about 3% of incident UVB radiation. Sand reflects about 25%, so that sitting under an umbrella on the beach can lead to sunburn both from scattered UVB from sky and reflected UVB from sand. It has been reported that fresh snow reflects up to 95% of incident sunlight, although reflectance of about 50% is probably more typical.

Ground reflectance from snow is important because reflected radiation exposes parts of the body normally shaded, such as eyes, which can lead to painful photokeratitis. In the case of skiing, there is the additional effect of altitude.

Contrary to popular belief, water reflects only about 5% of incident erythemal UVR. However, about 75% is transmitted through 2 m of clear ocean water, so swimming in either sea or open-air pools offers little protection against sunburn, since not only is water a good transmitter of UVR, but the swimmer may be exposed to a large area of sky and receive both direct radiation from the sun and a large part of the scattered radiation from sky.

Altitude: in general, each 300 m increase in altitude increases the sunburning effectiveness of sunlight by about 4%.

Intentional exposure

Sunbathing

Many people believe that sunlight is beneficial to their general well-being and, despite warnings about over-exposure, most of us enjoy relaxing in the sun. Sunbathing was practised by the Romans and Greeks 2000 years ago; enjoyment of sun has persisted.

Recreational sun exposure can result in an annual UV dose[1] of 20–100 multiples of an MED, often to a large fraction of the body surface area. In fact, the annual UV exposure of sun-loving indoor workers can result more from 2 or 3 weeks recreational exposure than from unintentional exposure during the remainder of the year.

In 1978, just under 1 million of 56 million residents of the UK went abroad for holidays. Ten years later, this figure had risen to 2.6 million (Department of Employment, personal communication, July 1989). Clearly, many more people are taking sunny holidays and this trend may be one reason for the increasing melanoma incidence.

Cosmetic UVR

The social desirability of a tanned skin is apparent and many people associate a bronzed body with good health. In northern Europe and America the lack of long periods of sunshine has led to the establishment of the 'suntanning industry', where artificial sources of UV radiation supplement sunlight exposure.

Prior to the late 1970s, the source of UVR was usually an unfiltered medium pressure mercury arc lamp mounted in a small table top unit. The units often incorporated one or more infra-red heaters and were commonly called 'sunlamps' or 'health lamps'. One disadvantage of this type of unit was that the area of irradiation was limited to a region such as the face and so whole body tanning was tedious. By incorporating several mercury arc lamps into a 'solarium', whole body exposure was achieved. Tanning devices based on mercury arc lamps emit relatively large quantities of actinic (UVB and UVC) radiation resulting in a significant risk of burning and acute eye damage.

The advent of high-intensity UVA fluorescent lamps in the 1970s coupled with the recognition that tanning could be induced by exposure to UVA radiation alone led to the development of sunbeds. These devices consist of a bed and/or canopy incorporating between 6 and 30 fluorescent lamps 150 or 180 cm in length. The most common type of UVA fluorescent lamp has a spectrum extending from 315 to 400 nm, peaking at around 352 nm. The UVA irradiance at the skin surface from a typical sunbed or suncanopy containing these lamps is between 50 and 150 W/m^2.

Surveys carried out in the Netherlands[2] and in the UK[3] in the mid-1980s showed that between 7 and 9% of the population in each country had used sunbeds in the previous 1–2 years. A more recent market survey in the UK,[4] with a sample of size of 5800, gave a slightly higher figure of 10% of the population having used a sunbed during the previous year (1988), with 19% of the sample admitting to using a sunbed at some time in the past. In these and other surveys in the UK[5] and the USA[6] women accounted for 60–85% of users, with about half the subjects being young women aged between 16 and 30 years. The most common reason for using tanning equipment is to acquire a pre-holiday tan; other reasons included the perceived health benefits, reduction of stress and improved relaxation, to achieve skin protection before going on holiday, to sustain a holiday tan and to treat skin diseases such as psoriasis and acne.

In the Dutch survey[2] about half the people interviewed used tanning equipment at home, and the other half used the facilities at commercial premises such as tanning salons, hairdressers, sports clubs, swimming pools, etc. Most people had used UVA equipment, with 24% using either mercury arc sunlamps or solaria. A more recent UK survey confirmed the Dutch findings that use at home or at commercial premises is split roughly equally. A survey carried out at commercial establishments only in the UK[5] inferred that all the equipment used emitted primarily UVA radiation, either fluorescent UVA lamps or optically filtered high-pressure lamps.

The mean number of tanning sessions per year was 24 in the Dutch survey and a half-hour session is the most popular.

Each tanning session with UVA equipment normally results in an erythemally weighted exposure of about 0.8 MED, whereas exposure with mercury arc lamps results in about 2 MED per session. From a survey of the use of artificial tanning equipment in the Netherlands[2] it was estimated that the median annual exposure was 24 MED with 10% of users receiving annual whole-body exposures from cosmetic tanning equipment in excess of 120 MED.

UVR in medicine

UVR has both diagnostic and therapeutic applications in medicine. The diagnostic uses are confined largely to fluorescence of either skin or teeth and the UVR source is normally an optically filtered medium pressure mercury arc lamp producing radiation mainly at 365 nm (Wood's lamps). Radiation exposure is limited to small areas (<15 cm diameter) and UVA radiation doses per examination are probably no more than 5 J/cm^2.

The therapeutic uses of UVR, which results in considerably higher UVR doses, are mainly concerned with the treatment of skin diseases and, occasionally, with the symptomatic relief of pruritus.

Phototherapy

The skin disease which responds most readily to UVR therapy is psoriasis, whilst other conditions which are sometimes treated by this technique are acne, eczema, alopecia, pityriasis rosea, superficial ulcers and pressure sores. Standard hospital phototherapy of psoriasis normally includes the use of tar or related derivatives, or other substances such as anthralin to the skin.

The therapeutic radiation for treating psoriasis lies principally within the UVB waveband and the cumulative UVB dose required for clearing is typically 200–300 MED,[7] usually delivered over a course consisting of 10–30 exposures over 3–10 weeks.[8]

Annual doses received by 90% of patients receiving UVB phototherapy for psoriasis range from about 60 to 670 MED with a median value of 240 MED.[9]

Psoralen photochemotherapy

This form of treatment, known colloquially as PUVA, involves the combination of the photoactive drugs, psoralens (P), with longwave UVR (UVA) to produce a beneficial effect. Psoralen photochemotherapy has been used to treat many skin diseases in the past decade, although its principal success has been in the management of psoriasis. The psoralens may be applied to the skin either topically or systemically; the latter route is generally preferred and the psoralens are administered as 8-methoxypsoralen (8-MOP). The patient ingests the 8-MOP tablets and, 2 h later, when the photosensitivity of the skin is at a maximum, is exposed to UVA radiation, normally from banks of fluorescent lamps. Values of UVA irradiance in clinical treatment cubicles have been found to range from 16 to 140 W/m^2, although an irradiance of 80 W/m^2 is probably typical. The UVA dose per treatment session is generally in the range 1–10 J/cm^2.

Treatment is given two or three times weekly until the psoriasis clears. The total time taken for this to occur will obviously vary considerably from one patient to another and, in some cases, complete clearing of the lesions is never achieved. However, it would be fair to say that something like 25 treatments are required to clear the psoriatic lesions in many patients over a period of between 6 and 12 weeks with a cumulative UVA dose of 100–250 J/cm^2.[10]

Unintentional exposure

Most people are unintentionally exposed to UVR. Exposure to natural UVR is unavoidable, whereas artificial UVR exposure occurs largely in the workplace.

Natural UVR exposure

Occupation is the prime determinant of unintentional exposure to solar UVR. Workers exposed to sunlight include farmers, construction workers, fishermen, gardeners, oil-field workers, road workers, police officers, sailors, and ski instructors. Representative values of annual, unintentional natural UV exposures of indoor and outdoor workers in midlatitudes (40–60° N) are given in Table 1. The ratio of UVA exposures between the two groups is less than that of UVB because window glass absorbs UVB radiation but transmits UVA.

There are groups, such as housebound elderly, some Asian immigrants and submariners, who receive almost no natural UV exposure and, as a consequence, may suffer vitamin D deficiency.

Occupational exposure from artificial UVR sources

Artificial sources of UVR are used in many different applications in the working environment. In some cases the UV source is well contained within an enclosure and, under normal circumstances, presents no risk of exposure to personnel. In other applications of UVR it is inevitable that workers will be exposed to some radiation, normally by reflection or scattering from adjacent surfaces. Under these conditions it is important that exposures be kept below maximum permissible limits for occupational exposure published by national regulatory authorities, either by administrative and engineering controls or by the use of protective clothing, eyewear and faceshields.

Industrial photoprocesses

Many industrial processes involve a photochemical component. The large-scale nature of these processes often necessitates the use of high-power (several kilowatts) lamps such as high-pressure metal-halide lamps.

Sterilization and disinfection

The bactericidal effects of sunlight were first noted by Downes and Blunt in 1877 and this property of UVR has been exploited for many years. Radiation with wavelengths in the range 260–265 nm is most effective since this corresponds with an absorption maximum in the DNA absorption spectrum. For this reason low-pressure mercury discharge tubes are often used as the radiation source as more than 90% of the radiated energy lies in the 253.7-nm line. These lamps are often referred to as 'germicidal lamps', 'bactericidal lamps', or simply 'UVC lamps'.

UVC has been used to disinfect sewage effluents, drinking water, water for the cosmetics industry and bathing pools. Germicidal lamps are sometimes used inside microbiological safety cabinets to inactivate airborne and surface micro-organisms. The combination of UVR and ozone has a very powerful oxidizing action and is capable of reducing the organic content of water to extremely low levels.

Welding

Welding equipment falls into two broad categories: gas welding and electric arc welding. Only the latter process produces significant levels of UVR, the quality and quantity of which depend primarily on the arc current, shielding gas and the metals being welded.

Welders are almost certainly the largest single occupational group exposed to artificial sources of

Table 1 Annual, unintentional natural UV exposures of indoor and outdoor workers in midlatitudes (40–60° N).

	UVB (MED)	UVA (J/cm^2)
Outdoor workers	250	3000
Indoor workers	70	1000

UVR. It has been estimated that there may be as many as half a million welders in the USA alone. The levels of UV irradiance around electric arc welding equipment are high[11] and it is not surprising that most welders at some time or other experience 'welder's flash' (photokeratitis) and skin erythema.

A survey of electric arc welders in Denmark[12] showed that 65% of those questioned had experienced erythema, although no indication of the frequency of skin reactions was reported and so it is not possible to make an estimate of annual exposure.

Phototherapy

Many of the lamps used to treat skin diseases are unenclosed, emit high levels of actinic UV radiation, and can present a marked UV exposure hazard to staff;[13] at 1 m from these lamps the recommended 8 h occupational exposure limits can be exceeded in less than 2 min.

From the results of a study of the occupational exposure to staff in hospital phototherapy departments,[14] it was shown[15] that the annual UV exposure of staff can be estimated from the number of occasions per year on which they experienced at least a minimal erythema. The estimated annual occupational UV exposures were 15, 92 and 200 MED corresponding to a frequency of erythema of once per year, once per month and once per week, respectively.

Operating theatres

UVC lamps have been used since the 1930s to decrease the levels of airborne bacteria in operating theatres. The technique is not widely used, filtered air units generally being preferred.

Fluorescence in cutaneous and oral diagnosis

Wood's light — a source of UVA obtained by optically filtering a mercury arc lamp with 'blackglass' — is used by dermatologists as a diagnostic aid in those skin conditions that produce fluorescence.

Irradiation of the oral cavity with a Wood's lamp will produce fluorescence which may prove useful in the diagnosis of various dental disorders, such as early dental caries, the incorporation of tetracycline into teeth, dental plaque and calculus.

Polymerization of dental resins

The restoration of pits and fissures in both deciduous and permanent teeth is often accomplished by using an adhesive resin polymerized with UVA. The resin is applied to the surfaces to be treated with a fine brush and is hardened by exposure to the UVA radiation at a minimum irradiance of 100 W/m^2 for 30 s or so. The restoration of teeth by resinous sealants is not only more aesthetically acceptable to patients than repair using conventional materials, but offers greater protection against tooth decay at the sites of pits and fissures. There is very little risk to the skin from the use of these appliances, but protective eyewear is recommended.

Research laboratories

Sources of UVR are commonly used by most experimental scientists engaged in aspects of photobiology and photochemistry. These applications, in which the effect of UV irradiation on the biological or chemical species is of primary interest to the researcher, can be differentiated from UV fluorescence or absorption techniques where the effect is of secondary importance.

Ultraviolet photography

There are two distinct forms of UV photography: reflected or transmitted UV photography; and UV fluorescence photography. In both applications the effective radiation lies within the UVA waveband.

Insect traps

Many flying insects are attracted to UVA radiation, particularly radiation in the wavelength region around 350 nm. This phenomenon is the principle of electronic insect traps in which a UVA fluorescent lamp is mounted in a unit containing a high-voltage grid. The insect, attracted by the UVA lamp, flies into the unit and is electrocuted in the air gap between the high-voltage grid and an earthed metal screen. Units such as these are commonly found in areas where food is prepared and sold to the public.

Sunbed salons and shops

The continuing popularity of UVA sunbeds and suncanopies for cosmetic tanning has resulted in a large number of salons, where the public go to use sunbeds, and shops selling sunbeds for use at home. Some shops may have 20 or more UVA tanning appliances all switched on exposing members of the public and, more importantly, staff to high levels of UVA radiation.

Discotheques

UVA 'blacklight' lamps are sometimes used in discotheques to induce fluorescence in the skin and clothing of dancers. The UVA levels would normally be low (<10 W/m^2).

Offices

Signature verification is commonly performed by exposing a signature, obtained previously with a colourless ink, to UVA radiation under which it fluoresces.

General lighting

Fluorescent lamps used for general lighting in offices and factories emit small quantities of both UVA and UVB. For typical levels of illuminance of 500 lux from bare fluorescent lamps found in the UK, measurements have indicated[16] UVA and UVB irradiances of about 30 mW/m^2 and 3 mW/m^2, respectively. These UV levels give rise to an annual exposure of no more than 5 MED to indoor workers, and this dose can be reduced appreciably by the use of plastic diffusers. A study of the personal UV doses received by workers in the car manufacturing industry who were engaged in inspecting paintwork of new cars under bright fluorescent lamps indicated a similar annual UV exposure.[17]

However, spectroradiometric measurements of the UV levels from indoor lighting fluorescent lamps carried out in the USA[18] indicated much higher annual doses for persons occupationally exposed for 2000 h/year. Typical estimates were about 18 MED per year for an illuminance level of 500 lux.

Desk-top lamps which incorporate tungsten halogen lamps may emit levels of UVR which can result in exposure to the hands and arms of a person using the lamps in excess of recommended occupational exposure levels.[19]

References

1. Diffey BL, Human exposure to ultraviolet radiation, *Sem Dermatol* (1990) **9**: 2–10.
2. Bruggers JHA, deJong WE, Bosnjakovic BFM et al, Use of artificial tanning equipment in the Netherlands. In: Passchier WF, Bosnjakovic BFM, (eds). *Human exposure to ultraviolet radiation: risks and regulations*, Amsterdam: Excerpta Medica, 1987, pp. 235–9.
3. The truth about tanning, *Which?*, London: Consumers Association, 1987, 214–6.
4. McLauchlan R, UK population attitude to tanning, unpublished data, 1989.
5. Diffey BL, Use of UV-A sunbeds for cosmetic tanning, *Br J Dermatol* (1986) **115**: 67–76.
6. Dougherty MA, McDermott RJ, Hawkins MJ, A profile of users of commercial tanning salons, *Hlth Values* (1988) **12**: 21–9.
7. Larkö O, Phototherapy of psoriasis — clinical aspects and risk evaluation, *Acta Dermatol Venereol (Stockh)* (1982) (suppl 103).
8. van der Leun JC, van Weelden H, Phototherapy: principles, radiation sources, regimens. In: Hönigsmann H, Stingl G, (eds). *Therapeutic photomedicine*, Basel: Karger, 1986, pp. 39–51.
9. Slaper H, Skin cancer and UV exposure: investigations on the estimation of risks, Ph.D. thesis, Utrecht, 1987, pp. 40–2.
10. Hensler T, Wolff K, Hönigsmann H et al, Oral 8-methoxypsoralen photochemotherapy of psoriasis. The European PUVA study: a cooperative study among 18 European centers, *Lancet* (1981) **i**, 853–7.
11. Cox CWJ, Ultraviolet irradiance levels in welding processes, In: Passchier WF, Bosnjakovic BFN, (eds). *Human exposure to ultraviolet radiation: risks and regulations*, Amsterdam: Excerpta Medica, 1987, pp. 383–6.
12. Eriksen, P. Occupational applications of ultraviolet radiation: risk evaluation and protection techniques. In: Passchier WF, Bosnjakovic BFM, (eds). *Human exposure to ultraviolet radiation: risks and regulations*, Amsterdam: Excerpta Medica, 1987, pp. 317–30.

13 Diffey BL, Langley FC, *Evaluation of ultraviolet radiation hazards in hospitals*, London: Institute of Physical Sciences in Medicine, 1986.
14 Larkö O, Diffey BL, Occupational exposure to ultraviolet radiation in dermatology departments, *Br J Dermatol* (1986), **114**: 479-84.
15 Diffey BL, Ultraviolet radiation and skin cancer: are physiotherapists at risk? *Physiotherapy* (1989) **75**: 615-6.
16 McKinlay AF, Whillock MJ, Measurement of ultraviolet radiation from fluorescent lamps used for general lighting and other purposes in the UK. In: Passchier WF, Bosnjakovic BFM, (eds). *Human exposure to ultraviolet radiation: risks and regulations*, Amsterdam: Excerpta Medica, 1987, pp. 253-8.
17 Diffey BL, Larkö O, Meding B et al, Personal monitoring of exposure to ultraviolet radiation in the car manufacturing industry. *Ann Occup Hyg* (1986) **30**: 163-70.
18 Cole C, Forbes PD, Davies RE et al, Effect of indoor lighting on normal skin, *Ann NY Acad Sci* (1985) **453**: 305-16.
19 McKinlay AF, Whillock MJ, Meulemans CCE, Ultraviolet radiation and blue-light emissions from spotlights incorporating tungsten halogen lamps, *Report NRPB-R228*, Didcot, National Radiological Protection Board, 1989.

2
Ozone depletion: historical review and prospects for the twenty-first century

Robin Russell Jones
St John's Dermatology Centre, St Thomas' Hospital, London, UK

Concern about the ozone depleting potential of man-made chemicals was first expressed in 1974, when *Nature* published a paper by Molina and Rowland predicting catalytic destruction of stratospheric ozone by free radicals generated by the action of sunlight on long-lived chlorine and bromine bearing compounds.[1] Of chief concern were chlorofluorocarbons (CFCs), widely used at that time in aerosols, food packaging, insulation, refrigeration and air conditioning. However, these warnings were not heeded except in the USA, where CFC propellants were banned in aerosols. Unfortunately, other uses were not curtailed; other applications were found, such as the cleaning of electronic circuitry, so that by 1985 annual production of the three main CFCs (CFCs 11, 12 and 113) was running at 1000 million kg/year. Since CFCs have very long atmospheric residence times (110 years in the case of CFC 12) atmospheric levels were increasing by between 5% and 10% per annum. Production of bromine bearing compounds such as Halons 1211 and 1301 was much less, only 10 million kg/year for each compound. However, halons are widely used in fire-extinguishing systems and are of particular concern since their ozone-depleting potential is approximately 10 times greater than the most damaging of the fully halogenated CFCs, atmospheric levels are rising more rapidly, at over 20% per annum, and a large pool is now banked in fire-extinguishing systems worldwide, awaiting release at some future date. Furthermore, there are indications that gas-phase reactions involving bromine monoxide and chlorine monoxide are synergistic, and that bromine bearing compounds account for up to 25% of the ozone losses observed over Antarctica.[2]

The United Nations Environment Programme (UNEP) was established in 1972 following an international conference in Stockholm on the state of the world environment. Ozone depletion was one of the first issues which UNEP addressed, but it was not until 1985 that the Vienna Convention for the Protection of the Ozone Layer was drawn up.[3] This coincided with the publication in *Nature* by the British Antarctic Survey of huge ozone losses over Antarctica during springtime.[4] The extent of the depletion and its rapidity made natural perturbations unlikely, and this observation transformed the status of ozone depletion from a peripheral issue to the centre stage of scientific enquiry.

It was recognized early on that large reductions in CFC emissions would be needed merely to stabilize CFC levels in the atmosphere. As stated in an article in the *Lancet* in August 1987,[5] 'Under U.N. auspices most of the major industrial nations have now signed the Vienna Convention for the protection of the ozone layer, but specific targets have been more difficult to achieve... For CFCs with atmospheric residence times of more than a century, only an 85% cut in output will stabilize atmospheric concentrations at their present level. ... Failure to agree further measures may yet impose grave burdens on future generations'.

In September 1987, the world's prime consumers and manufacturers of CFCs met in Montreal and agreed a cut in CFC consumption of 50% by the year 2000. Production, however, would be cut by only 35% to make allowance for developing and low consumer countries that might want to import more CFCs as their economies develop. Halon production was to be frozen at 1986 levels.[3] Needless to say, the Montreal Protocol did little to allay anxiety, and in October 1987 the results of a multinational scientific study in Antarctica provided unequivocal evidence of the primary role of man-made chemicals in depleting ozone over Antarctica.[6] It has been observed with some justification that the only reason why the Montreal Protocol was agreed so quickly was that much stricter measures would have been necessary once the results of the Antarctica survey became available.

In March 1988, the Ozone Trends Review Panel published a report showing that ozone depletion was not confined to extreme latitudes in the southern hemisphere, but that modest and significant losses of ozone were occurring in northern latitudes, overlying heavily populated areas of the globe. Since 1970, for example, there had been a year-round loss of 2–3% in total column ozone at latitudes 53°–64°N with maximum depletion of 8% occurring in mid-winter.[6] These data could not unequivocally identify man-made chemicals as the cause, but the observations were certainly consistent with the effects of man-made releases and were greater than had been predicted by the two-dimensional models of ozone depletion available at that time.

In November 1988, an international conference on ozone depletion was held in London which brought together for the first time the politicians, scientists and environmentalists in a public arena. The conference proceedings were subsequently published.[7] In the week preceding the conference the British Prime Minister, Margaret Thatcher, had stated that she herself would host a UN conference on ozone depletion in London in March 1989. Whether the timing of Margaret Thatcher's announcement was fortuitous or deliberate, it had a dramatic effect on the media, who poured journalists, television crews and radio reporters into the conference. Over the course of 2 days, more than 30 reports appeared in major national newspapers and 13 interviews took place on national radio and television. Other environmental issues had never attracted such attention in the UK and it marked the beginning of a major shift in public awareness on the environment. For perhaps the first time people became aware of the destructive power of uncontrolled industrial activity, and the fragility of the world's ecosystems. This concern was reflected in the results of the European elections the following year when the British Green Party, having polled less than 1% at the previous elections, achieved 15% of the total vote — more than in any other country within the European Community.

Meanwhile, in the USA the Environmental Protection Agency was producing some uncompromising predictions on future levels of chlorine in the atmosphere.[8] Under Phase I of the Montreal Protocol, chlorine levels were set to rise from below 3 ppb to 14 ppb by the year 2100. Since natural chlorine levels are below 0.6 ppb, and since the ozone hole over Antarctica had appeared between 1.5 and 2 ppb, the idea of allowing chlorine levels to reach 14 ppb caused considerable dismay. Even industrial giants such as Du Pont and ICI expressed concern. Simultaneously, UNEP was working hard to tighten the Protocol and in June 1990, Phase II of the Protocol was drawn up in London. Under the new agreement, fully halogenated CFCs, halons and carbon tetrachloride will be phased out by the year 2000, and methylchloroform by the year 2005. Limits on chemical substitutes such as HCFCs, which have limited ozone depleting potential, were discussed but not included in the agreement. However, this is unlikely to be the end of the story. Even under the terms of the new Protocol, chlorine levels will reach 4.5–5 ppb by the beginning of the next century, will stay above 3 ppb until the middle of the next century and will not fall below 2 ppb until the end of the next century. This means that the ozone hole over Antarctica will remain for at least the next century. Furthermore, there is still a 10 year derogation for developing nations and compliance may be incomplete. India and China in particular have yet to sign Phase II of the Protocol.

The issue has again been thrown into sharper focus by the recent data from NASA, showing that ozone depletion is occurring globally and progressing even faster than previously realised.[9] A Lancet editorial on the subject suggested that the phase-out date for CFCs carbontetrachloride and methylchloroform should be brought forward to 1995 and that halons should be banned immediately for all but the most essential uses.[10] This seems particularly important since halons are currently sold for use in the home, large quantities are released during routine fire-fighting practices, and there are no schemes to recycle or destroy existing stocks. Halons do offer considerable advantages over alternative fire retardants in the sense that they are relatively non-damaging to equipment and relatively non-toxic to humans, but their use should be severely restricted to situations where alternatives are unusable, i.e. in aircraft, tunnels and the control rooms of nuclear reactors, where personnel cannot or should not abandon their positions.

There is also an urgent need to examine the environmental impact of the chemical substitutes now being developed by industry. These fall into two main groups: hydrochlorofluorocarbons (HCFCs) which have limited ozone depleting potential, and hydrofluorocarbons (HFCs) which have no ozone depleting potential.[11] Unfortunately, both groups of chemicals are greenhouse gases, not as powerful as the fully halogenated CFCs but nonetheless significant. If CFC emissions were uncontrolled they would contribute 30% of the global warming effect due to carbon dioxide alone by the year 2030.[12] If HCFC 22 is used to substitute CFCs, it could contribute 15% by the year 2030. Similar, though less immediate, considerations apply to HFC 134a, industry's favourite substitute for CFC 12 in fridges and air-conditioning systems. Using a 20-year time frame, CFC12 has a global warming potential of 6200,[13] that is, 6200 times greater than an equivalent weight of carbon dioxide. HFC 134a has a global warming potential of 2800, and could contribute 15% or 20% of the global warming effect of carbon dioxide alone by the end of the next century.[14]

At present industry is reluctant to abandon these substitutes, partly because they are an improvement on the existing CFCs, but also because they wish to protect their commercial interests. It is important that the world community understands the dangers of these substitutes and develops alternative technologies, rather than substitute chemicals.

CFCs are not the only link between ozone depletion and global warming. Tropospheric, i.e. ground-level ozone, is a powerful greenhouse gas and contributes up to 10% of the global warming effect of carbon dioxide alone. Ozone production at ground level is driven photochemically, so as stratospheric ozone declines more ultraviolet radiation (UVB) penetrates the lower atmosphere, thus enhancing production of tropospheric ozone. Ozone is a powerful respiratory irritant and commonly exceeds World Health Organization (WHO) guidelines in many parts of the UK. At lower levels it is known to affect plant growth, reduce crop production and has been incriminated as one of the main causes of forest damage in Central Europe and tree die-back in the UK. Increasing UVB also affects crop production adversely, so any plant growing in the early part of the next century will already be under considerable stress.[15] Consider, in addition, the effect upon marine ecosystems. Some plankton are highly UV sensitive. Since plankton photosynthesize carbon dioxide, reduced viability from increased UVB will compound global warming by depleting a major oceanic sink of carbon dioxide. Extremes of temperature, drought and violent storms will become the norm for agricultural crops struggling to survive in a soil impoverished by years of acidification, pesticide use and over-production. It is the combined effect of several environmental insults acting simultaneously that will be so damaging to the integrity of terrestrial and marine ecosystems. Predictions as to the effects of stratospheric ozone depletion on human health relate mainly to skin cancer and cataract formation, since this is where most of the scientific certainty lies and likely increases are relatively easy to predict.[5,16] I am not alone, however, in thinking that global food production may collapse in the early part of the next century.[17] Unless there are major changes in attitude by governments world-wide, skin cancer and cataract formation will be two of the least important effects on human health resulting from ozone depletion in the stratosphere.

References

1 Molina MJ, Rowland FS, Stratospheric sink for chlorofluorocarbons: chlorine atom catalyzed destruction of ozone, *Nature* (1974) **249**: 810–14.
2 Anderson JG, Brune WH, Lloyd SA et al, Kinetics of O_3 destruction by ClO and BrO within the antarctic vortex: an analysis based on in situ ER-2 data, *J Geophys Res* (1989) **94**: D9: 11480–11520.
3 Usher P, The Montreal Protocol on substances that deplete the ozone layer: its development and likely impact. In: Russel Jones R, Wigley T (eds). *Ozone depletion: health and environmental consequences*, Wiley, Chichester, 1989.
4 Farman JC, Gardiner G, Shanklin JD, Large losses of total ozone in Antarctica reveal seasonal ClO_x/NO_x interaction, *Nature* (1985) **315**: 207–10.
5 Russell Jones R, Ozone depletion and cancer risk, *Lancet* (1987) **ii**: 443–6.
6 Watson RT, Present state of knowledge of the ozone layer. In: Russell Jones R, Wigley T (eds). In: *Ozone depletion: health and environmental consequences*, Wiley, Chichester, 1989.
7 Russell Jones R, Wigley T, (eds), *Ozone depletion: health and environmental consequences*, Wiley, Chichester, 1989.
8 Report of the Technology Review Panel, *Technical progress on protecting the ozone layer*. United Nations Environment Programme, 30 June 1989, UN, Geneva.
9 National Aeronautics and Space Agency, Ozone observations, press statement prepared by Watson RT, Process Studies Program Office, Earth Science and Application Division, NASA, April 1991.
10 Anonymous, Ozone depletion quickens, *Lancet* (1991) **337**: 1132–3 (editorial).

11 Tane CE, Alternatives to CFCs. In: Russell Jones R, Wigley T, (eds). *Ozone depletion: health and environmental consequences*, Wiley, Chichester, 1989.
12 Wigley T, Future CFC concentrations under the Montreal Protocol and their greenhouse-effect implications, *Nature* (1988) **335**: 333.
13 Atomic Energy Research Establishment, *Trace gases and their relative contribution to the greenhouse effect, AERE 13716*, HMSO: London, 1990.
14 Shine KP, The greenhouse effect. In: Russell Jones R, Wigley T, (eds). *Ozone depletion: health and environmental consequences*, Wiley, Chichester, 1989.
15 Worrest RC, Grant LD, Effects of ultraviolet-B radiation on terrestrial plants and marine organisms. In: Russell Jones R, Wigley T (eds). *Ozone depletion: health and environmental consequences*, Wiley, Chichester, 1989.
16 Russell Jones R, Consequences for human health of stratospheric ozone depletion. In: Russell Jones R, Wigley T (eds). *Ozone depletion: health and environmental consequences*, Wiley, Chichester, 1989.
17 Sir Crispin Tickell demands action to avoid ecological disaster, *The Times*, 27 April 1991, p2.

3
The epidemiology of malignant melanoma

Rona M. MacKie
Department of Dermatology, University of Glasgow, Glasgow, UK

At present the number of patients with melanoma of the skin increase steadily each year. The annual rate of increase is of the order of 5–8%[1] in most countries, and melanoma is increasing in incidence faster than most other malignancies, exceeded only by lung cancer in women. Mortality is also increasing, and in young men death from melanoma is exceeded only by death from road traffic accidents, leukaemias, and, more recently, AIDS. These depressing statistics are unfortunately not accompanied by any effective new therapy in the management of advanced melanoma. For this reason, a number of countries in Europe have embarked on educational exercises aimed both at encouraging earlier recognition of established disease,[2] and also at encouraging a more cautious approach to sun exposure, which is believed to be the prime aetiological factor.

In both these educational approaches it is important to target the educational message to the appropriate section of the population, so it is necessary to define the high-risk group. To achieve this aim, the epidemiological tool of the case-control study has been used. These are deceptively simple, but in reality surprisingly powerful, techniques comparing features of melanoma patients with those of age and sex-matched local control individuals. These studies have recently been carried out in Scotland,[3] Denmark,[4–6] Western Canada[7,8] and Germany.[9] In most case-control studies the population includes only superficial spreading and nodular melanoma patients, but as these two histogenetic types comprise around 70% of all melanomas in most series, they still gave valuable information relevant to the majority of patients.

Melanoma is a disease of white-skinned individuals, and in the USA the incidence is about one-tenth as common in blacks who live the same lifestyle in the same areas as whites. Furthermore, it is a problem of white-skinned peoples of northern European descent, so the incidence is higher in Scandinavians and Scots than in Spaniards and Italians.

There is a 5–8% incidence of second primary tumours, so the patient who has already had one melanoma is at risk of a second tumour. This has implications for follow-up, as the entire integument should be examined, not just the scar and nodal drainage area. About 5% of all melanomas are found in a familial setting, commonly but not exclusively in patients with multiple naevi, so first-degree relatives of melanoma patients are at increased risk, and should be educated on the features of early curable melanoma.

The large case control study carried out by Gallagher and Elwood[7] in Western Canada indicated that intermittent intense sun exposure of normally covered skin resulting in burning was a very strong risk factor for melanoma. The Canadian study attempted to quantify hours of sunlight exposure over a lifetime, and concluded that for melanoma the risk is associated with relatively brief but intense and burning sun exposure, in contrast to non-melanoma skin cancer. Indeed, this study suggested that an outdoor occupation and very high numbers of hours of exposure were actually mildly protective against melanoma.

The work of Østerlind and colleagues from Denmark has also emphasized the importance of intense intermittent rather than regular continuous sun exposure as a risk factor, and has further emphasized the importance of sun exposure early in life before the age of 25 years. Østerlind's studies were among the first to identify the importance of large numbers of banal or ordinary non-dysplastic naevi as a powerful risk factor. As trained interviewers who were not dermatologists carried out the counting, this was only conducted on the upper arms, and palpable naevi on this site were counted. The presence of five or more such naevi was a powerful risk factor.

The most recent case-control study from Scotland has used a study population all of whom were patients with cutaneous melanoma first diagnosed in Scotland in the year 1987, and from the data obtained a risk-factor chart has been devised. Using the log rank test to place risk factors in order of importance while allowing for the effect of the other risk factors, the most powerful risk factor by a considerable margin is the total number of banal, non-dysplastic naevi. This is based on total body naevus counts all carried out on both melanoma and control patients by one trained dermatologist. The second most powerful but independent risk factor is a tendency to freckle. For the study, complex maps of sites of freckles and of intensity of freckling were devised, but the risk was not affected by this and was related simply to the presence or absence of any freckles. The third most important risk factor was the presence of three or more clinically atypical naevi defined as naevi with a diameter of 5 mm or greater, and having at least one of an irregular edge, irregular colour, or inflammation. Many naevi with such characteristics will be pathologically dysplastic naevi, but as the purpose of the study was to derive a risk-factor chart which would be of clinical relevance, there was no requirement for biopsy in the study. The fourth most important risk factor was a history of three or more episodes of severe sunburn at any time prior to developing melanoma. These four features taken together gave a useful distinction between melanomas and controls, and the risk-factor chart (Figure 1) derived from it is currently being validated on a separate melanoma population from the same geographical area.

The strongest consistent risk factor to emerge from all the case-control studies to date is the presence of large numbers of banal non-dysplastic naevi or moles. This can be determined either by total body naevus counts or by counting the number of palpable naevi on the upper arms. The presence of five or more such naevi is a strong risk factor. The tendency to freckle is a risk factor independent of naevi, and is an additional risk factor. In addition, clinically atypical naevi, which are frequently but not always pathologically dysplastic naevi, are a third independent risk factor. The presence of three or more such naevi increases the melanoma risk.

Fair or red hair and blue or green as opposed to brown eyes are also additional but weak risk factors in some series.

The history of past sun exposure and the individual's response to that sun exposure also produce a group of additional risk factors. At present the evidence indicates that short sharp episodes of intense sun exposure rather than lifetime cumulative sun exposure is important in the evolution of melanoma. Thus, in most studies melanoma is a problem of the indoor worker who enjoys sunny holidays, rather than of the outdoor worker. The Danish studies have emphasized the role of outdoor activities such as bathing and boating as additional risk factors. Individuals who burn rather than tan on sun exposure are also at increased risk, and a history of sunburn in childhood, or of severe sunburn at any time is an additional risk factor. Studies from both Australia and Israel show that those who have spent their childhood in a sunny country are at greater risk than those who emigrated there as young adults, emphasizing the importance of protecting the skin of children from strong sun exposure.

Factors which are not associated with an increased risk include use of the oral contraceptive, dietary habits, and smoking. In the early 1980s Beral et al[10] suggested, on the basis of an Australian case-control study of females, that exposure to fluorescent light was a risk factor, but no large study since that time has confirmed this observation. A second isolated and interesting observation is the higher than expected incidence of melanoma at the Lawrence Livermore atomic energy research laboratory in California.[11] Workers have a higher incidence of melanoma than those in the same geographical area, but no other atomic research centre records a higher than expected number of melanoma cases, so the reason for the Livermore excess remains to be clarified.

In summary, the individual at greatest risk of melanoma is a Caucasian with fair skin which burns rather than tans in the sun. He or she may have spent their childhood in a sunny country, and may have a history of severe burning. They will have large numbers of naevi and also freckles. Such individuals urgently need advice about recognizing early melanoma and also about limiting further damaging sun exposure. However, the exact role

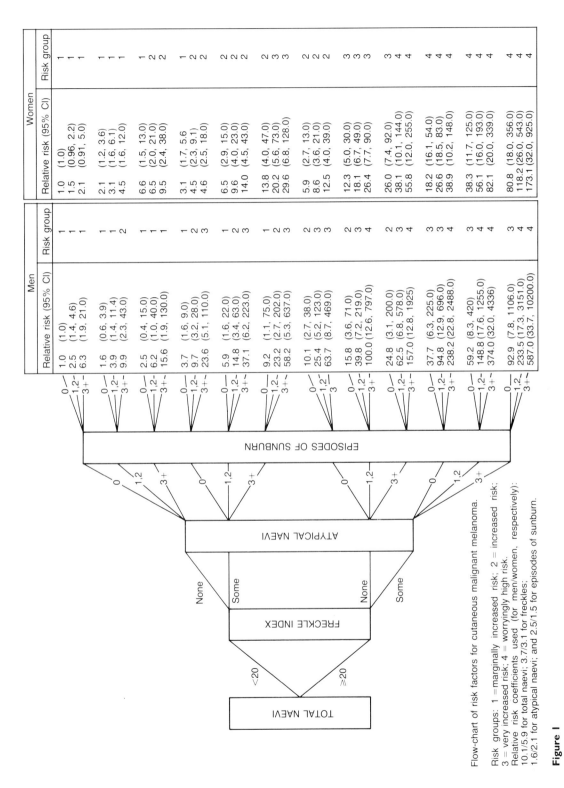

Figure 1

Flow chart of risk factors for cutaneous malignant melanoma. Risk groups: 1 = marginally increased risk; 2 = increased risk; 3 = very increased risk; 4 = worryingly high risk. Relative risk coefficients used (for men/women, respectively): 10.1/5.9 for total naevi; 3.7/3.1 for freckles; 1.6/2.1 for atypical naevi; and 2.5/1.5 for episodes of sunburn. (Reproduced with permission.[3])

of environmental sun exposure in initiating and progressing the molecular changes which result in melanoma is not yet established. This information would give valuable data and possibly help to define a group of individuals with precursor stages of fully developed melanoma. The current lack of a biologically relevant animal model is a major problem in this area.

References

1. Moller Jensen O, Esteve J, Moller H et al, Cancer in the European Community and its member states, *Eur J Cancer* (1990) **26**: 1167–256.
2. Doherty VR, MacKie RM, Experience of a public education programme on early detection of cutaneous malignant melanoma, *Br Med J* (1988) **297**: 388–91.
3. MacKie RM, Freudenberger T, Aitchison TC, Personal risk-factor chart for cutaneous melanoma, *Lancet* (1989) **ii**: 487–90.
4. Osterlind A, Tucker MA, Hou-Jensen K et al, The Danish case-control study of cutaneous malignant melanoma. I. Importance of host factors, *Int J Cancer* (1988) **42**: 200–6.
5. Østerlind A, Tucker MA, Stone BJ et al, The Danish case-control study of cutaneous malignant melanoma. II. Importance of UV-light exposure, *Int J Cancer* (1988) **42**: 319–24.
6. Østerlind A, Tucker MA, Stone BJ et al, The Danish case-control study of cutaneous malignant melanoma. IV. No association with nutritional factors, alcohol, smoking or hair dyes, *Int J Cancer* (1988) **42**: 825–8.
7. Elwood JM, Gallagher RP, Davison J et al, Sunburn, suntan and the risk of cutaneous malignant melanoma — the Western Canada Melanoma Study, *Br J Cancer* (1985) **51**: 543–9.
8. Elwood JM, Williamson C, Stapleton PJ, Malignant melanoma in relation to moles, pigmentation, and exposure to fluorescent and other lighting sources, *Br J Cancer* (1986) **53**: 65–74.
9. Garbe C, Wiebelt H, Orfanos CE, Change of epidemiological characteristics of malignant melanoma during the years 1962–1972 and 1983–1986 in the Federal Republic of Germany, *Dermatologica* (1989) **178**: 131–5.
10. Beral V, Evans S, Shaw H et al, Malignant melanoma and exposure to fluorescent lighting at work, *Lancet* (1982) **ii**: 290–3.
11. Schneider JS, Moore DH II, Sagebiel RW, Early diagnosis of cutaneous malignant melanoma at Lawrence Livermore National Laboratory, *Arch Dermatol* (1990) **126**: 767–9.

4
The epidemiology of non-melanocytic skin cancer in Australia

Robin Marks
Anti-Cancer Council of Victoria, Carlton South 3053, Victoria, Australia

In 1988, Australians celebrated the bicentenary of British settlement of this hot, sunny country in the antipodes. Just over 200 years since the first colony was established, subsequent immigration (for a large proportion of that time as a result of a selective immigration policy) has led to a population in Australia in which over 90% are classified as white. This legacy, plus a change in fashion in the last 60 years which dictated that a suntan is desirable, has led to skin cancer becoming a major public health problem in Australia.

The exact extent of the problem has only become clear following recent population-based cross-sectional and longitudinal epidemiological studies. Prior to these studies, considerable under-reporting of non-melanocytic skin cancer (NMSC) occurred because the vast majority of patients with these tumours were treated in private practice from which there is no reporting mechanism to cancer registries, and in which in many cases there was no histological confirmation of the clinical diagnoses.[1]

Recently, a number of community-based studies in localized areas in Queensland (Nambour), Western Australia (Geraldton) and Victoria (Maryborough) have revealed that the prevalence proportion of NMSC is now of the order of 2–5% of people aged 40 years and over who have at least one tumour.[2–4] The ratio of basal cell carcinoma (BCC) to squamous cell carcinoma (SCC) ranges from 2:1 to 5:1 in these studies in which all tumours recorded have been histologically confirmed.

The incidence rate of new tumours in these community-based studies has varied from 870 per 100 000 per year in Victoria to over 1300 per 100 000 per year in Queensland.[5,6] A national 12-month incidence survey of 31 000 people by Gallup Poll interview revealed an annual incidence rate of 823 per 100 000 for the whole country in 1985.[7] This varied from 489 per 100 000 in those people living south of latitude 37°S to 1242 per 100 000 in those living north of 29°S. The age-standardized incidence rates for BCC and SCC in the national study were 657 and 166 per 100 000, respectively. This survey sought only people who had received treatment within the 12 month incident period, and there may have been under-reporting of the true incidence rate for that period if it missed some people who did not seek treatment for a tumour which had developed during that period. Despite this, the method is satisfactory and reproducible for determining trends in incidence and has been repeated on 60 000 people in 1990, 5 years after the initial study.

The site distribution of tumours in these studies has been changing, particularly for BCC, in recent years. In the past, it has been suggested that up to 90% of BCCs occur on the head and neck. The study from Geraldton in Western Australia reported 53% of BCCs in men and 43% in women on the trunk. Most of these occurred on the upper back and shoulders. This figure is quite substantially different from the 81% of BCCs found to occur on the head and neck in a recent incidence study done in West Glamorgan, South Wales.[8] In the National Australian survey, 66% of BCCs were on the head and neck and 18% on the trunk. In the survey from Nambour in Queensland, the prevalence of BCCs on the trunk and limbs was over twice that on the maximal exposure sites of the head, neck, hands and forearms.

This change in the distribution of BCC has not been accompanied by a similar change in the distribution of SCC. However, in the Nambour study, 61% of people who had a full body examination had solar keratoses (SKs) on sites other than the head and neck, hands and forearms. If the change in distribution of BCC is attributed to changing bathing and exposure habits, then more work is necessary to explain why this has not been followed by a similar pattern in SCC. It may mean that BCCs require less exposure to induce a lesion than SCCs. This could partly explain why the highest proportion of BCCs occurring on the trunk are being reported from areas of high insolation, i.e. Nambour in Queensland and Geraldton in Western Australia, compared to areas such as the National Australian survey which includes southern Australia and the West Glamorgan, South Wales study. However, it must be borne in mind that not only are the radiation levels different in these different areas, but the temperature is also different. In the north of Australia, including Geraldton and Nambour, high temperatures may induce people to expose far more of their body to sunlight for longer periods than the colder parts of Australia or the UK.

The data from all recent studies confirm the risk factors for NMSC, including increasing age; sex (men greater than women); work patterns (outdoor workers greater than indoor workers); and skin type (greater in those who burn only and never tan when exposed unprotected to strong sunlight compared with those who tan only and never burn). On the latter point, although the rate ratio for those people who say they burn only when exposed unprotected to the strong sunlight compared to those who tan only is between 2 and 3, the absolute incidence rate for those who in the National survey said they tan only was 616 per 100 000. This rate is higher than previously reported for a population in any other country in the world. It suggests that the ability to tan in fair-skinned people certainly does not prevent NMSC. It suggests also that it may not be necessary to be exposed to doses of sunlight sufficient to cause burning to be at risk of these tumours.

Another major risk factor for both BCC and SCC is the presence of one or more solar keratoses.[6,9] The prevalence of SKs in the community surveys was of the order of 50–60% of people aged 40 years and over. The age-specific prevalence rates varied from 7.3% of 20–29 year olds to 73.6% of 60–69 year olds in Queensland. The incidence rates are even higher in people aged over 69 years.

The incidence rate of NMSC is significantly higher for people born in Australia than those who have migrated from the UK at some stage in their life.[7] Using SK as a surrogate for NMSC, a study comparing Australian born people to British migrants who came to Australia at different ages revealed that exposure to Australian sunlight in childhood and adolescence (less than 20 years) was a major risk factor for SK and, by implication, NMSC in adulthood.[10]

A prospective study on the rate of malignant transformation of SK to SCC has revealed that probably less than 1 in 1000 of these lesions transforms to SCC within 1 year.[11] A similar prospective study showed that a substantial proportion of SKs may remit spontaneously within a 12 month observation period, particularly in those who have the ability to reduce their sunlight exposure.[12]

A follow-up study of 291 people with 297 SCCs revealed a metastasis rate of 2% overall, and 1.6% for tumours arising in light exposed areas, excluding the lip, within 2 years.[13] This confirmed the results of other studies that the risk of metastasis from SCC arising in light exposed areas, although real, is relatively small.[14,15] It also confirmed that it is necessary to follow-up patients with SCC for at least 2 years in an attempt to detect secondary tumours as they become clinically apparent.

Finally, we still do not know the exact amount of sunlight necessary to cause NMSC. A study comparing the prevalence of SK in populations in Melbourne and Maryborough, one degree of latitude north of Melbourne, showed a greater than 50% increase in the age-adjusted prevalence rate in Maryborough which has 14% more UVB compared to Melbourne.[16] Transposing the national survey data on to ultraviolet radiation (UVR) grid maps of Australia reveals that for each 1% increase in UVR received over a lifetime, there would be a 1.41% increase in NMSC in southern Australia and a 2.36% increase in the north of the country.[17,18] These estimates, plus the above epidemiological data, are a warning of the need to take steps to protect our population today and prevent further ozone depletion in the future.

References

1 Ponsford MW, Goodman G, Marks R, The prevalence and accuracy of diagnosis of non-melanotic skin cancer in Victoria, *Aust J. Dermatol* (1983) **214**: 79–82.

2. Green A, Beardmore G, Hart V et al, Skin cancer in a Queensland population, *J Am Acad Dermatol* (1988) **19**: 1045–52.
3. Kricker A, English DR, Randell PL, Skin cancer in Geraldton, Western Australia: a survey of incidence and prevalence, *Med J Aust* (1990) **152**: 399–407.
4. Marks R, Ponsford MW, Selwood TS et al, Non-melanotic skin cancer and solar keratoses in Victoria, *Med J Aust* (1983) **2**: 619–22.
5. Marks R, Jolley D, Dorevitch AP et al, The incidence of non-melanocytic skin cancer in an Australian population: results of a five year prospective study, *Med J Aust* (1989) **150**: 475–8.
6. Green A, Battistutta D, Incidence and determinants of skin cancer in a high-risk Australian population, *Int J Cancer* (1990) **46**: 356–61.
7. Giles GG, Marks R, Foley P, Incidence of non-melanocytic skin cancer treated in Australia, *Br Med J* (1988) **296**: 13–17.
8. Lloyd-Roberts D, Incidence of non-melanoma skin cancer in West Glamorgan, South Wales, *Br J Dermatol* (1990) **122**: 399–403.
9. Marks R, Rennie G, Selwood TS, The relationship of basal cell carcinomas and squamous cell carcinomas to solar keratoses, *Arch Dermatol* (1988) **124**: 1039–42.
10. Marks R, Jolley D, Lecatsas S et al, The role of childhood sunlight exposure in the development of solar keratoses and non-melanocytic skin cancer, *Med J Aust* (1990) **152**: 62–5.
11. Marks R, Rennie G, Selwood TS, Malignant transformation of solar keratoses to squamous cell carcinoma in the skin: a prospective study, *Lancet* (1988) **i**: 795–7.
12. Marks R, Foley P, Goodman G et al, Spontaneous remission of solar keratoses: the case for conservative management, *Br J Dermatol* (1986) **115**: 649–55.
13. Nixon RL, Dorevitch AP, Marks R, Squamous cell carcinoma of the skin: accuracy of clinical diagnosis and outcome of follow-up in Australia, *Med J Aust* (1986) **144**: 235–9.
14. Lund HZ, How often does squamous cell carcinoma of the skin metastasize? *Arch Dermatol* (1965) **92**: 635–7.
15. Moller R, Reymann F, Hou-Jensen K, Metastases in dermatological patients with squamous cell carcinoma, *Arch Dermatol* (1979) **115**: 703–5.
16. Marks R, Selwood TS, Solar keratoses — the association with erythemal ultraviolet radiation in Australia, *Cancer* (1985) **56**: 2332–6.
17. Barton IJ, Paltridge GW, The Australian climatology of biologically effective ultra-violet radiation, *Aust J Dermatol* (1979) **20**: 68–74.
18. Marks R, Possible effects of increased ultra-violet radiation on the incidence of non-melanocytic skin cancer. In: *Health effects of ozone layer depletion: A report of the NHMRC Working Party, Melbourne, 1989*, Commonwealth Government Printer: Canberra, 1989, pp. 70–81.

5
Sun exposure and solar damage in a Welsh population

S. D. Shalom, R. Marks and I. Harvey*

*Department of Dermatology, and *Department of Community Medicine, University of Wales College of Medicine, Cardiff, UK*

Introduction

Out-patient data from the University Hospital of Wales (UHW), Cardiff, show a surprisingly high rate of referral for solar keratoses and non-melanoma skin cancer. Clinic-based figures showed that these disorders comprised 8% of all new dermatology referrals.[1]

Since it is widely assumed that people of Celtic origin are more prone to photodamage and UVR skin cancer,[1-3] and because South Wales is not a 'sun blessed' region but likely to have a large population of Celtic origin, the present survey was planned in order to characterize the extent of the problem.

In essence it was decided to perform a community-based study to assess both the prevalence and incidence of solar keratoses and skin malignancy in South Glamorgan, and to relate this data to likely predisposing factors such as age, sex, skin type, sun exposure, sunscreen usage and directness of Celtic lineage. Most previous studies of this type have relied on clinical criteria for diagnosis, but in this study it was decided to employ two validation procedures: close-up photography of all suspected lesions were taken for subsequent evaluation by a panel of experts and histological examination of a proportion of lesions.

The natural history of solar keratoses and their rate of transformation to squamous cell carcinomas was also assessed.

Method

A computerized random sample of subjects over the age of 60 years was taken from the South Glamorgan family practitioner register. The general practitioners of 1044 subjects were contacted and of these 793 subjects proved contactable (i.e. alive and living in South Glamorgan). Of these 559 (71%) were seen. A year later 501 of these 559 subjects could be contacted and 396 (79%) were seen again by the same surveyor.

On both occasions that the subjects were interviewed the light-exposed areas of skin were carefully examined. In addition to photography of suspected solar keratoses (SKs), polaroid photographs were also taken on the first visit to gauge the position of lesions for subsequent assessment of their natural history. Biopsy of a proportion of lesions was performed on the second visit; lesions that did not appear to be clinically certain SKs were predominantly sampled.

Two methods of measuring directness of Celtic lineage were employed. The first method used parental Welsh surnames as described in a paper from workers in West Glamorgan.[4] The other method was based on parental birthplace in regions considered to have a high prevalence of Celtic ancestry (Wales, Ireland and Scotland).

For validation, 160 of the close-up slides were chosen at random and shown to a panel of three experienced dermatologists who recorded their clinical diagnoses blind and without data or consultation. These diagnoses were compared with those of the surveyor, and the results analysed statistically using Cohen's kappa (κ) calculation which allows for chance agreement between observers.

Results

Photographic validation

Significant agreement ($P = 0.04$, $\kappa = 22.1\%$) was found between all four observers. The κ value for the surveyor compared to the majority panel decision was very similar ($\kappa = 21.5\%$) but just failed to reach formal significance. This implied a degree of over-diagnosis and suggested the estimated total number of lesions should be reduced to 89%.

Histological validation

Of 38 lesions biopsied, 20 were definite SKs, 16 were lentigos or seborrhoeic warts. The diagnosis was uncertain with the remainder. Hence only 56% were SKs, but as the lesions sampled were difficult to diagnose clinically, and since less than 10% of lesions were biopsied anyway, further correction is very difficult. Clearly the most pessimistic correction is a further 44% but in view of the type of lesion biopsied, it is suggested that not more than a further 20% reduction is justifiable. The results presented below are based on the surveyor's figures prior to validation.

Age, sex, skin type and life-time daylight exposure

There was a significant increase in the prevalence of lesions with age, male sex and lower numerical skin type (Boston classification) (Tables 1 to 3). During interview questions were asked which allowed an assessment to be made of each subject's cumulative sun exposure (in hours). There was a highly significant relationship between this and the prevalence of SKs (Table 4).

Table 2 Prevalence of SKs and skin type

Skin type*	Total no. of SKs	No. of subjects with SKs	Proportion of subjects with SKs (%)
I	47	20	43
II	193	56	29
III	240	45	19
IV	74	6	8
V	3	0	
VI	2	0	

* Boston classification.

Table 3 Sex distribution of subjects with SKs

Sex	Total no. of subjects seen	No. of subjects with lesions	Proportion of subjects with lesions (%)
Male	232	76	33
Female	327	51	16
Total	559	127	22.7

Table 1 Age distribution of subjects with SKs*

Age (years)	Total No. SKs detected	No. of subjects with SKs	Proportion of subjects with SKs (%)
60–65	135	18	13
65–70	164	23	18
70–75	89	25	28
75–80	89	32	36
80–85	50	16	32
85–90	24	7	29
90–95	6	4	67
95–100	2	2	100

* The total number of SKs observed on initial visits was 395 lesions.

Table 4 Lifetime sun exposure and SK prevalence

Total exposure (hours $\times 10^3$)	Subjects with SKs (%)
0–10	0
10–20	0
20–30	7
30–40	16
40–50	30
50–60	21
60–70	22
70–80	33
80–90	30
>90	40

The Chi squared test for trend shows that there is a significant trend toward there being a greater proportion of solar keratoses in those who have been more sun exposed ($P = 0.0007$).

Sunscreen usage

Sunscreens were used regularly by 188 subjects (34%). No relationship was found between the skin type and sunscreen usage (χ^2 test for trend, $P = 0.8$). Of those who used sunscreens, 18.9% had SKs. Of those who did not 30.3 had lesions. This implied that usage seemed to confer significant protection against development of lesions (χ^2 test, $P = 0.03$).

Celtic origin

No significant relationship was found between 'Celticity' measured by parental Welsh surnames and the presence of SKs ($P = 0.77$), or with skin type ($P = 0.71$), or with degree of solar damage as assessed by using the visual analogue scale assessment ($P = 0.43$).

Using the birthplace index, no significant relationship was found of this with solar damage ($P = 0.30$) or with the presence of SKs ($P = 0.15$), although had there been larger numbers in the study it is likely that this relationship would have reached significance.

Natural history of solar keratoses

Expressed as a percentage of lesions present at the second visit, 31% of lesions had remitted and 42% of those lesions present at the second visit were judged as 'new' as they had not been recorded at the first visit. During the survey no cases of transformation from SKs to squamous cell carcinoma were found.

Discussion

The results tend to support our clinic-based data in that the prevalence of SKs in South Wales appears high and comparable to some estimates made in sunnier climates.[5] However there is no available data for elsewhere in the UK with which to make a valid comparison. The relationships of the prevalence with age, sex and skin type support the findings made in previous studies.[5]

The apparent protection conferred by sunscreens found in this survey is surprising since, apart from limited clinical use of early products containing titanium dioxide, effective sunscreens have only been generally available in the last 20 years. If the conclusion is valid, and the results not confounded by other variables, this could suggest that 10 years of sunscreen usage in this age group significantly reduces the risk which would tend to modify the generally accepted 'cumulative sun exposure' model. Further multivariate analysis is in progress to 'harden' the data and take into account such factors as age, sex and sun-exposure habits. (Our data suggested that skin type is highly unlikely to be a confounding variable.)

It was disappointing not to confirm our strong clinical suspicion that individuals of Celtic ancestry were not especially prone to SKs or solar damage. The weak correlation between the presence of SKs and one of our indices of 'Celticity' which failed to reach formal significance levels suggests that further work is needed. It could be that intermarriage and geographical mobility have vitiated the results. One could also postulate that colonial populations in New World communities tend to retain a greater degree of genetic homogeneity, but this would not explain the apparent predilection for sun-induced skin damage noted in the Welsh population.

The natural history of SKs showing remission of some lesions and *de novo* lesions on follow-up supports previous work done in Maryborough.[6] Our figures show surprising agreement in the proportion of lesions that 'come and go' despite the differences in population and climatic environment. The very low tendency toward malignant change of solar keratoses to squamous cell carcinomas was first observed during a 5-year follow-up study in Australia.[7] This observation is supported by our results, which has important implications for the clinical management of SKs.

Acknowledgement

S. D. S. was supported by grants from the "Welsh Scheme", Roche, UK, Ltd, and Sandoz, UK, Ltd.

References

1 Marks R, Premalignant disease of the epidermis, *J R Coll Phys (London)* (1986) **20**: 116–21.

2 O'Beirn SF, Judge P, Urbach F et al, Skin cancer in County Galway, Ireland, *Proceedings of the National Cancer Conference, Philadelphia* (1970) **6**: 489–500.
3 Lane Brown MM, Sharpe CAB, Macmillan DS et al, Genetic predisposition to melanoma and other skin cancers in Australians, *Med J Aust* (1971) **i**: 852–3.
4 David JB, Ashley H, Davies D, The use of the surname as a genetic marker in Wales, *J Med Genet* (1966) **3**: 203–11.
5 Harvey I, Shalom SD, Marks R et al, Non-melanoma skin cancer, *Br Med J* (1989) **299**: 1118–20.
6 Marks R, Foley P, Goodman G et al, Spontaneous remission of solar keratoses: the case for conservative management, *Br J Dermatol* (1986) **115**: 649–55.
7 Marks R, Rennie G, Selwood TS, Malignant transformation of solar keratoses to squamous cell carcinoma, *Lancet* (1988) **i**: 795–7.

6
Photodysplasia: significance and measurement

R. Marks, A. D. Pearse, P. Laidler* and A. Knight
*Department of Dermatology, and *Department of Pathology, University of Wales College of Medicine, Heath Park, Cardiff CF4 4XN, UK*

Persistent exposure to solar ultraviolet irradiation (UVR) results in a series of changes in the skin that have come to be known collectively as photoaging. Non-melanoma skin cancer and solar keratoses are not infrequent components of this clinical picture even in temperate zones not renowned for the dangers of sunburn, such as the region in which the Cardiff group of dermatologists practice.[1,2] The incidence of such problems appears to be increasing in the affluent West as a result of the social trends to increased leisure time and the popularity of outdoor activities. In some parts of the world, such as Australia, all forms of skin cancer, including melanoma skin cancer, have become a major health problem in the community.[3,4]

The most obvious clinical consequences of long continued sun exposure and solar damage to the skin are due to solar elastotic degeneration of the dermal connective tissue in which the exposed skin becomes finely lined, yellowish and inelastic (Figure 1). It is also commonplace for individuals who show extensive changes of this sort to have solar keratoses on exposed sites. These small, scaling or horny lesions are classified as 'premalignant', although it is now evident that it is extremely uncommon for any particular solar keratosis to transform into a frank squamous cell carcinoma. But even if solar keratoses are not clinically evident, biopsy of apparently normal but exposed skin will frequently show minor morphological abnormalities in the epidermis. Accompanying these alterations there is thickening of the epidermis and a significantly raised rate of epidermal cell production as judged by the tritiated thymidine autoradiographic labelling index.[5] Further witness to this subclinical epidermal disturbance may be demonstrated cytochemically by alterations in glucose-6-phosphate dehydrogenase and succinic dehydrogenase activities in the epidermis.[6]

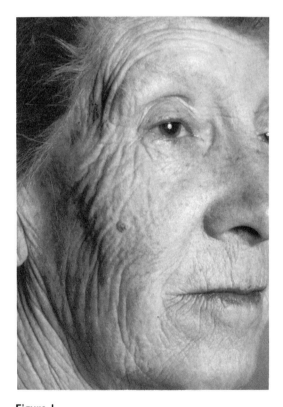

Figure 1

Solar elastotic degenerative change in a woman of late middle age with marked wrinkling of the skin and a yellowish discolouration.

The changes in keratinocyte morphology are not dissimilar to premalignant alterations seen in other epithelia including the uterine cervix, the bronchial mucosa and the epithelial lining of the gastrointestinal tract — particularly the colon and oesophagus. These are known collectively as dysplasia — literally meaning disordered growth.

Cytological alterations evoked in keratinocyte morphology by chronic exposure to UVR (photodysplasia) include heterogeneity in cell size and shape and loss of the normal vertical orientation in the process of epidermal differentiation (sometimes known as loss of polarity) (Figures 2 and 3). Changes are subtle and may be called 'minimal dysplastic change' with some justification as they are usually unaccompanied by marked alteration to the epidermal architecture or the presence of dyskeratotic cells, or even a marked subepidermal lymphocytic cellular infiltrate, such as are seen in solar keratoses.

The extent of such minor changes appears to be related to the degree of solar injury but their exact relationship to frank neoplasia is uncertain as has already been pointed out with regard to solar keratoses. It is also unclear as to whether these changes are reversible and, if so, whether any particular therapy is more or less effective in causing improvement than any other. These and related questions are not readily answerable without some form of quantitative assessment of the degree of dysplasia present. Similar considerations have led to the development of techniques for scoring the degree of dysplasia present in bronchial mucosa[7] and in the uterine cervical mucosa.[8] Classifications also exist for quantifying the degree of malignancy and invasiveness for frank epithelial cancers such as the Duke system for classification of colonic tumours[9] and the Breslow and Clarke[10,11] methods for categorizing the 'degree of malignancy' of malignant melanomata. Although the general purpose of all these techniques is quite similar, the measurement of the degree of dysplasia is somewhat different from the assessment of the degree of malignancy and invasiveness for at least three reasons. In the first place the alterations being assessed are important prognostically as in the Duke system for colonic carcinoma, but we have no quantitative idea as to the clinical significance of the degree of dysplasia present in the epidermis. Secondly, in photodysplasia the abnormalities are confined to the epidermis. In addition, the dysplastic changes are for the most part much more subtle to the eye and training is required in order to detect and assess them as well

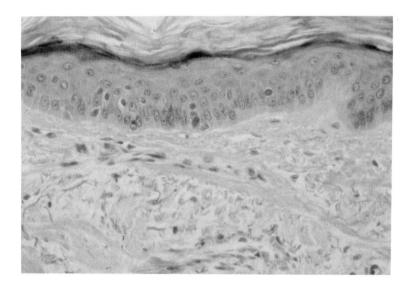

Figure 2

Minimal dysplastic change with some loss of cell polarity and irregularity of epidermal profile. There is also some heterogeneity of cell size.

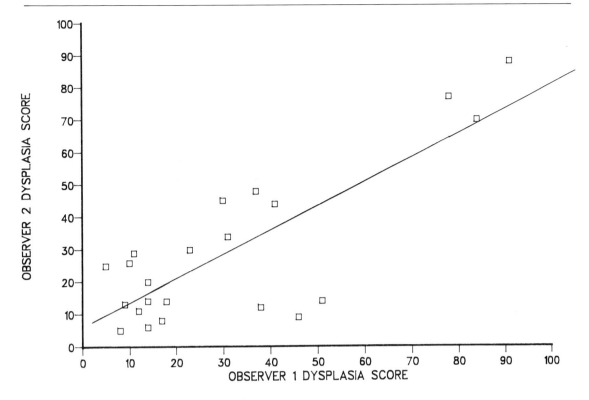

Figure 3

Inter-observer correlation of dysplasia scores of histological sections of biopsies using visual analogue scales (inter-observer correlation, Spearman's rho = 0.52, $P = <0.01$).

as the development of novel parameters and criteria.

We have assessed three approaches. The first of these uses a subjective visual scoring technique in which visual analogue scales (VAS) are used. The second was an attempt to make the assessment as objective as possible by deriving a dysplasia index using histometric and image analysis techniques. Both of the above methods have been described elsewhere, but recently we have again evaluated the VAS method alongside a further subjective technique.

Visual analogue scale scoring method

In this simple technique, representative histological sections from punch biopsies, stained with haematoxylin and eosin, are examined microscopically without the observer knowing their origin, and the degree of dysplasia marked off on a 10 cm line (zero representing no dysplasia and 10 representing the severest degree of dysplasia imaginable).

In a previous study,[12] we found surprisingly good interobserver reproducibility ($P < 0.01$) (Figure 3) as well as excellent intraobserver repeatability. Our group have used this VAS technique for the evaluation of dysplasia on several occasions previously. For example, we measured the degree of dysplasia in solar keratoses during the VAS method before and after intralesional injection of interferon α 2β in order to correlate the degree of dysplasia with other histological features in the lesion.[13] We have also employed the VAS method in studies of the Darier-like keratoses[14] and of lichenoid solar keratoses.[15]

In the present study the three observers concerned (A.K., P.L. and R.M.) saw all histological sections without knowledge of each others' VAS scores. The sections examined in this recent investigation came from 20 fair-skinned (types I and

II) Caucasian subjects (10 men, 10 women, mean age 67.4 years) who showed signs of moderate or severe photodamage. The subjects, all of whom had given their written, witnessed informed consent, had minor localized skin disorders (such as seborrhoeic warts) and were without significant systemic disease. Disease-free (but photodamaged) skin on the back of the wrist or lower forearm was sampled using local infiltration anaesthesia and a 4 mm punch biopsy technique. After routine formalin fixation and histological preparation the sections were stained with haematoxylin and eosin. The results were quite similar to those obtained previously and are set out in Tables 1 and 2. Clearly the three investigators had a similar ranking system for severity of dysplasia, although the absolute scores were somewhat different for one member of the team compared to the other two.

Table 1 Mean, median and standard error of mean (SEM) for VAS scores of dysplasia in biopsies from 20 photodamaged subjects by three observers.

	Observer		
	P.L.	A.K.	R.M.
Mean	31.0	29.2	19.4
Median	20.5	22.5	8.5
SEM	5.4	5.1	4.3

Table 2 Correlation between the VAS scores of dysplasia in biopsies from 20 photodamaged subjects by three observers.

	Correlation
A.K. versus P.L.	$r^2 = 0.639$, SE $= 16.665$ $y = 0.75x + 5.97$ Spearman's $\rho = 0.518$, $P = 0.0136$
A.K. versus R.M.	$r^2 = 0.657$, SE $= 11.99$ $y = 0.68x - 0.46$ Spearman's $\rho = 0.550$, $P = 0.008$
R.M. versus P.L.	$r^2 = 0.776$, SE $= 9.69$ $y = 0.69x - 2.05$ Spearman's $\rho = 0.667$ $P = 0.006$

SE, standard error.

'Digital' scoring method

In this system an attempt was made to rank dysplasia by its extent across the biopsy as well as by using a severity score. The same biopsies were used as in the recent VAS scoring experiment described above. Ten microscope slides were prepared from across the diameter of each biopsy. Each slide had five sections (each 5 μm) and the first and last of each slide were evaluated by each of the three observers who assessed them independently. The three observers scored each section as follows: 0, no significant abnormality; 1, irregular epidermal thickening with slight loss of polarity and minor nuclear abnormalities; or 2, heterogeneity in cell and nuclear size, shape and staining and the presence of dyskeratotic cells or multinucleate cells or parakeratosis. A mean score was computed for each biopsy; the numbers of biopsies that fell into the various categories are given in Table 3. It can be seen that, although two observers scored similarly, the other scored significantly differently. Furthermore, the scoring for individual biopsies bore no relationship to the VAS score for that biopsy (Figure 4).

Table 3 Means ($\pm$ sd) of numbers of times each dysplasia category was scored using the digital scoring method.

Observer	Grade		
	0	1	2
P.L.	1.91 $\pm$ 2.57	12.36 $\pm$ 5.23	5.76 $\pm$ 6.11
A.K.	6.11 $\pm$ 5.16	11.69 $\pm$ 6.04	2.20 $\pm$ 6.11
R.M.	6.61 $\pm$ 4.74	10.95 $\pm$ 5.06	2.43 $\pm$ 5.93

Dysplasia index determination

In the previous study referred to above,[12] an attempt was made to obtain an entirely objective measure of dysplasia by employing image-analysis techniques. The formula derived was

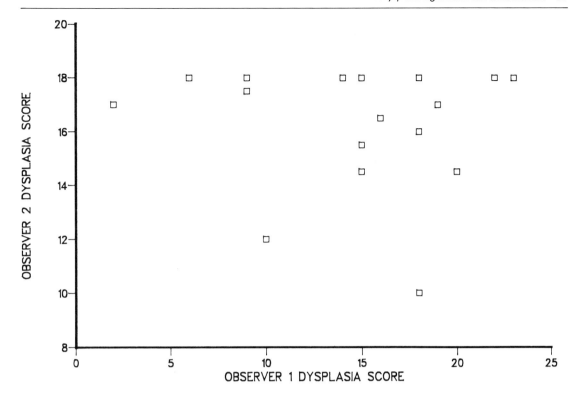

Figure 4

Inter-observer correlation of dysplasia scores using a digital method (inter-observer correlation, not significant).

Dysplasia index =

$$\frac{\text{mean epidermal thickness (MET)} + \text{nuclear area}}{\text{nuclear fraction (\%)} + \text{standard deviation of MET} + \text{'a form factor'}}$$

This index required the use of careful histological techniques with a specialized (gallocyanin) staining method and lengthy study using an image analysing device (Optomax V. image analyser, Analytical Measuring Systems Ltd). The dysplasia index obtained in this way did appear to correlate with the VAS scores for the same histological samples (Kendall's $W = 0.79$, $P < 0.001$) (Figure 5).

Current status and future needs

The present availability of new treatment regimens and the bright prospects of novel therapies for severe photodamage, including oral retinoids, topical retinoids, efficient sunscreens, abrasives and antioxidants, requires methods of assessment for the degree of epidermal dysplasia. It will be apparent from the above that no entirely satisfactory method exists. It would appear that the objective image analysis method can be made to 'match' the pathologist's eye but the enormous effort and resources required do not make the effort 'cost-effective'. The simplest and most reproducible method available seems to be the VAS scoring method. However, because this technique is subjective it is certainly not beyond criticism, and we will continue to explore other approaches.

References

1. Serrano H, Scotto J, Shornick G et al, Incidence of nonmelanoma skin cancer in New Hampshire and Vermont, *J Am Acad Dermatol* (1991) **24**: 574–9.
2. Shalom SD, Marks R, Harvey I, Sun exposure and solar damage in a Welsh population. In: Marks R, Plewig G, (eds). *The Environmental Threat to the Skin*, Martin Dunitz, London, 1992.

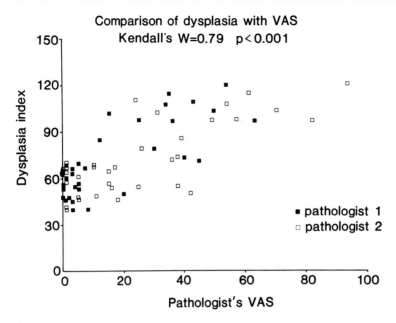

Figure 5

Correlation of dysplasia index with pathologist's visual analogue scale score of histological samples (Kendall's W = 0.79, P <0.001).

3 Marks R, The epidemiology of non-metallic melanocytic skin cancer in Australia. In: Marks R, Plewig G, (eds). *The Environmental Threat to the Skin*, Martin Dunitz, London, 1992.

4 Marks R, From slip! slop! slap! to sunsmart — the public health approach to skin cancer. In: Marks R, Plewig G, (eds). *The Environmental Threat to the Skin*, Martin Dunitz, London, 1992.

5 Pearse AD, Marks R, Actinic keratoses and the epidermis on which they arise, *Br J Dermatol* (1977) **96**: 45–50.

6 Pearse AD, Marks R, A quantitative histochemical study of three oxidative enzymes in solar keratoses and Bowen's disease, *Histochem J* (1978) **10**: 621–56.

7 Gouviea J, Mathé G, Hercend T et al, Degree of bronchial metaplasia in heavy smokers and its regression after treatment with a retinoid, *Lancet* (1982) **1**: 710–12.

8 Govan ADT, Haines RM, Langley FA, Taylor CW, Woodcock AS, The histology and cytology of changes in the epithelium of the cervix uteri, *J Clin Pathol* (1969) **22**: 383–95.

9 Dukes CE, Classification of cancer of rectum, *J Path & Bact* (1932) **35**: 323–32.

10 Breslow A, Tumor thickness, level of invasion and node dissection in stage I cutaneous melanoma, *Ann Surg* (1975) **182**: 572–75.

11 Clark WH, From L, Bernadino EA, Mihm MC, The histogenesis and biologic behaviour of primary human malignant melanomas of the skin, *Cancer Res* (1969) **29**: 705–26.

12 Barton SP, Pearse AD, Marks R, Derivation of a dysplasia index for epidermal neoplasia, *Dermatologica* (in press).

13 Shuttleworth D, Marks R, A comparison of the effects of intralesional interferon α-2b and topical 5% 5-fluorouracil cream in the treatment of solar keratoses and Bowen's disease, *J Dermatol Treat* (1989) **1**: 65–8.

14 Lever L, Marks R, The significance of the Darier-like solar keratotis and acantholytic change in preneoplastic lesions of the epidermis, *Br J Dermatol* (1989) **120**: 383–89.

15 Tan CY, Marks R, Lichenoid solar keratoses: Prevalence and immunological findings. *J Invest Dermatol* (1982) **79**: 365–67.

7
The effects of ultraviolet-B irradiation on proto-oncogene expression in normal human epidermis

S. Takahashi, A. D. Pearse and R. Marks
Department of Dermatology, University of Wales College of Medicine, Heath Park, Cardiff, UK

Introduction

It is well documented that proto-oncogenes play an important role in cell proliferation and carcinogenesis.[1] It is also known that neoplastic transformation may take place when these oncogenes are activated. Because proto-oncogenes are activated by point mutation, gene amplification and translocation, it is suggested that there may be a direct link between exposure to carcinogenic agents and genetic change leading to malignancy.[2]

It is also well documented that ultraviolet radiation (UVR) causes the formation of pyrimidine dimers. It has been suggested that this damage may lead to errors of DNA replication and gene mutations.[3] UVR is thought to be the main cause of non-melanoma skin cancer,[4] and DNA damage due to UVR may be attributed to the activation of proto-oncogenes. Recently, transient overexpression of c-Ha ras and c-myc has been observed in a human keratinocyte cell line after UVR in vitro.[5] It has also been reported that overexpression of c-Ha ras occurs in an in vivo model of UVR induced carcinogenesis.[6] Although these reports suggest that UVR may induce activation of proto-oncogenes, it is still unknown whether similar activation occurs in human skin after UVR in vivo. In order to research this issue we investigated c-Ha ras and c-myc proto-oncogene expression in normal human skin before and after UVR in vivo and related the findings to DNA synthesis in normal human skin before and after UVR.

Materials and methods

UV irradiation and skin biopsies

The buttock skin of six normal human volunteers was irradiated with 0.5 and 2.0 times their respective minimal erythema dose (MED) of UVB (300 ± 5 nm) using a 1000 W xenon arc lamp coupled to a grating monochromator. The UVR was delivered to each subject's skin using a 5 mm diameter liquid light guide. Biopsies of unirradiated skin and of irradiated skin were taken 5 h post-irradiation.

Anti-sense RNA probes

Anti-sense RNA probes were obtained after in vitro transcription of linealized template DNA fragments using SP6 RNA polymerase (Promega) with 800 Ci/mmol [^{35}S]UTP (Amersham International) and alkaline hydrolysis. The template DNA fragments used were: (i) C-myc — a linealized pSP64 vector whose EcoRI-Hind III site 1.5 kb c-DNA fragment was inserted into (Amersham International) (ii) c-Ha ras — a linealized pSP64 vector whose SacI site 3.0 kb c-DNA fragment was inserted (Amersham International) into (iii) a mixture of three linealized pGEM plasmid DNA fragments in which 11, 172 or 1386 bases of λϕ DNA fragments were subcloned (Promega).

In situ hybridization

The in situ hybridization study was done as reported previously.[7] The specimens were fixed with 4% paraformaldehyde for 3 h at 4°C and processed and embedded in paraffin wax. Sections (5 μm) were prepared and, after deparaffinization, the sections were treated with diluted hydrochloric acid and glycine and then acetylated with acetic anhydride. Prehybridization was performed in a solution of 50% formamide, 2 × sodium chloride–sodium citrate (SSC) at 50°C for 30 min. Hybridization was carried out in a solution of 50% formamide and 2 × SSC with 50 000 dpm/ml RNA probe at 42°C. After washing with 50% formamide and 2 × SSC, the sections were treated with RNase for 30 min. The sections were washed with 0.1 × SSC at 50°C and air dried. The sections were then dipped in the Ilford K-2 emulsion and stored at 4°C. After 6 days exposure the slides were developed, fixed and counter-stained through the emulsion using haematoxylin and eosin.

Grain counting

The number of grains per cell in basal, malpighian, and granular layers was counted using a microscope attached to an Optimax image analyser.

In order to count the number of grains per cell, we defined the area to be counted using a graphics tablet and 'a mouse'. After counting the cell number in each area, each grain was spotted electronically and the resulting yellow points in each defined area were counted. The number of grains in the background in each area was also measured and subtracted from the values in the defined areas. In order to know how many fields were required to obtain representative data, we measured the cumulative standard error in several specimens; we concluded that it was necessary to measure five fields.

BrdU incorporation to label DNA synthesis

The biopsy specimens were incubated in minimum essential medium containing 33 μm of BrdU for 4 h at 37°C. The specimens were then immediately quenched in hexane at −70°C and stored in liquid nitrogen until used. The sections were cut and fixed with acetone for 10 min. After treatment with hydrochloric acid, the incorporated BrdU was detected by the avidin–biotin complex method using mouse monoclonal antibody to BrdU (Amersham International).

Measurement of labelling index

The number of labelled cells and unlabelled basal cells were counted microscopically. Approximately 1000 basal cells were counted in order to calculate the labelling index (LI) as follows:

$$LI(\%) = \frac{\text{No. of labelled cells} \times 100}{\text{No. of labelled cells and unlabelled basal cells}}$$

Results

c-myc expression in non-irradiated and irradiated normal human skin

C-myc transcripts were detected throughout the epidermis in irradiated and non-irradiated skin. The values obtained for each of the three layers of the epidermis were almost identical (Table 1). The signals for c-myc RNA throughout the epidermis of irradiated skin following 2 × MED were stronger than those of non-irradiated skin (Figures 1 and 2). According to the Friedmann and Wilcoxon non-parametric test, the value for 2 × MED was significantly different from that of non-irradiated sites. The values for 0.5 × MED were not significantly different from the non-irradiated sites. The sections stained with λφ RNA probe showed very little background (data not shown).

Table 1 The c-myc expression before and after UVR

	0 MED*	0.5 MED*	2 MED†
Basal layer	11.8	13.5	17.5‡
Malpighian layer	12.4	12.4	19.1‡
Granular layer	13.3	12.9	18.9‡

* Mean value of six volunteers (grains/cell).
† Mean value of five volunteers (grains/cell).
‡ Significantly different from the value for non-irradiated sites ($P < 0.05$).

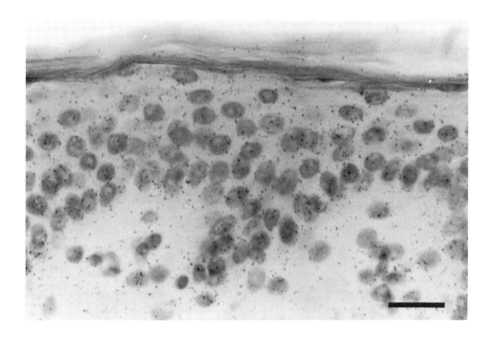

Figure 1

The c-myc expression in non-irradiated normal human skin.
Bar: 10μm.

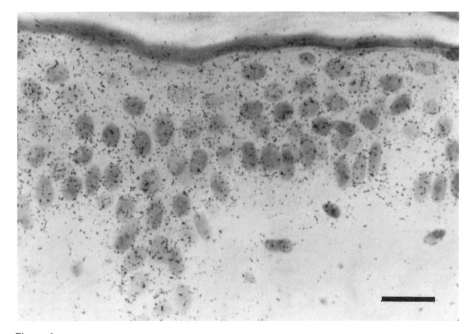

Figure 2

The c-myc expression of normal skin 5 h after UVB irradiation by 2 × MED. Bar: 10μm.

c-Ha ras expression of non-irradiated and irradiated normal human skin

C-Ha ras transcripts were detected in whole layers of non-irradiated and irradiated skin (Table 2). The intensity of signals in the irradiated skin was almost identical to that for non-irradiated skin. There was no statistically significant difference between the value for non-irradiated skin and that for irradiated skin (Friedmann test).

Table 2 The c-Ha ras expression before and after UVR

	0 MED*	0.5 MED*	2 MED†
Basal layer	13.2	12.7	13.7
Malpighian layer	14.0	12.9	15.6
Granular layer	13.2	11.8	11.5

* Mean value of six volunteers (grains/cell).
† Mean value of five volunteers (grains/cell).

DNA synthesis of non-irradiated and irradiated human skin

Most labelled cells were seen in the basal layer (Figure 3). The mean LI value for irradiated skin was lower than that for non-irradiated skin (Figure 4). According to the Friedmann test, the value for $2 \times$ MED irradiation sites was significantly different from that for non-irradiated skin. The value for the $0.5 \times$ MED sites was not significantly different from that of non-irradiated skin.

Correlation between the expression of c-myc oncogene in the basal layer and DNA synthesis

We also investigated the correlation between the value for c-myc expression in the basal layer and the LI of the same specimen. The data from five of six volunteers studied were clearly correlated (Figure 5). Subsequently, it was found that the volunteer whose data differed from the others was

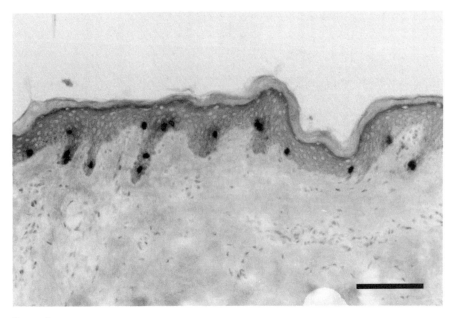

Figure 3

BrdU incorporation by non-irradiated human skin. Bar: 50 μm.

not normal. There was a previous history of thyrotoxicosis and treatment with radioactive iodine which may well explain the discrepancy in this patient.

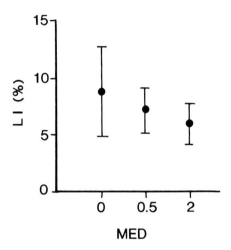

Figure 4

Changes in labelling index after UVR.

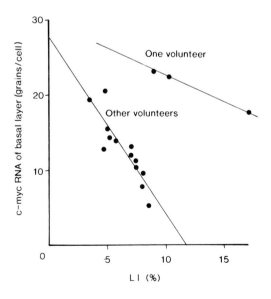

Figure 5

Correlation between c-myc expression in basal cells and labelling index (LI).

Discussion

A previous study using an in vitro system has shown that expression of c-myc and c-Ha ras in a human keratinocyte cell line were both increased 7 h after irradiation with 15 J/m^2 of UVB.[5] In this study c-myc expression was induced after 2 × MED of UVB irradiation, but the signals for c-Ha ras transcripts remained unchanged after UVR in vivo. This difference may reflect the difference between in vivo and in vitro studies. The changes in labelling index were very similar to those given in a previous report.[8]

This study has shown that c-myc expression is induced and DNA synthesis is inhibited 5 h after UVB irradiation of 2 × MED. If the results from the abnormal volunteer with a previous history of radioactive iodine treatment are excluded, then there is a negative correlation between c-myc expression in the basal layer and DNA synthesis in both non-irradiated and irradiated normal human skin 5 h after UVB irradiation. The function of c-myc is thought to be closely related to DNA synthesis.[9] One possible mechanism for the induction of c-myc expression by UVR is the inhibition of DNA synthesis. However, this theory does not explain why c-myc transcripts were detected not only in the basal layer but also in the upper epidermis — the differentiating compartment. Another possible mechanism is an increase in the half-life of c-myc RNA due to stabilization and the inhibition of synthesis of putative repressor proteins as suggested by Ronai et al.[5] Clearly further studies are required to elucidate the precise mechanism.

In conclusion, c-myc and c-Ha ras transcripts were detected throughout normal human epidermis before and after UVR. The c-myc expression was increased significantly in the whole epidermis 5 h after irradiation by 2 × MED but not by 0.5 × MED. DNA synthesis was decreased significantly in normal human skin 5 h after UVB irradiation by 2 × MED but not by 0.5 × MED. C-Ha ras expression remained unchanged in normal human epidermis 5 h after UVB irradiation.

References

1. Bishop JM, The molecular genetics of cancer, *Science* (1987) **235**: 305–11.
2. Quintanilla M, Brown K, Ramsden M et al, Carcinogen-specific mutation and amplification of Ha-ras during mouse skin carcinogenesis, *Nature* (1986) **322**: 78–80.

3 Haseltine WA, Ultraviolet light repair and mutagenesis revisited, *Cell* (1983) **33**: 13–17.

4 Marks R, Premalignant disease of the epidermis (Parkes Weber Lecture 1985), *J R Coll Phys (London)* (1986) **20**: 116–21.

5 Ronai ZA, Okin E, Weinstein IB, Ultraviolet light induces the expression of oncogenes in rat fibroblast and human keratinocyte cells, *Oncogene* (1988) **2**: 201–4.

6 Husain Z, Yang Q, Biswas DK, cHa-ras proto-oncogene, amplification and overexpression in UV-B-induced mouse skin papillomas and carcinomas, *Arch Dermatol* (1990) **126**: 324–30.

7 Mariani-Costantini R, Escot C, Theilett C et al, *In situ* c-myc expression and genomic status of the c-myc locus in infiltrating ductal carcinomas of the breast, *Cancer Res* (1988) **48**: 199–205.

8 Epstein WL, Fukuyama K. Epstein JH, Early effects of ultraviolet light on DNA synthesis in human skin *in vivo*, *Arch Dermatol* (1969) **100**: 84–9.

9 Rayter SI, Iwata KK, Michitsch RW et al, Biochemical properties of the c-myc gene product. In: Glover DM, Hames BD, (eds). *Oncogenes*, Oxford University Press: Oxford, 1989, pp. 157–8.

8
From Slip! Slop! Slap! to SunSmart — the public health approach to skin cancer control in Australia in the 1990s

Robin Marks
Anti-Cancer Council of Victoria, Carlton South 3053, Australia

Australia has the highest incidence of skin cancer in the world. A combination of four factors has led to this major public health problem which has reached the state where now two out of three people who live their life in Australia will require treatment for at least one skin cancer at some stage during that time. The first factor is that Australia has a hot, sunny climate with high levels of insolation, being greatest in the summer period, but present all year round. The second factor is that over 90% of the Australian population can be classified as white. The third factor is the fashion for a suntan which dictates the increased status, health and well-being apparently enjoyed by those people who are able to attain this environmentally induced change in their skin colour. The last factor is the change in clothing fashions and public attitudes which now promote and tolerate wearing of very brief clothing and removal of clothing in public. This facilitates the practice in which a vast proportion of the body is exposed to the sun in pursuit of a tan.

The first two of these factors are geophysical, about which little can be done. The next two are behavioural factors, which are subject to change and thus are obvious targets for a skin cancer prevention programme. Whilst prevention is the long-term and ideal approach to skin cancer control, there is a need to deal with those skin cancers that are occurring now and those that escape the preventive net in the future. Early detection, therefore, is an important part of the public health approach to skin cancer control. Although early detection programmes can be run concurrently with primary prevention programmes, they are not the same, and in a number of countries have been run quite independently.

With the extent of the problem in Australia, both prevention and early detection programmes have been running for many years. What started as public and professional education programmes on the early detection of melanoma in Queensland in the 1970s, evolved into the national Slip! (on a shirt) Slop! (on a sunscreen) Slap! (on a hat) prevention approach of the early 1980s and has now become increasingly sophisticated in both prevention and early detection under the banner of SunSmart in the 1990s.

Once current scientific knowledge has determined the target groups for interventions, behavioural research becomes an integral part of the programmes which are now delivered in Australia. This research is essential in formulating an approach to the target groups, pretesting concepts and materials, and evaluating outcomes. Running a skin cancer control programme without this vital component is analogous to placing a shotgun out of a window, closing both eyes and pulling the trigger in the hope that it will hit something. Having not even initially understood the target of this approach, after the exercise it is impossible to determine what effect it had. Although more often than not it is likely to hit an innocent bystander — a very costly result indeed!

On the basis of evidence suggesting that childhood sunlight exposure is critical in the development of both melanoma and non-melanoma skin cancer, a large proportion of the primary prevention programmes in Australia have targeted children, adolescents, and those responsible for their care. Public education material has developed along lines such as 'Kids Cook Quick', 'Is your child old enough for the sun?', 'Sunburn — SunSmart'.

These have been delivered through a large number of networks including the media (television, radio, billboards with 24-sheet posters), community health centres, pharmacies, maternal and child health centres, child care agencies, sporting groups, and local government agencies responsible for community health programmes. Particular attention has been paid to schools, with extensive materials being developed and inserted into curricula at various levels in the education framework. School Council Policy documents are produced which set guidelines for all the ways in which a reduction in sunlight can be achieved in a school for both the children and the staff. These include changes within the curriculum as well as changes within the structure of the school environment and schedules, e.g. providing shade in the playgrounds and rescheduling sporting and other outdoor activities away from the middle of the day.

Adolescents, a particularly difficult group with whom to communicate at the best of times, have been targeted in special ways. Their sporting heroes have been involved in promotions which highlight 'how to have fun in the sun', promoting a very positive approach to a reduction in sunlight exposure. The beach lifeguards are sponsored by the skin cancer programme and they set role models for their peers. Hats, shirts, lifeguard shelters with canopies providing shade, rescheduling of surf and swimming carnivals away from the middle of the day all set an example to the young people around these lifeguards on the beach and at swimming pools. The lifesaving clubs are provided with their own sun protection factor (SPF) $\geqslant 15$ broad spectrum (UVA blocking) sunscreen to sell on the beaches and at swimming pools as a fundraiser for their own club. Thus, they promote the use of as much of this product as possible! State Championships are sponsored, e.g. the Victorian State SunSmart Life Saving Championships, which give out prizes, including SunSmart jackets for winners of events. The desire by the young winners to promote their victory by wearing such clothing also promotes our messages.

Although we focus particularly on protection in childhood and adolscence, we do not neglect adults in our programmes. Sporting clubs and other activities in which adults are involved become networks for delivering our messages through brochures, posters and exemplar behaviours. Unions, employers and government departments of labour and industry have been targeted which has allowed the development of mutually acceptable guidelines on ways to reduce sunlight exposure in the workplace.

In all these programmes, several basic approaches are used. The first is that the natural approach to reduction of sunlight is the best approach. Sunscreens are adjunct to natural protection, not a substitute for it. Avoiding sunlight and seeking shade in the 2 h either side of midday is the major lynch pin of our approach. We use themes like 'Between 11 and 3 slip under a tree, the best sunscreen of all is absolutely free — shade'. We have developed tree planting programmes — 'Pick up a spade and plant some shade'. Trees which provide a dense canopy are promoted for planting in school playgrounds, parks, beach foreshores and other public open spaces. Other man-made canopies are also produced and promoted for public open space, as well as around the home.

Clothing and hats are widely promoted as natural protection. Fashion/design awards are made for clothing which is attractive, practical and also useful in reducing sunlight exposure. Some manufacturers are now promoting their clothing on the basis of its ability to protect from Australian sunlight. Testing is done at the Australian Radiation Laboratory.

Finally, in prevention, comes the use of sunscreens. We do not know the amount of sunlight necessary to cause skin cancer. Until we do, we promote the use of maximum protection products (SPF $\geqslant 15$, broad spectrum UVA blocking) regardless of skin type. We recommend that they be used on the areas of skin which cannot be protected naturally, e.g. face, neck, hands and forearms if sleeves are short. Manufacturers are only able to promote an SPF number greater than 15 as 15+, regardless of whether it is 16 or 60. This is to prevent the misleading advertising of the value of very high SPF numbers which we believe are unnecessary. The production of high SPF numbers increases the price of products, increases the need for more and greater concentration of sunscreen actives in the products, and inevitably leads to increased risk of short- and long-term side-effects, all for relatively little increase in protection. When all the natural approaches we recommend are used, there is little to be gained by use of a product with an SPF of greater than 15 (94% reduction of UVB).

The desire for a suntan is the obvious target for a skin cancer prevention programme. In Australia, we have been concentrating on the facts which show that a tan is not healthy, it does not increase social status, it does not provide adequate protection from skin cancer and it is a sign that sufficient sunlight is being received to lead to long-term damage of the skin.

All the above preventive approaches are incorporated in both education programmes and structural changes designed to reduce sunlight exposure. Structural changes include such things as ensuring easy availability of cheap and adequate sunscreen; legislating to remove sales tax from sunscreens; planting trees in open spaces; shade design incorporated in public and domestic architecture; rescheduling sport and outdoor work away from the middle of the day; legislating to prevent the manufacture and release of ozone depleting substances.

Short-term measures of outcome include changes in knowledge, beliefs and attitudes, and then changes in behaviour. The long-term measures of outcome are a reduction of the incidence of and mortality rates from these cancers. In Australia, our behavioural research programmes monitoring the short-term changes are showing substantial changes in all the early parameters. The desire for deep suntans is decreasing; people's knowledge of skin cancer is increasing; hat and sunscreen use is increasing; hat and sunscreen sales are increasing substantially. The most potent measure of behaviour changes has been a continuing decrease in the proportion of the population who are sunburnt in the weekends in the summer each year for the last three years to 1990. It is too early, as yet, to demonstrate an effect of these prevention programmes on the incidence rates of skin cancer.

Early detection programmes in Australia have concentrated on highlighting to the public and the professions the features of skin lesions which suggest that they need to be seen by a doctor. Although we promote the fact that individuals should 'know their own and their partner's skin', as yet we have not promoted a specific skin self-examination technique, or recommended a specific frequency with which this should be performed. There are no published reports demonstrating any satisfactory value of any particular technique. Research is underway currently in Australia looking specifically at these questions.

Similarly, we do not recommend that the normal public be screened by a doctor on an annual or any other regular basis. There are no data as yet which demonstrate that this is a cost-effective way of dealing with the problem. We certainly recommend the practice of opportunistic screening by medical practitioners, i.e. taking the opportunity to examine patients' skin when they seek a consultation about another problem. Randomized community-based trials are necessary to determine the role of screening by professionals in the control of skin cancer.

There have been extensive public and professional education programmes in Australia on features of early skin cancer, methods of diagnosis and management of these tumours. These have used many of the networks available, including media, community health centres, medical practitioners' waiting rooms, pharmacies, nurses, physiotherapists, podiatrists, hairdressers/beauty therapists and many other people who are likely to notice abnormalities on people's skin. Brochures, posters and other written, visual and spoken methods have been used to transmit the educational messages required.

Free screenings for the public have been offered, particularly during the summer. These are staffed by dermatologists, surgeons and general practitioners. They occur in city centres, workplaces, beaches and other public areas. They are offered mainly for their publicity value, rather than as a continuing or effective screening service. They offer to screen either a particular lesion about which a person is concerned, or to screen the whole body in an apparently normal person. The former is less likely to lead to the medico-legal complications of having missed a lesion on a person who is seen during a busy publicity event.

Extensive educational material has also been developed for medical practitioners specifically. This is both written and audio-visual. It is distributed in undergraduate and postgraduate training programmes and other sources from which medical practitioners receive their continuing education. At the end of 1990, a new booklet on diagnosis and management of skin cancer was distributed to every general practitioner in the country. This was associated with update seminars run by dermatologists, articles placed in all the local medical journals that are sent to general practitioners and a variety of other educational activities at that time. One of these was the dermatologists opening their clinics at the major teaching hospitals to general practitioners who were able to attend to see patients with skin tumours and the dermatologists' approach to them. Future research is continuing on what facilities and approaches are perceived to be useful by general practitioners and how these can be supplied.

Evaluation of early detection programmes relies on assessment of the stage at which people are now presenting for diagnosis and management of skin tumours. Data from cancer registries are showing that a very large proportion of melanomas are now being removed when they are still 1.5 mm or less in thickness. The short-term effect on incidence rates of these programmes is to lead to an initial rise as people with existing tumours prevalent in the community present at an earlier stage for management. If tumours can be treated in the pre-invasive phase, then the incidence rate will eventually decline with the continuing success of these programmes.

The long-term effect is continued diagnosis of tumours in the early curable phase and thus a reduction in mortality rate. At the moment, the mortality rate is not rising at the same rate as the incidence rate in Australia, and this is probably attributable to the effect of tumours being treated at an earlier stage. However, the mortality rate still remains high for elderly men who are presenting with thick or late tumours. This group of people need to be included in targetting in future programmes.

In summary, extensive prevention and early detection programmes have been running in Australia for a number of years. Research is demonstrating that the programmes are having some success. Behavioural research is being used increasingly to underpin our programmes. With the improvement in targetting, delivery and measure of effect, more specific designs will enable us to maintain the work on what is a major and continuing public health problem. We still have a long way to go.

9
What do children know about the effects of sun on their skin?

S. Blackford and D. Roberts
Department of Dermatology, Singleton Hospital, Swansea, West Glamorgan, UK

Introduction

The incidence of skin cancer has been rising over the last 30 years, and the incidence of malignant melanoma has doubled in the last decade alone.[1] There is strong evidence to link the aetiology of non-melanoma skin cancer with exposure to sunlight, and, perhaps more significantly, studies have shown an association between episodes of sunburn during childhood and adolescence and increased risk of cutaneous melanoma.[2] This is important as children have many more summer days available for exposure to the sun than do working adults, and their daily routine is such that they are more likely to be exposed to the midday sun. It has been estimated that the average child receives three times more annual UVB than the average adult.[3] With the continual depletion of the earth's protective layer of ozone, we can expect the increase in skin cancer incidence to continue.[4] Public health initiatives to heighten awareness of skin cancer and promote preventative measures have been aimed primarily at adults. Health education may be more effective when aimed at younger people who have not become entrenched in their habits.[5] However, a suntan is still perceived as a desirable and healthy social symbol. Young people are generally more influenced by fashion and peer group pressure, so simply informing children of the harmful effects of the sun may not lead to changes in behaviour.

We undertook a survey of local schoolchildren aged 11–16 years, to determine their attitudes to sunbathing and their knowledge of skin cancer and the aging effects of sun exposure.

Methods

A simple 'yes/no' questionnaire was sent to five comprehensive schools in the Swansea area. The pupils were asked to complete the questionnaire during class at the end of the summer term, July 1990.

Results

A total of 1308 completed questionnaires (Table 1) were received (four were excluded because details of sex had not been given): 739 boys (56%) and 569 girls (44%) took part in the survey, the mean age of subjects was 13.3 years (SD = 0.95).

A majority of the schoolchildren surveyed enjoy sunbathing (80% of girls and 68% of boys). The association between female sex and enjoyment of sunbathing was statistically significant ($\chi^2 = 6.85$, df = 1, $P < 0.001$). Girls were also more likely to use sunscreens when in the sun ($\chi^2 = 19.4$, df = 1, $P < 0.001$) and more girls than boys feel better when they have a tan (80.5% girls and 64.8% boys; $\chi^2 = 11.12$, df = 1, $P < 0.001$). A total of 49% of subjects reported having a tan at the time of the survey, with no significant differences between the sexes. As expected, the majority of those questioned (73%) thought a tan made them more attractive, but it seems that these children were aware of the sun's harmful effects. Only 14% thought a tan improves health, 93% knew that the sun can cause damage to the skin, and 95% that the sun may cause skin cancer. However, a much

Table 1 Results of the questionnaire.

		Yes (%)	No (%)
Do you enjoy sunbathing?	Male	68	31*
	Female	80	19
Do you usually use sunscreens when out in the sun?	Male	58	41†
	Female	78	21
Do you feel better with a suntan?	Male	65	34†
	Female	81	18
Have you got a suntan now?	Male	51	48
	Female	47	50
Do you think a suntan makes you look more attractive?	Male	72	27
	Female	73	25
Do you think a tan improves your health?	Male	15	84
	Female	13	85
Do you think the sun can damage your skin?	Male	94	6
	Female	92	7
Do you believe that the sun can age your skin, leading to early wrinkles?	Male	61	38*
	Female	73	25
Do you believe that the sun may cause skin cancers?	Male	95	5
	Female	96	3
Does skin cancer only happen in people who live in hot climates?	Male	18	79
	Female	10	87
Does skin cancer ever happen in people who live in this country all their lives?	Male	65	33
	Female	73	24
Does skin cancer ever occur in younger people (under 35 years)?	Male	81	17
	Female	84	13
Are skin cancers commoner than other forms of cancer?	Male	52	46
	Female	57	39
Can ordinary moles and birthmarks ever turn into cancer?	Male	52	46*
	Female	66	29
Have you been sunburnt (skin red and sore) this year?	Male	50	49
	Female	47	52
Have you heard of the type of skin cancer known as malignant melanoma?	Male	24	75
	Female	24	75
If you were told that sunbathing and sunburn can definitely lead to premature aging of the skin would you be put off sunbathing?	Male	55	44
	Female	49	48
If you were told that the sun definitely causes skin cancer would this put you off sunbathing?	Male	70	28
	Female	70	26

* $P < 0.01$.
† $P < 0.001$.

smaller proportion (66%) knew about the aging effects of sun exposure, with girls (415 = 73%) more likely than boys (449 = 61%) to know that the sun causes early aging and wrinkles ($\chi^2 = 7.16$, df = 1, $P < 0.01$).

Despite their being well informed about skin cancer, only 24% of the children surveyed had heard about malignant melanoma, although 58% knew that ordinary moles could become malignant. Once again girls had better knowledge than boys, and this association was statistically significant ($\chi^2 = 11.9$, df = 1, $P < 0.001$). When asked about changing sunbathing habits in the future, 70% of those surveyed thought that being told 'the sun definitely causes skin cancer' would put them off sunbathing, but only 52% would be put off by being told that sunbathing can lead to premature aging of the skin.

Discussion

The schoolchildren in our survey were generally well informed about the harmful effects of sunlight on the skin, most notably the risk of skin cancer. Girls knew more about the aging effect of sun exposure than boys, possibly due to extensive coverage of the topic in women's magazines in recent years. Girls were also more likely to apply sunscreens than boys who may consider this 'sissy'.

Our survey also shows that schoolchildren enjoy sunbathing, and feel better and more attractive with a tan. Despite the fact that they are aware of the sun's harmful effects, nearly half the children in our survey (634, 48.5%) had been sunburnt in the year of the survey. Previous studies have shown an association between smoking status and failure to use sunscreen in adolescents. This is thought to show that failing to use sunscreen is part of a constellation of risk-taking behaviour.[6] The long-term consequences of behaviour are not as important to adolescents as the perceived rewards of a deep suntan, especially improved standing within their peer group. Therefore, simply increasing knowledge about skin cancer among adolescents is unlikely to be effective on its own. We should attempt to make the practice of using sunscreen and covering-up more fashionable. By emphasizing the positive aspects of the healthy option and perhaps using sporting or television personalities to glamourize the process, we can achieve this goal.

Many female pop stars already seem to promote a 'pale and interesting' image and film of Gazza applying sunscreen prior to a football match would do more to project sunscreen use in boys than any amount of government promoted scare posters.

References

1. Roush GC, Schymura MJ, Holford TR, Patterns of invasive melanoma in the Connecticut tumour registry, *Cancer* (1988) **61**: 2586-95.
2. Holman CDJ, Armstrong BK, Heenan P et al, The causes of malignant melanoma: results from the West Australian Lions melanoma project, *Rec Res Cancer Res* (1986) **102**: 18-37.
3. Hurwitz S, The sun and sunscreen protection: recommendations for children, *J Dermatol Surg Oncol* (1988) **14**: 657-60.
4. Mackie R, Rycroft MJ, Health and the ozone layer, *Br Med J* (1988) **297**: 369-70.
5. Sanson-Fisher RW, Redman S, The Challenge of community health. In: King NJ, Remeny A, (eds), *Health care, a behavioural approach*. Grune and Stratton: Sydney, 1986.
6. Cockburn J, Hennrikus D, Scott R et al, Adolescent use of sun-protection measures, *Med J Aust* (1989) **151**: 136-40.

10
Ultraviolet radiation and the immune system

Warwick L. Morison
Associate Professor of Dermatology, The Johns Hopkins Medical Institutions, 600 N. Wolfe Street, Baltimore, MA 21205, USA

Exposure to non-ionizing radiation, predominantly in the ultraviolet (UV) region, can induce alterations in immune function in humans and experimental animals and this area of research is termed photoimmunology. The first experimental observations were made only about two decades ago but already there is considerable information at both a descriptive and a mechanistic level and this has been recently reviewed.[1-6] This chapter will focus on a few areas to demonstrate that exposure to UV radiation (UVR) does influence immune responses, that this effect is involved in the pathogenesis of a disease in an experimental system, that photoimmunology may be involved in the pathogenesis and therapy of human disease and, finally, to review briefly the potential for further investigation.

Contact hypersensitivity

The influence of UVR on contact hypersensitivity (CHS) in experimental animals has received more attention than any other photoimmunologic effect and, consequently, it is the most well understood. Exposure of mice and other rodents to UVB (290–320 nm) radiation produces both local suppression of CHS when the sensitizer is applied through exposed skin and systemic suppression when the sensitizer is applied to a distant non-exposed site. These two effects are mediated by the generation of hapten-specific T suppressor cells that act on the induction but not the elicitation of CHS. However, the mechanisms involved in the generation of these cells are probably different.

Local suppression of CHS requires only a low dose of UVR and the most effective wavelengths for inducing suppression are <300 nm. Suppression appears to be initiated by a UV-induced alteration of antigen-presenting (A-P) cell function in the exposed skin. Initially, attention was focused on an alteration of Ia$^+$ Langerhans cells but two other cells have now been identified as playing a role and keratinocytes may also be involved. Thy-1$^+$ dendritic epidermal cells which down-regulate CHS responses are not affected by low doses of UV radiation and may preferentially activate a suppressor cell pathway in the absence of an effector pathway mediated by Langerhans cells. Functional studies have identified a population of I-J$^+$ A-P cells which are Thy-1$^-$ and Ia$^-$ that are also resistant to low doses of radiation and preferentially activate suppressor cells. Finally, exposure to UVR diminishes production of thymocyte activating factor by keratinocytes and this can lead to a defect of A-P cell function.

Systemic suppression of CHS requires a much higher exposure dose of UVR in comparison with the dose required to produce local suppression, and the most active wavelengths are around 265–275 nm. Attempts have been made to identify the chromophore molecule responsible for absorbing radiation and two candidates, i.e. urocanic acid and DNA, have been suggested based on the similarity of their absorption spectra to the action spectrum for the effect. A recent observation that systemic suppression can be photoactivated in the opossum *Monodelphis domestica* provides good evidence for involvement of pyrimidine dimers in the pathway to suppression. Therefore, DNA may or may not be the chromophore but certainly it appears to be involved at some point in the pathway to suppression. The next steps in the pathway are not clear. Several lines of evidence indicate that local alterations in A-P cells at the site of exposure are not important. Recently, attention has been focused on the possibility that soluble mediators are released from irradiated skin and result in the generation of suppressor cells in a distant organ. Serum collected from mice 2 h after exposure to UVB and supernatant from epidermal cells exposed in vitro to UVB can initiate the pathway to suppression and in both cases a low molecular weight protein may be the active mediator.

There is no clear-cut evidence that exposure to UVR produces either local or systemic suppression of CHS in humans, but this is due to a lack of experimentation rather than findings to the contrary. Presuming these effects do occur raises the teleologic purpose of the responses. The most likely explanation is a defence against immune responses to UV-altered self-antigens and consequent autoimmune disease.

Skin cancer

Photocarcinogenesis in the mouse has been used as an experimental model of non-melanoma skin cancer for decades, but it has only recently been observed that UVR-induced alterations of immune function are central to the pathogenesis of these tumors. The observation that most UVR-induced tumors in mice are highly antigenic and are rejected upon transplantation into normal syngeneic recipients, but not in immunosuppressed recipients, prompted interest in the role of immunologic alterations in photocarcinogenesis. The specific immunologic rejection of these transplanted tumors is mediated by T lymphocytes. The question that arises from these observations is: Why do the tumors grow in the primary host? The answer is that exposure of mice to a subcarcinogenic dose of UVR results in the generation of suppressor T lymphocytes that prevent normal immunologic rejection of the tumors. The function of these suppressor cells is specific in that they do not alter the growth of tumors produced by other carcinogens. Two lines of evidence indicate that these suppressor cells are important in the development of primary neoplasms: there is accelerated development of UVR-induced tumors in mice previously exposed to UVR at a distant site, and if suppressor cells are present from the time of commencement of irradiation, the latency period of tumor development is shortened and tumor yield is increased.

The 270–315 nm region is the most active in producing tumor susceptibility but UVC (essentially 254 nm) radiation, large doses of UVA (320–400 nm) radiation and sunlight can also induce this effect. The appearance of tumor-associated antigens and tumor-specific antigens on epidermal cells along with alterations of A-P cell function in the dermis are thought to be early steps in the pathway to suppressor cells and the $I\text{-}J^+$ A-P cell may be involved. Suppressor factors may also play a role since serum from irradiated mice has been shown to contain a protein which can cause generation of suppressor cells in naive syngeneic mice.

The evidence that UVR-induced alterations of immune function play a role in the development of skin cancer in humans is much less compelling than it is in experimental systems. The observation that sun-related tumors are more common than expected in renal transplant recipients on immunosuppressive therapy is probably the best evidence. However, non-immunologic effects of the therapy or the activation of latent oncogenic viruses could also explain this observation. The finding of impaired development of contact allergy in patients with xeroderma pigmentosum, a condition characterized by increased susceptibility to skin cancer, is another indirect piece of evidence that sunlight-induced immunosuppression may be important in the pathogenesis of skin cancer.

Photodermatoses

The first interest in the interactions between UVR and the immune system was stimulated by observations on the pathogenesis of certain photodermatoses. Some cases of solar urticaria have an immunologic basis and involve an antigen–antibody reaction leading to the degranulation of mast cells and the production of urticarial lesions. The role of UVR in this disease is to produce the antigen which may be a normal photoproduct produced in all exposed people or a photoproduct unique to affected patients. Photoallergy to exogenous chemicals is the aetiological basis of another group of photodermatoses involving a photoimmunologic pathogenesis, and in this instance a cell-mediated immune response is triggered by exposure to UVR in the presence of the chemical. Again, UVR acts by inducing the formation of the antigen either by photochemical alteration of the hapten or by causing interaction of the hapten with a protein to form the complete antigen. Finally, certain autoimmune diseases, the most notable example being lupus erythematosus, are characterized by photosensitivity which probably has a photoimmunologic basis. The mechanism is incompletely understood but probably involves the formation of new antigens from exposure to UVR and these photoproducts initiate the autoimmune reaction.

Phototherapy of disease

There is evidence that therapeutic exposure to photons results in alterations in immune function and that selective manipulation of such functions may be the basis for some of the beneficial effects of modalities such as UVB phototherapy and psoralen/UVA (PUVA) photochemotherapy. This was suggested by the finding that some diseases, for example atopic eczema, which are thought to have an immunologic pathogenesis respond to these treatments. More direct evidence for this suggestion has been provided by the observation that graft-versus-host (GVH) disease can be suppressed by treatment with PUVA therapy. GVH disease following allogeneic bone-marrow transplantation is mediated by an immune response initiated by immune-competent cells in the graft directed at host tissues including the skin. The chronic lichenoid form of cutaneous GVH disease is characterized by a lymphocyte infiltrate in the skin and elimination of this infiltrate by PUVA therapy is associated with regression of the disease. The most interesting aspect of this observation is that long-term apparent 'cures' of the disease can be induced, suggesting that selective cytotoxicity by the treatment might result in elimination of a pool of sensitized cells responsible for the disease. It is very possible that similar mechanisms might underlie the therapeutic effect of UVR in other diseases such as lichen planus, vitiligo and some photodermatoses.

The future

The recent advances in our understanding of the effects of UVR on immune responses and how they interact with contact allergy and immunological mechanisms in skin cancer appear significant until they are compared with what is still to be learnt. For example, infectious diseases involve immune responses that are quantitatively and qualitatively more important than any of those mentioned and virtually nothing is known of the influence of UVR on immunity to these diseases. A few preliminary observations suggest that such effects may be very important. Experimental infections with herpes simplex virus in mice are exacerbated by exposure to UVB radiation and this is associated with suppression of delayed hypersensitivity (DHS) to the virus due to the generation of antigen-specific suppressor T lymphocytes. The doses of radiation required to produce these effects were small and quite within human tolerance to UVB radiation. Exposure of mice to UVB radiation also alters the immunity and the outcome of infections induced by the protozoan *Leishmania*. Radiation abrogates the development of DHS to the organism so that a second inoculation is treated as a primary infection which may have importance for our understanding of leishmaniasis in humans. Finally, UVB radiation also suppresses DHS to *Candida albicans* in mice and this can involve the generation of suppressor cells.

Taken together, these reports indicate that infectious diseases due to a variety of organisms can be influenced, at least in experimental systems, by exposure to UVB radiation and that this is often due to a systemic effect on immune function. Perhaps most importantly, in each instance the exposure to radiation has resulted in a suppression of natural defence mechanisms and there are no reports of either a failure to detect an effect of radiation or of a positive beneficial influence from such exposure. Clearly much more needs to be known about how exposure to UVR influences infectious disease both in experimental systems and in vivo in humans. A related issue is the effect of irradiation on vaccine effectiveness. Does exposure to sunlight around the time of vaccination effect subsequent development of immunity to the disease vaccinated against? This is a question that has not even attracted a preliminary observation to suggest a likely answer, despite its obvious importance. The critical importance of this issue is magnified when it is considered that the prevalence of many infectious diseases, and hence requirements for vaccination, are highest in tropical areas with high solar fluence of radiation with people who spend much time outdoors.

Another global and very important question is the role of melanin in protecting against the suppressive effects of UVR on immune function since whether or not it is protective will determine the susceptibility of different populations to such suppression. The location of Langerhans cells above melanocytes and the suggestion that urocanic acid in the stratum corneum might be the chromophore for UVR-induced immune suppression, imply that melanin might not protect against this effect. The observations that Langerhans cells are similarly susceptible to the damaging effects of UVR in Australian aboriginals and fair-skinned Celts and in people with and without a UVR-induced tan gives the only preliminary insight to the answer to this important question.

Finally, there is an urgent need for studies in humans to learn whether observations already made in experimental animals are relevant. There has not been a convincing demonstration that exposure to UVR alters an immune response in normal human subjects in a manner similar to that observed in rodents. Since most is known about the effects of UVR on the induction of CHS in mice, and this immune response is readily quantitated in humans, it appears to provide the best model for exploring this question. From a medical viewpoint it is also essential to determine whether photoimmunologic effects are involved in the pathogenesis of non-melanoma skin cancer in humans. Such information may offer scope for the selective manipulation of the immune system for therapeutic benefit.

References

1. Parrish JA, Kripke ML, Morison WL, *Photoimmunology*, Plenum Medical: New York, 1983.
2. Morison WL, Photoimmunology, *Photochem Photobiol* (1984) **40**: 781–7.
3. Morison WL, Kripke ML, Photoimmunology and skin cancer, *Photobiochem Photobiophys* (1987) (Suppl.): 467–74.
4. Cruz PD, Bergstresser PR, The low-dose model of UVB-induced immunosuppression, *Photodermatology* (1988) **5**: 151–61.
5. Krutmann J, Elmets CA, Recent studies on mechanisms in photoimmunology, *Photochem Photobiol* (1988) **48**: 787–98.
6. Morison WL, Effects of ultraviolet radiation on the immune system in humans, *Photochem Photobiol* (1989) **50**: 515–24.

11
Photoallergens and photosensitivity: current problems

Ian R. White
St John's Dermatology Centre, St Thomas' Hospital, London SE1 7EH, UK

Numerous contact photoallergens have been described but in most instances reports of these photoallergens causing problems are sporadic and rare. However, some groups of compounds and particular substances have been responsible for causing significant numbers of cases of contact photosensitivity. In the decade before 1975 the halogenated salicylanilides, used as antibacterial agents in soaps for instance, caused an epidemic of photosensitivity reactions. The problem was first identified by Wilkinson[1] who described the clinical sign of sparing of a small area of skin behind the ears in those photosensitive individuals with eczematous changes on their faces; this sign is known as Wilkinson's triangle. Once halogenated salicylanilides had been removed from the domestic environment the epidemic settled, although a very few affected individuals have remained with persistent light reactivity (PLR).

In 1978 musk ambrette, used primarily as a fragrance fixative in toiletries, was identified as a photoallergen by Larsen.[2] During the next few years musk ambrette became an important and common photoallergen, with allergic contact dermatitis also occurring. Again, following the identification of the problem and the lowering of the quantities of musk ambrette used in toiletries, the incidence of new cases of musk ambrette photosensitivity has fallen dramatically.

During more recent years there has been appreciably greater population exposure to a number of ultraviolet radiation (UVR) screening agents, brought about by the greater awareness of the carcinogenic potential of sunlight and its effect of causing premature aging of the skin. Contact and photocontact sensitivity to these sunscreens has started to become a problem.

The use of UVR absorbing substances has increased considerably recently and, with the consequent increase in skin contact, there has been an increase in reports of adverse reactions.[3] The worldwide campaign warning populations of the association of excessive sunlight exposure with the development of malignant melanoma has been one reason for the increased use of these agents. A second reason has been the more frequent incorporation of UVR absorbers in facial toiletries and cosmetics, and especially those which claim an anti-wrinkle effect, because of the public's awareness that excessive sunlight exposure is a cause of premature aging of the skin. The third reason has been the incorporation of UVR absorbers into toiletries to increase the shelf-life of the product, by protecting against photodegradation.[4]

The main groups of UVR absorbers are p-aminobenzoic acid (PABA) and its derivatives, the cinnamates, benzophenones and dibenzoylmethanes. The latter, with excellent long-wave UVR absorbing properties, are being used increasingly in Europe.[5–7]

UVR absorbing agents can cause an allergic contact dermatitis which may present acutely and have features of an allergic contact dermatitis, similar to those of the more common cosmetic allergens. However, because UVR screening cosmetics will generally be applied liberally to the skin before exposure to sunlight, allergic or photoallergic contact reactions to the UVR absorbing susbstance may be misinterpreted as an idiopathic light sensitivity response. In addition, some individuals using sunscreens to treat an idiopathic photodermatosis may acquire allergy or photoallergy to the UVR absorbing substance, which may exacerbate the pre-existing condition. Such an example has been demonstrated with photoallergy to 2-ethoxy-*p*-methoxycinnamate in an Asian, using the screen, who had chronic actinic dermatitis (CAD) with negative previous photopatch tests.[8] In such cases the sunscreen may appear to cause 'persistence' of the light-related dermatosis.

Care needs to be taken when evaluating contact and photocontact reactions to some UVR absorbing substances, and especially to PABA and its derivatives. The reactions may be caused by contaminants in the product.[9]

The results of patch and photopatch testing with a series of UVR absorbing substances at St John's Dermatology Centre are given in Table 1.

Table 1 UVR absorbers as (photo)allergens.*

Compound	Allergens	Photoallergens
Benzophenone-3	3	1
Benzophenone-10	25	2
Butylmethoxydibenzoylmethane	2	1
2-Ethoxyethyl-*p*-methoxycinnamate	2	2
4-Isopropyldibenzoylmethane	5	6
3-(4-Methylbenzylidine)-camphor	1	2
Octyldimethyl-PABA	3	1
Octylmethoxycinnamate	1	1
PABA	9	4

* Cohort of 600 individuals; 1986–90.

Diagnostic difficulties

Chronic eczema on light-exposed areas may be due to true 'idiopathic' light sensitivity and also to other factors. Musk ambrette can present with a pattern of photosensitivity identical to such idiopathic light sensitivity. More commonly, however, a chronic eczema on exposed areas is not due to photosensitivity but is the result of airborne contact allergy. In the UK this is seen with phosphorus sesquisulphide present in some matches, but more globally it occurs with *Compositae* (*Asteraceae*) dermatitis. Although airborne allergic contact dermatitis characteristically involves the eyelids, and extends to involve the skin under the chin and behind the ears, this is not always so; and, conversely, in CAD/PLR there may be involvement of these shaded areas which are typically spared in these light-related conditions.

Compositae

Allergic contact dermatitis to *Compositae* can mimic CAD morphologically[10,11] and, in addition, both are worse in the summer months when there is both increased exposure to sunlight and to *Compositae* allergens. Furthermore, it is accepted that *Compositae* sensitivity predisposes to the development of photosensitivity[12] and the clinical evolution of this process has been described.[13]

Patch testing with leaves or flowers of *Compositae* will not always detect *Compositae* dermatitis because of ranges in species content of the allergens and seasonal variation. Occlusive patch tests performed with some commercially available oleoresin extracts have caused false-positive irritant reactions. Open tests with these oleoresins may give false-negative results in *Compositae* sensitive subjects.

The development of a sesquiterpene lactone mix by Ducombs et al[14] has given reliability in the detection of *Compositae* sensitivity. This mix consists of a 0.1% dilution of an equal mixture of alantolactone, costunolide, and dehydrocostuslactone. The latter two substances are the more important allergens in the mix (White, personal observation). This mixture is not irritant and active sensitization is rare at this concentration. As an alternative to this mix, 1% costus oil may detect the majority of *Compositae* sensitive individuals, but the oil contains a variable amount of allergen and may be sensitizing. A *Compositae* mix developed by Hausen[15] contains the oleoresins of five species of *Compositae*.

A cohort of 120 individuals allergic to the sesquiterpene lactone mix has been identified at the St John's Dermatology Centre. This cohort represents 1.8% of all individuals subjected to routine patch testing during the course of data collection. Of the 120, 41 have been further investigated by monochromator light testing and of this number 66% had abnormal tests. This data confirms the association between sesquiterpene lactone sensitivity and light sensitivity. The mean age of all individuals subjected to routine patch testing was 38 years, of those who were lactone sensitive 58 years, and those who were both lactone and light sensitive 69 years (Figure 1).

Photopatch testing

It is clear that there can be diagnostic difficulties between allergic contact dermatitis, photoallergic

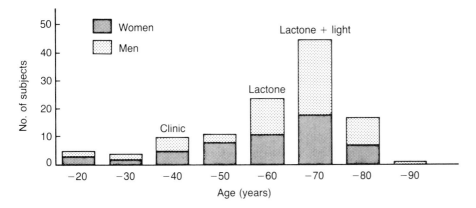

Figure 1
Age distribution of sesquiterpene lactone sensitivity.

contact dermatitis and a photodermatitis of the PLR/CAD type. The purpose of a protocol of photopatch testing is, therefore, to provide an adequate screen of those allergens which can mimic photoallergic reactions as well as being able to detect true photoallergens.

Changes in importance of photoallergens

There are both temporal and geographical variations in those photoallergens to which an individual is likely to be exposed. New cases of halogenated salicylanilide photosensitivity amongst the population of the UK are unlikely to be found, as there has been no exposure to these compounds for nearly two decades. However, these compounds may still be in use in some developing countries and the possibility remains of contact to them from imported goods (E. Hölzle, personal communication). The incidence of new cases of photoallergy to musk ambrette rapidly decreased as population exposure was reduced. The banning of 6-methylcoumarin from fragrances removed exposure to this photoallergen. In the UK, photocontact dermatitis to fentichlor has not been reported from domestic exposure to it for more than a decade,[16] whilst more recent domestic use in Scandinavia has meant more recent reports of photoallergy to it in these countries. Reactions from UVR absorbing compounds is increasing as the population exposure is increasing. Different UVR absorbing agents have more popular use in some countries than others and the sunscreen formula for a branded product may change seasonally.

Because of these factors, there is no single simple series of allergens which will be a good screen for photoallergy in all countries, whilst an excessively comprehensive series may be appropriate for use in specialized centres only.

Standard light series

At the St John's Dermatology Centre in the UK, the photopatch test series is reviewed regularly and changed at intervals. The current series appears to suit the UK domestic exposure to photoallergens, and to detect those allergens which may mimic photosensitivity or must be considered in evaluating an eczema on light-exposed areas (Table 2).

UVA radiation dose

As a rule, photoallergens are active in UVA radiation (315–400 nm), but there are rare exceptions to this and sulphanilamide and diphenhydramine are examples of compounds with their action spectra involving UVB. For normal investigations UVA is used for photopatch testing.

There are differences in the amount (dose, measured in joule per square centimetre) of UVA radiation which various centres consider appropriate to use during photopatch testing to elicit allergic photocontact reactions. In the series

Table 2 Scheme of allergens for photopatch testing used at St John's Dermatology Centre, 1991.

Not for irradiation:
Extended European standard series of contact allergens
A series of facial and cosmetic contact allergens including (in 0.5% petroleum):
    sesquiterpene lactone mix,[14]
    phosphorus sesquisulphide,
    light series
Drugs, as appropriate: suitable dilution
Other contact substances, as appropriate: suitable dilution

For irradiation (light series)	% in petroleum
Benzocaine	2
Chlorpromazine	0.1
Musk ambrette	5
Promethazine	1
Benzophenone-3 (Oxybenzone)	2
Benzophenone-10 (Mexenone)	2
Butylmethoxydibenzoylmethane (Parsol 1789)	2
2-Ethoxyethyl-*p*-methoxycinnamate (Cinoxate)	2
4-Isopropyldibenzoylmethane (Eusolex 8020)	2
3-(4-Methylbenzylidene)-camphor (Eusolex 6300)	2
Octyldimethyl-PABA (Escalol 507)	2
Octylmethoxycinnamate (Parsol MCX)	2
PABA	2

Drugs, as appropriate: suitable dilution
Other contact substances, as appropriate: suitable dilution

reported by Cronin[17] the photoallergic contact reactions to musk ambrette were elicited by 1 J/cm² UVA. The photoallergic contact reaction to 2-ethoxy-*p*-methoxycinnamate[8] in an Asian was elicited by 2 J/cm² UVA. The threshold dose of UVA to produce a photoallergic contact reaction to isopropyldibenzoylmethane was 2 J/cm² UVA, determined by incremental exposures from 0.5 to 5 J/cm².[18] At the St John's Dermatology Centre 5 J/cm² is now used for routine photopatch testing, but this may be reduced for individuals with a low minimum erythemal dose (MED) or increased for dark skinned subjects.

The dermatologist undertaking photopatch testing will not generally know the MED of his patients and this is usually unimportant. However, exposure to 5 J/cm² of UVA can give a very severe sunburn-type reaction to exposed skin in very light-sensitive individuals. If required, the MED can be determined by irradiating defined, small areas of the skin on the back in sequence, with increasing doses of UVA from the same radiation source to be used for photopatch testing.

Source of UVA

Any artificial source of radiation with a good broad spectral output of UVA (315–400 nm) is suitable for photopatch testing. A small unit used for giving hand and foot PUVA is an example. If significant amounts of UVB are present this needs to be filtered with window glass as it is significantly more erythemogenic than UVA. The energy output of the radiation source needs to be known and monitored at intervals as there may be fluctuation. The Waldmann Lichttechnik UV meter may serve as a standard monitoring device. At the St John's Dermatology Centre the light source is a bank of Philips TL 44D 25/09 fluorescent tubes. There is now available the Philips TLK 40W/09N fluorescent tube which is free from UVB contamination.

Allergen application and readings — recommended methods

Individuals undergoing photopatch testing should also be patch tested with a standard series of contact allergens, allergens which cause contact reactions on the face and, if appropriate, cosmetics. Patch testing to these allergens may take place at the same time as photopatch testing. Substances for photopatch testing are applied in duplicate as parallel series on either side of the back. Additional substances for photopatch testing may include drugs such as thiazide diuretics,[19] or benzydamine[20] and occupational contactants such as thiourea, used as an antioxidant in photocopying paper.[21]

After 2 days, the sites are examined for reactions which are recorded in the usual manner. The photoallergens which are not for irradiation are masked with an opaque material. The second series of photo-allergens are irradiated with the UVA and then covered with opaque material. After a further 2 days the opaque covers are removed and any reactions are again recorded.

In order to produce positive photopatch test reactions to methylcoumarin, the substance must be applied shortly before irradiation.

Interpretation of results

No reaction at an unirradiated site but a reaction at an irradiated site signifies a photoallergic response. The situation when equal reactions are found at both sites is interpreted as simple contact allergy alone. Reactions at both sites but with the irradiated site showing a significantly greater reaction may indicate that both contact and photocontact allergy exists.

Although positive photoallergic contact reactions are usually quite clear, as with ordinary patch testing, it may sometimes be necesssary to differentiate between a phototoxic and a photoallergic reaction. One method is to do a serial dilution series of the suspected photoallergen and also vary the dose of irradiation. This technique has been called photopatch test mapping.[22] A positive response at a very low concentration and/or very low light dose points to photoallergy rather than phototoxicity.

References

1. Wilkinson DS, Patch test reactions to certain halogenated salicylanilides, *Br J Dermatol* (1962) **74**: 302–6.
2. Larsen W, Photoallergy to musk ambrette found in aftershave lotion. Presented at the American Academy of Dermatology meeting, San Francisco, 1978.
3. Thune P, Contact and photocontact allergy to sunscreens, *Photodermatology* (1984) **1**: 5–9.
4. English JSC, White IR, Cronin E, Sensitivity to sunscreens, *Contact Dermatit* (1987) **17**: 159–62.
5. English JSC, White IR, Allergic contact dermatitis from isopropyl dibenzoylmethane, *Contact Dermatit* (1986) **15**: 94.
6. Schauder S, Ippen H, Photoallergic and allergic contact dermatitis from dibenzoylmethanes, *Photodermatology* (1986) **3**: 140–7.
7. Schauder S, Ippen H, Lichtschutzfilterhaltige Präparate in der Bundesrepublik Deutschland 1988, *Z Hautkrank* (1988) **63**: 707–63.
8. Murphy GM, White IR, Photoallergic contact dermatitis to 2-ethoxy-p-methoxycinnamate, *Contact Dermatit* (1987) **16**: 296.
9. Bruze M, Gruvberger B, Thune P, Contact and photocontact allergy to glyceryl *para*-aminobenzoate, *Photodermatology* (1988) **5**: 162–5.
10. Hjorth N, Roed-Petersen J, Thomsen K, Airborne contact dermatitis from *Compositae oleoresins* stimulates photodermatitis, *Br J Dermatol* (1976) **95**: 613–20.
11. English JSC, Norris P, White I et al, Variability in the clinical patterns of *Compositae* dermatitis, *Br J Dermatol* (1989) **121** (suppl 34): 27.
12. Frain-Bell W, Johnson BE, Contact sensitivity to chrysanthemum and the photosensitivity dermatitis and actinic reticuloid syndrome, *Br J Dermatol* (1979) **101**: 491–501.
13. Murphy GM, White IR, Hawk JLM, Allergic airborne contact dermatitis to *Compositae* with photosensitivity — chronic actinic dermatitis in evolution, *Photobiology* (1990) (in press).
14. Ducombs G, Benezra C, Talaga P et al, Patch testing with the 'sesquiterpene lactone mix': a marker for contact allergy to *Compositae* and other sesquiterpenelactone-containing plants, *Contact Dermatit* (1990) (in press).
15. Wrangsjö K, Ros AM, Wahlberg JE, Contact allergy to *Compositae* plants in patients with summer exacerbating dermatitis, *Contact Dermatit* (1990) **22**: 148–54.
16. Norris P, Hawk JLM, White IR, Photoallergic contact dermatitis from fentichlor, *Contact Dermatit* (1988) **18**: 318–20.
17. Cronin E, Photosensitivity to musk ambrette, *Contact Dermatit* (1984) **11**: 88–92.
18. Murphy GM, White IR, Cronin E, Immediate and delayed photocontact dermatitis to isopropyl dibenzoylmethane, *Contact Dermatit* (1990) **22**: 129–31.
19. White IR, A positive photopatch test with hydrochlorothiazide, *Contact Dermatit* (1983) **9**: 237.
20. Frosch PJ, Weickel R, Photokontaktallergie durch Benzydamin (Tantum), *Hautarzt* (1989) **40**: 771–3.
21. Dooms-Goossens A, Chrispels MT, De Veylden H et al, Contact and photocontact sensitivity problems associated with thiourea and its derivatives: a review of the literature and case reports, *Br J Dermatol* (1987) **116**: 573–9.
22. Takashima A, Yamamoto K et al, Allergic contact and photocontact dermatitis due to psoralens in patients with psoriasis treated with topical PUVA, *Br J Dermatol* (1991) **124**: 37–42.

12
Drug and chemical photosensitization

B. E. Johnson
Department of Dermatology, University of Dundee, Level 8 Polyclinic Area, Ninewells Hospital and Medical School, Dundee DD1 9SY, UK

Photosensitization

Solar radiation and chemicals, either naturally occurring or products of a complex industrial society, are two major components of the human environment which pose a threat to the skin. Low levels of exposure to ultraviolet (UV) or visible radiation or to chemicals alone, may be harmless but, with increasing incidence, a combination of the two may produce damage through a process of photosensitization.[1-4] This is a process in which radiation, particularly UVA (315–400 nm) and visible, is absorbed by the chemical in the skin, the absorbed energy producing damage at cell and tissue levels through a variety of photochemical, molecular and biochemical pathways (Figures 1 and 2). In some instances, photosensitization may be so efficient that UVB wavelengths (280–315 nm) may produce skin reactions with exposures lower than those required for sunburn. Immediate and/or delayed inflammatory reactions of varying severity resulting directly from photosensitization at the cellular or tissue level are included in a broad category of 'phototoxicity'; where the immune system, cell mediated delayed hypersensitivity type reactions in particular are involved, the term 'photoallergy' is used. This useful classification is complicated slightly by the finding that complement activation, more often associated with the immune system, is induced by the phototoxic action of substances such as chlorpromazine, demethylchlortetracycline and porphyrins.[5] Both phototoxicity and photoallergy are more or less acute, short-term effects. However, repeated exposure to pho-

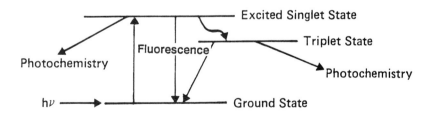

Figure 1

Simple molecular electron energy level diagram illustrating events after exposure to UV or visible radiation ($h\nu$). Ground-state electrons are raised to the short-lived (10^{-9}–10^{-6} s) excited singled state. From here, photochemistry may occur or the energy may be re-emitted as fluorescence. Alternatively, an intersystem crossing gives rise to the triplet state with a relatively long lifetime ($>10^{-3}$ s) during which photosensitization may occur.

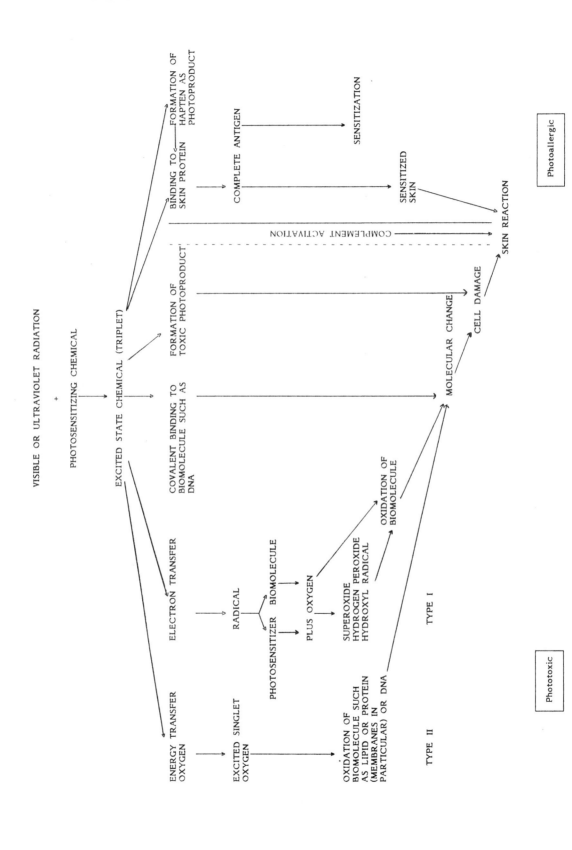

Figure 2
Diagrammatic illustration of various pathways for the photosensitization process in skin.

totoxic insult with agents such as coal tar and psoralens may give rise to skin cancer in experimental animals.[6] The benefits of psoralen + UVA (PUVA) as a treatment for psoriasis and other dermatoses are well established but evidence is accumulating that 8-methoxypsoralen (8-MOP) photosensitized skin cancer may also be induced in humans.[6]

Although the mechanisms are not understood, in some cases photoallergy appears to be part of a process in which a state of persistent light reaction arises in the skin of an affected subject where an exquisite sensitivity is observed, the wavelength dependency is shifted towards the UVB away from that of the original photosensitization, and an exogenous photosensitizer is no longer required.

Where the molecular mechanisms of photosensitization are oxygen dependent, the term 'photodynamic action' is applied. Type I reactions, through electron or hydrogen transfer, involve radical species of the photosensitizer or substrate molecule which may react directly with oxygen, or given rise to the damaging superoxide, hydrogen peroxide and hydroxyl radicals. Type II reactions involve the formation of the highly reactive excited singlet state of oxygen. In both types of reaction, lipid, protein and guanine in nucleic acids may be oxidized but biomembranes appear to be the major cellular target.[7]

Some part of the photosensitization due to furocoumarins may be oxygen dependent, but the major biological effects appear to be mediated through oxygen independent reactions. Of these, the most important are the UVA-induced covalent binding of, in particular, the psoralens, to DNA resulting in monoadducts and, with sequential exposure, cross-link formation.[8] Part of the photosensitization due to chlorpromazine, α-terthienyl, anthracene and polycyclic hydrocarbons generally may also be mediated through photobinding to DNA and other target biomolecules. An apparent photosensitization, due to toxic photoproduct formation, is seen in chlorpromazine induced cytotoxicity[9] and photohaemolysis with both chlorpromazine[10,11] and protriptylene.[12] Photoproducts of benoxaprofen and demethylchlortetracycline may also be important, both compounds being photosensitizers in their own right.[13] Photosensitization at cell and tissue levels, mediated variously through changes in lipid, protein and nucleic acid may produce membrane damage, inhibition of macromolecular synthesis, mutation and cell death. It is evident that for any photosensitizer, although its molecular structure may indicate a preferred mode of action, the overall biological effect obtained may be mediated through a number of pathways rather than one well-defined process. This is especially true for cutaneous photosensitization where the location of the photosensitizer in the skin also plays a major role in the type of reaction produced.

Photosensitizers and their place in the environment

Drugs, plant materials, perfume and cosmetic constituents, dyestuffs, polycyclic hydrocarbons in wood preservatives, coal tars, pitch and pollutants, sunscreen and printing ink materials and even metal salts are exogenous photosensitizers, agents which enter the skin from the surface or through parenteral administration in a domestic (Table 1), recreational (Table 2), industrial/working place (Table 3), or therapeutic setting (Table 4).

Table 1 Photosensitizers in the domestic environment.

Bacteriostats in soaps	Halogenated salicylanilides; bithional; hexachlorophene
Wood preservative	
Vegetables	Psoralens in celery and parsnips

Table 2 Photosensitizers in the recreational environment.

Garden and countryside	
Plants:*	
Umbelliferae:	giant hogweed (*Heracleum mantegazzianum*)
	cow parsnip (*Heracleum sphondylium*)
	wild parsnip (*Pastinaca sativa*)
	tromso palm (*Heracleum laciniatum*)
Rutaceae:	common rue (*Ruta graveolens*)
	gas plant (*Dictamnus alba*)
	Bergamot orange (*Citrus bergamia*)
Moraceae:	fig (*Ficus carica*)
Furocoumarins:	psoralen, 8-methoxypsoralen, 5-methoxypsoralen, pimpinellin, sphondin, angelicin.
General	
Perfumes and cosmetics:	5-methoxypsoralen (Bergapten) in oil of Bergamot, musk ambrette, 6-methylcoumarin.
Sunscreens:	p-aminobenzoic acid (PABA), ethoxyethyl-p-methoxycinnamate, isopropyldibenzoylmethane, butylmethoxydibenzoylmethane
Tattoos:	cadmium sulphide

* See also Table 7.

Table 3 Photosensitizers in the industrial/working environment.

Anthraquinone based dyestuffs: benzanthrone; Disperse Blue 35.

Polycyclic hydrocarbons: pitch, coal tar, wood preservatives, anthracene, fluoranthrene.

Drugs: chlorpromazine

Plants: giant hogweed, psoralens

Printing ink: amyl-o-dimethylaminobenzoic acid

Animal feed supplement: quinoxaline-n-dioxide

Table 4 Major photosensitizers in the therapeutic environment.

Drugs
Antibacterial:	tetracyclines, sulphonamides, nalidixic acid, 4-quinolones
Tranquillizer:	phenothiazines (chlorpromazine)
Antidepressant:	protryptiline
Diuretic:	chlorthiazides, frusemide
Antiarrhythmic/antihypertensive:	amiodarone, methyldopa, quinidine, propranolol
Anti-inflammatory:	benoxaprofen, ibuprofen, azapropazone, naproxen piroxicam, tiaprofenic acid
Antifungal:	grizeofulvin
Bacteriostat:	halogenated salycilanilides, bithionol, buclosamide
Topical antifungal:	fentichlor, hexachlorophene
Anticramp:	quinine

Therapies
Photochemotherapy:	8-methoxypsoralen, 5-methoxypsoralen, trimethylpsoralen, khellin
Photodynamic therapy:	photofrin II

Abnormal metabolites such as uro- and coproporphyrin, and normal metabolites in excess, such as protoporphyrin, bilirubin, kynurenic acid and riboflavin, are classified as endogenous photosensitizers. An atypical interaction of chemical and radiation insult to the skin is seen in the cases of 'porphyria turcica' in which hepatotoxicity due to hexachlorobenzene ingestion led to the production of excess porphyrins and cutaneous photosensitization.[14] This situation is familiar in sheep and cattle where hepatotoxins lead to abnormal chlorophyll metabolism and the build up of photosensitizing phylloerythrin in the skin.[15]

Phototoxicity

Phototoxicity should be produced in any individual where sufficient photosensitizer is present in the skin which is exposed to high enough doses of the appropriate radiation. A photosensitizer distributed evenly throughout the skin will produce a reaction at any level, depending on the penetration of the active wavelengths. In experimental erythropoietic protoporphyria, where the photosensitizer is restricted to the blood, damage is confined to the vascular endothelium.[16] Mast cells are particularly sensitive targets when photosensitizer is free in the dermis, but when the photosensitizer is applied to the skin surface the epidermis is preferentially damaged. Photosensitized reactions in the dermis result in immediate phase reactions, while epidermal effects alone give rise to the delayed, sunburn type of response.[17] Complex patterns of phototoxic reaction should therefore be expected. Nonetheless, it is possible to classify cutaneous phototoxicity into four major reaction types (Table 5).[18]

Prickling and burning

Coal tar, pitch and a number of their constituent polycyclic hydrocarbons combined with exposure to sunlight or UVA alone, produce prickling or burning in the exposed skin and, as in erythropoietic protoporphyria, there may be no physical signs of photosensitization. Longer exposures increase the intensity of the 'pitch smarts' and elicit erythema and a wheal and flare reaction which subsides an hour or so after the exposure to leave erythema restricted to the exposed area of skin. The early phase erythema may also fade but develops again, reaching a maximum between 24 and 48 h. Hyperpigmentation, presenting in a bizarre pattern if due to splashing with wood preservative for instance, may succeed the various inflammatory reactions.

The dyestuffs, benzathrone and Disperse Blue 35, drugs such as benoxaprofen, amiodarone and in some instances, chlorpromazine when taken orally and the printing ink material amyldimethylaminobenzoate produce similar reactions. Methylene blue, eosin and rose bengal, the polyacetylenes and α-terthienyl from plants of the *Compositae* applied to intact skin have no effect but produce a typical coal tar phototoxicity when injected intradermally or applied to scarified skin.

Table 5 The major reaction patterns of cutaneous phototoxicity.

Type	Skin reactions	Photosensitizers or diseases
1	Prickling or burning during exposure, immediate erythema, oedema/urticaria with higher doses, sometimes delayed erythema/hyperpigmentation	Coal tar, pitch, anthraquinone based dyestuffs, benoxaprofen, amiodarone, chlorpromazine, erythropoietic protoporphyria
2	Exaggerated sunburn	Drugs such as chlorpromazine, chlorthiazides, quinine, demethylchlortetracycline
3	Late onset erythema, blisters with slightly higher doses, hyperpigmentation only with low exposures	Psoralens, phytophotodermatitis, Berloque dermatitis
4	Increased skin fragility giving blisters with trauma	Nalidixic acid, frusemide, tetracylcine, naproxen, amiodarone, porphyria cutanea tarda

This phototoxic reaction pattern appears to be the major manifestation of photodynamic, i.e. oxygen dependent, membrane damage mediated, action in the skin.

Exaggerated sunburn

An exaggerated sunburn reaction is associated with a number of systemic drugs, but typically with moderate doses of demethylchlortetracycline or high doses of other tetracyclines such as doxycycline and chlorpromazine. Sunlight exposures which are normally harmless produce mild sunburn and those which are normally just erythemogenic result in severe reactions. With chlorpromazine, the reaction pattern is complex and an early phase response is common.

Blistering

The third class of reaction appears to be specific for the UVA dependent psoralen type of photosensitization seen in phytophotodermatitis. Typically, the reactions are initiated by contact with the sap from a psoralen containing plant (Table 6) and exposure

Table 6 Plants commonly reported to cause phytophotodermatitis and containing psoralens.*

Order	Botanical name	Common name
Leguminocae	Psoralea corylifolia	Bavachee
Umbelliferae	Ammi majus	Aatrillal
	Angelica archangelica	Angelica
	Anethum graveolene	Dill
	Apium graveolens	Celery
	Daucus carota	Wild carrot
	Daucus sativa	Garden carrot
	Foeniculum vulgare	Fennel
	Heracleum gigantum	Garden parsnip
	Heracleum mantegazzianum	Giant hogweed
	Heracleum sphondylium	Cow parsnip
	Heracleum laciniatum	Tromso palm
	Pastinaca sativa	Wild parsnip
	Peucedanum oreoselium	Parsley
	Peucedanum ostruthium	Masterwort
Rutaceae	Ruta graveolens	Commun rue
	Citrus aurantifolia	Bergamot lime
	Citrus aurantium	Persian lime
	Dictamnus alba	Gas plant
	Phebalium argentum	Blister bush
Moraceae	Ficus carica	Fig

* This limited table is based on that of Pathak et al.[55] Further information is given in Mitchell and Rook.[56]

to sunlight on a hot, humid day. Erythema, possibly painful, distributed in a pattern clearly related to contact with the plant, is seen first some 24 h later. Blisters develop during the next 24 h which may coalesce to produce a bizarre pattern of response, but subside relatively quickly. Where the skin damage is not too severe, intense hyperpigmentation develops which may persist for months. The intensity of erythema and blistering depend on exposure dose and amount of photosensitizer in the skin. When these are low, only erythema may occur with a latent period of 72 h or more, followed by hyperpigmentation. With minimal exposures, the reaction may consist of pigmentation alone, often the case in Berlock dermatitis due to 5-methoxypsoralen in perfumes.

For the severe reactions of phytophotodermatitis, the molecular mechanism involved is probably covalent binding of the psoralen to DNA and the cross-linking reaction may be required. However, other reaction pathways are available, including binding to RNA, protein and fatty acids and there is evidence for an oxygen dependent reaction with lipid.

Skin fragility and blistering

Acute photosensitivity reactions may be observed in porphyria cutanea tarda, but the major feature of this condition is an increased fragility in exposed skin leading to blistering after trauma. Frusemide and nalidixic acid produce a similar reaction and the photosensitization might be considered as chronic rather than acute, repeated exposures being required. This drug-induced 'pseudoporphyria' also accompanies high-dose tetracycline, naproxen and amiodarone.

In addition to these four major reaction types, less common drug-induced photosensitivity reactions are photo-onycholysis with tetracyclines and benoxaprofen for instance. More chronic reactions occur such as milia with benoxaprofen, a slate grey or purple hyperpigmentation with chlorpromazine and, as well as a greyish pigmentation, a bronze appearance in some cases of amiodarone-induced photosensitivity.

Photoallergy

The terms phototoxicity and photoallergy[19] were introduced by Stephan Epstein in 1939 to differentiate between the reactions obtained with intradermal sulphanilamide and exposure to sunlight.[20] A first, phototoxic reaction occurred in all subjects tested and resembled sunburn. A second reaction, occurring in a limited number of subjects, appeared 10 days later after a second test and resembled contact allergic dermatitis. The histopathology of the test sites was typically eczematous and clearly differed from that of primary phototoxicity.

Topically applied phenothiazines, especially chlorpromazine, 3,4'5'5-tetrachlorosalicylanilide (TCSA) introduced into soaps as a bacteriostat, 3,4'5-tribromosalicylanilide, bithionol, hexachlorophene, bromochlorosalicylanilide (Multifungin) fentichlor and 4-chloro-2-hydroxybenzoic acid-N-n-butylamide (Jadit)[21] featured in subsequent reports of photoallergy, the incidence of which fell dramatically after the withdrawal of halogenated phenolic compounds from the toiletries market.[22] More recently, photoallergy has been associated with quinoxaline-n-dioxide (Quindoxin) a feedstock animal-growth promoter and the fragrance materials, musk ambrette and 6-methylcoumarin.[23,24]

Experimental studies have provided unequivocal evidence for the cell-mediated photoallergic potential of sulphanilamide, chlorpromazine, TCSA and musk ambrette.[25–27] A contact allergic reaction to a photoproduct of the parent compound may be obtained with sulphanilamide, tolbutamide and chlorpromazine,[28,29] but for TCSA a UVA-induced protein binding is required for complete antigen formation.[30]

In mice, systemic chlorpromazine and sulphanilamide[31] produce photoallergy and there is clinical evidence at least for a photoallergic reaction in subjects taking drugs such as quinidine, enoxacin and with thiazides. Photoallergy is also recorded as a part of phytophotodermatitis due to Umbelliferae,[32] but with the minimally phototoxic compounds sphondin and isobergapten rather than 8-MOP and photoallergic responses are not observed when a repeated form of mild bergapten (5-MOP) phototoxicity is obtained with perfumes. Finally, it should not be surprising to find that preparations designed to be applied to the skin to protect it against sun damage by abosrbing the damaging radiation, may turn out to be photosensitizing themselves. Both apparent photoallergic and contact allergic reactions have been reported with sunscreen materials such as p-aminobenzoic acid (PABA), cinnamates, oxybenzone and benzoylmethanes.[33]

Dealing with the threat

Government regulation of photosensitizing substances is limited. In the USA, the quantity of 5-MOP in perfumes and toiletries is the subject of a Hazardous Substances Act.[34] In a number of countries, incorporation of 5-MOP in sunscreening agents to promote suntanning has been banned, although initial fears regarding this threat of photosensitized mutation and carcinogenesis may not be merited.[35] Governmental interest in control of photosensitizing plants is raised only if livestock are threatened and Safety at Work legislation does not appear to take account of this possible industrial injury with dyestuffs.[36] Drug-induced photosensitization is one area in which regulation through legislation is possible. The high incidence of cutaneous phototoxicity due to benoxaprofen and its use in litigation processes[37,38] shows that, although little attention has been paid to this aspect of safety of medicines, it may be very important. In the majority of countries in which cutaneous photosensitization by drugs is recognized clinically, reports of the incidence of this adverse effect in clinical trials or post-market surveys are all that is required.[36] Advice may then be sought for confirmation and certification may be withdrawn. It is not certain that photosensitization of the skin is good reason for banning or withdrawing from the market a drug of proven and superior value unless an equally efficacious, non-photosensitizing substitute is available. If drugs are identified as photosensitizing and information about their action is available, it should be possible to continue their use by a combination of judicious prescribing, advice about avoiding exposure to sunlight when drug concentrations in the skin are high and applications of appropriate protection in the form of clothing and sunscreens. However, the requisite information should be available and legislation directed at the product licencing stage of drug development in terms of acquisition of knowledge of hazard and provision of advised warning. The formulation of regulations is an ongoing process, but procedures for product licencing in the UK required by the Medicines Act of 1968, revised according to European Council Directive 83/570/EEC, show that detailed toxicological tests at in vitro, animal model and clinical trial levels are established and recognized as valuable in assessing the safety of a new drug. At each stage, these tests can be adapted for photosensitization as an adverse effect which may then be treated on a risk/benefit basis in the same way as any other side-effect. Some companies already operate in-house phototoxicology testing to a certain extent, but formalized procedures are still required.

Numerous tests have been developed to study the mechanisms of photosensitization and to screen for phototoxic potential. These should logically extend from simple photochemistry such as absorption spectrum studies through complex flash photolysis techniques to provide information on triplet-state and excited-singlet oxygen yields, for instance; simple models such as the photosensitized destruction of histidine, killing of *Candida albicans* and photohaemolysis, more complex cell models such as mouse peritoneal macrophages, human peripheral lymphocytes in short-term culture and established cell lines such as the Chinese Hamster V79, to animal models and finally clinical trials.[39–44] The simple models are useful in that they may be used to differentiate two distinct forms of phototoxicity. The major phototoxic psoralens are positive against *Candida albicans* but negative in photohaemolysis and histidine tests. Extracts from the *Compositae* are negative against *C. albicans* but positive in the photohaemolysis and histidine tests and these tests are usually useful for photodynamic agents. It is clear that one of these tests alone is not sufficient as a screening test and, obviously, where a specific intracellular target is involved such as DNA, photohaemolysis is inadequate. Moreover, with the new-generation 4-quinolone broad-spectrum antibiotics, both *C. albicans* and photohaemolysis fail to demonstrate a phototoxic potential which is unequivocally revealed with more sophisticated mammalian cell models such as the lymphocyte and CHV79 tests. A requirement for a standardized and validated test model remains and the published work should provide a good foundation for this. Whatever system is used, testing of drug metabolites should be included. Drugs which are highly phototoxic in vitro such as trimethylpsoralen and the non-steroidal anti-inflammatory ketoprofen, prove to be poorly photosensitizing when taken orally. The reverse may be seen with the non-phototoxic vitamin A analogue etretinate, the major metabolite of which is positive. The phototoxic anti-arrhythmia drug, amiodarone, is metabolized to desethylamiodarone which is 10 times as phototoxic, while with chlorpromazine the desmethyl metabolites are more phototoxic than the parent drug, but others such as chlorpromazine sulphoxide are inactive.

Photoproducts of suspected photosensitizers should also be tested in these models, not only because they may be toxic but also because they may be phototoxic in their own right, benoxaprofen for example produces a more lipid soluble phototoxic photoproduct.[13] The photoproduct of demethylchlorotetracycline is also phototoxic but with an action spectrum shifted from that of the parent drug and more closely resembling the action spectrum obtained in skin.[45]

Animal models for phototoxicity include the flank skin of hairless mice or plucked haired mice, guinea-pigs, rabbits and miniature swine.[46] While mouse ear swelling may be useful for quantitative work, the most reliable model appears to be the mouse tail test in which increase in tail weight is related to phototoxic potential.[47]

There are good protocols for testing suspect photoallergic substances using both mice[26,48] and guinea-pigs.[49] Photopatch and intradermal injection techniques[50] have a place in the testing of phototoxic agents in human skin, but are of limited use for drug-induced photosensitivity for which good clinical trial protocols are required. Field trials have used volunteer subjects given usual prescribed doses of drug and exposure to natural sunlight.[51] Alternatively, subjects already taking the suspect drug are phototested under controlled conditions, results being compared with those from a large sample size normal population.[52-54] However, this form of trial may only reveal a strongly photosensitizing drug and more detailed protocols have been devised. In these, phototesting of volunteers is done before, during and after a prescribed course of drug treatment so that each subject provides his/her own control; drug dose is varied to produce a concentration effect; the pharmacokinetic profile of the drug governs the time after dosing of the phototesting and plasma levels of the drug are assayed at that time; the trial is blind with placebo and positive controls built in.[44] The use of such a trial procedure should allow the identification of any phototoxic drug unless the mechanism of cutaneous phototoxicity requires a build up of phototoxic insult through repeated exposure.

Conclusion

As with the environmental threat of UV radiation alone, the major approach to protection against photosensitized damage is through obtaining knowledge of the threat and education of the threatened population.

References

1 Blum HF, *Photodynamic action and diseases caused by light*, Hafner Publishing Company: New York, 1964.
2 Lamola AA, Fundamental aspects of spectroscopy and photochemistry of organic compounds; electronic energy transfer in biologic systems; and photosensitization. In: Fitzpatrick TB, (ed.). *Sunlight and man*, University of Tokyo Press: Tokyo, 1974, pp17–55.
3 Johnson BE, Light sensitivity associated with drugs and chemicals. In: Jarrett A, (ed.). *The physiology and pathophysiology of the skin*, Academic Press: San Diego, 1987, pp2541–606.
4 Harber LC, Bickers DR, *Photosensitivity diseases: principles of diagnosis and treatment*, 2nd edn, B. C. Decker Inc.: Toronto, 1989.
5 Lim HW, Gigli I, Complement-derived peptides in phototoxic reactions. In: Daynes RA, Spikes JD, (eds). *Experimental and clinical photoimmunology*, CRC Press: Boca Raton, FL, 1983, pp81–93.
6 Epstein JH, Topical therapeutic agents and photocarcinogenesis. In: Marks R, Plewig G, (eds). *Environmental threat to the skin*, Martin Dunitz: London, 1992.
7 Spikes JD, Photosensitization. In: Smith KC, (ed.). *The science of photobiology*, Plenum: New York, 1977, pp87–110.
8 Averbeck D, Recent advances in psoralen phototoxicity mechanism, *Photochem Photobiol* (1989) **50**: 859–82.
9 Carraz G, Beriel H, Photosensibilisants et radiosensibilitants. 2e memoire: les photomimetiques (Photosensitizers and radiosensitizers. Part 2: The photomimetics), *Therapie* (1962) **17**: 195–202.
10 Johnson BE, Chlorpromazine phototoxicity: a non-classical mode of action, *Br J Dermatol* (1983) **89** (suppl 9): 16–17.
11 Kochevar IE, Hom J, Photoproducts of chlorpromazine which cause red blood cell lysis, *Photochem Photobiol* (1983) **37**: 163–8.
12 Kochevar IE, Possible mechanisms of toxicity due to photochemical products of protriptyline, *Toxicol Appl Pharmacol* (1980) **54**: 258–64.
13 Kochevar IE, Mechanisms of UVA photosensitization. In: Urbach F, Gange RW, (eds). *Biological effects of UVA radiation*, Praeger: New York, 1986, pp87–97.
14 Cripps DJ, Peters HA, Gocmen A et al, Porphyria turcica due to hexachlorobenzene—a 20–30 year follow-up study on 204 patients, *Br J Dermatol* (1984) **111**: 413–22.
15 Pathak MA, Phytophotodermatitis. In: Fitzpatrick TB, Pathak MA, Harber LC et al, (eds). *Sunlight and man*, University of Tokyo Press: Tokyo, 1972, pp495–513.
16 Gschnait F, Wolff K, Konrad K. Erythropoietic protoporphyria—submicroscopic events during the acute photosensitivity flare, *Br J Dermatol* (1975) **92**: 545–57.
17 McGrae JD Jr, Perry HG, Relationship of photodynamic action to phototoxicity, *Arch Dermatol* (1963) **87**: 252–7.
18 Johnson BE, Photosensitization. In: Cronly-Dillon J, Rosen ES, Marshall J, (eds). *Hazards of light*, Pergamon: Oxford, 1986, pp41–56.
19 Epstein JH, Photoallergy—a review, *Arch Dermatol* (1972) **106**: 741–8.

20 Epstein S, Photoallergy and primary phototoxicity to sulfanilamide, *J Invest Dermatol* (1939) **2**: 43–51.
21 Herman PS, Sams WM Jr, *Soap photodermatitis, photosensitivity to halogenated salicylanilides*, Charles C. Thomas: Springfield, IL, 1972.
22 Smith SZ, Epstein JH, Photocontact dermatitis to halogenated salicylanilides and related compounds, *Arch Dermatol* (1977) **113**: 1372–4.
23 Raugi GJ, Storrs J, Larsen WG, Photoallergic contact dermatitis to men's perfumes, *Contact Dermatit* (1979) **5**: 251–60.
24 Wojnarowska F, Calnan CD, Contact and photocontact allergy to musk ambrette, *Br J Dermatol* (1986) **114**: 667–75.
25 Takigawa M, Miyachi Y, Mechanisms of contact photosensitivity to tetrachlorosalicylanilide under genetic restrictions of the major histocompatability complex, *J Invest Dermatol* (1982) **78**: 108–15.
26 Maguire HC Jr, Kaidbey K, Experimental photoallergic contact dermatitis; a mouse model, *J Invest Dermatol* (1982) **79**: 147–52.
27 Granstein RD, Morison WL, Kripke ML, The role of UVB radiation in the induction and elicitation of photocontact hypersensitivity to TCSA in the mouse, *J Invest Dermatol* (1983) **80**: 158–62.
28 Burckhardt W, Photoallergische Ekzeme durch Sulfanilamidsalben (Photoallergic eczema due to sulfanilamide), *Dermatologica* (1948) **96**: 280–92.
29 Maguire HC, Kaidbey K, Studies in experimental photoallergy. In: Parrish JA, (ed.). *The effect of ultraviolet radiation on the immune system*, Johnson and Johnson Baby Products Co: Skillman NJ, 1983, pp181–92.
30 Barratt MD, Goodwin BFJ, Lovell WW, Induction of photoallergy in guinea pigs by injection of photoallergen-protein conjugates, *Int Arch Allergy Appl Immunol* (1987) **84**: 385–9.
31 Giudici PA, Maguire HC, Experimental photoallergy to systemic drugs, *J Invest Dermatol* (1985) **85**: 207–11.
32 Kavli G, Volden G, Raa J, Accidental induction of photocontact allergy to *Heracleum laciniatum*, *Acta Dermatovenereol (Stockh)* (1982) **62**: 435–38.
33 Dromgoole SH, Maibach HI, Contact sensitization and photocontact sensitization of sunscreening agents. In: Lowe NJ, Shaath NA, (eds). *Sunscreens development, evaluation and regulatory aspects*, Marcel Decker: New York, 1990, pp313–40.
34 Marzulli FN, Maibach HI, Perfume phototoxicity, *J Soc Cosmet Chem* (1970) **21**: 695–715.
35 Young AR, Potten CS, Chadwick CA et al, Inhibition of UV radiation-induced DNA damage by a 5-methoxypsoralen tan in human skin, *Pigment Cell Res* (1988) **1**: 350–4.
36 Johnson BE, Cutaneous photosensitization... hazard and regulation. In: Riklis E, (ed.). *Photobiology: the science and its applications*, Plenum Press: New York, 1991, in press.
37 Anonymous, Benoxaprofen, *Br Med J* (1982) **285**: 459–60 (editorial).
38 Gerber P, Mass product-liability litigation. *Med J Austr* (1988) **148**: 485–8.
39 Oppenlander T, A comprehensive photochemical and photophysical assay exploring the photoreactivity of drugs, *Chimia* (1988) **62**: 331–42.
40 Johnson BE, Walker EM, Hetherington AM, In vitro models for cutaneous phototoxicity. In: Marks R, Plewig G, (eds). *Skin models, models to study function and disease of skin*, Springer-Verlag: Berlin, 1986, pp264–81.
41 Lock SO, Friend JV, Phototoxicity testing in vitro: evaluation of mammalian cell culture techniques, *Food Chem Toxicol* (1986) **24**: 789–93.
42 Duffy PA, Bennett A, Roberts M et al, Prediction of photoxic potential using human A431 cells and mouse 3T3 cells, *Mol Toxicol* (1987) **1**: 579–87.
43 Maurer T, Phototoxicity testing in vivo and in vitro, *Food Chem Toxicol* (1987) **25**: 407–14.
44 Ferguson J, Johnson BE, Double blind, controlled study to investigate the photosensitizing potential of norfloxacin in human volunteers, *J Am Acad Dermatol* (1991) (in preparation).
45 Hasan T, Kochevar IE, McAuliffe DJ et al, Mechanism of tetracycline phototoxicity, *J Invest Dermatol* (1984) **83**: 179–83.
46 Forbes PD, Urbach F, Davies RE, Phototoxicity testing of fragrance raw materials, *Food Cosmet Toxicol* (1977) **15**: 55–60.
47 Ljunggren B, The mouse tail phototoxicity test, *Photodermatology* (1984) **1**: 96–100.
48 Brown WR, Shivji GM, Furukawa D et al, Studies of the action spectrum for induction of photosensitivity to tetrachloro salicylanilide, *Photodermatology* (1987) **4**: 196–200.
49 Maurer T, *Contact and photocontact allergens*, Marcel Decker: New York, 1983.
50 Kligman AM, Kaidbey KH, Human models for identification of photosensitizing chemicals, *J Natl Canc Inst* (1982) **69**: 269–72.
51 Blank H, Cullen S, Catalano P, Photosensitivity studies with demethylchlortetracycline and doxycycline, *Arch Dermatol* (1968) **97**: 1–2.
52 Kaidbey KH, Mitchell FN, Phototesting potential of certain nonsteroidal anti-inflammatory agents, *Arch Dermatol* (1989) **125**: 783–6.
53 Bjellerup M, Ljunggren B, Double blind cross over studies on phototoxicity to three tetracycline derivatives in human volunteers, *Photodermatology* (1987) **4**: 281–7.
54 Ferguson J, Addo HA, Johnson BE et al, Quinine-induced photosensitivity. Clinical and experimental studies, *Br J Dermatol* (1987) **117**: 631–40.
55 Pathak MA, Fitzpatrick TB, Daniels Jr F, Presently known distribution of furocoumarins (psoralens) in plants, *J Invest Dermatol* (1962) **39**: 225–39.
56 Mitchell J, Rook A, *Botanical dermatology*, Greengrass Ltd: Vancouver, BC, 1979.

13
Ultraviolet radiation and the photosensitivity disorders

J. L. M. Hawk
Photobiology Unit, St Thomas' Hospital, London SE1 7EH, UK

Photosensitivity disorders, or photodermatoses, are common and often disabling skin diseases induced by exposure to ultraviolet radiation (UVR) and visible radiation from sunlight or artificial sources, particularly sunbeds. Although not so well recognized as normal photosensitivity reactions affecting all exposed persons such as sunburn, skin aging and skin cancer, these disorders affect a surprisingly large number of individuals. Perhaps 10% of persons in Boston, Massachusetts,[1] 23% in Scandinavia,[2] 5% in Australia and 15% in the UK may be affected.

The photosensitivity disorders are listed below.

(1) Acquired photodermatoses with a possible immunological basis:
 (a) polymorphic light eruption,
 (b) actinic prurigo,
 (c) hydroa vacciniforme,
 (d) solar urticaria, and
 (e) chronic actinic dermatitis.
(2) Metabolic photodermatoses:
 (a) the porphyrias
  (i) hepatic porphyrias (porphyria cutanea tarda, variegate porphyria, and hereditary coproporphyria),
  (ii) erythropoietic porphyrias (congenital erythropoietic porphyria (Günther's disease), and erythropoietic protoporphyria); and
 (b) xeroderma pigmentosum and other genophotodermatoses.
(3) Drug and chemical photosensitivity.
(4) UVR-exacerbated dermatoses.

Acquired photodermatoses with a possible immunological basis

Polymorphic light eruption

Polymorphic light eruption (PLE) is a common, long-lasting disorder which affects about 15% of the population in temperate climates, mostly young women.[1,2] Its aetiology is probably immunological. Induction occurs following exposure to summer or snow-reflected sunlight or solar simulated radiation, other artificial sources generally being ineffective. The dermal cellular infiltrate contains predominantly $CD4^+$ T cells at the onset of eruption, but by the 72 h mostly $CD8^+$ cells are present.[3] Epidermal and dermal antigen presenting cells are also increased in number. This is consistent with a delayed type hypersensitivity reaction, perhaps to a dermal UVR-induced neoantigen, a hypothesis made more likely by the fact that keratinocyte intercellular adhesion molecule-1 (ICAM-1), perhaps a specific marker for delayed type hypersensitivity,[4] is expressed during the reaction.[5]

The eruption occurs within hours after minutes, hours, or rarely a day or two of constant exposure, in black or white subjects, and fades after hours, days or, often with continuing exposure, weeks. The nose, the malar regions of the cheeks or chin, the sides and back of the neck, the upper chest, the backs of the hands and dorsolateral aspects of arms and other exposed areas may be affected, with sharp cut-off at lines of clothing. Exposed areas are usually symmetrically affected, and in any patient, certain, often normally exposed sites, such as the face and the backs of the hands, are frequently spared. Lesions may be micropapular, pinhead-sized, confluent, erythematous, whitish or yellowish papules on an erythematous background or macropapular, separate or confluent 2–3 mm flat or rounded, clustered lesions on normal skin. Occasionally there are vesicles, confluent plaques, irritation without rash and, particularly on the face, confluent eyrthema and swelling. Eczematization may sometimes occur during resolution. Solar urticaria is differentiated by its wealing, onset within 5–10 min of exposure, and resolution over an hour or two after covering up. Actinic prurigo, possibly a variant of PLE, usually affects children with persistent excoriated papules of exposed sites, sometimes in association with typical PLE. Erythropoietic protoporphyria (EPP) demonstrates painful tingling within half an hour or so of exposure and elevation of red blood cell protoporphyrin concentration. Lupus erythematosus is distinguished by abnormal circulating titres of antinuclear factor, or anti-SSA (Ro) and anti-SSB (La) antibodies. UVR-exacerbated atopic and seborrhoeic eczemas have differing morphologies and distributions.

Diagnosis is made from the clinical appearance if the eruption is present. Histology shows focal epidermal spongiosis and a dermal perivascular lymphocytic infiltrate. Irradiation skin tests with monochromator or broad-band UVB and UVA sources often show abnormal erythemal or papular responses to UVB or UVA, while solar simulated irradiation of previously affected sites, especially in suberythemogenic doses, commonly induces the rash.

Treatment is by restriction of UVR exposure and use of high protection absorbent sunscreens, preferably also effective against UVA. Low-dose psoralen photochemotherapy (PUVA) or UVB phototherapy 2–3 times weekly for 3–6 weeks or less before spring or vacation are very effective for patients who can conveniently attend a treatment centre. β-Carotene, chloroquine and hydroxychloroquine therapy may rarely prevent the eruption, or in severe cases a 3–5 day course of oral prednisolone may rapidly clear it.

Actinic prurigo

Actinic prurigo (AP), perhaps a persistent, excoriated PLE variant, predominantly affects children until adolescence, but occasionally adults, usually female; native American Indians are also afflicted by a similar condition, frequently into adulthood.

The disease is generally worse in summer, clearing slowly in winter, a variation often not noted by the patient. It may deteriorate after sun exposure, sometimes as typical PLE. There are excoriated, sometimes crusted, papules or nodules on the upper chest, upper back, face and limbs, more profuse distally, often accompanied by shallow, linear, punctate or irregular scars on the face, and usually sparing under the hair fringe. The sacrum and buttocks may also be affected in some patients.

Atopic eczema and prurigo, insect bites, prurigo nodularis, occasionally scabies and, because of the facial scarring, erythropoietic protoporphyria must be differentiated. Diagnosis, which is difficult in mild cases, is based primarily on history and clinical appearance. Irradiation monochromator tests, only sometimes positive, may assist diagnosis.

Treatment is by minimizing UVR exposure and using high protection broad spectrum sunscreens. Low dose PUVA and UVB phototherapy as for PLE may be helpful, but for severely affected patients intermittent courses of low dose thalidomide 50–100 mg daily are usually very effective,[6] although teratogenicity and tendency to induce peripheral neuropathy in around 15% of subjects necessitate careful supervision.

Chronic actinic dermatitis

Chronic actinic dermatitis (CAD) is a rare, light-induced eczematous disorder, particularly affecting middle-aged and elderly men who are often outdoor enthusiasts.[7] It encompasses the severe actinic reticuloid variant, the milder photosensitive eczema, and the photosensitivity dermatitis and actinic reticuloid (PD/AR) syndrome. It is induced by UVB radiation and, in addition, sometimes by UVA and occasionally also short visible irradiation. The clinical, histological and immunohistochemical features of the eruption resemble those of persistent allergic contact dermatitis, perhaps to an endogenous photoallergen.[8] This theory is supported by the fact that irradiated histidine in albumin may convert to weak antigen in vitro, particularly in the presence of a photosensitizer, and that CAD is well recognized to occur following contact photosensitization or in the presence of contact sensitization to photoactive substances. Furthermore, persons who are frequently outside are continuously sun-exposed as well as being exposed to such photoactive substances, for example *Compositae* oleoresins, thus perhaps facilitating photoallergen formation; in addition, older skin may also conceivably permit easier penetration of such substances.

Both black and white subjects, sometimes with a history of other eczema, may be affected, more in summer and after sun exposure, a fact often not recognized by patients. Widespread eczema, often lichenified, or associated with infiltrated, erythematous, shiny papules or plaques, affects the exposed skin of the face, scalp, back and sides of the neck, upper chest and backs of arms and hands, occasionally leaving irregular areas of sparing. Skin contours may be accentuated and skin folds or creases often spared, particularly on the forehead and face, in the groins and fingerwebs, and on the upper eyelids. Palmar and plantar eczema may occur. Eyebrows and eyelashes may be stubbly or absent. Irregular areas of hypo- or hyperpigmentation are not uncommon on exposed or covered sites. In severe cases there may be progression to generalized erythroderma, not always accentuated on exposed areas. Patients are thus frequently severely disabled by the condition, unless there is spontaneous remission, which is an occasional event.

CAD must be distinguished from airborne contact dermatitis which is unrelated to light sensitivity by the distribution of the rash, and in subjects with infiltrated plaques from cutaneous T-cell lymphoma, the histology of which may be virtually the same. The severe light sensitivity of CAD is the major distinguishing factor, cutaneous T-cell lymphoma being associated only occasionally with mild light sensitivity. In addition, in CAD the dermal infiltrate contains a higher proportion of $CD8^+$ T lymphocytes. Erythrodermic CAD resembles the Sézary syndrome, large numbers of circulating Sézary cells being present in both disorders, but the light sensitivity of CAD and a predominance of circulating $CD8^+$ rather than $CD4^+$ T lymphocytes are differentiating features.[9] Erythrodermic CAD must also be distinguished from other non-Sézary forms of erythroderma.

Irradiation skin tests are essential to establish the diagnosis, as well as the inducing wavelengths in order to facilitate treatment. Lower than normal minimal erythema doses induce erythema or eczema following UVB, and also UVA and occasionally in addition visible light irradiation. Such tests may sometimes be normal for some months after disease onset and should be repeated if clinical suspicion of CAD persists. Skin histology shows eczematous changes associated with a deep dermal lymphohistiocytic infiltrate and sometimes epidermal invasion by Pautrier-like epidermal cell collections reminiscent of those that occur in cutaneous T-cell lymphoma. Patch tests may be positive to a variety of allergens such as airborne plant sensitizers and sunscreen constituents. Photopatch tests may sometimes indicate an excerbating or predisposing photosensitizer such as a sunscreen constituent or musk ambrette in toiletry preparations.

Treatment requires marked restriction of UVR exposure. This is assisted by the use of commercially available plastic film blinds over windows which filter most UVR and short visible radiation while allowing reasonable yellowish lighting. Broad spectrum non-irritating sunscreens are also helpful but seldom totally effective. Orally administered azathioprine is very effective in many CAD patients in a dose of about 1.5–2.5 mg/kg/day for up to several months, leading to gradual onset of remission which may last for months to years.[10] White cell and platelet counts and liver function should be monitored after 1 week and monthly throughout treatment; abnormalities of these tests or adverse gastrointestinal effects in around 10–20% of patients may necessitate termination of therapy. If azathioprine is ineffective, PUVA therapy two or three times weekly for several weeks under oral and topical steroid cover may induce clearing, although some patients cannot tolerate it.

Solar urticaria

Solar urticaria (SU) is a rare disorder of young and middle age and more common in women, is often immunologically based, apparently following mast cell degranulation induced by IgE-mediated allergic hypersensitivity to cutaneous UVR-induced allergen.[11] Rare cases are associated with the presence of a chemical photosensitizer. Any waveband of UVR or visible radiation, relatively constant for any patient, may induce the eruption. Tingling occurs 5–10 min after exposure on irradiated sites, although sometimes not on regularly uncovered areas such as face and backs of hands, followed rapidly by erythema and wealing, often with sharp demarcation at lines of clothing. The eruption lasts for an hour or two after covering up, following which temporary lack of reactivity may persist for up to 24 h. Rarely PLE, systemic lupus erythematosus, erythropoietic protoporphyria and photosensitization to topically applied agents such as tar, pitch and dyes may be associated with SU.

The time course of SU may occasionally suggest PLE, lupus erythematosus or chemical or drug photosensitivity, but SU is more rapid, and its morphology is different. SU is most reliably diagnosed following induction of lesions by solar or artificial irradiation. Monochromatic tests are less certain to evoke the eruption, but better define the action spectrum, thereby assisting treatment.

UVB-sensitive SU may respond to restricted UVR exposure and the use of a high-protection sunscreen. The non-sedative H_1 antihistamines, perhaps slightly more effective with an H_2 agent, often give good protection in other cases.[12] Regular exposure to the inducing wavelengths from sunlight or artificial sources may lead to useful tolerance, while PUVA may also be effective in some patients.

Hydroa vacciniforme

Hydroa vacciniforme is a very rare, recurrent eruption of unknown aetiology, perhaps conceivably a scarring variant of PLE, which affects mainly children and young adults.[13] UVA radiation seems primarily responsible in most patients. Within hours of summer sun exposure, particularly on the face and backs of the hands, groups of 2–3 mm stinging, erythematous macules progress into discrete or confluent vesicles or bullae, umbilicate in a day or so, crust and heal to form pitted scars. The condition must be differentiated from PLE, actinic prurigo, herpes simplex and hepatic porphyria by the history, severe scarring and histology. Diagnosis is from the clinical features and histology, which shows mid-epidermal necrosis and dermal, predominantly perivascular, lymphocytic infiltration. UVR avoidance and UVA protective sunscreens are helpful, whilst oral chloroquine, PUVA and UVB phototherapy have also been used with occasional success. Remission frequently develops during adolescence.

Metabolic photodermatoses

The hepatic porphyrias

The hepatic porphyrias include particularly porphyria cutanea tarda, variegate porphyria and hereditary coproporphyria, all of which are associated with deficient function of haem biosynthetic enzymes.[14] As a result excessive accumulated porphyrinogen in skin is converted to the photosensitizer porphyrin, leading to the clinical abnormalities.

Exposed skin, particularly in summer, of the backs of hands and occasionally the forehead, face and scalp very readily forms erosions and bullae after minor injury, often followed by crusting or infection. Healing then slowly occurs, sometimes with superficial scarring, milia, hypertrichosis, irregular pigmentation and, rarely, scarring alopecia and reversible scleroderma-like changes of exposed sites.

Systemic attacks with abdominal pain and neurological and psychiatric abnormalities, sometimes fatal, may also sometimes occur in variegate porphyria and hereditary coproporphyria. Many drugs can precipitate such attacks, relatively few being safe.

Treatment is by restriction of light exposure and avoidance of precipitating drugs and alcohol. Porphyria cutanea tarda usually also remits with recurrent venesection or very low dose oral chloroquine over about 6–12 months. Systemic attacks also need appropriate general medical supervision.

Erythropoietic porphyrias

The erythropoietic porphyrias are also associated with deficient function of haem biosynthetic enzymes but, in addition, there are markedly elevated porphyrin levels in circulating erythrocytes, and more severe cutaneous clinical features than the hepatic porphyrias.[14] Only erythropoietic protoporphyria is relatively common. Painful skin irritation occurs after minutes to an hour or two of summer sun exposure followed, if exposure continues, by oedematous skin-coloured swelling that persists for days. Purpura, erythema, wealing and blistering may also rarely occur. Chronic signs often present are waxy, linear, punctate or irregular shallow scars on the face or nose, sometimes with furrows radiating from the lips. Exposed skin may have a coarse, dry texture, and the skin of the knuckles may also show thickening with accentuation of skin markings.

Restriction of light exposure and occasionally the use of UVA-protective sunscreens may be helpful in treatment. β-Carotene up to 200 mg daily in summer also significantly improves many patients, according at least to many uncontrolled studies.

The genophotodermatoses

Xeroderma pigmentosum is a rare, autosomal recessive disorder often characterized by marked susceptibility to sunburning, generally first noted in infancy, and by the early onset of degenerative and malignant cutaneous and ocular changes, predisposed to by defective repair of UVB-induced cellular DNA damage.[15] Diagnosis is by clinical assessment, by irradiation skin testing which often shows enhanced, delayed erythemal responses to UVB, and by assessment of cellular DNA repair. Natural killer cell function and, as a result, natural immunity are also apparently impaired. Treatment is by assiduous restriction of UVR exposure and use of high-protection sunscreens.

Bloom's, Cockayne's and Rothmund–Thomson syndromes are other rare genophotodermatoses with multiple congenital defects, the first two also being associated with defective DNA repair.

Drug and chemical photosensitivity

Drug or chemical photosensitivity occurs following exposure to environmental, therapeutic or cosmetic photosensitizing agents. Several clinical reactions are possible. These are: painful skin irritation within minutes of exposure, often followed by erythema, oedema, vesiculation or, rarely, wealing; skin fragility and formation of subepidermal bullae, followed by crusting, superficial scarring and appearance of milia; localized eczema which may very rarely progress to resemble CAD; or onycholysis. Irradiation skin tests are usually normal but may occasionally show abnormal irritation, erythema, wealing or papules following UVA or rarely UVB or visible irradiation. Photopatch tests to topical photosensitizers are often negative except in eczematous reactions. Photosensitizer avoidance is the most effective treatment, or failing this avoidance of light exposure. Broad-spectrum high-protection sunscreens may also help.

UVR-Exacerbated dermatoses

Dermatoses of non-photosensitive aetiology may be precipitated or aggravated in some patients by UVR exposure, even though in other subjects there may be no effect, or else improvement.[17] Such disorders include acne, rosacea, atopic eczema, seborrhoeic eczema, psoriasis, herpes simplex, lupus erythematosus (discoid or systemic), dermatomyositis, lichen planus, keratosis follicularis, cutaneous T-cell lymphoma, pemphigus foliaceus and pemphigus erythematosus. UVB exposure is usually responsible for disease exacerbations, perhaps often as a non-specific irritant effect, but exact mechanisms are largely unknown. Either exposed sites or the areas of predilection for the condition under normal circumstances are affected. Diagnosis is as for the underlying condition. Treatment is by restriction of UVB exposure, use of high-protection sunscreens and therapy of the underlying dermatosis.

References

1 Morison WL, Stern RS, Polymorphous light eruption: a common reaction uncommonly recognized, *Acta Dermat Venereol (Stockh)* (1982) **62**: 237–40.
2 Ros A, Wennersten G, Current aspects of polymorphous light eruptions in Sweden, *Photodermatology* (1986) **3**: 298–302.
3 Norris PG, Morris J, McGibbon DM et al, Polymorphic light eruption: an immunopathological study of evolving lesions, *Br J Dermatol* (1989) **120**: 173–83.
4 Vejlsgaard GL, Ralfkiaer E, Arnstorp C et al, Kinetics and characterisation of intercellular adhesion molecule-1 (ICAM-1) expression on keratinocytes in various inflammatory skin lesions and malignant cutaneous lymphomas, *J Am Acad Dermatol* (1989) **20**: 782–90.
5 Norris PG, Hawk JLM, Polymorphic light eruption, *Photodermatol Photoimmunol Photomed* (1990) **7**: 186–91.
6 Lovell CR, Hawk JLM, Calnan CD, Thalidomide in actinic prurigo, *Br J Dermatol* (1983) **108**: 467–71.
7 Ferguson J, Photosensitivity dermatitis and actinic reticuloid syndrome (chronic actinic dermatitis), *Sem Dermatol* (1990) **9**: 47–54.
8 Norris PG, Hawk JLM, Chronic actinic dermatitis. A unifying concept, *Arch Dermatol* (1990) **126**: 376–8.
9 Chu AC, Robinson D, Hawk JLM et al, Immunologic differentiation of the Sezary syndrome due to cutaneous T-cell lymphoma and chronic actinic dermatitis, *J Invest Dermatol* (1986) **86**: 134–7.
10 Murphy GM, Maurice PDL, Norris PG et al, Azathioprine in the treatment of chronic actinic dermatitis: a double blind controlled trial with monitoring of exposure to ultraviolet radiation, *Br J Dermatol* (1989) **121**: 639–46.
11 Leenutaphong V, Holzle E, Plewig G, Pathogenesis and classification of solar urticaria: a new concept, *J Am Acad Dermatol* (1989) **21**: 237–40.
12 Michell P, Hawk JLM, Shafrir A et al, Assessing the treatment of solar urticaria: the dose response as a quantifying approach, *Dermatologica* (1980) **160**: 198–207.
13 Sonnex TS, Hawk JLM, Hydroa vacciniforme: a review of ten cases, *Br J Dermatol* (1988) **118**: 101–8.

14 Elder GH, The cutaneous porphyrias. In: Hawk JLM, Maibach HI, (eds). *Seminars in dermatology*, vol 9, W. B. Saunders: Philadelphia, 1990, pp. 63–9.

15 Lehmann AR, Norris PG, DNA repair deficient photodermatoses. In: Hawk JLM, Maibach HI, (eds). *Seminars in dermatology*, vol 9, W. B. Saunders: Philadelphia, 1990, pp. 55–62.

16 Johnson BE, Ferguson J, Drug and chemical photosensitivity. In: Hawk JLM, Maibach HI, (eds). *Seminars in dermatology*, vol 9, W. B. Saunders: Philadelphia, 1990, pp. 39–46.

17 Kerker BJ, Morison WL, The photoaggravated dermatoses. In: Hawk JLM, Maibach HI, (eds). *Seminars in dermatology*, vol 9, W. B. Saunders: Philadelphia, 1990, pp. 70–7.

14
Ultraviolet irradiation and thiazides: in vitro effects

Edgar Selvaag, Thomas Bergner and Bernhard Przybilla
Dermatologische Klinik und Poliklinik der Ludwig-Maximilians-Universität München, Frauenlobstraße 9–11, D-8000 München 2, Germany

Photosensitivity reactions due to the thiazides chlorothiazide and hydrochlorothiazide were described shortly after their introduction in the treatment of hypertension in the 1950s.[1–3] Several reports on light-induced drug reactions have been published, the mechanism of action proposed being sometimes phototoxic[4] and sometimes photoallergic.[3] We screened a number of thiazides for their phototoxic properties using a haemolysis test. Of the 19 compounds studied, 16 exhibited phototoxic effects.

Material and methods

UVR sources

A UVASUN 5000S (Mutzhas, Munich, Germany), which emits radiation in the wavelength range 340–450 nm (maximum at about 370 nm), was used. The UVA irradiance at a distance of 40 cm was 34 mW/cm^2. TL 20W/12 light bulbs (Philips, Hamburg, Germany), which emit radiation in the wavelength range 275–375 nm (maximum at about 300 nm) was used. The UVB (UVA) irradiance at a distance of 40 cm was 1 mW/cm^2 (0.3 mW/cm^2). In addition, a SOL 3 sunlight simulating lamp equipped with an h2 filter (Hönle, Martinsried, Germany), with emission from 300 to 800 nm (maximum in the range of 400–600 nm) was used. The UVA (UVB) irradiance at a distance of 40 cm was 13 mW/cm^2 (1.2 mW/cm^2).

Dosimetry

Both the UVR intensity and dose were measured using an integrating instrument (Centra-UV, Osram, Munich, Germany).

Test substances

The following substances were used: bemetizide, bendroflumethiazide, benzthiazide, benzylhydrochlorothiazide, butizide, chlorazanile, chlorothiazide, chlortalidone, clopamide, cyclopenthiazide, cyclothiazide, hydrochlorothiazide, hydroflumethiazide, indapamide, mefruside, metolazone, polythiazide, trichlormethiazide and xipamide. The test substances were dissolved in organic solvents (acetone, methanol or ethanol), and diluted with TCM buffer (pH 7.4; 280 mosm/kg).

Photohaemolysis assay

The photohaemolysis assay was modified from the procedure described previously.[5–7] Human erythrocytes were prepared by washing the cells three times with TCM buffer, and resuspending the cells in TCM buffer containing 0.03% albumin (1 : 200). Aliquots (0.4 ml) of these suspensions were incubated in polystyrene tissue culture dishes (plain bottom, opening area 1.75 cm^2) in the dark (1 h at 37°C) with 0.1 ml of the test substance solutions at final concentrations of 10^{-3}, 10^{-4} or 10^{-5} M, or with buffer alone (blank).

Erythrocyte-free test samples were prepared in order to consider the effects of irradiation on the absorbance characteristics of the test compounds (erythrocyte-free samples).

After UV irradiation (0–200 J/cm² UVA with UVASUN 5000S, 0–2000 mJ/cm² UVB with TL 20, or 0–120 J/cm² UVA with SOL 3) incubation was continued for another 30 min. The supernatant liquid was then recovered by centrifugation, incubated for 15 min with Drabkin's solution, and the absorbance was measured using a microplate reader.

The 100% haemolysis values were obtained by adding distilled water to the test solutions (hypotonic shock). Haemolysis was calculated on the basis of the absorbance data according to:

$$\text{Photohaemolysis (\%)} = 100 \times \frac{(\text{test sample}) - (\text{blank}) - (\text{erythrocyte-free sample})}{(100\% \text{ value}) - (\text{blank})}$$

For each compound, complete testing was performed with erythrocytes from three donors; the results are given as the median value. A photohaemolysis of >5% was regarded as a positive finding.

Results

Irradiation with TL 20W/12 light bulbs did not cause significant photohaemolysis with any of the test substances. After exposure to UVASUN 5000S, only bendroflumethiazide caused significant photohaemolysis (median 27%). With the exception of chlorazanile, clopamide and indapamide, all compounds caused phototoxic haemolysis at the 10^{-3} M concentration. The degree of haemolysis was dependent on the UV-dose and the concentration of the test substance.

Bemetizide, bendroflumethiazide, benzylhydrochlorothiazide, butizide, cyclothiazide, hydroflumethiazide, mefruside, metolazone and xipamide also showed phototoxic properties at the 10^{-4} M concentration. None of the substances showed photohaemolysis at the 10^{-5} M concentration. For detailed results see Figure 1.

Discussion

In our study, 16 of 19 thiazides exhibited a phototoxic action, dependent on the UV dose and the concentration of the test substance. All of the thiazides tested had one absorbance maximum at 200 nm, and other maxima between 200 and 320 nm. Our investigations indicate that the action spectrum of these substances is at the longer wavelengths of the UV spectrum, despite their absorbance characteristics. Other factors, e.g. membrane binding or molecule alterations, may also be important in the mechanism of thiazide phototoxicity. The most prominent photohaemolysis was found after exposure to SOL 3, a sunlight simulating lamp, which emits both shortwave UV and visible light in addition to UVA. Augmentative effects between the different wavelengths may play a role in the phototoxicity mechanism.

Phototoxicity due to hydrochlorothiazide has been demonstrated in vitro using human peripheral mononuclear cells,[8] human red blood cells,[9,10] human laryngeal carcinoma cells[11] and fungus.[12] Using fungi,[12] chlorothiazide, methiclothiazide and trichlormethiazide, have also induced phototoxic reactions. Penfluthizide is another thiazide that has been shown to cause phototoxic haemolysis.[9] Chlorothiazide has been demonstrated to induce phototoxic skin reactions in mice[13] and guinea-pigs.[14] However other investigators[15-17] could not confirm this observation.

Chlorothiazide administered intradermally to human skin caused intense erythema and oedema after exposure to UVA and solar simulating irradiation.[18] In a study of subjects who were treated with thiazides, phototesting yielded skin changes due to hydrochlorothiazide after exposure to UVA, UVB and visible light. Bendroflumethiazide and cyclopenthiazide induced similar skin changes in this study.[19]

Monochromatic testing at 330 nm in several subjects on hydrochlorothiazide or bendroflumethiazide therapy showed an increase in erythemal sensitivity.[20] UVA photoprovocation testing demonstrated a phototoxic action of hydrochlorothiazide.[21]

The underlying mechanism of thiazide phototoxicity has also been studied.[9] It was concluded that membrane lipids may be one of the target molecules in thiazide phototoxicity. This is one of the mechanisms which is thought to initiate phototoxic reactions.[22]

In contrast to these findings, clinical photosensitivity reactions after the administration of thiazides has been reported for only three compounds: chlorothiazide, hydrochlorothiazide and chlorhalidone.[1-4, 23-26] This could point to a lack of major photosensitivity potential in vivo.

However, since the thiazides are widely used, photosensitivity reactions should arise more often. Further investigations are necessary to evaluate the actual risk of photosensitization due to these agents in vivo. In any case it seems

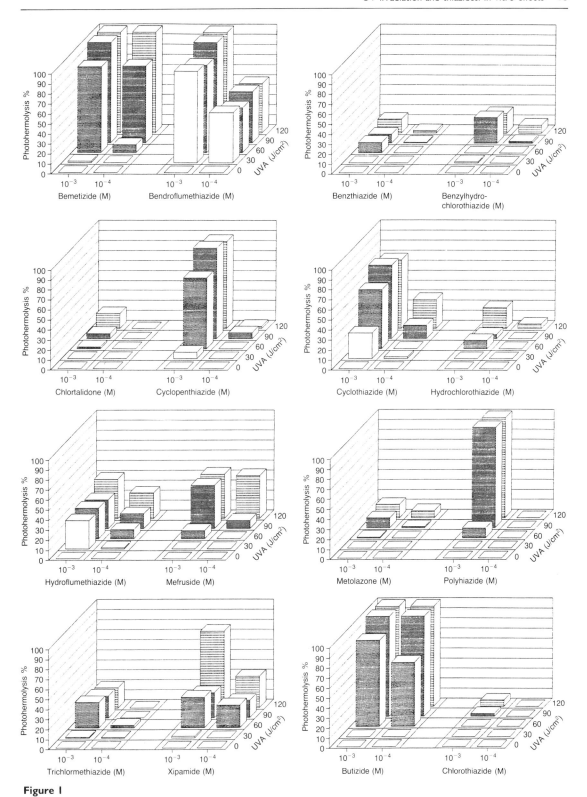

Figure 1

Results obtained with the photohaemolysis test for the 16 thiazides which revealed phototoxic effects after exposure to incremental doses from the SOL 3 apparatus.

advisible to avoid intense light exposure during thiazide therapy.

References

1. Norins AL, Chlorothiazide drug eruption involving photosensitization, *Arch Dermatol* (1959) **79**: 592.
2. Harber LC, Lashinsky AM, Baer RL, Skin manifestations of photosensitivity due to chlorothiazide and hydrochlorothiazide, *J Invest Dermatol* (1959) **33**: 83–4.
3. Harber LC, Lashinsky AM, Baer RL, Photosensitivity due to chlorothiazide and hydrochlorothiazide, *New Engl J Med* (1959) **261**: 1378–81.
4. Torinuki W, Photosensitivity due to hydrochlorothiazide, *J Dermatol (Jpn)* (1980) **7**: 293–6.
5. Kahn G, Fleishaker B, Red blood cell hemolysis by photosensitizing compounds, *J Invest Dermatol* (1971) **56**: 85–90.
6. Hetherington AM, Johnson BE, Photohemolysis, *Photodermatology* (1984) **1**: 255–60.
7. Przybilla B et al, Demonstration of quinolone phototoxicity in vitro, *Dermatologica* (1990) **181**: 98–103.
8. Morison WL, McAuliffe DJ, Parrish JA et al, In vitro assay for phototoxic chemicals, *J Invest Dermatol* (1982) **78**: 460–3.
9. Matsuo I, Hayakawa K, Ohkido M, Lipid peroxidative potency of photosensitized thiazide diuretics, *J Invest Dermatol* (1986) **87**: 637–41.
10. Freeman RG, Interactions of phototoxic compounds with cells in tissue culture, *Arch Dermatol* (1970) **102**: 521–6.
11. Freeman RG, Murtishaw W, Knox JM, Tissue culture techniques in the study of cell photobiology and phototoxicity, *J Invest Dermatol* (1970) **54**: 164–7.
12. Horio T, Evaluation of drug phototoxicity by photosensitization of Trichopyton mentagrophytes, *Br J Dermatol* (1981) **105**: 365–70.
13. Ison A, Blank H, Testing drug phototoxicity in mice, *J Invest Dermatol* (1967) **49**: 508–11.
14. Mitchell W, Epstein JH, The experimental production of drug phototoxicity in guinea-pigs, *J Invest Dermatol* (1967) **48**: 89–94.
15. Ison A, Davis CM, Phototoxicity of quinoline methanols and other drugs in mice and yeast, *J Invest Dermatol* (1969) **52**: 193–8.
16. Ljunggren B, Möller H, Drug phototoxicity in mice, *Acta Dermatovenereol (Stockh)* (1978) **58**: 125–30.
17. Ljunggren B, The mouse tail phototoxicity test, *Photodermatology* (1984) **1**: 96–100.
18. Kaidbey KH, Kligman AM, Identification of systemic drugs by human intradermal assay, *J Invest Dermatol* (1978) **70**: 272–4.
19. Addo HA, Ferguson J, Frain-Bell W, Thiazide-induced photosensitivity: a study of 33 subjects, *Br J Dermatol* (1987) **116**: 749–60.
20. Diffey BL, Langtry J, Phototoxic potential of thiazide diuretics in normal subjects, *Arch Dermatol* (1989) **125**: 1355–8.
21. Rosen K, Swanbeck G, Phototoxic reactions from some common drugs provoked by a high-intensity UVA-lamp, *Acta Dermatovenereol (Stockh)* (1981) **62**: 246–8.
22. Nilsson R, Swanbeck G, Wennersten G, Primary mechanisms of erythrocyte photolysis induced by biological sensitizers and phototoxic drugs, *Photochem Photobiol* (1975) **22**: 183–6.
23. Baker EJ, Reed KD, Dixon SL, Chlorthalidone-induced pseudoporphyria: clinical and microscopic findings of a case, *J Am Acad Dermatol* (1989) **21**: 1026–9.
24. White IR, Photopatch test in a hydrochlorothiazide drug eruption, *Contact Dermatit* (1983) **9**: 237.
25. Darken M, McBurney EI, Subacute cutaneous lupus erythematosus-like drug eruption due to combination diuretic hydrochlorothiazide and triamterene, *J Am Acad Dermatol* (1988) **18**: 38–42.
26. Parodi A, Romagnoli M, Rebora A, Subacute cutaneous lupus erythematosus-like eruption caused by hydrochlorothiazide, *Photodermatology* (1989) **6**: 100–2.

15
Mechanisms of cutaneous photoaging

Karin Scharffetter-Kochanek, Meinhard Wlaschek, Klaus Bolsen, Gernot Herrmann, Percy Lehmann, Günter Goerz, Cornelia Mauch* and Gerd Plewig

*Department of Dermatology, University of Düsseldorf, Moorenstrasse 5, 4000 Düsseldorf 1, Germany, and *Department of Dermatology, University of Cologne, Joseph-Stelzmann-Str. 9, 5000 Köln 41, Germany*

Introduction

Photoaging secondary to chronic ultraviolet radiation (UVR) exposure overlaps and probably accelerates the intrinsic aging process, finally resulting in wrinkle formation, increased fragility and impaired wound healing of the skin. The clinical manifestations collectively known as photoaging are thought to be due to quantitative and qualitative alterations of dermal extracellular matrix proteins. Histologically basophilic degeneration of the dermis is a constant feature.[1] Besides an accumulation of elastotic material[2,3] and proteoglycans,[4,5] a reduction of interstitial collagen fibrils and hydroxyproline has repeatedly been observed in actinically damaged skin.[4,6,7] However, the underlying mechanisms for the UVR-induced loss of interstitial collagen has only been partly characterized. UVB does not penetrate into the mid-dermis, even though profound actinic alterations have been observed in these areas of the dermis after UVB-irradiation.[3] For this reason, UVB-induced epidermal factors were postulated to mediate UVB effects to fibroblasts which reside in the mid-dermis. As has been recently reviewed,[8] a variety of growth factors are induced by UVB irradiation, among them tumour necrosis factor α (TNFα). In this study we addressed the regulatory role of TNFα in modulating collagen metabolism of the dermal fibroblast. Following treatment of fibroblasts with TNFα, a dose-dependent induction of collagenase was detected, while type I collagen was found to be reduced, indicating that TNFα may play an important role in the epidermis mediated UVR damage of the dermis.

Since UVA irradiation reaches fibroblasts in the deep reticular dermis, we studied the direct effects of UVA on the collagen metabolism of dermal fibroblasts. Our data indicate that collagenase mRNA levels were induced in a dose-dependent manner following UVA irradiation, while steady-state levels of type I collagen remained unaffected.

Material and methods

Cell culture and incubation with TNFα

Human skin fibroblasts obtained from healthy 25-year-old volunteers were grown to confluency in monolayer culture as described previously.[9] Fibroblast monolayer cultures in the fifth passage were incubated with various concentrations (1, 10, 100 ng/ml) of recombinant human TNFα (specific activity 8.5×10^6 U/mg, BASF, Ludwigshafen, Germany) in Dulbecco Modified Eagles Medium (DMEM), supplemented with 10% fetal calf serum (FCS), 50 µg/ml ascorbate, 300 µg/ml glutamine, 50 µg/ml streptomycin and 400 U/ml penicillin for 24–48 h.

RNA extraction, dot blot and Northern blot analysis

Total RNA was isolated from cells (confluent monolayers) following established procedures.[10] For Northern blot analysis, 3 µg total RNA per lane was resolved by gel electrophoresis in 1% agarose gel under denaturing conditions. RNAs were then blotted onto nictrocellulose (Bio-Rad, Munich, Germany). For dot blot analysis serial dilutions of total RNA (3, 1.5, 0.75, 0.375 and 0.15 µg/ml) were dotted onto nitrocellulose. Filters were baked at 80°C for 2 h. After prehybridization at 42°C in 50% formamide, 5 × SSC (1 × SSC is 0.15 M sodium chloride plus 0.015 M tris(sodium citrate)), 50 mM sodium phosphate (pH 6.5), 5 × Denhardt's (1 × Denhardt's is 0.02% bovine serum albumin, 0.02% polyvinylpyrrolidone and 0.02% ficoll) and 0.5% sodium dodecylsulphate (SDS) for 12 h, hybridization was carried out using deoxyadenosine-5′[^{32}P]triphosphate-oligolabelled cDNA probes (Multiprime DNA Labelling System, Amersham Buchler, Braunschweig, Germany) in 50% formamide, 50 mM sodium phosphate (pH 6.5), 5 × SSPE (1 SSPE is 0.18 M sodium chloride, 10 mM sodium phosphate (pH 7.7) and 1 mM EDTA), 5 × Denhardt's and 250 µg/ml salmon sperm DNA at 55°C for 24 h. For oligolabelling the following clones were used: a 1200 base pair long Eco RI fragment of the original cDNA clone hf677 coding for the α_1(I) collagen chain;[11] a 920 base pair long fragment of the original clone K4 corresponding to the 3′ terminal end of the coding sequence and the 3′ untranslated portion of collagenase RNA;[12,13] and a 450 base pair long cDNA fragment of human β-actin.[14] Following hybridization, filters were washed twice in 2 × SSC, 0.1% SDS at room temperature for 15 min and twice in 0.1 × SSC, 0.1% SDS at 50°C to 60°C for 15 min. Filters were then exposed to X-ray film (Kodak X-Omat AR) at −80°C. After development, the intensity of dots was measured by densitometry and calculated as a percentage of control values derived from RNA of mock irradiated cells.

In situ hybridization

In order to localize the cells that synthesize collagenase mRNA in human UVA-irradiated skin (50–60 J/cm^2), in situ hybridization was performed on biopsies of healthy human volunteers as described previously.[15] In vitro transcription was carried out using Gem 3 Koll K4, a cDNA fragment coding for human collagenase which has been subcloned into a Gemini vector.[16] Cells containing specific collagenase mRNA were identified by means of autoradiography and hematoxylin–eosin staining.

Measurement of newly synthesized collagen

Confluent monolayers were preincubated for 36 h in DMEM supplemented with 10% fetal calf serum and TNFα (1–1000 ng/ml). After washing the cultures twice with phosphate buffered saline (PBS), cell layers were labelled for 12 h with L-[2.3-^{3}H]proline (0.74 MBq/ml) in serum free DMEM containing TNFα as above and β-aminopropionitrile (50 µg/ml). After 48 h, incubation was stopped and the enzyme inhibitors p-chloromercuribenzoate (3 µg/ml; Sigma, Deisenhofen, Germany) and phenylmethylsulphonyl fluoride (3 µg/ml; Sigma, Deisenhofen, Germany) were added. Cells and medium were combined and dialysed against 1 M CaCl$_2$ and 0.05 M Tris-HCl (pH 7.4), followed by several changes of 0.5% acetic acid. The material was lyophilized and hydrolysed with 6 N HCl (plus mercaptoethanol) at 110°C for 24 h under nitrogen atmosphere. The samples were dissolved in 0.1 M sodium citrate (pH 3.2), and [^{3}H]proline and [^{3}H]hydroxyproline were separated on an amino acid column (Beckmann Spherogel, TM).

Zymography

Collagenase activity in conditioned media was assayed by means of a gelatin substrate enzymogram. Gelatin (type I collagen) (Bio-Rad, Munich, Germany) was incorporated in 8% polyacrylamide gels to a final concentration of 1 mg/ml. The serum-free conditioned medium was mixed with a sodium dodecylsulphate (SDS) sample buffer without heating. Following electrophoresis, the SDS was removed from the gels by 2.5% Triton X-100 for 1 h at room temperature. The gels were incubated in 0.05 M Tris-HCl buffer (pH 8.0) containing 5 mM CaCl$_2$, and 10^{-6} M ZnCl$_2$ at 37°C for 16 h and then stained with Coomassie blue.

UVA irradiation

UVA irradiation was performed as described previously.[16] Briefly, cells were irradiated at a distance of 40 cm with a high intensity UVR source (UVA SUN 3000^R) emitting wavelengths in the range of 340–450 nm (Mutzhas, Munich, Germany).[17] Dose rates in the range 15–35 J/cm^2 during irradiation of the cells were determined with a combined UVA/UVB ultravioletmeter (Centra-UV-dosimeter, Osram, Munich, Germany). During irradiation, the cells were incubated in PBS and maintained at 35–37°C in a thermostatically controlled water bath.

Results

Effects of TNFα on steady-state levels of type I collagen and collagenase mRNAs

Northern blot analysis was carried out using total RNA from fibroblasts treated with TNFα at a concentration of 100 ng/ml. No difference in the densitometric values of the β-actin band could be detected with and without TNFα (Figure 1(A)). The densitometric values of the two type I collagen mRNA species decreased following TNFα treatment as compared to controls without TNFα (Figure 1(B)). Collagenase mRNA of 2.4 kb length was increased five-fold (Figure 1(C)).[18]

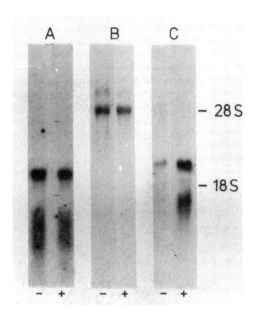

Figure 1

Determination of specific mRNAs by Northern blot analysis. Total RNA was isolated from fibroblast monolayer cultures after incubation with (+) and without (−) TNFα at a concentration of 100 ng/ml for 48 h. Total RNA was then fractionated by electrophoresis under denaturing conditions and blotted onto nitrocellulose. The filter was sequentially hybridized with cDNA probes for human β-actin (A), human α_1 (I) collagen (B) and human collagenase (C).

Quantification of newly synthesized collagen

To study whether the TNFα mediated reduction of collagen mRNA steady-state levels are reflected at the protein level, the rate of synthesis of collageneous proteins was evaluated. Synthesis of collagen was reduced to 50% at 0.1 ng/ml of TNFα. This inhibition was specific for collageneous proteins, as indicated by the reduction of collagen relative to total protein synthesis (Table 1).

Induction of collagenase following TNFα treatment

In order to monitor whether TNFα induced collagenase mRNA levels result in increased translation, enzymograms with supernatants of TNFα treated cells using collagen containing 8% polyacrylamide gels were prepared. At a size of about 50 kDa a clear band becomes visible, indicating that collagen was degraded by collagenase (data not shown).

Effect of UVA irradiation on steady-state levels of type I collagen and collagenase mRNA in vitro

As shown in Figure 2(A), β-actin mRNA appears to be reduced after UVA irradiation. This is due to unequal amounts of total RNA loaded onto the gel, since densitometric evaluation of dot blot analysis (Table 2) did not reveal any regulation of β-actin mRNA levels after UVA irradiation of corresponding dose rates. Following UVA irradiation, no specific alteration of collagen mRNA levels was

Table 1 Influence of TNFα on newly synthesized collagen and on total protein.*

TNFα (ng/ml)	cpm Hyp/cell	% Collagen/ total protein
0	31.3 ± 6.0	8.3 ± 0.2
0.1	17.2 ± 1.1	6.4 ± 0.2
1	18.2 ± 0.96	6.6 ± 0.5
10	17.8 ± 0.7	6.6 ± 0.8
100	16.2 ± 1.7	6.4 ± 0.2
1000	16.8 ± 2.4	5.5 ± 0.7

* After incubation of confluent fibroblast monolayer cultures with [³H]proline, as detailed in the text, collagen was calculated by measuring non-dialysable [³H]hydroxyproline (Hyp) in combined medium and cell layer. Synthesis is expressed as percentage collagen of total protein and represents the average as cpm/cell of triplicate determinations.

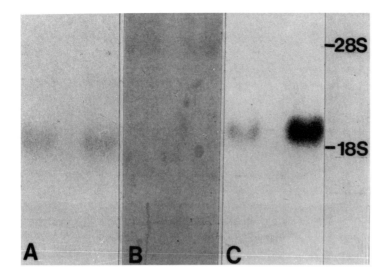

Figure 2

Northern blot analysis of β-actin (A), collagen (B) and collagenase mRNA (C) from fibroblast monolayer cultures following UVA irradiation (35 J/cm^2). Northern blot analysis was carried out as described in the legend to Figure 1.

Table 2 Quantification of α_1 (I) collagen, collagenase and β-actin mRNA levels in fibroblast monolayers following UVA irradiation.*

	Control	\\ UVA dose (J/cm^2) \\ 5	10	30
Collagenase/β-actin	1	1.5	2.8	5.2
Collagen/β-actin	1	0.9	1.2	0.8

* Identical blots were sequentially hybridized with α_1 (I) collagen, collagenase and β-actin cDNA probes. Dot blot analysis was carried out as described in the text. The amounts of mRNA were quantified using densitometric analysis and expressed as ratio of collagenase to β-actin or as α_1 (I) collagen to β-actin.

detected (Figure 2(B)), whereas collagenase mRNA increased in a dose-dependent manner following UVA irradiation (Figure 2(C), Table 2).

Effect of UVA irradiation on dermal fibroblasts in vivo

In situ hybridization was performed in order to localize collagenase mRNA containing fibroblasts in UVA irradiated human skin. Unirradiated skin did not reveal any specific signal (data not shown), indicating that remodelling of collagen was almost absent in normal adult human dermis. In contrast, after UVA irradiation specific labelling was observed in dermal fibroblasts providing evidence that UVA irradiation induces collagenase mRNA in vivo (Figure 3).

Discussion

Photoaging is due to chronic sun exposure or therapeutic/cosmetic irradiation and is characterized by profound alterations in the dermal connective tissue. Several extracellular dermal proteins are involved (for reviews see Uitto et al,[3] Oikarinen et al[6] and Oikarinen[19]), among them collagen which constitutes the major structural component of the dermis. Collagen has been found to be reduced in actinically damaged skin.[4,6,7]

The net accumulation of collagen is a balance of the rate of synthesis and the rate of degradation. Therefore, understanding the UVR-induced loss of collagen requires knowledge about the ways in which UVR affects these fibroblast-controlled processes. Furthermore, the skin is a rather complex tissue consisting of several histogenetically distinct cell compartments. Hence, UVR effects might be mediated from one cell species to another by

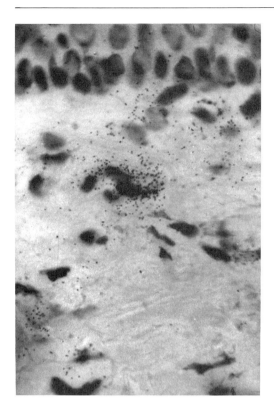

Figure 3

Location of specific mRNA in human skin following UVA irradiation. Biopsies of UVA-irradiated skin (50–60 J/cm^2) were taken 24 h following irradiation and processed for in situ hybridization as described in the text. An antisense collagenase RNA-probe (1.5 × 10^6 cpm/section) was used for hybridization. Magnification: ×250.

UVR-induced soluble factors. This is of particular importance in the actinic damage of the mid-dermis following UVB irradiation which is known to be mainly absorbed by the epidermis. We have reported earlier[18] on the coordinate effect of TNFα in reducing type I collagen, while inducing collagenase synthesis under the same experimental conditions. This indicates that TNFα has a complex impact on collagen metabolism controlling synthesis and degradation. In conjunction with the recent observation that UVB induces TNFα in epidermal cells[8,20] and also in mast cells,[21] TNFα appears to be an important signalling molecule which mediates UVB effects on dermal fibroblasts and thus profoundly modulates its collagen metabolism, finally resulting in a loss of interstitial collagen. Interestingly, UVA irradiation is not able to induce TNFα in human mast cells (R. M. Lavker, personal communication), providing some evidence that different wavelengths

act via different mechanisms. In contrast to UVB, UVA irradiation penetrates into the deep dermis making fibroblasts a direct target. Since the steady-state levels of collagen mRNA and collagenase mRNA play an important regulatory role in the synthesis of the corresponding proteins,[22–26] we monitored the UVA effects on collagen and collagenase mRNA levels in fibroblast cultures in vitro by hybridization techniques suitably reflecting the pretranslational level. Our results indicate that procollagen type I mRNA levels remain unaltered following irradiation of fibroblast monolayers, providing sufficient evidence that the synthetic pathway of collagen metabolism at the pretranslational level is not affected following short-term UVA irradiation. Collagenase mRNA levels increased following UVA irradiation of fibroblast monolayer cultures. This is not due to TNFα induction in fibroblasts (data not shown). The underlying molecular mechanism for the UVA induction of collagenase has not yet been clarified. Our in vitro data are supported by in vivo studies. Using in situ hybridization, moderately increased collagenase mRNA levels were detected in dermal fibroblasts of UVA irradiated skin. Dose rates of 35 J/cm^2 of UVA, as used in this study, represent a physiological dose easily acquired during a 3 h sun exposure in June at 40°N latitude.[27] In addition, upregulation of collagenase mRNA in monolayer cultures was observed at a radiation dose rate as low as 15 J/cm^2.

The results of this study provide initial evidence that UVR at different wavelengths affects collagen metabolism profoundly and by different mechanisms and thus may be responsible for the loss of interstitial collagen in the photodamaged dermis.

Acknowledgements

The clone for the α$_1$ (I) collagen was kindly supplied by Drs D. Prockop and F. Ramirez, the clone for the human collagenase was a gift from Dr P. Herrlich. We are grateful to Dr P. Gunning for giving us the clone for human β-actin. Recombinant TNFα was kindly provided by BASF, Ludwigshafen, Germany. This work was supported by the Deutsche Forschungsgemeinschaft (Scha 411/1–2).

References

1 Lever WF, Schaumburg-Lever G, *Histopathology of the skin*, 6th edn, Philadelphia: JB Lippincott Company, 1983, pp271–89.

2. Kligman LH, Kaidbuy KH, Hitchins VM et al, Long wavelength (>340 nm) ultraviolet-A induced skin damage in hairless mice is dose dependent. In: Passchier WF, Bosnjakovic BFM, (eds). *Human exposure to ultraviolet radiation: risks and regulations*, Elsevier: Amsterdam, 1987, pp77–81.
3. Uitto J, Fazio MJ, Olsen DR, Molecular mechanisms of cutaneous aging, *J Am Acad Dermatol* (1989) **21**: 614–22.
4. Smith JG, Davidson EA, Sams WM et al, Alterations in human dermal connective tissue with age and chronic sun damage, *J Invest Dermatol* (1962) **39**: 347–50.
5. Sams WM, Smith JG, The histochemistry of chronically sun-damaged skin, *J Invest Dermatol* (1961) **37**: 447–52.
6. Oikarinen A, Karvonen J, Uitto J et al, Connective tissue alterations in skin exposed to natural and therapeutic UV-radiation, *Photodermatol* (1985) **2**: 115–26.
7. Trautinger F, Gruenwald C, Trenz A et al, Influence of natural vitamin E and UV-irradiation on dermal collagen content in hairless mice, *Arch Dermatol Res* (1991) (abstract) (in press).
8. Schwarz T, Luger TA, Effect of UV-irradiation on epidermal cell cytokine production, *Photochem Photobiol* (1989) **4**: 1–13.
9. Fleischmajer R, Perlish JS, Krieg T et al, Variability in collagen and fibronectin synthesis by scleroderma fibroblasts in primary culture, *J Invest Dermatol* (1981) **76**: 400–3.
10. Maniatis T, Frisch EF, Sambrook J, *Molecular cloning: a laboratory manual*, Cold Spring Harbor Laboratory: Cold Spring Harbor, NY, 1989.
11. Chu ML, Myers JC, Bernard MP et al, Cloning and characterization of five overlapping cDNAs specific for the human proα$_1$(I) collagen chain, *Nucl Acid Res* (1982) **10**: 5925–34.
12. Angel P, Pöting A, Mallick U et al, Induction of metallothionein and other mRNA species by carcinogens and tumor promoters in primary human skin fibroblasts, *Mol Cell Biol* (1986) **6**: 1760–6.
13. Angel P, Rahmsdorf HJ, Pöting A et al, 12-O-Tetradecanoylphorbol-13-acetate (TPA)-induced gene sequences in human primary diploid fibroblasts and their expression in SV 40-transformed fibroblasts, *J Cell Biochem* (1985) **29**: 351–60.
14. Gunning P, Poute P, Okayama H et al, Isolation and characterization of full-length cDNA clones for human alpha-, beta-, and gamma-actin mRNAs: Skeletal but not cytoplasmic actins have an amino-terminal cysteine that is subsequently removed, *Mol Cell Biol* (1983) **3**: 787–95.
15. Scharffetter K, Lankat-Buttgereit B, Krieg T, Localization of collagen mRNA in normal and scleroderma skin by in-situ hybridization, *Eur J Clin Invest* (1988) **18**: 9–17.
16. Scharffetter K, Wlaschek M, Hogg A et al, UVA-irradiation induces collagenase in human dermal fibroblasts in vitro and in vivo, *Arch Dermatol Res* (in press).
17. Mutzhas M, Hölzle E, Hofmann C et al, A new apparatus with high radiation energy between 320–460 nm: physical description and dermatological application, *J Invest Dermatol* (1981) **71**: 42–7.
18. Scharffetter K, Heckmann M, Hatamochi A et al, Synergistic effect of tumor necrosis factor alpha and interferon gamma on collagen synthesis of human skin fibroblasts in vitro, *Exp Cell Res* (1989) **181**: 409–17.
19. Oikarinen A, The aging of skin: chronoaging versus photoaging, *Photodermal Photoimmunol Photomed* (1990) **7**: 3–4.
20. Oxholm A, Oxholm P, Staberg B et al, Immunohistological detection of interleukin 1-like molecules and tumor necrosis factor in human epidermis before and after UVB-irradiation in vivo, *Brit J Dermatol* (1988) **118**: 369–79.
21. Lavker RM, Walsh LJ, Kaidbey K et al, Mast cell degranulation results in endothelial activation after acute exposure of human skin to ultraviolet irradiation. *The Environmental Threat to the Skin*. An international symposium, 14–17 April 1991, Cardiff, UK.
22. Mauch C, Hatamochi A, Scharffetter K et al, Regulation of collagen synthesis in fibroblasts within a three-dimensional collagen gel, *Exp Cell Res* (1988) **178**: 493–503.
23. Mauch C, Adelmann-Grill B, Hatamochi A et al, Collagenase gene expression in fibroblasts is regulated by a three dimensional contact with collagen, *FEBS Lett* (1989) **250**: 301–5.
24. Rowe LB, Schwarz RI, Role of procollagen mRNA levels in controlling the rate of procollagen synthesis, *Mol Cell Biol* (1983) **3**: 241–9.
25. Uitto J, Perejda AJ, Abergel RP et al, Altered steady state ratio of type I/III procollagen mRNAs correlates with selectively increased type I procollagen biosynthesis in cultured keloid fibroblasts, *Proc Natl Acad Sci* (1985) **82**: 5938–9.
26. Werb Z, Tremble PM, Behrendtsen O et al, Signal transduction through the fibronectin receptor induces collagenase and stromelysin gene expression, *J Cell Biol* (1989) **109**: 877–89.
27. Kligman LH, Kligman AM, The nature of photoaging: its presentation and repair, *Photodermatol* (1986) **3**: 215–27.

16
Assessment of actinic elastosis by means of high-frequency sonography

K. Hoffmann, T. Dirschka, S. el-Gammal and P. Altmeyer
Dermatology Department, Ruhr University, Bochum, Germany

In routine dermatological diagnosis technical equipment is of minor importance. The assessment of chronic but dynamic processes of the skin is mainly based on clinical and subjective evaluations. Nevertheless, innovations in the field of microelectronics have made available ultrasound scanners for use in dermatology which have significant advantages over those available only a few years ago.[1,2] These scanners work at frequencies of 20 MHz and above and enable one to see into the skin as dermal and subcutaneous structures are presented in high resolution. These new scanners have been used mainly to investigate benign and malignant skin tumours. Moreover, using these scanners the thickness of the skin can be evaluated precisely and the increase in collagen fibres that occurs in the course of wound healing or in the progression or regression of scleroderma can also be observed.[3,4]

Equipment

A digital ultrasound scanner (DUB 20, Taberna pro medicum, Lüneburg, Germany) was used which consists of a Panametrics 20 MHz transreceiver, a digital Tectronic 2430 oscilloscope with GPIB interface and a Tandon 80286 personal computer with a 40 Mbyte hard disc. (The Dermascan C (Cortex Technology, Hansund, Denmark) is also suited to dermatological investigations.) Both scanners are shown in Figure 1.

The DUB 20 works as follows. A pulse-motor drive moves the transducer 12.8 mm through a defined water path over the area to be examined. The lateral resolution is 200 μm and the axial resolution 80 μm.

The scanner permits evaluation of structures situated at a depth of up to 7 mm below the surface of the skin and the images are depicted in eight-fold lateral and 24-fold axial magnification on the monitor. Both A-mode and B-mode imaging are possible. The computer converts the echo signals into a 255-colour false colour code according to the amplitude. This coding permits better differentiation of structures than the grey-scale representation usually used in ultrasonography. Light colours correspond to strong reflections and dark colours to weak reflections.

Images are obtained as follows. The coupling water path is echo free. A dense, highly reflecting line represents the entry echo and arises from the change in impedance from water to epidermis. The following region with medium and high reflections relates to dermal structures. Depending on the location, follicles and sharply delimited blood vessels can be found. Subcutaneous fat is almost echo free and shows up as stripy internal lines which represent muscle fascias. A sonogram of healthy skin is shown in Figure 2.

Actinic elastosis

Actinic elastosis is a chronic aging process of the skin which results from ultraviolet (UV)A (UVA), UVB and infra-red radiation.[5,6] Clinically, pale yellow, sometimes elevated indurated areas develop in the exposed regions, especially on the temples, the forehead and the back of the neck; the skin is wrinkled, lax, and sometimes scaling.

This paper contains significant material from the thesis of T. Dirschka

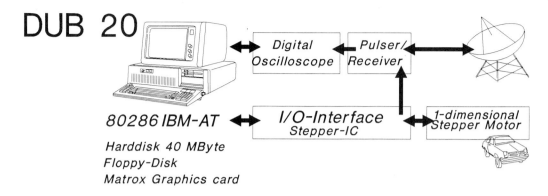

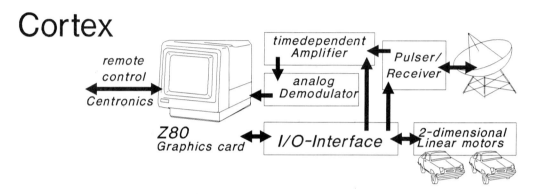

Figure 1

The DUB 20 and Cortex Dermascan C digital ultrasound scanners.

Histology

Histological examination of skin with chronic actinic damage shows a thin epidermis, a reduction in the subepidermal elastic plexus with fragmentation and clumping of fibres in the upper dermis which stain as do elastic fibres. An increase and alteration in this elastotic material indicates quite early on that significant actinic damage has occurred.[7]

Ultrastructural examination shows that this elastotic material is a three-component system. It comprises (1) an elastotic matrix, (2) microfibrils, and (3) electron-dense inclusions.[8] It can be assumed that the formation of the elastotic material is an active process with a tendency, as elastotic fibre formation progresses, towards degenerative changes such as irregular fibre arrangements and, later, vacuolar disintegration. At the same time the production of collagen fibres declines. In the upper dermis, and less often also in the epidermis, there is a sparse inflammatory cell infiltrate. This complex process of fibre restructuring results in complete dermal metamorphosis which appears as a tangle of haphazardly arranged fibres and finally as an amorphous disorganized mass.

B-scan sonography

We first became aware of the changes due to actinic elastosis during our research on skin tumours. Basal cell carcinoma sometimes shows ill-defined lateral delimitation. The echo-poor, but rarely echo-lucent, tumour was sonographically embedded in echo-lucent linear structures. Histology revealed these structures to be actinically transformed dermal connective tissue.[9]

Therefore, in B-scan sonography actinic elastosis appears between the entry echo and the dermal reflexes as a hypoechoic, frequently echolucent band containing inhomogeneously distributed, ill-defined internal echoic structures. The boundary with the entry echo is usually sharp. The basal boundary can be indistinct. In particularly severe elastosis, the lower margin of the hypoechoic band is frequently 'serrated', whilst in less severe elastosis the boundary is usually sharp. We refer to this as the echolucent band (ELB). The severity of the elastosis, i.e. the width of the zone of elastotic transformation in the upper dermis, can be measured directly on the ultrasound scan using a scale which can be displayed on the screen. Because of this indistinct upper demarcation, it is sometimes difficult to determine the depth of the band. In such cases the thickness of the band can be measured using a so-called 'summated A-scan'. Here all the reflex lines composing the B-scan are shown as a single average amplitude image. The simultaneous presentation of this summated A-scan and the corresponding B-scan permits highly accurate measurement of the visualized structures. In general, there is no interexaminer variation in measurements obtained using this procedure. The software integrated into the scanner permits densitometric quantification of the number and intensity of the echoes in particular areas.

Relationship of the histological picture to the sonographic findings

The conclusion that the ELB is the ultrasonic correlation of actinic elastosis is supported by the following evidence.

The hypoechoic (to echolucent) band below the entry echo is found only in areas of the skin exposed to light (forehead, cheek, outer aspect of the forearm, etc.). It is not found in the gluteal region, i.e. in regions of the skin protected from sunlight. The ELB in its typical formation cannot be found in children; the development of the collagen network is not complete in children and, consequently, all dermal structures are hypoechoic.

The dermal echoes are produced mainly by bundles of collagen fibres. As a result of actinic exposure the subepidermal elastic plexus is destroyed and the upper and middle parts of the dermis are homogenized into an amorphous structure so that there is a depletion of interfaces in the dermis. The frequently present sparse inflammatory infiltration is also hypoechoic.

Thus high-frequency B-scan sonography permits exact quantification of the actinically transformed dermis and permits a non-invasive evaluation of the damage. These findings are illustrated in Figures 2–7.

Clinical investigation

Thirty patients (aged 40 to 68 years) were evaluated for the degree of elastosis at three different sites (forehead, temporal region and gluteal region). In addition, patients were treated topically with a hyaluronic acid creme for 3 months on the face. Hyaluronic acid is a constituent of the dermal matrix and it has been shown to affect fibroblast proliferation in wound healing.[10] It is already used in a number of cosmetics.

The aim of the study was to determine whether ultrasound studies are suitable for the detection of even small changes in the skin. Patients were examined on days 0, 14, 30, 60 and 90. The gluteal region was examined on days 0 and 90 only. All patients showed some clinical elastosis on the forehead and temporal regions.

Results

At the beginning of the study the thickness of the dermis was 1743 μm (forehead) and 1740 μm (temporal region) (average of 30 patients). At the end of the study the dermal thickness had increased slightly in both regions (1784 μm forehead, 1868 μm temporal region). The increase in the temporal region was statistically significant (Figure 8).

All patients showed an ELB associated with the actinic elastosis in these locations. During the course of the study the thickness of the ELB decreased in the temporal region from 735 μm to 716 μm (Figure 9). A non-significant increase in the ELB of the forehead was observed. In contrast, the gluteal region showed no ELB at any time during the study and the thickness of the dermis at this site remained static.

Discussion

The ELB beneath the entry-echo is correlated with actinically transformed dermal connective tissue. Nevertheless, it should be borne in mind that a number of dermatoses can also produce an ELB. It has been shown by our working group that psoriasis, lichen planus, type IV reactions and rosacea also demonstrate an ELB. It can be particularly difficult

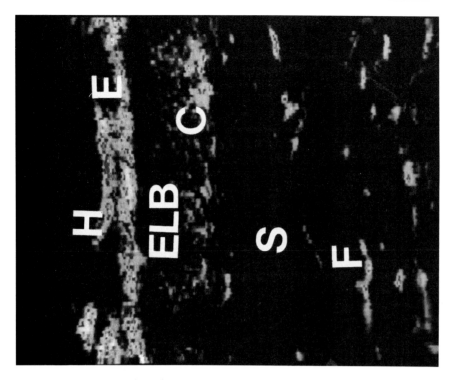

Figure 3

Outer aspect of the forearm of the same 65-year-old man as in Figure 4. The region was sun exposed and shows a distinct difference in the ELB compared to the inner aspect of the forearm (see Figure 6). There are hairs lying tangentially (H) above the entry echo (E). The entry echo itself is echo rich. An echo lucent band in the upper dermis represents a marked solar elastosic change (ELB). A limited number of punctuate echoes delimit the dermis (C) from the subcutaneous fat (S). Linear structures within the subcutaneous fat represent muscle fascia (F).

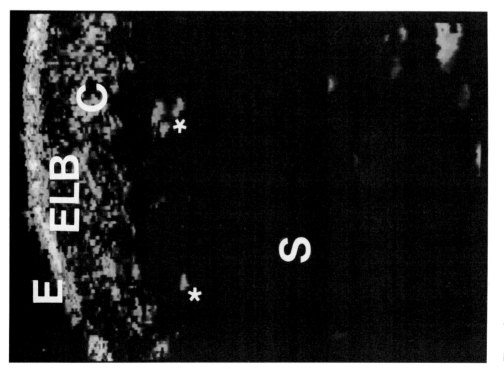

Figure 2

Forehead of a 34-year-old woman. Only limited actinically transformed dermal connective tissue can be detected as an ELB underneath the entry echo (E). Dermal structures (C) are echo rich with homogeneously distributed echoes. The subcutaneous fat (S) is echo lucent with single highly reflecting spots (*).

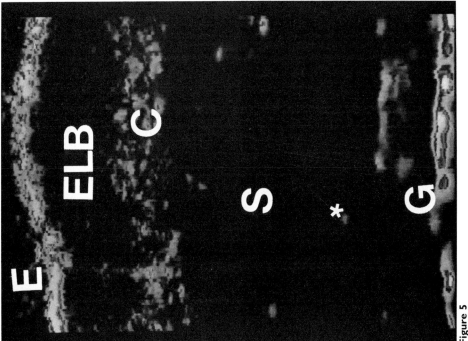

Figure 5

Forehead of a 72-year-old woman. Marked actinic damage can be expected in the upper dermis. The entry echo (E) is wider than usual. A strong ELB represents an actinically destroyed dermis. Only about 25% of the dermis shows regular dermal echoes (C). The subcutaneous fat is echo lucent (S). Single echo-rich spots can be seen (*). In the lower parts of the image the scalp aponeurosis has been hit tangentially (G) and is presented as an echo rich linear structure.

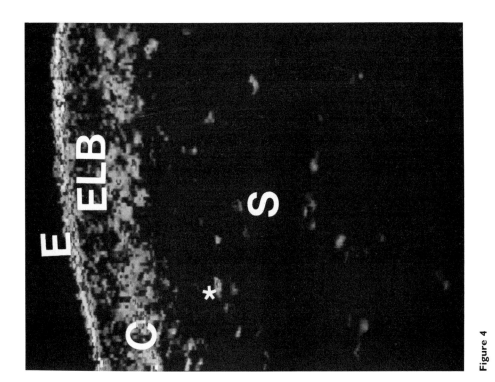

Figure 4

Inner aspect of the forearm of a 65-year-old man. The region was only slightly exposed to sunlight during life. The relatively small entry echo (E) shows a typical echo-rich pattern. A small band of poor echos in the upper dermis (ELB) corresponds to early actinic transformation of the dermal connective tissue. Deeper dermal structures are echo rich (C). The subcutaneous fat (S) is echolucent with single echo-rich spots (*).

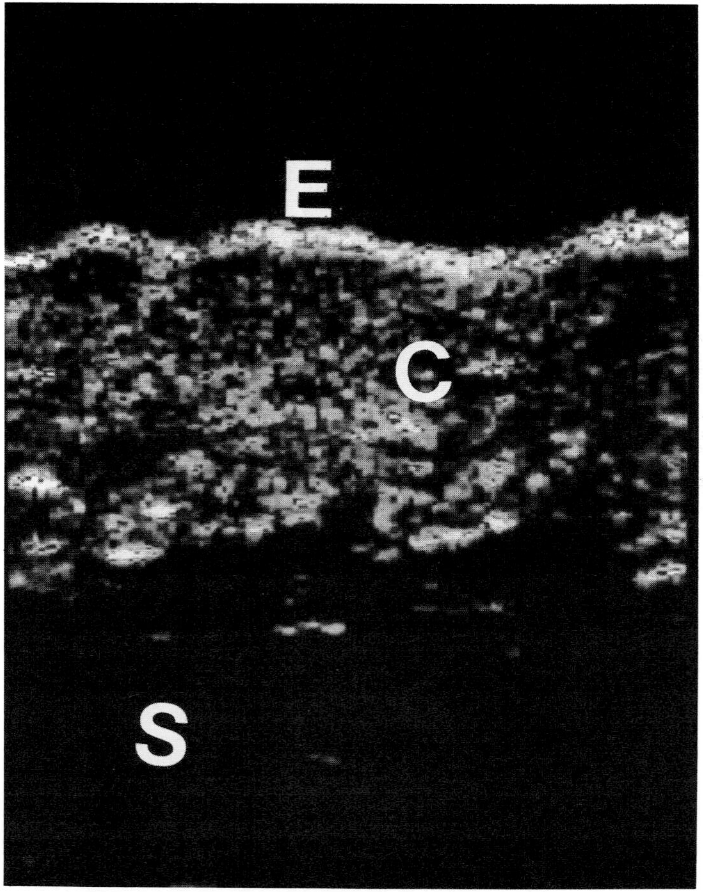

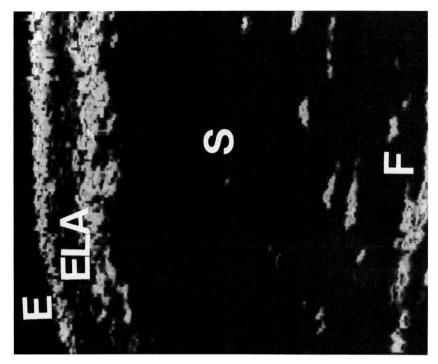

Figure 7

Inner aspect of the forearm of a 3-year-old child. Actinic damage cannot be expected, but the sonogram demonstrates the typical echo pattern of a child with an echo-lucent area within the dermis. The entry echo (E) shows a regular echo rich pattern. The underlying dermis is an echo-lucent area (ELA) because the collagen network is not fully developed. Only in the lower regions of the dermis is there a highly reflecting linear band which represents the so-called 'inferior reflex arch'. The subcutaneous fat is echo poor (S). Muscle fascial planes (F) are linear structures embedded in the subcutaneous fat.

Figure 6

Gluteal region of a 56-year-old man. The region was not exposed to sunlight during life. The entry-echo (E) is undulated and echo rich. The structure is fairly homogeneous. Underlying dermal structures (C) show mainly high echos with partial echo-poor areas which result from deposits of fatty tissue. The dermis–subcutis border is well defined. In some regions the subcutaneous fat (S) arches into the dermis. The subcutaneous fat itself is echo lucent.

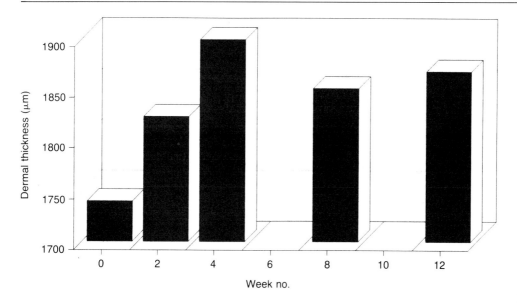

Figure 8

The change in the thickness of the dermis at the temporal region over the 3 months of the study.

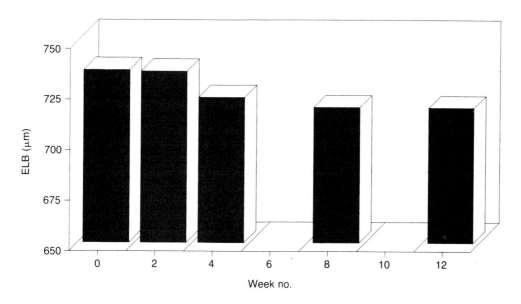

Figure 9

The change in the ELB in temporal region over the 3 months of the study.

to distinguish between elastosis and the changes that occur in rosacea.

The resting tension of the skin can influence the echogenicity of the sonogram. Regional differences in areas with only limited fixation of the skin to underlying structures were found. The cheek, for example, is not suitable for ultrasound evaluation because the variable skin tension influences the ultrasonic image. The appearance of the ELB in children has been discussed above. The echo pattern in children can be distinguished from sonograms which show actinic elastosis. A so-called 'lower reflex arch' (high tension in the fibre network of the lower dermis causing strong echoes) delimits the ELB sharply in children's sonograms and does not show the usual serrated demarcation of the ELB in elastosis.

If patients with inflammatory skin diseases are excluded, only regions with defined skin tensions are examined, and only take into account the special echo pattern in children, ultrasound seems to be a reliable method for investigating degenerative skin processes, such as actinic elastosis, and allows evaluation of treatment for this disorder.

Further progress in microelectronics offers new possibilities in the use of high-frequency sonography. We have already constructed a prototype 50 MHz scanner with which it is possible to look into epidermal structures.[11] Interpretation of sonograms by image analysis will provide further diagnostic possibilities, and differential diagnosis of several skin processes (which is at present still a subjective matter) will become more objective.

References

1. Altmeyer P, Dermatologische Ultraschalldiagnostik—geganwärtiger Stand und Perspektiven (Dermatologic ultrasound diagnostics—the present state and diagnostics), *Z Hautkr* (1989) **64**: 727–8.
2. Altmeyer P, Hoffmann K, el-Gammal S, Sonographie der Haut (Sonography of the skin), *MMW* (1990) **132**: 14–22.
3. Winkler K, Hoffmann K, el-Gammal S et al, The repair process of a wound healing model under sonographic control, *Zbl Haut* (1990) **157**: 327–8.
4. Hoffmann K, Gerbaulet U, el-Gammal S et al, 20 MHz b-scan Sonographie bei der circumskripten Sklerodermie und Psoriasis vulgaris (20 MHz B-scan sonography for circumscribed sclerodema and psoriasis), *Acta Dermat Venereol* (1991) (in press).
5. Braun-Falco O, Plewig G, Wolff HH, *Dermatologie und Venerologie*, Springer-Verlag: Berlin, 1984.
6. Kligman AM, Early destructive effects of sunlight on human skin, *J Am Med Assoc* (1969) **210**: 2377–80.
7. Kligman LH, Photoaging. Manifestation, prevention and treatment, *Dermatol Clin* (1986) **4**: 517–28.
8. Braun-Falco O, Die Morphogenese der senil aktinischen Elastose (The morphogenesis of senile actinic elastosis), *Arch klin exp Derm* (1969) **235**: 138–60.
9. Hoffmann K, Stücker M, el-Gammal S et al, Digitale 20-MHz-Sonographie des Basalioms im b-scan (Digital 20 MHz sonography of the basal cell carcinoma in B scan), *Hautarzt* (1990) **41**: 333–9.
10. Alexander SA, Donoff RB, The glycosaminoglycans of open wounds, *J Surg Res* (1980) **29**: 422–9.
11. el-Gammal S, Experimental approaches and new developments with high frequency ultrasound in dermatology, *Zbl Haut* (1990) **157**: 327.

17
Pigmented facial macules: a sign of photoaging?

L. Lever and R. Marks
Department of Dermatology, University of Wales College of Medicine, Cardiff CF4 4XN, UK

Introduction

Brown spots on the face, forearms and backs of hands, sometimes called 'liver spots' or 'cemetery medals', are a common feature of cutaneous aging. Clinical differential diagnoses include lentigo senilis, seborrhoeic keratosis, solar keratosis and lentigo maligna. Although 'brown spots' have been said to be a sign of chronic exposure to ultraviolet radiation there appears to be no evidence to support this contention. Indeed, the exact histological nature of these lesions does not seem to have been described. The aims of this study were to characterize the histological features of lesions on the face presenting as brown macules or plaques and to determine whether they were related to chronic photodamage.

Methods

Patients attending dermatology clinics at the University Hospital of Wales, Cardiff, with brown macules or flat brown plaques on the front or sides of the face were entered into the study after giving written, witnessed informed consent. Some lesions were the presenting problem, others were noted in the clinic. Lesions that were obviously lentigo maligna or seborrhoeic warts were excluded.

Assessment of photodamage

The extent of lifetime sun exposure and the likelihood of photodamage were assessed in four ways: history of sun exposure (outdoor work or hobbies, holidays or residence in sunny countries); Boston skin classification (sun reactivity); the presence of the changes of solar elastotic degenerative change (photodamage) assessed by the extent of coarse and fine wrinkling and yellowish discoloration; and history of previous solar keratoses, Bowen's disease or skin cancer.

Measurements

If lesions were multiple, the largest was examined, measured and photographed. Skin surface contours were recorded by taking lesional and perilesional silicone rubber impressions.[1] Profilometry was performed using a Hommel tester. Skin surface biopsies were taken from lesional and perilesional skin using a cyanoacrylate adhesive (Powabond).[2]

Biopsies

A 4 mm punch biopsy under local anaesthesia was taken from the centre of the lesion. If the lesion was irregular the biopsy was taken from the darkest or thickest area.

Results

Clinical

Thirty-six subjects (12 men, 24 women) were entered into the study. The age range was 35–88 years (mean age 64 years). Lesions varied in size from 4 to 25 mm diameter and occurred on the forehead, temples, cheeks and nose. Appearance ranged from pale, evenly pigmented macules (Figure 1) to dark, irregularly pigmented dark brown plaques (Figure 2). Precise clinical diagnosis was impossible in most cases.

Histology

An exact histological diagnosis could not be made in all cases. There was one nodular malignant melanoma (probably arising in a lentigo maligna), one lentigo maligna, three solar keratoses and three seborrhoeic warts. The remaining cases showed features most in keeping with a diagnosis of lentigo senilis,[3,4] but there was a wide range of appearances within each lesion. Appearances included: regular budding with slight melanocytic hyperplasia (Figure 3); irregular downgrowth of strands of epidermal cells and basaloid cell hyperplasia (Figure 4); irregular acanthosis; budding, melanocyte hyperplasia and acanthosis; and epidermal irregularity and keratinocyte atypia.

In order to quantify the relative frequency of each type of change, the specimens were assessed subjectively for the following features (scored on visual analogue scales): (i) budding and melanocyte hyperplasia ('lentigo-like' change); (ii) irregular epidermal downgrowths and basaloid cell hyperplasia (seborrhoeic wart-like change); (iii) epidermal irregularity and keratinocyte atypia (dysplastic change); and (iv) inflammatory infiltrate. Twenty eight lesions were scored in this way. Highest scores were for 'lentigo-like' change in 70%; for 'wart-like' change in 13%; for dysplastic change in 9%; and inflammation in 9%.

Skin surface profilometry

The mean roughness (RA) of lesional skin in lesions diagnosed histologically as seborrhoeic warts was 41.0 ± 15.5 (perilesional skin RA = 7.4 ± 3.2). The

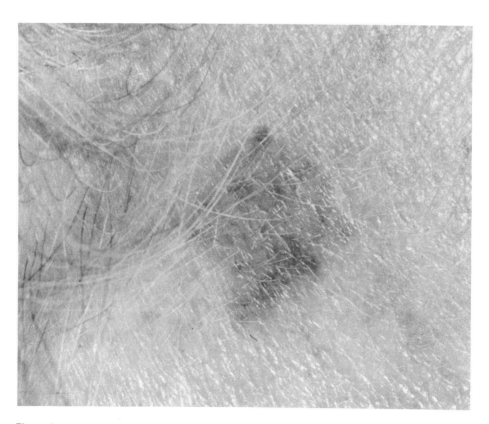

Figure 1

Pale brown macule (histology: lentigo senilis).

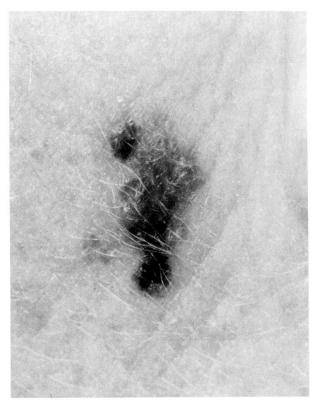

Figure 2
Dark brown plaque (histology: nodular malignant melanoma).

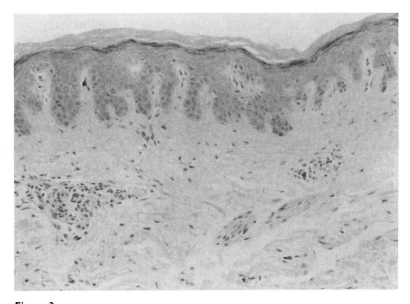

Figure 3
Senile lentigo.

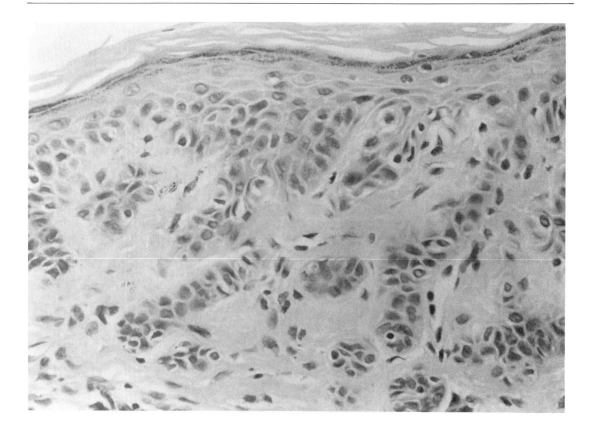

Figure 4

Senile lentigo with extensive budding.

remaining pigmented macules had a normal RA (7.8 ± 3.9) compared with perilesional skin (RA = 7.6 ± 1.1).

Skin surface biopsy

Skin surface biopsies were examined unstained then stained with haematoxylin and eosin. The unstained specimens mostly showed a normal stratum corneum pattern. However, the seborrhoeic warts showed a 'honeycomb appearance' (Figure 5). Stained skin surface biopsies showed parakeratotic stratum corneum in two specimens from solar keratoses but the rest of the specimens were unremarkable. In four specimens (two 'lentigo senilis' lesions, one seborrhoeic wart, one atrophic solar keratosis) follicular hyperkeratosis or plugging were also visible on skin surface biopsies and in vivo when the lesions were examined through a fibreoptic skin surface microscope (Scopeman). The significance of these stratum corneum patterns remains uncertain, but they must represent a form of hyperkeratosis which passes unnoticed on vertical skin sections.

Relationship to solar damage

Seven patients were judged to have had excessive sun exposure because they had lived or worked in sunny countries for more than 6 months or took regular sunbathing holidays, six had moderate sun exposure and the remainder had very little sun exposure (lifetime exposure to sun outside Wales of less than 2 weeks).

The distribution of Boston skin types is shown in Table 1. The mean degree of photodamage (on a 0 to 100 visual analogue scale) was 65.2 ± 22.

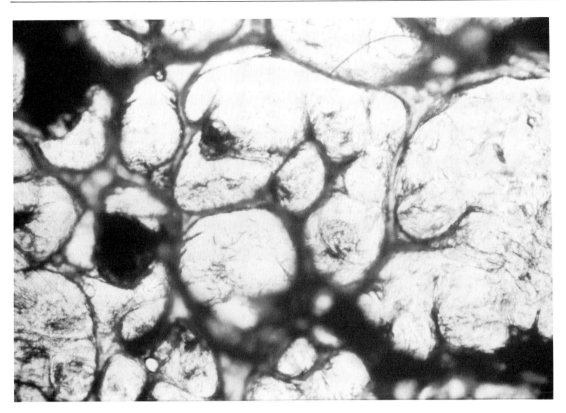

Figure 5

Skin surface biopsy of seborrhoeic wart ('honeycomb' appearance).

Table 1 Boston skin classification and degree of photodamage.

Skin type	Frequency (%)	
	Patients	Controls
1	17	50
2	45	38
3	31	12
4	7	0
Degree of photodamage (0–100)	65 ± 22	59 ± 23

As controls, a group of 16 individuals, without facial brown spots and without a personal or family history of malignant or premalignant skin disease, were assessed for sun damage in a similar way (Table 1). Two had excessive sun exposure, five moderate exposure and nine had minimal exposure (as defined above).

Other evidence of malignant or premalignant skin disease

If the group of patients with a past history of solar keratosis, Bowen's disease or skin cancer were separated, they were on average 10 years older and had much more sun damage (visual analogue scale score for solar elastosis 75 ± 16) than the patients with no previous skin cancer (visual analogue scale score for solar elastosis 53 ± 23). The histological features of the lesions from the two groups did not differ. The patients with a previous history of malignant or premalignant skin disease gave a similar history of lifetime sun exposure, although they were more likely to have skin type 1 (35%) than the group without previous skin cancer (0%).

Conclusion

Examination of flat brown spots on the face does not often result in a firm clinical diagnosis unless there are other accompanying physical signs. The histological picture of such lesions allows a definite diagnosis in only a quarter of cases and the remainder are difficult to classify. The pathological term 'lentigo senilis' has been used[3,4] to describe the finding of melanocyte proliferation with epidermal budding but, as Mehregan has pointed out,[3] there is considerable overlap between the features of 'lentigo senilis', seborrhoeic keratosis, solar keratosis and lichenoid solar keratosis. Patients with brown flat spots on the face are not distinguished with regard to previous sun exposure, skin type, degree of photodamage or previous malignant or premalignant skin disease. Apart from lentigo maligna and solar keratosis, it is not clear whether any of the other forms of pigmented macule signify an increased risk of skin cancer.

As clinical examination does not even appear to permit significant lesions to be distinguished from trivial ones with certainty, it would be helpful if non-invasive methods of assessment could be employed. The studies performed here suggest that skin surface biopsy and profilometry as well as skin surface microscopy[5] may be helpful, although no single technique is likely to provide the answer in every case. The major problem may be that the lesions themselves appear not to have 'decided' which particular biological route to take.

References

1 Sarkany I, Caron G, Microtopography of the skin, *J Anat* (1965) **99**: 359–64.
2 Marks, R, Dawber RPR, Skin surface biopsy, *Br J Dermatol* (1971) **84**: 117–20.
3 Mehrigan AM, Lentigo senilis and its evolutions, *J Invest Dermatol* (1975) **65**: 429–33.
4 Montagna W, Hu F, Carlisle K, A reinvestigation of solar lentigines, *Arch Dermatol* (1980) **116**: 1151–4.
5 Bahmer FA, Fritsch P, Kreusch J et al, Terminology in surface microscopy, *J Am Acad Dermatol* (1990) **23**: 1159–62.

18
Differences between basal cell carcinomas arising in light-exposed and non-light-exposed skin

Richard J. Motley and Ronald Marks
Department of Dermatology, University of Wales College of Medicine, Cardiff, UK

Introduction

Basal cell carcinoma (BCC) is the commonest malignant tumour in humans and most frequently arises on sun-damaged skin; more than 99% of affected individuals are white, and 95% are between the ages of 40 and 79 years. Eighty five per cent of all BCCs appear in the head and neck region with 25–30% occurring on the nose alone.[1,2] BCCs may, however, also develop on non-light-exposed body sites. The aim of the present study was to assess whether these lesions differ in nature from those arising on sun-exposed sites.

Patients and methods

The names of all patients who had a BCC removed from a non-light-exposed area of the body were obtained from the departmental surgical records for the years 1980–90. Forty six patients were identified. Thirty four patients were excluded from further analysis because of a history of or clinical evidence of previous excessive sun exposure at the BCC site. Twelve nodular lesions arising in 11 patients (4 male, 7 female; mean age 55 years, range 30–82 years) were considered unlikely to be sun induced. Three BCCs were from the back, three from the chest (one in the inframammary crease), one from the abdomen, one from the scalp, one from the axilla, one from the buttock, one from the vulva and one from a finger. Two of the patients had the basal cell naevus syndrome. None of the patients had a history of arsenic exposure.

The pathological features in these 12 lesions were compared with 12 nodular BCCs excised from 12 randomly selected patients (7 male, 5 female; mean age 69 years, range 48–85 years). The locations were: three on the nose, three on the forehead, two on the neck, two on the temple, one on the lip and one on the lower eyelid (Table 1). In order to quantify the pathological features of these lesions the degree of solar damage, the extent of colloid degeneration, the amount of fibroplasia, the density of inflammatory cell infiltrate, the degree of peripheral pallisading and the amount of artefact retraction were assessed and recorded using 10 cm visual analogue scales. The mean values obtained for these parameters were compared for statistical significance using Student's t test.

Table 1 Details of patients.*

Non-exposed patients			Control patients		
Age (years)	Sex	Site	Age (years)	Sex	Site
64	M	Back (BCNS)	58	M	Nose
32	F	Scalp (BCNS)	65	M	Lip
68	F	Inframammary	80	M	Neck
30	M	Chest	66	F	Forehead
70	M	Finger	75	F	Forehead
37	M	Chest	48	M	Nose
38	F	Back	85	M	Temple
65	F	Buttock	67	F	Neck
62	F	Shoulder	71	F	Temple
53	F	Abdomen	72	F	Forehead
82	F	Axilla	69	M	Nose
82	F	Vulva	73	M	Eyelid

* BCNS, basal cell naevus syndrome.

Results

As would be anticipated, there was a highly significant greater degree of solar elastosis in the control skin than in skin from non-light-exposed sites ($p < 0.001$) (Table 2). The degree of artefact retraction was significantly less ($p < 0.001$), and the extent of the peripheral pallisade increased, although not significantly so ($p = 0.07$, in non-exposed BCCs compared with controls. There was no difference between the two groups in the degree of colloid degeneration, fibroplasia, or in the type or amount of inflammatory cell infiltrate seen.

Table 2 Results obtained for non-light-exposed and light-exposed sites.

Parameter	Visual analogue scale scores			
	Mean	Median	S.D.	Range
Non-light-exposed sites				
Solar damage	0.800	0.200	1.814	0.0–6.4
Colloid degeneration	1.908	0.150	2.745	0.0–7.5
Fibroplasia	1.542	0.850	1.693	0.0–5.5
Inflammation	2.292	1.750	1.654	0.4–5.7
Peripheral pallisade	5.392	5.650	2.313	0.3–8.6
Artefact retraction	0.700	0.200	0.839	0.0–2.7
Light-exposed sites				
Solar damage	4.342	5.300	2.551	0.0–7.7
Colloid degeneration	1.875	1.450	1.785	0.1–6.4
Fibroplasia	1.767	0.900	1.662	0.1–4.7
Inflammation	2.750	1.750	2.370	0.2–7.0
Peripheral pallisade	3.700	3.750	2.144	1.0–7.5
Artefact retraction	3.483	2.950	2.368	0.3–8.1

Discussion

Retraction spaces are a characteristic feature of BCCs in paraffin-embedded sections, the so-called 'artefact retraction'. These spaces are thought to result from decreased numbers of hemidesmosomes resulting in impaired tumour cell to basement membrane attachments: a local decrease in dermal collagen due to collagenase production by peritumoural fibroblasts and an increase in peritumoural fibroblast production of mucopolysaccharide may also play a part.[2] The formation of a peripheral pallisade of tumour cells is a further typical feature of BCCs and is helpful in distinguishing these tumours from other basaloid proliferations. BCCs arise from cells whose function it is to interact with the basement membrane to form the dermo-epidermal junction.[3] BCCs which show loss of the peripheral pallisade and increased retraction spaces may be considered to be 'less differentiated' than those lesions which preserve these basal cell functions. A study of incompletely excised BCCs found that the risk of tumour recurrence was lower in those lesions having a well-formed peripheral pallisade.[4,5] Thus it would appear from this study that BCCs arising in non-light-exposed sites may be more differentiated than those arising in solar damaged skin. Although we found a significantly greater degree of solar damage in the light-exposed skin than in the non-exposed skin, the range of solar damage observed in 'non-exposed' skin was considerable. This raises the possibility that some of these patients had received significant unrecognized sun exposure at these sites.

The development of BCCs on non-light-exposed body sites may be an indication of an underlying genetic predisposition or previous arsenical therapy.[6] Two patients in this study with BCCs arising in non-light-exposed sites had basal cell naevus syndrome, an inherited condition which gives rise to multiple BCCs. The finding of a BCC arising on non-light-exposed skin raises the possibility of unusual environmental or genetic influences and it would seem prudent to investigate these patients accordingly. Despite their rarity, there appears to be no evidence that BCCs arising in non-light-exposed skin differ fundamentally in structure or natural history from those arising at solar-damaged sites.

References

1 Diwan R, Skouge JW, Basal cell carcinoma, *Curr Prob Dermatol* (1990) **May/Jun**: 75–91.
2 Miller SJ, Biology of basal cell carcinoma (I), *J Am Acad Dermatol* (1991) **24**: 1–13.
3 Reidbord HE, Wechsler HL, Fisher ER, Ultrastructural study of basal cell carcinoma and its variants with comments on histogenesis, *Arch Dermatol* (1971) **104**: 132–40.
4 Dellon AL, DeSilva A, Connolly M et al, Prediction of recurrence of incompletely excised basal cell carcinoma, *Plast Reconst Surg* (1985) **75**: 860–71.
5 Sexton M, Jones DB, Maloney ME, Histologic pattern analysis of basal cell carcinoma, *J Am Acad Dermatol* (1990) **23**: 1118–26.
6 Miller SJ, Biology of basal cell carcinoma (II), *J Am Acad Dermatol* (1991) **24**: 161–75.

19
Objective assessment of intra- and inter-individual skin colour variability: an analysis of human skin reaction to sun and UVB

S. el-Gammal, K. Hoffmann, P. Steiert, J. Gaßmüller,* T. Dirschka and P. Altmeyer

*Dermatologische Klinik der Ruhr-Universität, D-4630 Bochum, Germany, and *Humanpharmakologie II, Schering AG, D-1000 Berlin, Germany*

Introduction

Perceived skin colour is influenced by many factors including the skin surface (e.g. humidity, oiliness and scaling), the blood perfusion of the skin, structures in the corium and the corium/subcutis interface (e.g. blue nevus), skin temperature,[1] previous sun exposure,[2] and, quite importantly, the ambient light conditions during examination. It has therefore been good practice in dermatology to judge skin colour under standard natural illumination conditions, i.e. indirect sunlight.

Skin colour changes, resulting from drug effects (e.g. corticosteroids and sunscreens) in experimentally induced erythema and/or different skin diseases has been one of the major concerns of clinical and experimental skin colorimetry. Many authors have used experimental set-ups, where a pigmentation was not expected to occur, thereby avoiding the problems of exact colour measurement and determining only the redness.[3-6]

It must be emphasized, however, that a precise, reproducible and objective colour measurement is quite difficult to perform. Different skin-colour measuring systems using filters or colour plates have been proposed in the past, promising a better classification of colours (for a review see Bode[7]). Correspondingly, industry has suggested a colour table for hairs (e.g. hair parts) and eye colours (e.g. eye prostheses).

In the present study we used the Minolta CR200 colorimeter, which is supposed to measure like the human eye. The aim of the study was to analyse the skin colour of a representative group of the German population and to find a system of clinically relevant skin type classification.

Historical overview

According to Hausmann,[8] the English surgeon Everard Home postulated in 1820 that there was an interrelationship between eyrthema and the sun exposure in the white population. Home exposed his hands to the sun, one covered with a black cloth, the other one uncovered. He remarked an erythema on the uncovered hand and a persisting pigmentation a few days later. He concluded that the skin pigmentation of the coloured human races protects them from light irritation. In 1828, the Chemist John Davy confirmed these findings and noted that skin pigmentation could also be observed after diffuse light exposure without previous eyrthema. The effects on skin of ultraviolet radiation (UVR) were discovered by accident. In 1858 two chemists experimented with a carbon arc lamp in the Charcot laboratory and observed skin changes resembling sunburn the following day. Charcot showed that, when the light of the carbon arc lamp was filtered by a uranium glassplate, skin erythema did not occur.[8]

Niels Finsen[9] introduced light therapy into medicine. His new concepts for the treatment of lupus vulgaris were honoured with the Nobel prize in 1904. About two decades later, Hausser and Vahle[10] studied the erythema reaction of the skin using quartz spectral equipment and a very powerful mercury arc lamp. The erythema curve exhibited a high narrow peak at about 300 nm followed by a

---

This publication contains substantial results from the dissertation of Mrs P. Steiert.

depression at 280 nm and a relative minimum at 250 nm. These workers showed that in the visible and the long UV spectrum no erythema occurred. These findings have found application in the division of the UV spectrum into UVA, UVB and UVC.[11] The boundary between UVB and UVC is at 280 nm. The UVB/UVA boundary was fixed at 315 nm (1% below the maximum at 297 nm). The findings of Hausser and Vahle[10] were later confirmed by Uhlmann,[12] Fetz[13] and Anders et al,[14] the latter authors used a dye laser.

In 1934, Bode[7] published light remission curves of the skin under different experimental conditions. Using a Zeiss photometer and monochromator, he separated a white light source into the colour spectrum and measured the grey-filter adjustment which was necessary to render the colour of the skin and a Baryt white plate identical. He needed about 7 min to measure 22 points between 400 and 700 nm. All remission curves showed a peak at 500 and 630 nm and a third small peak at 560 nm. Deep depressions were observed at 545 and 575 nm, due to the absorption bands of oxyhaemoglobin. In normal skin, he observed a higher peak at 630 nm (46% remission) then another at 500 nm (35.5%). In less pigmented, red skin he observed a shift of the 500 nm peak to lower levels (26%) and remarked that this greater absorption in the blue–green spectrum is responsible for the red colour shift. In another experiment he compared the remission curves of white, anaemic skin and pigmented skin. According to Bode,[7] pigmentation is characterized by a relative shift of the entire curve to lower levels; i.e. the total light reflection is diminished. These observations led to the theory that skin pigmentation behaves like a grey-filter. 'Erythrometers' and 'melanometers' are based on this theory.

Until 1970, ultraviolet radiation was widely accepted as being dangerous and harmful. In those days, the standard equipment used for therapeutic ultraviolet radiation emitted in the entire UV-spectrum (including UVC). Skin tuberculosis, acne vulgaris and conglobata and the parapsoriasis en plaques were considered to be an indication for this kind of therapy. After the rediscovery and spread of photochemotherapy for psoriasis vulgaris[15–18] and the development of UVA-selective lamps, which were supposed to tan without danger, the general opinion about UVR changed radically. This development culminated in the use of aggressive phototherapy in dermatology using very powerful equipment.[19] Since then, new developments in light therapy have shown that powerful lamps with a narrow emission spectrum are able to bring about sufficient therapeutic effects without prior-sensitization (PUVA). This therapy is known as SUP.[19]

The assessment of human skin sensitivity to UVR is important in photo(chemo)therapy, photodermatoses, photoaging, photocarcinogenesis and photoprotection. Today it is standard practice to determine the minimal erythema dose (MED) experimentally and to extrapolate the degree of light sensitivity. Wucherpfennig[20] was one of the first to describe a technical set-up for a mechanically working UVR provocation apparatus. He noted that skin patches, where the radiation increases geometrically in steps of 20%, is well suited to defining the MED. The test protocol which is used today (e.g. to test sunscreens) is highly standardized[21] and is essentially based on the findings of Wucherpfennig.[20]

Methods

Colorimetry

Colour-measuring instruments which analyse the whole colour spectrum are suitable for dermatology when they comply to the following conditions: they should perceive the skin colour like the human eye (Figure 1(a)); different standard colour systems should be available; they must have a very stable light source, which is controlled by the measuring system; the measured skin region should be small and must not be submitted to pressure or tangential forces during measurement; the surrounding temperature must not be influenced; and the measurements should be registered quickly and automatically.

The Minolta CR 200 Colorimeter (Minolta, Japan) (Figure 2) complies to these conditions. It uses a pulse xenon arc lamp and six silicon photocells, three for measuring the source illumination, and three for measuring the reflected light (Figure 1(b)). Different filters select the value pairs for blue (450 nm), green (550 nm) and red (600 nm) light. A microcomputer corrects the three measured value pairs according to the Comission Internationale d'Eclairage (CIE) Colorimetric Standard Observer Curve (Figure 1(c)). Wilhelm and Maibach[22] observed a low variability in measuring different skin surfaces repeatedly. They found, however, a considerable variation in measuring untreated skin from day to day. For this reason it is

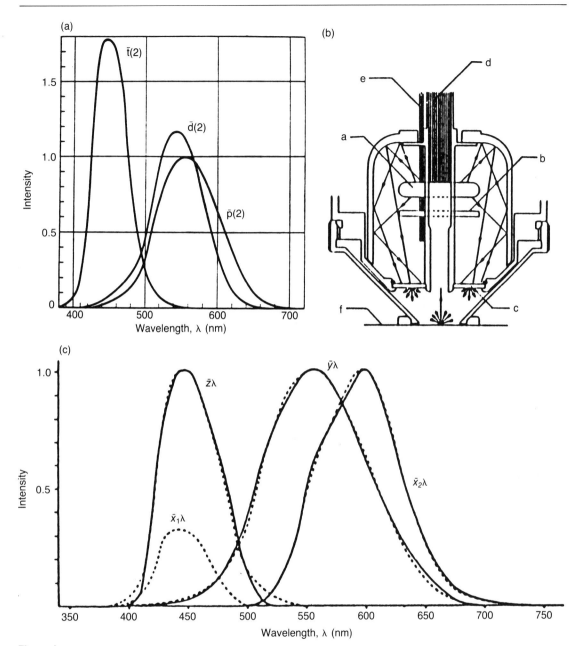

Figure 1

(a) The spectral response of the three different cone-shaped light receptors of the human retina. (b) Schematic diagram of the optical set-up of the Minolta CR200 Chroma Meter probe head: a, pulsed Xenon arc lamp; b, baffle; c, diffusing plate; d, optical cable for receiving reflected light; e, optical fibre for monitoring illumination; f, sample surface. (c) Spectral response of the Minolta Chroma Meter (continuous line) compared to that of the CIE Colorimetric Standard Observer curves (dotted line): $\bar{x}_1 \lambda$ is calculated from $\bar{z}\lambda$ to move the CIE Yxy colour triangle into the positive quadrant of the coordinate system.

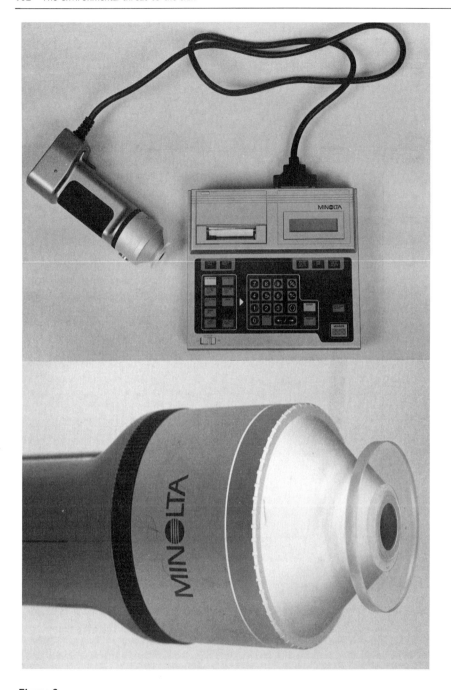

Figure 2

(a) The Minolta tristimulus Chroma Meter CR200. The equipment consists of a microprocessor controlled panel and a hand-held probe (weight 1032 g). By pressing the button at the base of the probe, a xenon arc lamp light pulse is emitted. (b) Close-up view of the probe head, which has a round measuring field of 8 mm diameter at its tip. The transparent plastic ring should be changed for skin-colour measurements (see text).

advisable to change the plastic ring (Figure 2(b)) for a thinner, black ring which has 6–8 tiny feet (2 mm thick, 5 mm diameter) on the far periphery of the ring, in order to reduce direct contact with the skin and to minimize the pressure of the measuring window on the skin.[23]

The three measured values are reassembled to form a colour which can be described by three parameters: the colour lightness (brightness) or 'grey value'; the basic colour or 'hue'; and the colour saturation (vividness) or 'chroma'. The three colour parameters can be converted to different colour representation systems, such as the CIE Yxy colour triangle, the Munsell notation or the 'Lab' system. Whatever colour system is used, the cluster of all colour combinations forms a three-dimensional structure.

A common and comprehensive system for representing colours is the 'Lab' system. 'L' stands for the lightness (brightness) of the colour, 'a' for its hue (oriented circularly) and chroma (oriented radially) on the green–red axis, and 'b' for the same aspects on the blue–yellow axis (Figure 3). The green–red and blue–yellow axes are oriented horizontally, the vertical axis represents the lightness factor, which varies from 0 (dark) to 100 (white).

UVB provocation

Erythema and tanning are the cardinal macroscopic responses of human skin to UVR. Using photoprovocation procedures, the skin reaction to UVR can be studied under standardized conditions. Different systems have been proposed in the past, using covering-plates (e.g. Waldmann), wire-frames and grey-filters (e.g. Saalmann) or a rotating sector wheel.[20] While some devices reduce the energy dose in the different skin patches (e.g. Saalmann) whilst keeping the time constant, other systems keep the energy constant and reduce the exposure time (e.g. Waldmann). All methods have in common that the cumulative UVA and/or UVB dose varies between the different skin patch areas (100% to 0% of the primary emitted energy).

We used a photoprovocation apparatus which uses wire frames (the relation between the wire thickness and the meshes varies) to reduce the energy prior to UVA or UVB filtering. This equipment emits different energies through the seven rows of holes in the UVA and UVB spectrum (Figure 4(b)). Two separate lamps are used for the UVA and UVB spectrum. In this study we concentrated on UVB provocation. After applying twice the MED in the UVB spectrum, the skin colour within the seven patch areas was measured after 7, 12, and 24 h. A few volunteers with sensitive skin exhibited a slight oedema in several skin patch areas after 24 h. As discussed later, the 24-h colour values were then rejected.

Volunteers

A total of 500 volunteers (230 men, 270 women; 8–86 years old) were studied in the winter period. The skin colour was measured several times in two UVR exposed regions (forehead and back of the hand) and two non-UVR-exposed regions (gluteal region and back of the foot). In addition, the colour of the hair in the temporal region was measured. An average of three measurements at the same spot was taken.

The group of central Europeans ($n = 450$) was classified further into different 'sun-reactive' skin types I–IV (Table I). This working classification of sun-reactive skin types, as introduced by Fitzpatrick et al,[24] is based on the history of an

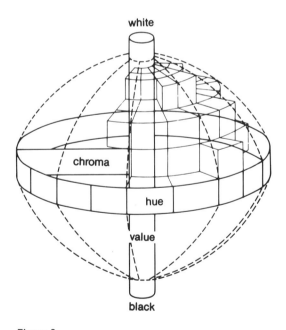

Figure 3

The 'Lab' colour representation system forms a three-dimensional ovaloid, where all possible colours are included (see text). By moving in a radial direction the chroma of the colour changes, by moving in a circular fashion the hue changes.

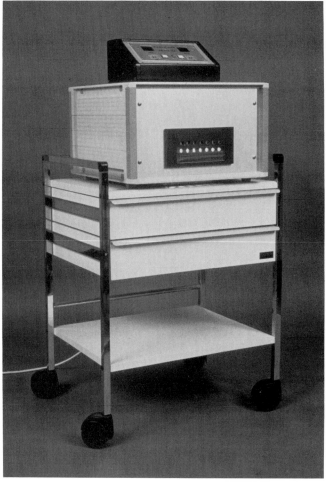

Field	Factor
1	1.00
2	0.87
3	0.75
4	0.60
5	0.45
6	0.32
7	0.18

a b

Figure 4

(a) Photoprovocation apparatus. Two lamps (UVA and UVB) with separate timing circuits are used. Each lamp emits its light through seven holes arranged in a row. Before reaching the skin patch area, the energy has been reduced stepwise by grids and has been filtered appropriately. (b) The cumulative total energy for each patch area is calculated by multiplying the cumulative emitted light energy with the corresponding field factor. For example, for UVB 0.177 J/cm^2/min for 20 s: field 1 = 0.059 J/cm^2, field 2 = 0.0513 J/cm^2, field 3 = 0.0443 J/cm^2, etc.

individual's tendency to sunburn and to tan (Table 1), along with some racial parameters.

From the group of central Europeans, 20 volunteers were subjected to UVB photoprovocation to study the effect of erythema on skin colour.

Chroma 3D software

In order to visualize skin colour changes, we used the three-dimensional 'Lab' colour ovaloid. The computer program CHROMA3D is an add-on for

Table 1 The working classification of sun-reactive skin types introduced by Fitzpatrick et al[24] is based on the tendency to sunburn and to tan as remembered by the individual along with some racial parameters. The skin type classes I–IV were sufficient to classify our central European volunteers ($n = 450$).

Sun-reactive skin type	Sunburn	Tanning
I	Always	Never
II	Always	Sometimes
III	Sometimes	Always
IV	Never	Always

the program ANAT3D.[25,26] Precise colour determination is essential for an exact analysis, especially when complex changes occur simultaneously along several axes in space (three-dimensional vector).

Results

To interpret skin-colour changes, it is important to know the depth penetration of the light source used for UVR provocation or for colour measurements. Figure 5 shows that the energy spectrum of interest (100–3000 nm) has a maximum penetration in the visible and infra-red (IR-A) range. This non-linear effect is to a great extent due to the energy absorption curve of water, which shows a steep minimum between 400 and 550 nm.[27] Moreover, because the penetration of light varies at different wavelengths, the perceived colour of deep lying structures can be modified, a typical example being the 'blue' aspect of the blue naevus.

Natural skin colours

The natural skin colour arising due to UVR exposure in the winter was studied in 500 volunteers.

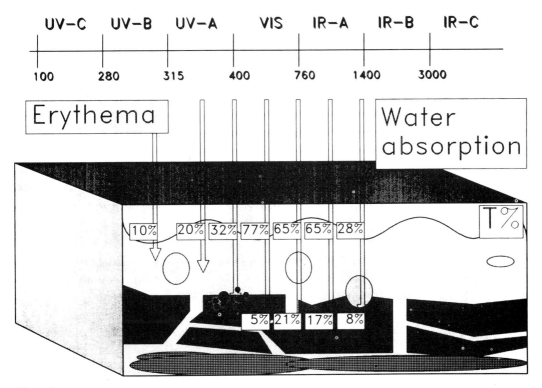

Figure 5

The light transmission of the skin at different wavelengths. Ultraviolet (UV), visible (VIS) and infrared (IR). Note the penetration of visible light to deep skin layers; at 760 nm, 21% of the light energy reaches the corium/subcutis border. In the UVC and UVB ranges, the energy is absorbed in the upper skin layers. At wavelengths above IR-B the energy is largely absorbed by water. (Modified from Müller and Müller-Stolzenburg.[28])

Their natural skin colour ('L'; 'a'; 'b') exhibited the following mean values: forehead (59.16; 13.81; 14.80), back of the hand (57.72; 11.63; 16.99), gluteal region (66.22; 8.28; 14.67), back of the foot (62.91; 8.25; 13.49) and hair in the temporal region (34.77; 3.77; 7.89). In the UVR-exposed regions (forehead and dorsum of the hand) the 'L' value was lower than in the non-exposed regions (gluteal region and dorsum of the foot), whereas the 'a' value was significantly higher. The 'b' values showed no statistically significant changes.

Central European skin colours

The natural skin colour of the hand and gluteal region of 450 central European volunteers classified into skin types I–IV is shown in Figure 6. It can be seen that the lightness factor 'L' of the hand is lower than that for the gluteal region since it is more sun exposed. The red saturation is higher on the dorsum of the hand than in the gluteal region. Furthermore, the 'L' grey value decreases from skin type I to IV, whereas 'a' and 'b' increase.

The measured values within each type (I–IV) are shown in Figure 7, in which the 'a' values are plotted against the 'L' values (Figure 7 (a)) and 'b' values (Figures 7 (b)). Note the strong overlap of the point-cloud regions of skin types I–IV, making a classification into skin types by simple colour measurement impossible. A different classification approach is necessary.

Photoprovocation and UVB erythema

As has been shown by Hausser and Vahle,[10] the ability of UVR to induce 'sun-burn' erythema is maximum in the UVB range. Since skin tanning is known to have a protective effect against sunburn, we tried to characterize the energy filtering capabilities of natural and tanned skin under UVB exposure by studying the colour changes. Figure 8 shows the skin colour changes which occurred after UVB exposure in summer and in winter on the back of the same volunteer. The skin colour was measured in the different skin patch areas after 7, 12, and 24 h. All values were found to fit a

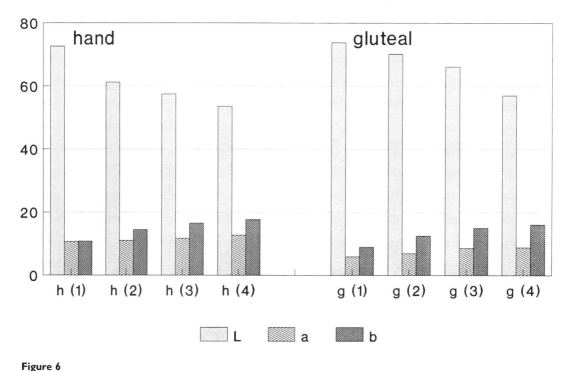

Figure 6

Comparison between one of the sun-exposed regions (hand) and a non-sun-exposed region (gluteal) in winter, for central Europeans ($n = 450$) divided into the four skin type groups (cf. Figure 5). The 'L' value decreases from skin type I to IV; the 'a' and 'b' values increase from I to IV.

Objective assessment of intra- and inter-individual skin colour variability 107

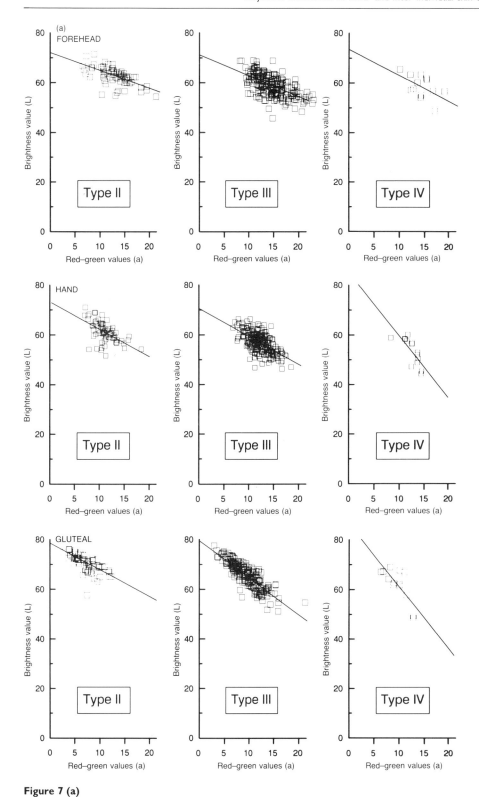

Figure 7 (a)
Natural skin colour of 450 central Europeans in winter. Skin colour measurements as plots of 'a' values versus 'L' values. The point clusters of the skin type classes II–IV overlap. The regression lines exhibit different slopes.

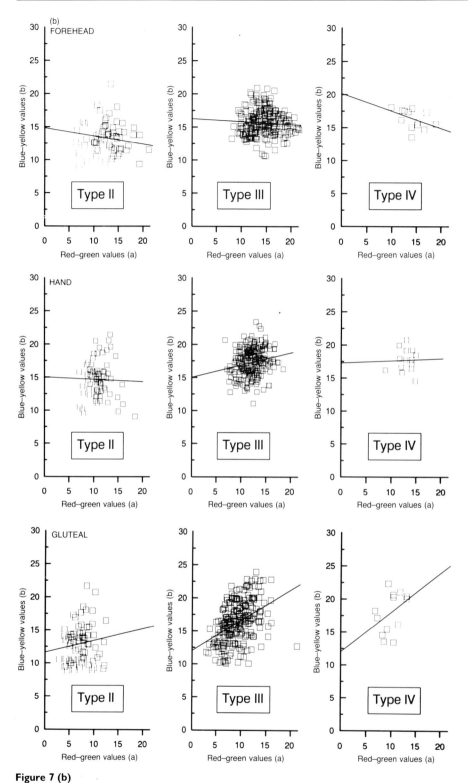

Figure 7 (b)

Natural skin colour of 450 central Europeans in winter. Skin colour measurements as plots of 'a' values versus 'b' values.

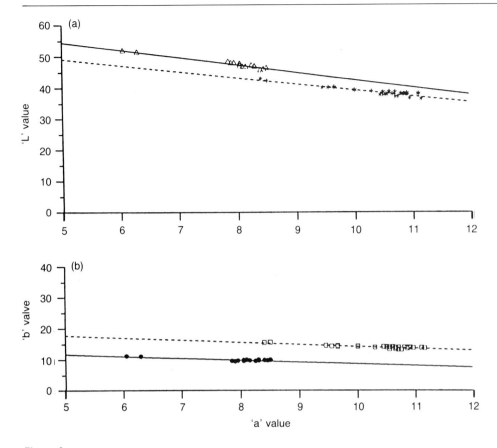

Figure 8

Colorimetric dose–response curve to UVB provocation of a single volunteer in winter (continuous line) and summer (dotted line). (a) Plot of the 'a' value versus the 'L' value. Note, that the regression line is shifted parallel downwards whereas its slope remains almost constant. (b) Plot of the 'a' value versus the 'b' value. The regression line is shifted parallel upwards.

regression line oriented in space. Two orthogonal side projections of this line ('aL' and 'ab' diagram) are shown in Figure 9. When comparing skin reactions in summer and winter, only a parallel shift of the line was observed, whereas the slope of the line remained nearly constant.

The regression lines of the other central European volunteers, which were determined in winter, were entered into the computer program (Chroma3D) using different colours to distinguish skin types I–IV (Figure 9). By rotating the 'Lab' colour ovaloid, it can be shown that the four 'sun-reactive' skin types exhibit regression lines which have a specific slope and shift. The exact spatial orientation of the regression lines can be studied in different projections (Figures 9(a)–9(e)). A projection similar to a 'bL' diagram shows that the regression lines have a positive slope which varies between 90° and 0° (Figure 9(d)). The slope angle of the slope decreases in going from skin type I to IV.

The colorimetric dose–response regression lines for the sun-reactive skin types I–IV, assessed from a perspective corresponding to the 'ab' diagram, did not exhibit any apparent order (Figure 9(e)).

The colorimetric dose–response values to UVB provocation, when plotted in a projection corresponding to an 'aL' diagram, are all located on a regression line having a negative slope angle (arctan x). This slope angle decreases in going from skin

110 *The environmental threat to the skin*

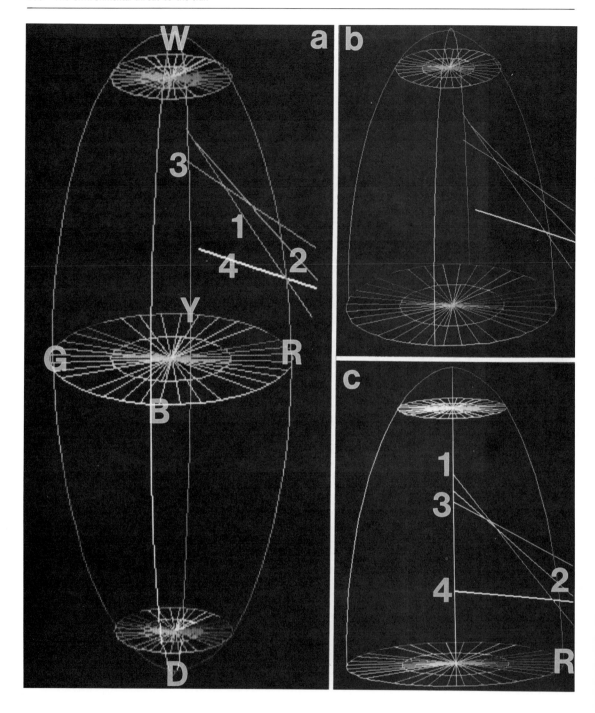

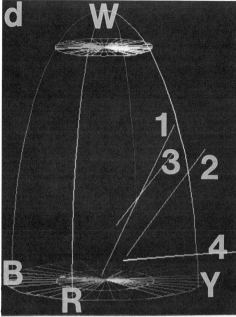
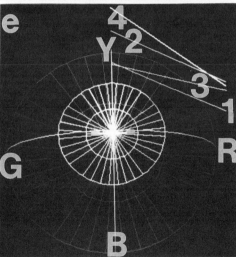

Figure 9

Colorimetric dose–response curve to UVB induced erythema in volunteers of sun-reactive skin types I–IV: the three-dimensional 'Lab' colour representation ovaloid created with the program Chroma3D. The ovaloid is represented in full colours on the monitor and is depth shaded to improve the perspective impression. The colour wheel gives the basic colours green (G), yellow (Y), red (R) and blue (B). The lightness factor varies between black (D) and white (W). Representative regression lines of sun-reactive skin types I (1), II (2), III (3) and IV (4) from a pool of 20 volunteers. (a) The two concentric rings in the middle, upper and lower level correspond to 'a' and 'b' values of 10 and 20. The vertical lines move along the contour of value 20. Note that the slopes of the regression lines for skin types I–IV differ. (b) The upper part of the 'Lab' ovaloid, represented in the same perspective as in (a). (c) Perspective projection corresponding to an 'a' versus 'L' diagram (see Figure 8(a)). Note that the slopes of the regression lines for skin types I–IV differ. (d) Perspective projection corresponding to a 'b' versus 'L' diagram. Note that the slopes of the regression lines for skin types I–IV differ. (e) Top view down onto the 'Lab' ovaloid. This view corresponds to an 'a' versus 'b' diagram (see Figure 8(b)). Note, that there is no apparent order in this perspective.

types I to IV (Figure 9(c)), varying between 0° (never sunburn) and 90° (always sunburn).

In most cases, the subjective classification into sun-reactive skin types by the volunteer corresponded to our classification using the slope angle in the 'aL' diagram. However, some volunteers obviously gave incorrect answers, particularly those with skin type II or III.

Discussion

The results can be summarized as follows: (1) In central Europeans, a clinically relevant classification into skin types is only possible using photoprovocation tests, since their natural skin colour is highly variable due to sun exposure and thus there is much overlap within the skin type groups. (2) The erythema observed after UVB provocation correlates well with changes in the 'a' value in the 'Lab' colour representation system. (3) The slope of the 'Lab' colour regression line in the 'aL' projection is well suited to defining skin sensibility to sunburn. The angle of the slope of this line is a good indicator for sun-reactive skin sensitivity and is better suited to clinical use than is the working classification of sun-reactive types introduced by Fitzpatrick et al.[24]

The erythema

It is generally accepted that the erythema is mainly due to accumulation of blood in the capillaries. Analysis of light remission curves has revealed that haemoglobin and oxyhaemoglobin contribute little to the absorbance in comparison to the other skin pigments.[7] Therefore, precise quantification of erythema has been difficult even with highly developed instrumentation. Many not too successful attempts have been made to develop spectrometers which can separate the haemoglobin and melanin components of the skin colour (e.g. Dermatospectrometer, Cortex Technology, DK[29]).

The pigmentation can cause a systematic error in quantitative erythema evaluation. Melanin, which is localized in the epidermis, interferes in the observation of skin vessels: in this case tanning can overlap erythema. Without further knowledge about this interference, pigmentation and erythema cannot be quantified. We also observed an interdependence between the three colour parameters since, with increasing cumulative energy, the skin redness ('a') increased, whereas the yellow component ('b') and colour lightness ('L') decreased. Our results confirm that the 'a' value recorded with the Minolta Chroma Meter is a good indicator of skin erythema.[30,31]

Wilhelm and Maibach[22] induced erythema by using sodium lauryl sulphate at six different concentrations. They observed the same interdependence between the 'Lab' values, stating that the 'a' value correlated best with the dose of the irritant and with the visual score.

Skin pigmentation

There has been some doubt as to whether skin pigmentation behaves like a grey filter or modifies the skin colour perception in a specific way. Using remission spectrophotometry, Bode[7] concluded that pigmentation behaves like a grey filter to skin colour.

To elucidate this problem, the absorption characteristics of 3,4-dihydroxyphenylalanine(DOPA)–melanin and of extracted natural melanins have been studied.[32–35] Melanin was put into solution before registering the absorbance by standard spectrophotometric techniques.[35] It has been proposed[33] and confirmed experimentally,[32] that when powdered melanin is formed into pellets it behaves like an amorphous semiconductor.[36] Attempts to characterize the melanin compounds chemically and physically were not very successful, because the UV–visible absorption spectrum of melanin shows no specific absorption bands.[33] Some research groups have assumed that epidermal melanin absorbs much like DOPA melanin, which is soluble in water, and is easily analysed. Extracted hair melanins have been solubilized in very strong basic solutions and their absorption spectrum was found to be similar to that of DOPA–melanin. Moreover, the same absorber was found in vitiliginous and normal volunteers.[37] Kollias and Baqer[36] have proposed that human melanin absorbs visible radiation through two distinct mechanisms: one that is in effect over the entire visible range and is linear with respect to wavelength, and a second one that is evident at wavelengths in the range 400–500 nm and is exponential with respect to frequency. By comparing the diffuse reflection spectra of DOPA–melanin in solution (low molecular weight) and in the powdered state (high molecular weight) Kollias and Baqer[36] concluded that melanin must exist in two distinct states in the skin.

Their model is further supported by measurements obtained from very dark individuals.[36] In

Africans and very dark Indians the straight line absorption curve dominated the absorption spectrum and the exponential deviation was very difficult to discern. According to Pathak et al[38] the melanin of these individuals is concentrated in thoroughly melanized melanosomes. In light skinned individuals, however, Kollias and Baqer[36] found a distinct deviation from the straight line absorption at wavelengths below 500 nm.

The cumulative UVB dose

In a recent study, Breit[39] analysed the spectral remission curves of the skin after UVA exposure. Although he concentrated on the mechanisms of UVA tanning, he published some spectral remission curves of general interest. He applied a collar used for blood pressure measurements on the upper arm and inflated it slowly up to 200 mmHg. Successively, first the venous pressure and later the arterial pressure was exceeded; blood volume was therefore trapped in the lower arm. This resulted in darkening, i.e. the entire remission curve moved downward (2–8%). After injection of physiological 0.9% NaCl solution into the upper corium and waiting for the reflex erythema to disappear, the remission curve moved upwards (2–8%). Breit then studied the changes of the skin remission spectrum observed after applying three times the minimal erythema dose (MED) of UVB after 2 and 7 h. After 2 h the remission curve had moved downwards by 5% in the region below 600 nm and exhibited two peaks at 545 and 575 nm (approximately the absorption spectra of oxyhaemoglobin). After 7 h the depression below 600 nm had become more prominent, whereas above 600 nm the remission values were even higher than on the contralateral normal skin. Breit explained this effect as the development of a local oedema. These findings emphasize that skin colour is highly sensitive to different physical effects, which must be kept constant when making measurements. Furthermore, since the oedema falsifies colour measurements, the applied cumulative UVB dose must either be below the dose that produces oedema, or the measurements have to be made within the first hours. We rejected those 24-h colour measurements after UVB provocation, where an oedema could be palpated. As has been shown by Breit,[39] an oedema can obviously modify the colour perception significantly.

Sun-reactive skin-type classification

Haake et al[40] studied a population consisting of skin types I to III and found no correlation between the UVR sensitivity (MED) and skin colour. The findings were confirmed by Westerhof et al,[41] who observed a greater than three-fold difference between the highest and lowest MED values in each skin type, reflecting the large variation in individual MED values. They speculated that either the skin type did not accurately estimate UVR sensitivity, or that the MED is not a sensitive measure of the skin response to UVR provocation. Westerhof et al.[40] concluded that the lack of a close relationship of Fitzpatrick's skin types with the dose–response curves for erythema and pigmentation shows that Fitzpatrick's skin types are an inadequate predictor of skin UVR reaction. These findings are further supported by the findings of Alsins et al,[42] who showed that the minimal blister dose (MBD) varies less between individuals than does the minimal erythema dose at 313 nm.

We therefore believe that the dose–response regression line to UVB provocation is of clinical relevance, because it measures the human skin reaction to UVR provocation over a longer time period. However, because skin colorimetry is not widely available at present, MED determination will continue to be used to obtain data on UVB skin sensitivity.

However, for sophisticated phototesting, such as the determination of the protection which is provided by sunscreens, the response curve of the skin better reflects changes in UVR sensitivity. We believe that the dose–response curves for erythema and pigmentation describe more accurately the tendency of an individual's skin to sunburn or to tan. The skin colour dose–response curve for evaluating sunburn can be easily determined 12 h after UVB radiation and should become a standard part of phototesting.

We proposed the use of the angle of regression line (arctan x) in the 'aL' diagram as a direct measure of the individual's sunburn sensitivity. This angle can vary between 0° (never sunburn) and 90° (sunburn at infinitely low energy).

Summary

The Minolta CR200 Chroma Meter is well suited for precise colour quantifications. Every colour can be described by a combination of three characteristics, the *hue* or basic colour, the *grey value* or colour lightness and the *chroma* or colour saturation. The 'Lab' colour representation system is a three-dimensional ovaloid where all colours are included: 'a' and 'b' are oriented horizontally, 'L' is represented vertically; 'a' determines the hue and chroma along the green–red axis, 'b' the same aspects on the blue–yellow axis.

We analysed the natural skin colour of 500 volunteers in two sun-exposed areas (forehead and dorsum of the hand) and in two non-sun-exposed areas (gluteal region and dorsum of the foot) in winter. The sun exposed areas exhibited significant lower 'L' values and higher 'a' values.

Furthermore, 450 central European volunteers were classified into skin type groups I-IV (after Fitzpatrick et al[24]). Although the mean values exhibited trends, the point clouds of the different skin regions exhibited a strong overlap for all four skin type groups. A classification of a single central European by simple skin colour measurement is therefore impossible in most cases.

To study the interdependance of skin types and sunburn, 20 volunteers were subjected to an UVB-provocation on the back. The colour changes observed on the different skin patch areas with increasing total energy exposure exhibited linear changes of the 'L', 'a' and 'b' values. Moreover, when the same volunteer was subjected to an UVB-provocation also in summer the lines had shifted nearly parallel to lower levels in the 'La' diagram and to higher levels in the 'ba' diagram. By comparing the skin type groups I to IV in the 'aL', 'bL' and 'ab' diagrams, it becomes apparent that the four sun-reative skin types differ mainly by their slope in the 'aL' diagram.

Since it is known from literature, that the 'a' value correlates well with the intensity of the erythema, we propose a new clinically relevant classification of sun-reactive skin types to predict sunburn sensitivity using the negative slope angle of the regression line in the 'aL' diagram after UVB-exposure which varies between 0° (never sunburn) and 90° (sunburn at infinitely low energy).

References

1 Little MA, Sprangel CJ, Skin reflectance relationships with temperature and skinfolds, *Am J Phys Anthropol* (1980) **52**: 145–51.
2 Clark P, Stark AE, Walsh RJ et al, A twin study of skin reflectance, *Ann Human Biol* (1981) **8**: 529–41.
3 Emden J, Schaefer H, Stüttgen G, Vergleich physikalischer Parameter von Hautdurchblutungsänderungen nach epikutaner Applikation von Nikotinsäurebenzylester, *Arch Dermatol Forsch* (1971) **241**: 353–63.
4 Zaun H, Altmeyer P, Ergebnisse reflexphotometrischer Bestimmungen der Vasokonstriktion nach topischer Steroidapplikation, *Arch Dermatol Forsch* (1973) **247**: 378–86.
5 Altmeyer P, Modification of experimental UV erythema by external steroids — a reflex photometric study, *Arch Dermatol Res* (1977) **258**: 203–9.
6 Rampini E, Rastelli A, Cardo P, Comparative study of the vasoconstrictor activity of halopredone acetate in a modified McKenzie test, *Eur J Clin Pharmacol* (1978) **14**: 325–9.
7 Bode HG, Über spektralphotometrische Untersuchungen an menschlicher Haut unter besonderer Berücksichtigung der Erythem- und Pigmentmessung, *Strahlentherapie* (1934) **51**: 81–118.
8 Hausmann W, *Grundzüge der Lichtbiologie und Lichtpathologie*, Urban und Schwarzenberg: Berlin, 1923.
9 Finsen NR, *Über die Anwendung von concentrierten chemischen Strahlen in der Medicin*, Vogel: Leipzig, 1899.
10 Hausser KW, Vahle W, Sonnenbrand und Sonnenbräunung. Wissenschaft, *Veröfftl des Siemens Konzerns* (1921) **6**: 101–20.
11 Deutsches Institut für Normung, Berlin, *DIN 5031*, Parts 7 and 10.
12 Uhlmann E, Über die Abhängigkeit der Pigmentbildung von der Wellenlänge der Strahlung, *Strahlentherapie* (1930) **35**: 361–8.
13 Fetz S, Untersuchungen zur Erythemwirksamkeitskurve, *Strahlentherapie* (1970) **140**: 236–42.
14 Anders A, Aufmuth P, Böttger EM et al, Investigation of the erythema effectiveness curve with tunable lasers, *Dermatol Beruf Umwelt* (1984) **32**: 166–70.
15 Mortazawi SAM, Oberste-Lehn H, Lichtsensibilisatoren und ihre therapeutischen Fähigkeiten, *Z Hautkr* (1973) **48**: 1–9.
16 Tronnier H, Schüle D, Zur dermatologischen Therapie von Dermatosen mit langwelligem UV nach Photosensibilisierung der Haut mit Methoxsalen. Erste Ergebnisse bei der Psoriasis vulgaris, *Z Hautkr* (1973) **48**: 385–93.
17 Parrish JA, Fitzpatrick TB, Tannenbaum L et al, Photochemotherapy of psoriasis with oral methoxsalen and long-wave ultraviolet light, *New Engl J Med* (1974) **291**: 1207–11.
18 Weber G, Combined 8-methoxypsoralen and black light therapy of psoriasis, *Br J Dermatol* (1974) **90**: 317–23.
19 Tronnier H, Heidbuchel H, Zur Therapie der Psoriasis vulgaris mit ultravioletten Strahlen, *Z Hautkr* (1976) **57**: 379–92.
20 Wucherpfennig V, Eine automatische Sektorentreppe zur genauen Bestimmung der Erythem-Schwellen des UV, *Strahlentherapie* (1933) **48**: 391–6.
21 Deutsches Institut für Normung, Berlin, *DIN 67501*.
22 Wilhelm KP, Maibach HI, Skin color reflectance measurements for objective quantification of erythema in human beings, *J Am Acad Dermatol* (1989) **21**: 1306–8.
23 Lees FC, Byard PJ, Relethford JH, Interobserver error in human skin colorimetry, *Am J Phys Anthropol* (1978) **49**: 35–7.
24 Fitzpatrick TB, Pathak MA, Parrish JA, Protection of human skin against the effects of the sunburn ultraviolet (290–320 nm). In: Fitzpatrick TB et al, (eds). *Sunlight and*

man—normal and abnormal photobiological responses, University of Tokyo Press: Tokyo, 1974, p751.

25 el-Gammal S, ANAT3D: On-line computer demonstrations of shaded three-dimensional models under Microsoft Windows. In: Elsner N, Roth G (eds). *Brain—perception—cognition*, Georg Thieme Verlag: Stuttgart, 1990.

26 el-Gammal S, Altmeyer P, Hinrichsen K, ANAT3D: Shaded three-dimensional surface reconstructions from serial sections. Applications in morphology and histopathology, *Acta Stereol* (1989) (suppl 2): 543–50.

27 Helfmann J (1989) Nichtlineare Prozesse. In: Berline HP, Müller G, (eds). *Angewandte Lasermedizin, Lehr- und Handbuch für Praxis und Klinik,* Ecomed Verlagsgesellschaft mbH: Landsberg, 1989; pII–3.4

28 Müller GJ, Müller-Stolzenburg N, Biologische Wirkung der Laserstrahlung—Potentielle Risken für Haut und Augen, *Biotronic* (1989) **1**: 55–60.

29 Diffey BL, Oliver RJ, Farr PM, A portable instrument for quantifying erythema induced by ultraviolet radiation, *Br J Dermatol* (1984) **111**: 663–72.

30 Babulak S, Rhein L, Scala DD et al, Quantification of erythema in a soap chamber test using the Minolta Chroma (Reflectance) Meter: comparison of instrumental results with visual assessments, *J Soc Cosmet Chem* (1986) **37**: 475–9.

31 Seitz JC, Whitmore CG, Measurement of erythema and tanning response in human skin using a Tristimulus Colorimeter, *Dermatologica* (1988) **177**: 70–5.

32 Crippa PR, Christofoletti V, Romeo N, A band model for melanin deduced from optical absorption and photoconductivity experiments, *Biochim Biophys Acta* (1978) **538**: 164–70.

33 Wolbarsht ML, Walsh AW, George G, Melanin, a unique biological absorber, *Appl Opt* (1981) **20**: 2184–6.

34 Bridelli MG, Crippa PR, Optical properties of melanin: a comment, *Appl Opt* (1982) **21**: 2669–70.

35 Menon IA, Persad S, Haberman HF et al, A comparative study of the physical and chemical properties of melanins isolated from human black and red hair, *J Invest Dermatol* (1983) **80**: 202–6.

36 Kollias N, Baqer AH, Absorption mechanisms of human melanin in the visible, 400–720 nm, *J Invest Dermatol* (1987) **89**: 384–8.

37 Kollias N, Baqer A, Spectroscopic characteristics of melanin in vivo. *J Invest Dermatoal* (1985) **85**: 38–42.

38 Pathak MA, Jimbow K, Szabo G et al, Sunlight and melanin pigmentation, *Photochem Photobiol Rev* (1976) **1**: 221–39.

39 Breit R, *Rötung und Bräunung durch UV-A. Spektrales Remissionsverhalten und farbmetrische Analyse der Hautreaktionen des Menschen unter UV-Bestrahlungsanlagen.* Habilitationsschrift, W. Zuckschwerdt-Verlag: Munich, 1976, pp36–110.

40 Haake N, Buhles N, Altmeyer P, Sensitivity of human skin to UV-light, practicability and limits in clinical diagnosis, *Z Hautkr* (1987) **62**: 1505–9.

41 Westerhof W, Estevez-Uscanga O, Meens J et al, The relation between constitutional skin color and photosensitivity estimated from UV-induced erythema and pigmentation dose–response curves, *J Invest Dermatol* (1990) **94**: 812–6.

42 Alsins J, Claesson S, Fischer T et al, Development of high intensity narrow-band lamps and studies of irradiation effect on human skin, *Acta Dermatovener (Stockh)* (1975) **55**: 261–71.

20
Ultraviolet radiation induced erythema: a proposal for a computerized quantification

G. C. Fuga, C. Spina, A. Di Palma, F. Acierno, G. F. Cirillo and W. Marmo
Istituto Dermatologico, S. Maria & S. Gallicano, Roma, Italia

The increase in acute actinic dermatitis observed in recent years has led several workers to search for a precise method of quantifying the erythema induced by ultraviolet radiation (UVR).

Measurement of changes in colour, even if attempted by the attentive and expert eye of the dermatologist shows great observer variation. Subjective assessment depends on a variety of physical and environmental conditions (including colour, temperature, the direction of the incident light, the amount of light, and the type of surface being examined) and on the sensory and perceptive characteristics of the observer which can also be influenced by psychological conditioning. The evaluation of UVR induced erythema was first attempted in 1927 by Hausser and Vahle[1] who used red cards as standards for comparison. Berger et al. used various red photographic filters, whilst Breit and Kligman[3] and Daniels et al.[4] obtained useful data using photoelectric reflectance meters. More recently, very good results were obtained by Dawson et al.,[5] Wan et al.,[6] by Diffey et al.,[7] Leonard et al.,[8] Thomas et al.,[9] and Andreassi et al.[10] using various types of spectrophotometers.

We have been interested in the UVR threat to the skin for many years. Last year in Glasgow at MIE 90[11,12] we presented a colour evaluation system comprising a light reflectance densitometer (X-Rite 404) which is able to quantify, using logarithmic values to the base 10, both the total optical reflectance density (visual, V) of an opaque circular surface (3.4 mm diameter), and the logarithmic values of the colours cyan, magenta and yellow that contribute to define V. The instrument can provide automatically the difference between two consecutive readings.

The intensity of erythema (IE) is due to vasodilatation of the cutaneous microcirculation with consequent increase in the quantity of red blood cells and, therefore, of haemoglobin. This haemaglobin absorbs the green light and reflects red light. Consequently the greater the quantity of haemaglobin in the skin, the greater is the absorption of green light with an increase in the reflected red colour.

The quantification of IE is obtained by subtracting the logarithm of the inverse reflectance (R) of the red light from that of the green light:

$$IE = \log(1/R_{green}) - \log(1/R_{red})$$

and then, using the scale of complementary colours

$$IE = \log R_{magenta} - \log R_{cyan}$$

The melanin content of the epidermis and the reflection of the light from the deep tissue layers do not affect the results of the equation.[7]

The difference between the IE of damaged skin and the IE of apparently healthy perilesional skin represents the gradient of erythema (GE).[8]

Since the degree of erythema depends on the number of open cutaneous microvessels, it was decided to compare the results of optical reflectance densitometry with those of computerized capillaroscopy.

A method of quantifying the capillaroscopic modifications induced by various physical, chemical or pharmacological factors has been presented previously.[13,14] Capillaroscopy on normal skin usually demonstrates only a few open capillaries per microscopic field. On erythematous skin the number of visible capillaries is closely related to the intensity of erythema. By calculating the number of open capillaries present per unit area of skin it is possible to obtain a measure of the degree of erythema.

We used a Zeiss OMPI-1 reflected light microscope with fixed lens ($f = 50$), magnifications of 0.4–0.6 and 1, enlargement of tube ($f_2 = 160$), and interfaced twice with a Sony CCD telecamera connected to a 3/4 in. videorecorder. The video image is run through a personal computer which, appropriately programmed with a graphics card, digitizes and visualizes the signal on a high-definition monitor. The system is suitably calibrated so that any magnification change in the microscopic field corresponds to a precise metric value of the pixel of the digital image: with the 0.4 magnification a pixel corresponds to 0.004 mm, with a 0.6 magnification to 0.0027 and with the 1.0 magnification a pixel corresponds to 0.0016 mm.

In the image obtained with the smaller microscopic enlargement, 1 mm^2 is represented by a square of 250 pixels per side and the videoscreen, therefore, represents a surface of the microscopic field equal to about 3 mm^2.

To evaluate the relationships between the two methods we exposed both forearms to UVR from an Original Hanau Psorilux 3060 lamp giving out UVA at 2.30 mW/cm^2 intensity (equal to 100 mJ/cm^2 in 43 s) and UVB at 0.80 mW/cm^2 intensity (equal to 100 mJ/cm^2 in 2 min). One forearm was protected by applying 3% bendazac cream three times daily for 5 days. The exposures were randomized using the following doses: 0, 50, 100, 150 mJ/cm^2 of UVB for sites designated A, B, C and D, respectively.

The capillaroscopic examination and reflected densitometry were carried out 24 h after irradiation at all skin sites.

The results are reported in Table 1. It can be seen that the increase in the number of open capillaries per square millimetre is correlated to the UVB dose. The treated areas showed significantly less open capillaries than the corresponding control areas.

The value of IE is also related to the UVB doses and was particularly high in control areas; it seems to be closely related to the number of open vessels.

The correlation (Table 2) between the two methods is significant only for the highest dose ($r = 0.65$). Doubling the number of observations would probably make the correlation significant for lower doses as well.

We employed topical bendazac because of its well-known photoprotective activity. This cream has been demonstrated to prevent the erythematous response to UVR exposure after topical application.[15–18] Capillaroscopic studies showed a sharp decrease in cutaneous microcirculatory damage.[19] The inhibition of UVR induced degranulation of rat mastocytes after isolation and incubation with bendazac is probably due to the drug's membrane protecting activity.[20] A lesser degree of erythema corresponds to a reduced release of vasoactive substances. It is of note that we irradiated five patients 30 min after a single application of bendazac observing only a very low photoprotective activity.

The above experiments are further confirmation of the validity of these two non-invasive methods

Table 1 Capillaries per square millimetre (CSM), intensity of erythema (IE) and gradient of erythema (GE) of skin exposed to UVR (absolute values)

Subjects (N = 10)	Parameters (means)	Intensity of radiation (mJ/cm^2)			
		0	50	100	150
Treated areas	CSM ± SE	25 ± 2.7	39 ± 3.0	61 ± 2.8	74.5 ± 3.2
	IE ± SE	0.11 ± 0.01	0.17 ± 0.03	0.25 ± 0.02	0.33 ± 0.02
	GE		1.5	2.3	3
Control areas	CSM ± SE	25 ± 2.7	37 ± 3.1	72 ± 2.9	92 ± 3.6
	IE ± SE	0.11 ± 0.01	0.16 ± 0.04	0.32 ± 0.02	0.41 ± 0.02
	GE		1.45	2.9	3.7

Table 2 Capillaries per square millimetre (CSM) and intensity of erythema (IE) of skin exposed to UVR (statistical data)

Subjects (N = 10)	Intensity of radiation (mJ/cm^2)		
	50	100	150
Student's t paired test (CSM)	2.050	2.298	3.651
P	NS	<0.05	<0.01
Student's t paired test (IE)	1.920	2.271	3.060
P	NS	<0.05	<0.05
Correlation test CSM vs. IE			
r	0.58	0.61	0.65
P	NS	NS	<0.05
Coefficient of regression CSM/IE			2.250
Coefficient of regression IE/CSM			0.005

NS, not significant.

for the study of the skin's reaction to various stimuli. The methods would be suitable for quantifying the activity of many drugs.

Acknowledgements

This work has been accomplished thanks to Banco di Santo Spirito-Cassa di Risparmio di Roma, ACRAF Angelini, CFA and Cinecitta.

References

1 Hausser KW, Vahle W, Sonnerbrad und sonnerbräunung, Wiessenschaft Veroff Siemens Konzern (1927) 6: 101–10.
2 Berger D, Urbach F, Davies RE, The action spectrum of erythema induced by ultraviolet radiation, Preliminary report on the XIII Congress Intern. Dermatologiae, Vol I, Springer-Verlag: Berlin, 1968.
3 Breit R, Kligman AM, Measurement of erythemal and pigmentary responses to ultraviolet radiation at different spectral qualities. In: The biologic effects of ultraviolet radiation with emphasis on the skin, Vol I Pergamon Press: Oxford, 1969.
4 Daniels F, Imbrie JD, Comparison between visual grading and reflectance measurements of erythema produced by sunlight, J Invest Dermatol (1958) 30: 295–301.
5 Dawson JB, Barker DJ, Ellis DJ et al, A theoretical and experimental study of light absorption and scattering by in vivo skin. Phys Med Biol (1980) 25: 695–700.
6 Wan S, Parrish JA, Jaenicke KF, Quantitative evaluation of ultraviolet induced erythema, Photochem Photobiol (1983) 37: 643–50.
7 Diffey BL, Oliver RJ, Farr PM, A portable instrument for quantifying erythema induced by ultraviolet radiation, Br J Dermatol (1984) 111: 663–72.
8 Leonard F, Kalis B, Demange L, Mesure quantitative de l'érythème cutané par photodensitométrie, Nouv Dermatol (1987) 6: 254–47.
9 Thomas P, Bocquet JL, Leplat J et al, La téléréflectométrie: une nouvelle technique d'exploration cutanée, Nouv Dermatol (1987) 6: 220–3.
10 Andreassi L, Simoni S, Casini L et al, Studio sull'attività depigmentante di un prodotto a base di Achillea millefoglie, Med Estet (1988) 12: 153–7.
11 Fuga GC, Spina C, Cavallotti C et al, Computerized reflected optical densitometry. A research on the colour of the skin. In: O'Moore R, Bengtsson S, Bryant JR, et al, (eds). Medical Informatics Europe '90, Springer-Verlag: Berlin, 1990, p. 791.
12 Fuga GC, Spina C, Cavallotti C et al, Computerized reflected optical densitometry. A research on the colour of the skin, J Appl Cosmet (1990) 8: 91–110.
13 Fuga GC, Spina C, Di Palma A et al, Microcirculation. Usefulness of informatics in capillaroscopy. In: Barber B, Cao D, Qin D et al, (eds). Medinfo '89 North Holland: Amsterdam, 1989, p. 1236.
14 Fuga GC, Marmo W, Di Palma A, Capillaroscopia computerizzata. Stato dell'arte e riflessi nello studio dell'angioneurosi da strumenti vibranti, Boll Coll Med Ital Trasport (1990) 11: 15–19.
15 Bessone L, Anselmi L, Photoprotective activity of Bendazac. In: Fuga GC, De Gregorio M, Milbradt R, (eds). New trends in skin therapeutics, Leonardo: Rome, 1975, p. 59.
16 Ippen H, Research of the erythema-preventing and erythema-inhibiting effects of anti-inflammatory drugs. In: New trends in skin therapeutics, Leonardo: Rome, 1975, p. 71.
17 Tronnier H, Experimental comparative studies on the topical action of bendazac and betamethasone. In: New trends in skin therapeutics, Leonardo: Rome, 1975, p. 11.
18 Fuga GC, Proto A, Considerazioni cliniche su una sperimentazione controllata con acido bendazolico in alcune dermatosi, Min Derm (1970) 45: 528–34.
19 Fuga GC, Barduagni O, De Gregorio M, Osservazioni sul potere fotoprotettivo dell'acido bendazolico, Ann Ital Derm Cl Sper (1970) 24: 204–10.
20 Fuga GC, De Gregorio M, Ippolito F et al, Bendazac's effect on mast cell degranulation. In: Fuga GC, De Gregorio M, Milbradt R (eds). New trends in skin therapeutics, Leonardo: Rome, 1975, p. 77.

21
Microcirculatory damage in subjects exposed to the risk of ionizing radiation: image analysis and statistics of a 5-year observation

G. C. Fuga, C. Cavallotti, A. Di Palma, F. Leonetti and W. Marmo

Istituto Dermatologico, S. Maria and S. Gallicano, Rome, Italy

Changes in small cutaneous vessels, particularly capillaries, represent the earliest damage induced in the skin by ionizing radiation in those individuals who administer X-rays. It is not necessary to describe the clinical and histopathological pictures of chronic radiodermatitis, but we would like to describe briefly the capillaroscopic patterns of the illness studied for the first time in 1932 by Turano.[1] Turano stressed the early damage to the microvasculature in cutaneous lesions. Initially, the calibre and length of the capillaries are reduced, the blood flow becomes sluggish and the vessel walls lose their elasticity. Later there is an increase in the calibre of vessels with the appearance of twists and tortuosities and the blood flow is further reduced. In areas that are not particularly atrophic, the calibre may be either reduced or increased, many twists and tortuosities are present and the subpapillary plexus is visible. In the most severe form represented clinically by atrophy, telangiectasia, keratoses and epitheliomas, the capillaroscopic pattern is very varied. In atrophic areas, there are a few slim, shorter comma-like capillaries, while in other telangiectatic areas the microvessels are greatly increased in calibre forming lakes in which the blood flow is very slow, discontinuous or almost static. Some haemorrhages are present.

Unfortunately, because of the technical difficulties, such as eye strain after prolonged use of the microscope, and photographic difficulties, capillaroscopy has been limited in the past to research purposes only. Recently, however, the technique has been improved by interfacing the microscope with a camera and a videorecorder. We have assembled a system which enables us to digitize images and calculate exactly some parameters which are recorded and memorized on a clinical card. Microcirculatory damage is quantified according to the scale which we proposed some years ago.[3]

We report there our observations made over the years 1985 to 1989 in a group of subjects professionally exposed to ionizing radiations. During these 5 years, of the 1872 capillaroscopic examinations performed, 819 (43.61%; 672 male and 147 female) were of subjects exposed to ionizing radiation for professional reasons (medical radiology for diagnosis and therapy, nuclear radiology, radioimmunology or industrial radiology, as shown in Table 1). The working period in the exposed and potentially hazardous areas was from a few months to over 30 years.

Table 1 Subjects ($N = 819$) professionally exposed to ionizing radiation subdivided by occupational class.

	No of subjects
Medical radiology	
Radiologists	122
Orthopaedic surgeons	68
Surgeons in other fields	64
Heart specialists	11
Dentists	5
Nurses	58
Technicians	422
Nuclear radiology or radioimmunology	
Doctors	9
Technicians	30
Industrial radiology	
Technicians	20

In 133 (16.24%) patients some type of dermatological disorder of the hands was present, either alone or in combination with onychodystrophy, keratoses, atrophy, dryness and scaling of the skin, lichenification, or eczema. In 280 subjects we observed alopecia of the fingers. We consider this disorder separately as we could not tell with certainty whether it was constitutional or attributable to the radiation exposure (Table 2).

It can be seen from Figure 1 that, of the 819 subjects, 227 (27.71%) did not show any capillaroscopic damage, 222 (27.10%) showed slight damage, 130 (15.87%) showed moderate damage, 144 (17.58%) showed severe damage, and 96 (11.72%)

Table 2 Macroscopic skin disorders in subjects professionally exposed to ionizing radiation.

	Degree of capillaroscopic damage					
	Absent	Light	Moderate	High	Very high	Total
Acroasphixia	3	—	2	1	4	10
Atrophy	—	—	—	—	14	14
Dryness	1	3	2	1	3	10
Eczema	1	3	—	—	—	4
Keratoses	—	3	1	6	20	30
Lichenification	—	—	—	1	—	1
Onychodistrophy	5	18	11	28	39	101
Scaling	—	—	2	1	1	4
Total	10	27	18	38	81	174
Alopecia	23	79	55	82	41	280

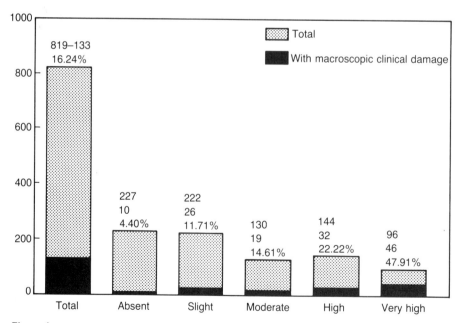

Figure 1

Results of capillaroscopic examinations carried out in 1985–89 on subjects occupationally exposed to ionizing radiation. Absolute and percentage values of capillary damage are given together with the symptomatology. Alopecia is excluded.

demonstrated very severe damage. The total area of each column in the histogram indicates the total number of patients in each group and the portion in black indicates the patients with clinical macroscopic skin damage of the hands.

The interpretation of this histogram becomes more interesting when we note the relationship between the total number of patients examined and the numbers of patients with macroscopic disorders at all levels of damage. It becomes suddenly clear that 10 or 4.40% of the 227 patients without any microcirculatory damage had macroscopic cutaneous disorders. If we include the cases with alopecia alone, the number rises to 33 (13.65%). As far as other degrees of damage are concerned, the percentage increases from 11.76% to 47.91% and, if alopecia is included, from 43.24% to 69.79%.

The groups with the highest prevalence of damage were orthopaedic surgeons and general surgeons who carried out intraoperative cholecystography. Many orthopaedic surgeons presented with serious disorders and this may be explained by the fact that, considering the safety of modern devices, they exposed their unprotected hands to a great deal of radiation. The working period and degree of damage are strongly related.

If we compare, unfortunately only by relying on memory, the results now presented with those of the first years in which we made capillaroscopic observations (1956), we can say that the number of subjects with severe damage has greatly reduced whether we express this in absolute figures or as a percentage. We have not seen any further cases of the serious radiodermatitis of the hands once seen in subjects administering ionizing radiation. This improvement is due to the protection now afforded by radiological devices, the elimination of the practice of radioscopy, increased awareness of the risk, the use of dosimetric devices and, we believe, periodic capillaroscopic examinations.

Acknowledgements

This work has been accomplished thanks to Banco di Santo Spirito-Cassa di Risparmio di Roma and ACRAF Angelini.

References

1 Turano L, L'importanza della capillaroscopia nelle lesioni da raggi X (Importance of capillaroscopy in X-ray-caused lesions), *Atti X Congr Ital Radiol Med* (1932) **2**: 198–9.
2 Fuga GC, Spina C, Di Palma A et al, Microcirculation. Usefulness of informatics in capillaroscopy, *Proc 6th Conf Med Informatics*, Singapore, 11–15 December 1989, Part 2, p. 1236.
3 Fuga GC, Osservazioni sulle alterazioni morfologiche e funzionali dei capillari in soggetti esposti al rischio di radiazioni ionizzanti (Observations on capillaroscopic morphological and functional alterations in subjects exposed to ionizing radiation risk), *Riv Microang Capillaroscop* (1984) **1**: 24–9.

22
Mast cell degranulation results in endothelial activation after acute exposure of human skin to ultraviolet irradiation

Robert M. Lavker, Michael S. Kaminer and George F. Murphy
Department of Dermatology, University of Pennsylvania School of Medicine, Clinical Research Building, Room 235A, 422 Curie Boulevard, Philadelphia, PA 19104, USA

Ultraviolet radiation (UVR) and its effects on human skin pose a significant health-care problem to a population that is currently enjoying a steadily increasing mean life-span. While the so-called 'graying' of the population has its obvious benefits, one of the results of this longer life-span is increased long-term sun exposure and its resultant complications. Although much is known about the long-term effects of chronic sun exposure, to date little has been done to delineate the initiating and propagating factors. While it is difficult to treat and correct the chronic damage of sun exposure, an understanding of the underlying mechanisms would enable researchers and clinicians to approach the problem in a more systematic and effective way.

The principal cause of 'sunburn' in human skin is UVR of wavelengths 290–320 nm (UVB). Clinical characteristics of the sunburn response include transient erythema and increased dermal vascular permeability within minutes after exposure to UVR, followed by more persistent erythema delayed in onset by 4–24 h.[1] Initial vascular leakage has been attributed to liberation of histamine by perivascular mast cells, whereas the appearance of delayed erythema correlates with the development of perivascular infiltrates of neutrophils and mononuclear cells.[2,3] Speculation that primary cutaneous targets of UVB radiation include the endothelium and its extensive network of associated cellular elements has arisen from these clinical and histological observations. Supporting this notion is the natural evolution of several clinical disorders (polymorphous light eruption, photo-induced cutaneous lupus erythematosus, and photoeczematous dermatitis). These disorders arise upon exposure of skin of predisposed individuals to sunlight, and are characterized by erythema and perivascular inflammatory infiltrates.

The histological correlate of the human sunburn reaction is the natural evolution of photo-independent inflammatory dermatoses. Initial histological findings include perivascular accumulation of leukocytes primarily about the post-capillary venule of the superficial miscrovascular plexus (the major site of leukocyte migration) as a result of directed movement of leukocytes into the skin. In certain naturally occurring dermatoses, these perivascular leukocytes subsequently migrate in the direction of the epidermis (psoriasis, contact dermatitis and atopic dermatitis).[4] To gain access to the dermis, circulating leukocytes must first pass through the barrier posed by endothelial cells of the post-capillary dermal venule (PCV).[5-7] Numerous studies have demonstrated morphological and ultrastructural endothelial cell alterations, referred to as 'endothelial cell activation', prior to inflammatory cell migration into the dermis from the luminal surface of the PCV. Endothelial cell activation facilitates binding of neutrophils, lymphocytes, monocytes, and eosinophils to specific ligands and recptors,[5] and correlates with the ability of affected microvascular beds to recruit and transpose circulating leukocytes into extravascular compartments.[8,9] Activation includes prominent bulging of the endothelial cells and expression of endothelial–leukocyte adhesion molecule-1 (ELAM-1).[10] ELAM-1 is a non-integrin, lectin-like cell surface glycoprotein that is an early indicator of EC activation and is associated with adhesion of leukocytes to the endothelial luminal membrane.[11-14]

ELAM-1 is induced in vivo during the early stages of hapten-specific cutaneous delayed hypersensitivity responses,[10,15] and in vitro by the immunoregulatory cytokines tumor necrosis factor-α (TNF) and interleukin 1 (IL-1).[11,13–14,16] The production of these cytokines by resident skin cells (TNF by perivascular monocytes and mast cells, and IL-1 by epithelial cells) in proximity to the dermal microvasculature is likely to facilitate ELAM-1 mediated leukocyte trafficking in physiological and pathological conditions.[4,17,18] In situ, ELAM-1 can be detected on the luminal surface of the PCV 2 h after induction with TNF.[10,14,16,17] This display peaks at 6 h, and is dissipated by 24 h after a single pulse of cytokine. This is in contradistinction to intercellular adhesion molecule-1 (ICAM-1) which is constitutively expressed on non-stimulated endothelial cells, and is up-regulated 24 h after endothelial stimulation.[12,19] Moreover, its up-regulation is mediated by γ interferon, a cytokine not found constitutively in normal skin.[20] Furthermore, ICAM-1 expression is maintained for 72 h, whereas ELAM-1 expression cannot be detected after 24 h. Vascular cell adhesion molecule (VCAM-1) is also expressed on cytokine-stimulated endothelial cells,[21] however, its expression is maintained for 48 h whereas ELAM-1 diminishes after 6 h. Furthermore, ELAM-1 interacts primarily with neutrophils in vitro, while VCAM-1 binds selectively to lymphocytes.[21] Recent evidence, however, suggests that ELAM-1 may interact with other inducible glycoproteins on endothelial cells to mediate T lymphocyte adhesion.[22] The early induction of ELAM-1 during endothelial cell activation suggests a role for this glycoprotein in the initial phase of cellular migration.

UVR-induced mast-cell degranulation, with resultant TNF release,[4,23–26] is a possible mechanism for ELAM-1 induction with consequent leukocyte infiltration. In a recent study, we investigated initiating events in the human sunburn response. Our approach was centered on the effects of UVR on dermal vascular ELAM-1 expression in biopsies obtained from human volunteers, and in skin organ cultures subjected to various experimental manipulations. Skin of three subjects exposed to a three times the minimum erythemogenic dose (MED) of solar simulated radiation (SSR, 290–400 nm waveband) or radiation restricted to the UVB spectrum (290–320 nm waveband) demonstrated marked ELAM-1 induction on endothelial cells lining superficial dermal venules. Time-course experiments in three additional subjects disclosed ELAM-1 expression to begin at 2 h and to peak at 6 h after irradiation, kinetics identical to those observed following exposure to endothelium to recombinant cytokines in vitro.[13,14,16] Elicitation of ELAM-1 was abrogated by topical application of a sun protection factor (SPF) 15 sunscreen prior to irradiation.

Whereas perivascular mast cells contained preformed mediators (TNF, tryptase, chymase) within cytoplasmic granules prior to irradiation and in irradiated skin protected by sunscreen, loss of mediators, indicative of degranulation, coincided with ELAM-1 expression after exposure of unprotected skin to SSR or UVB. Mast-cell degranulation following exposure to UVR was associated with externalization of mast-cell preformed mediators in a manner identical to that previously reported for morphine sulfate induced mast-cell degranulation in organ culture.[27] Moreover, routine microscopy confirmed loss of metachromatic granules and externalization of granules in these specimens. Throughout these studies, TNF immunoreactivity was not observed within epidermal cells either before or within 4 h following UVR exposure. Thus, while various epidermal cell types may be capable of TNF synthesis,[28,29] only mast cells appear responsible for the acute release of TNF in this in vivo system.

Low levels of ELAM-1 were evident even after exposure to sub-erythemogenic (1/2 MED) doses of radiation. These data suggest that casual exposure to UVB may result in endothelial activation even though clinical manifestations of 'redness' are absent. Exposure of skin of six subjects to varying doses of UVA or to visible plus infra-red (IR) radiation calculated to duplicate the levels of these wavelengths in the SSR waveband failed to induce significant ELAM-1 expression, suggesting that the action spectrum for ELAM-1 induction lies mainly in the UVB region.

To examine the possible direct effects of UVB radiation on endothelial cells, we exposed cultured human umbilical vein endothelial cells (HUVE) to three times the MED and then evaluated ELAM-1 expression after 4 h of culture. UVB did not induce ELAM-1 expression by HUVE, and did not alter cell viability. Moreover, irradiated HUVE subsequently cultured in the presence of TNF showed high levels of ELAM-1 glycoprotein, indicating intact biosynthetic capabilities. These findings support the notion that UVB-induced ELAM-1 expression is a mast-cell-dependent event which is not mediated by a direct effect of UVB on endothelium.

To formally exclude the possibility that UVB-induced ELAM-1 in vivo resulted from effects of systemic factors or cells circulating through the microvasculature, human noenatal foreskin explants were irradiated with UVB (three times the MED) and then cultured for 4 h. ELAM-1 expression was evaluated immunohistochemically. In foreskin organ cultures, UVB induced ELAM-1 in a manner similar to that observed in the in vivo experiments described above. ELAM-1 induction in vitro was also observed following exposure to recombinant TNF as described previously.[17,25] Topical preapplication of sunscreen that blocked UVB resulted in complete abrogation of UVB-induced ELAM-1 in foreskin explants. Moreover, preincubation of explants with the mast-cell inhibitor cromolyn sodium[17,30] markedly reduced UVB-induced ELAM-1. Pure dermal explants prepared by complete removal of the epidermal layer using EDTA[31] demonstrated similar results after UVB exposure, although abrogation of ELAM-1 induction by cromolyn sodium was now complete. Taken together, these findings indicate that ELAM-1 induction following UVB exposure (of dermal explants) is independent of epidermis and is cromolyn sensitive (i.e. mast-cell dependent). This view is consistent with the known propensity of UVB to induce mast-cell degranulation in vivo[26] and in vitro.[32] The observation that ELAM-1 induction in full-thickness explants is markedly reduced but not completely abolished by pretreatment with cromolyn sodium indicates that epidermally derived cytokines (e.g. IL-1)[33] may act in concert with mast-cell derived mediators to induce ELAM-1 in these cultures.

Recent studies have implicated mast-cell-derived TNF as a critical mediator of endothelial–leukocyte adhesive interactions in skin.[17,18,23–25] Previous studies have demonstrated that ELAM-1 induction following mast-cell degranulation is abrogated by neutralizing antisera to TNF (but not to IL-1) and is, therefore, a TNF-dependent event.[17,25] Our in vivo studies indicated that release of TNF from dermal mast cells was a consequence of UVB exposure. Accordingly, we then analysed supernatants of foreskin explants for TNF released as a consequence of UVB exposure in vitro. TNF was released both from UVB-irradiated intact explants (epidermis + dermis) and from UVB-irradiated pure dermal explants. Moreover, more TNF was liberated from pure dermal cultures, suggesting that the UVB effect is augmented when the overlying epidermis and its associated photoprotective pigment granules are removed. The quantity of TNF in supernatants of dermal explants exposed to three times the MED of UVB approximated that liberated by exposure of replicate cultures to the mast cell secretagogue, morphine sulfate. Moreover, preincubation of both intact explants and dermal explants with the mast cell inhibitor, cromolyn sodium, abolished UVB-induced TNF release. Taken together, these results indicate that the primary source of TNF was the dermal component of explants, specifically cromolyn-sensitive mast cells. Neither UVB-irradiated HUVE nor irradiated epidermal sheets released significant quantities of TNF, thereby excluding these cell types as the primary source of TNF in the explants. From these data, we conclude that mast cells, the only dermal cell type which contains preformed TNF,[25] are the principal, if not the sole, source of TNF in these cultures. While it is likely that epidermal cells and other cell types contribute to inflammation following chronic exposure to UVB,[33–35] degranulating mast cells, via liberation of TNF, appear to mediate ELAM-1 induction following acute UVB exposure. This is consistent with previous studies which have suggested that mast cells play an important role in UVB-induced inflammation.[36,37]

How the UVB region of the electromagnetic spectrum elicits the human sunburn reaction and initiates certain light-exacerbated dermatoses has until now been unclear. Our results suggest that UVB-induced mast cell degranulation and resultant release of TNF and expression of ELAM-1 by PCV endothelial cells may be critical early events in the genesis of these seemingly diverse conditions. Moreover, these findings add to a growing body of data suggesting that even subclinical exposure to UVB results in both cellular and molecular perturbations in skin that, with chronicity, may be harbingers of premature aging or neoplastic transformation. Therapeutic blockade of mast cells, cytokines, or adhesion molecules may therefore have a role as potential adjuncts in prevention of sunburn reactions, photo-induced dermatoses, and sequelae of persistent UVB exposure.

Conclusions

TNF-α release consequent to mast-cell degranulation represents an endogenous mechanism for the induction of endothelial cell–leukocyte adhesive interactions. This event may represent a critical first step in the migration of leukocytes from peripheral blood to the tissues. However, it is unlikely that the cascade of proinflammatory events is this simple, Evolving data indicate that mast cells are likely to contain a variety of proinflammatory cytokines, and that collaborative interaction of multiple adhesion molecules is responsible for endothelial–leukocyte interactions in vivo. Because mast cells are located in close proximity to vessels and are capable of releasing proinflammatory mediators in the immediate vicinity of post-capillary venular endothelium, they are ideally situated to serve as 'gatekeepers' of the dermal microvasculature. There is evidence for adhesive interactions between laminin receptors of the mast-cell membrane and the laminin component of vascular basement membrane,[38] which correlates with the preferential localization of mast cells about the dermal microvasculature. Furthermore, mast-cell degranulation may induce mast cells to 'release' from the vascular basement membrane and migrate freely into the dermis. Perhaps this represents an autoregulatory mechanism by which mast cells control the extent of their influence on vascular events.

Mast cells are a central participant in a wide array of physiological and pathological interactions, predominantly at the level of the post-capillary venule endothelial cell. Along with induction of endothelial–leukocyte adhesive glycoproteins by mast cell cytokines, mast cells may further influence leukocyte diapedesis through release of other granule contents. Histamine, serine proteases, and heparin within mast-cell granules may facilitate cell migration by forming inter-endothelial cell gaps, degrading basement membrane, and preventing microthrombi, respectively. As our understanding of the mechanisms involved in mast-cell induction and leukocyte migration expand, so will our ability to pursue the early events that lead to the visible lesions characteristic of these processes.

References

1 Parrish JA, Responses of skin to visible and ultraviolet radiation. In: Goldsmith LA, (ed.). *Biochemistry and physiology of the skin*, Oxford University Press: New York, 1983, pp713–33.

2 Gilchrest BA, Soter NA, Stoff J et al, The human sunburn reaction: histologic and biochemical studies, *J Am Acad Dermatol* (1981) **5**: 411–22.

3 Valtonen EJ, Janne J, Siimes M, The effect of the eyrthemal reaction caused by ultraviolet radiation on mast cell degranulation in the skin, *Acta Dermatol Venereol (Stockh)* (1964) **44**: 269–72.

4 Walsh LJ, Lavker RM, Murphy GF, Determinants of leukocyte trafficking in the skin, *Lab Invest* (1990) **63**: 592–600.

5 Cavender DE, Lymphocyte adhesion to endothelial cells in vitro: models for the study of normal lymphocyte recirculation and lymphocyte emigration into chronic inflammatory lesions, *J Invest Dermatol* (1989) **93s**: 88s–95s.

6 Gimbrone MA, Buchanan MR, Interactions of platelets and leukocytes with vascular endothelium: in vitro studies, *Ann NY Acad Sci* (1982) **401**: 171–83.

7 Harlan JM, Leukocyte–endothelial cell interactions, *Blood* (1985) **65**: 513–25.

8 Majno G, Palade G, Studies on inflammation II. The site of action of histamine and serotonin on vascular permeability: an electron microscopic study, *J Biophys Biochem Cytol* (1961) **11**: 571–605.

9 Willms-Kretschmer K, Flax MH, Cotran RS, The fine structure of the vascular response in hapten-specific delayed hypersensitivity and contact dermatitis, *Lab Invest* (1967) **17**: 334–49.

10 Cotran R, Gimbrone MA, Bevilacqua MP et al, Induction and detection of a human endothelial activation antigen in vivo, *J Exp Med* (1986) **164**: 661–6.

11 Bevilacqua MP, Pober JS, Mendrick DL et al, Identification of an inducible endothelial–leukocyte adhesion molecule, *Proc Natl Acad Sci USA* (1987) **84**: 9238–42.

12 Bevilacqua MP, Stengelin S, Gimbrone MA et al, Endothelial leukocyte adhesion molecule 1: an inducible receptor for neutrophils related to complement regulatory proteins and lectins, *Science* (1989) **243**: 1160–5.

13 Pober JS, Bevilacqua MP, Mendrick DL et al, Two distinct monokines, interleukin-1 and tumor necrosis factor, each independently induce biosynthesis and transient expression of the same antigen on the surface of cultured human vascular endothelial cells, *J Immunol* (1985) **136**: 1680–7.

14 Pober JS, Gimbrone MA, Lapierre LA et al, Overlapping patterns of activation of human endothelial cells by interleukin-1, tumour necrosis factor, and immune interferon, *J Immunol* (1986) **137**: 1893–6.

15 Waldorf HA, Walsh LJ, Schechter NM et al, Early cellular events in evolving cutaneous delayed hypersensitivity in humans, *Am J Pathol* (1991) **138**: 477–86.

16 Messadi DV, Pober JS, Fiers W et al, Induction of an activation antigen on postcapillary venular endothelium in human skin organ culture, *J Immunol* (1987) **139**: 1557–62.

17 Klein LM, Lavker RM, Matis WL et al, Degranulation of human mast cells induces an endothelial antigen central to leukocyte adhesion, *Proc Natl Acad Sci USA* (1989) **86**: 8972–6.

18 Matis WL, Lavker RM, Murphy GF, Substance P induces the expression of an endothelial leukocyte adhesion molecule by microvascular endothelium, *J Invest Dermatol* (1990) **94**: 492–5.

19 Lewis RE, Buchsbaum M, Whitaker D et al, Intercellular adhesion molecule expression in the evolving human cutaneous delayed hypersensitivity reaction, *J Invest Dermatol* (1989) **93**: 672–7.

20 Nickoloff BJ, Role of interferon-gamma in cutaneous trafficking of lymphocytes with emphasis on molecular and cellular adhesion events, *Arch Dermatol* (1989) **124**: 1835–43.

21 Osborn L, Hessian C, Tizard R et al, Direct expression cloning of vascular cell adhesion molecule-1, a cytokine-induced endothelial protein that binds to lymphocytes, *Cell* (1989) **59**: 1203–11.

22 Graber N, Gopal TV, Wilson D et al, T-cells bind to

cytokine-activated endothelial cells via a novel, inducible sialoglyocprotein and endothelial-leukocyte adhesion molecule, *J Immunol* (1990) **145**: 819–30.
23 Gordon JR, Galli SJ, Mast cells as source of both preformed and immunogically inducible TNF/cachectin, *Nature* (1990) **346**: 274–6.
24 Walsh LJ, Savage NW, Ishii I, The immunopathogenesis of oral lichen planus, *J Oral Pathol Med* (1990) **19**: 389–96.
25 Walsh LJ, Trinchieri G, Waldorf HA et al, Human dermal mast cells contain and release tumour necrosis factor alpha which induces endothelial leukocyte adhesion molecule-1, *Proc Natl Acad Sci USA* (1991) **88**: 4220–40.
26 Lavker RM, Kligman AM, Chronic heliodermatitis: a morphologic evaluation of chronic actinic dermal damage with emphasis on the role of mast cells, *J Invest Dermatol* (1988) **90**: 325–30.
27 Kaminer MS, Lavker RM, Walsh LJ et al, Extracellular localization of human connective tissue mast cell granule contents, *J Invest Dermatol* (1991) **96**: 1–8.
28 Larrick JW, Morhenn V, Chiang YL et al, Activated Langerhans cells release tumour necrosis factor, *J Leukocyte Biol* (1989) **45**: 429–33.
29 Oxholm A, Oxholm P, Staberg B et al, Immunohistochemical detection of interleukin-1 like molecules and tumour necrosis factor before and after UVB-irradiation in vivo, *Br J Dermatol* (1988) **118**: 369–76.
30 Theoharides TC, Sieghart W, Greengard P et al, Anti-allergic drug cromolyn may inhibit histamine secretion by regulating phosphorylation of a mast cell protein, *Science* (1980) **207**: 80–2.
31 Scaletta LJ, MacCallum DK, A fine structural study of divalent cation-mediated epithelial union with connective tissue in human oral mucosa, *Am J Anat* (1972) **133**: 431–53.
32 Gendimenico GJ, Kochevar IE, Degranulation of mast cells and inhibition of the response to secretory agents by phototoxic compounds and ultraviolet radiation, *Toxicol Appl Pharmcol* (1984) **76**: 374–82.
33 Barker JN, Mitra RS, Griffiths CE et al, Keratinocytes as initiators of inflammation, *Lancet* (1991) **337**: 211–4.
34 Granstein RD, Sander DN, Whole body exposure to ultraviolet radiation results in increased serum interleukin-1 activity in humans, *Lymphokine Res* (1987) **6**: 187–93.
35 Kupper TS, Chua AO, Flood P, Interleukin 1 gene expression in cultured human keratinocytes is augmented by ultraviolet radiation, *J Clin Invest* (1987) **80**: 430–6.
36 Fjellner B, Hagermark O, Histamine release from rat peritoneal mast cells exposed to ultraviolet light, *Acta Dermatol Venerol (Stockh)* (1982) **62**: 215–20.
37 Ikai K, Danno K, Horio T et al, Effect of ultraviolet radiation on mast cell deficient W/Wv mice, *J Invest Dermatol* (1985) **85**: 82–4.
38 Walsh LJ, Kaminer MS, Lazarus GS et al, Role of laminin in localization of human dermal mast cells, *Lab Invest* (in press).

23
Advances in sunscreen protection and evaluation

Nicholas J. Lowe
Skin Research Foundation of California, Santa Monica, CA 90404-2115, USA

Sunlight exposure to the skin may result in increased incidence of skin carcinogenesis, acceleration of skin aging, pigmentary changes and photosensitivity reactions.[1] There is therefore a need for sunscreen protection to reduce the damaging effects of ultraviolet (UV) radiation of the skin.

The most photoactive and photodamaging wavelengths for most skin reactions lie within the UVB range of 290–320 nm. However, more recently it has been shown that UVA wavelengths (320–400 nm) produce significant photodamage. This photodamage includes augmentation of the harmful effects of the UVB including sunburn erythema, and photocarcinogenesis in animals.[2-4] In addition, UVA produces significant photosensitivity reactions in susceptible individuals with different skin diseases[5,6] (see Table 1) as well as photosensitivity reactions in patients taking photosensitizing medication (see Table 2).[7]

A variety of sun-protection measures have been introduced and encouraged in recent years. The wearing of sun-protective clothing and hats, particularly between the most harmful hours of sunlight exposure, usually between 10 am and 2 pm, is now recommended.

Topical sunscreens were first developed as long ago as 1928. The early sunscreens were a combination of salicylate and cinnamate. More recent developments have produced p-aminobenzoic acid (PABA) and, subsequently, a number of PABA derivatives of which the most commonly used is octyldimethyl-PABA. These initial sunscreens were most effective at filtering UVB wavelengths.

Table 1 Some photosensitivity diseases, i.e. diseases that are either initiated or exacerbated by exposure to UV wavelengths.*

Polymorphous light eruption (PMLE) (290–365 nm)
Chronic actinic dermatitis (290–360 nm)
Actinic reticuloid (290–360 nm)
Lupus erythematosus (290–330 nm)
Solar urticaria (290–515 nm)
Persistent light reaction (290–400 nm)
Xeroderma pigmentosum (290–340 nm)

* From Lowe,[1] with permission of the publisher.

Table 2 Some photosensitizing medications.*

Drug	Wavelength range (nm)
8-Methoxypsoralen	320–400
Coal tar	340–430
Tetracycline	320–400
Piroxicam	320–400
Hydrochlorothiazide	320–400
Chlorpromazine	320–400
Griseofulvin	320–400
Amiodarone	290–400

* From Lowe,[1] with permission of the publisher.

Tables 1–4 are listed courtesy of Sun-screens —Development, Evaluation and Regulatory Aspects: Lowe, N.J. and Shaath, N.A. (Publisher: Marcel Dekker, New York, New York, 1990)

Because of the increasing awareness of the need for UVA protection, different, recent sunscreens have included benzophenones, anthranilates and more recently dibenzoylmethanes which protect more in UVA than UVB or, in the case of anthranilates, in both UVB and UVA. In this chapter the methods utilized for the evaluation of sunscreening chemicals are reviewed.

Ultraviolet B protection — sun protection factor determination

The sun protection factor may be defined as the ratio of the minimal erythema dose in sunscreen protected skin divided by the minimal erythema dose in non-sunscreen protected skin.[8] There are at present several differences in the methodology for sun-protection-factor (SPF) determinations between different countries. Some of these differences are as follows. In the USA the Federal Register[8] recommends application sunscreen quantity of 2 μl/cm². The German DIN standards currently recommend 1.5 ul/cm². In addition, differences exist between the amounts of incremental UV irradiance. In the USA, irradiances are increased by 25% over each previous irradiance, whereas in Germany there is a logarithmic increase in the amount of irradiance.[7]

A longer application time is allowed in Germany of 20 min sunscreen application prior to irradiance compared to the 15 min as recommended in the USA.

It is important to define the types of UV apparatus available for SPF evaluation. Probably an ideal UV source is an appropriately filtered xenon arc solar simulator. The xenon arc sources generally range between 150 and 5000 W of output. Appropriate filters are used to exclude undesirable UV wavelengths below 290 nm and above 400 nm. Many of the current machines use WG 320 3 mm thick filters to exclude wavelengths below 295 nm. Dichroic mirrors and UG11 filters to exclude the visible and infra-red wavelengths. Other sources used for SPF testing that are less satisfactory because of poor solar simulating spectrum include intermediate pressure mercury vapor sources, fluorescence sun lamp tubes and high pressure metal halide sources. It is to be noted, however, that the comparison of SPFs using two different light sources (filtered xenon arc and high pressure metal halide) have shown comparative SPF numbers and the Federal Register does allow at present for other sources to be used providing such correlation can be shown with xenon arc solar simulators.[7]

Outdoor testing — evaluation of sunscreen SPF

With most sunscreens outdoor SPF testing will lead to significantly lower SPF values than those achieved in an indoor laboratory setting. This relative over-prediction of SPF by indoor static laboratory solar simulators is probably the result of relatively short irradiance times in the indoor setting with an absence of infra-red irradiance with most sources. In the outdoor situation prolonged irradiance times in natural sunlight may lead to photodegradation of the sunscreen, sweat removal of the sunscreen, and percutaneous absorption of the sunscreen, and thus result in a relatively lower SPF than the indoor setting. A practical solution to indoor laboratory testing may be to add factors such as infra-red irradiance and change of humidity in an attempt to more accurately reproduce the natural outdoor environment.

In addition, water-resistant and waterproof claims of sunscreen SPF[8] are important to simulate more closely a situation of sunscreen use by individuals exercising, perspiring and swimming.

A revision of the USA Federal Register monograph on sunscreens[8] is currently expected to be published at some stage during 1991.

Evaluation of UVA protection

Because of the awareness of the potential hazards of UVA to the skin (see above) the development and testing of UVA protecting sunscreens has been recently pursued.[9-13] There are however, several unresolved questions about the optimum ways of evaluating UVA absorbing sunscreens.

It has now been suggested that the UVA region (320–400 nm) be separated into two different segments: UVA II (320–340 nm) and UVA I (340–400 nm). UVA II contains the most erythemogenic of the UVA wavelengths and may contribute significantly to sunburn erythema. UVA I is much less photoactive as regards sunburn erythema, but contains wavelengths that are clearly important in photosensitivity diseases and photosensitivity reactions to medications. In addition, because of the greater penetrance of UVA there are theoretical concerns that UVA I may enhance photoaging changes in the skin.

UVA protection factor

Present assays that have been used for UVA protectiveness include UVA induced erythema. Stanfield et al[10] have described a method using xenon arc solar simulators filtered with a 2 mm Schott WG 345 filter. The solar simulator beam was focused with a quartz lens to emit localized high intensity irradiance up to 250 mW/cm^2. Unwanted visible and infra-red energy were removed using a black glass (Schott UG II) filter, plus a circulating water filter. The studies showed that spectral irradiance of this system contained no clinically significant wavelengths from UVB. Prolonged irradiance times are needed with UVA protection factors using this system, particularly when evaluating sunscreens with UVA protection factors of 4 or greater.

Phototoxic protection factor

Phototoxic protection factors for evaluating UVA photoprotection have been in use recently. We have used topical methoxsalen photosensitization in healthy volunteers to determine UVA photoprotection factors.[9,11] These investigations utilized appropriately filtered xenon arc solar simulators, utilizing filters to remove wavelengths below 320 nm. The phototoxic protection factor was defined as the minimal phototoxic dose in protected skin divided by the minimal phototoxic dose in unprotected skin. Gange et al[12] using an oral methoxypsoralen photosensitization technique have shown that for similar sunscreens there is a good correlation with our topical methoxsalen method.[12]

Phototoxic protection factor assay utilizing topical methoxypsoralen as photosensitizer and an appropriately emitting broad UVA source appears to be a good means of evaluating UVA sunscreens in view of the short irradiation times that are required, localized skin photosensitization and no risk of systemic toxicity compared to the oral psoralen derivative. It can also be argued that there is clinical relevance for photoprotection in photosensitized individuals and in subjects taking photosensitizing medications.

UVA induced immediate pigment darkening for evaluating UVA sunscreens

There have been reports of the utilization of immediate pigment darkening (IPD) as a means of evaluating UVA sunscreens.[13] This may be a useful method if appropriate filtration of the UV sources are carefully performed to exclude visible and UVB wavelengths. Advantages of immediate pigment darkening are the short irradiance times and relatively small amounts of UVA energy required to produce the IPD. In addition, there is very little persistent tanning in volunteers compared to utilization of topical 8-methoxypsoralen. The clinical relevance, however, of immediate pigment darkening still remains to be determined.

Transmission protection factors

Other studies have utilized the ability of sunscreens to reduce the transmission of UV irradiance through both animal as well as human skin. In recent investigations on normal human volunteers, our laboratory utilized suction blisters to induce an epidermal substrate that then was subsequently used to evaluate the sunscreen's ability to reduce the transmission of UVA (N. J. Lowe et al, unpublished). We termed the assay the 'transmission protection factor'. This method in human skin should be able to be modified using different UV absorbing radiometers to selectively study absorption by sunscreens at different UV wavelengths. It has the advantage that it avoids direct irradiance of the skin as the irradiance occurs after the epidermal blister roofs are excised. Further studies are required to evaluate this method further and to determine the correlation of this method with other assays.

Conclusion

The currently approved sunscreens allowed in the USA are listed in Table 3. The only additional sunscreen allowed since the 1978 Federal Register monograph is that of Avobenzone, which is still the subject of new drug applications. It absorbs light of wavelengths between approximately 315 and 391 nm. In Europe, a greater number of sunscreens are currently approved, these are summarized in Table 4.

Table 3 Sunscreens allowed in the USA under FDA-OTC panel and their concentration range.*

Chemical	Approved (%)
UVA absorbers	
Oxybenzone	2–6
Sulisobenzone	5–10
Dioxybenzone	3
Menthylantranilate	3.5–5
Avobenzone†	
UVB absorbers	
Aminobenzoic acid	5–15
Amyldimethyl-PABA	1–5
2-Ethoxyethyl-*p*-methoxycinnamate	1–3
Diethanolamine-*p*-methoxycinnamate	8–10
Digalloyltrioleate	2–5
Ethyl-4-bis(hydroxypropyl)aminobenzoate	1–5
2-Ethylhexyl-2-cyano-3,3-diphenylacrylate	7–10
Ethylhexyl-*p*-methoxycinnamate	2–7.5
2-Ethylhexyl salicylate	3–5
Glyceryl aminobenzoate	2–3
Homomenthyl salicyate	4–25
Lawsone with dihydroxyacetone	0.25 with 3
Octyldimethyl-PABA	1.4–8
2-Penylbenzimidazole-5-sulfonic acid	1.4
Triethanolamine salicylate	5–12
Physical	
Red petrolatum	30–100
Titanium dioxide	2–25

* From Lowe,[1] with permission of the publisher.
† Subject of NDA submissions.

Table 4 Sunscreen chemicals used in Europe.

EEC Chemical Name	Maximum concentration (%)	EEC Chemical Name	Maximum concentration (%)
4-Aminobenzoic acid	5	Cinoxate	5
N,N,N-Trimethyl-4-(2-oxoborn-3-ylidene) methyl anilinium methyl sulphate	6	Digalloyl trioleate	4
		Mexenone	4
Homosalate	10	Sulisobenzone	5
Oxybenzone	10	2-Ethylhexyl-2-(4-phenylbenzoyl)benzoate	10
3-Imidazol-4-ylacrylic acid and ethyl ester	2	5-Methyl-2-phenylbenzoxazone	4
2-Phenylbenzimidazole-5-sulfonic acid and salts	8	Sodium 3,4-dimethoxphenylglyoxylate	5
Ethyl-4-bis(hydroxypropyl)aminobenzoate	5	1,3-bis(4-Methoxyphenyl)propane-1,3-dione	6
Ethoxylated 4-aminobenzoic acid	10	5-(3,3-Dimethyl-2-norbonylidene)-3-penten-2-one	3
Amyl-4-dimethylaminobenzoate	5	a'-(Oxoborn-3-ylidene)-*p*-xylene-2 sulfonic acid	6
Glyceryl-1-(4-aminobenzoate)	5	a'-(2-Oxoborn-3-ylidene)toluene-4 sulfonic acid and its salts	6
2-Ethylhexyl-4-dimethylaminobenzoate	8		
2-Ethylhexyl salicylate	5	3-(Methylbenzylidene)bornan-2-one	6
3,3,5-Trimethylcyclohexyl-2-acetamido benzoate	2	3-Benzylidenebornana-2-one	6
Potassium cinnamate	2	a-Cyano-4-methoxyclinnamic acid and its hexyl ester	5
4-Methoxycinnamic acid salts	8	1-*p*-Cumenyl-3-phenylpropane-1,3-dione	5
Propyl-4-methoxycinnamate	3	4-Isopropylbenzyl salicylate	4
Salicylic acid salts	2	Cyclohexyl-4-methoxycinnamate	1
Amyl-4-methoxycinnamate	10	1-(40-tert-Butylphenyl-3-(4-methoxyphenyl) propane-1,3-dione	5
2-Ethylhexyl-4-methoxycinnamate	10		

* From Lowe,[1] with permission of the publisher.

In view of the potential problems of irritancy, face stinging, eye stinging, allergy and photoallergy in different individuals it is desirable for the development of new sunscreens to continue. An ideal sunscreen would be one that binds well to the stratum corneum, resists rub-off, resists wash-off, is non-toxic, is non-staining, has low allergy, irritancy and photoallergic risks. In addition, the ideal sunscreen would absorb as far as possible throughout the UVB and UVA wavelength ranges. The quest for such an ideal sunscreen will hopefully continue and, when available, it will enable the public to protect themselves more rigorously from UV induced skin photodamage.

References

1. Lowe NJ, The need for photoprotection. In: Lowe NJ, et al, (eds). *Sunscreens — development, evaluation and regulatory aspects*, Marcel Dekker: New York, 1990, pp. 37–42.
2. Staberg B, Wulf HC, Poulsen T et al, The carcinogenic effect of sequential artificial sunlight + UVA irradiation in hairless mice. Consequences for solarium 'therapy', *Arch Dermatol* (1983) **119**: 641–2.
3. Paul BS, Parrish JA, The interaction of UVA and UVB in the production of threshold erythema, *J Invest Dermatol* (1982) **78**: 371–4.
4. Gilchrest BA, Soter NA, Hawk JLM et al, Histologic changes associated with ultraviolet A induced erythema in normal skin, *J Am Acad Dermatol* (1983) **9**: 213–9.
5. Gschnait F, Schwarz T, Ladich I, Treatment of polymorphous light eruption, *Arch Dermatol Res* (1983) **275**: 379–82.
6. McFadden N, UVA sensitivity and topical photoprotection in polymorphous light eruption, *Photodermatology* (1984) **1**: 76–8.
7. Lowe NJ, Sun protection factors. In: Lowe NJ, Shaath NA, (eds). *Sunscreens — development, evaluation and regulatory aspects*, Marcel Dekker: New York, 1990, pp. 379–94.
8. Sunscreen products for over-the-counter use, *Fed. Reg.* 43:28269 (1978).
9. Lowe NJ, UVA photoprotection. In: Lowe NJ, Shaath NA, (eds). *Sunscreens — development, evaluation and regulatory aspects*, Marcel Dekker: New York, 1990, pp. 459–68.
10. Stanfield JW, Feldt PA, Csortan ES et al, UVA sunscreen evaluations in normal subjects, *J Am Acad Dermatol* (1989) **20**: 744–8.
11. Lowe NJ, Dromgoole SH, Sefton J et al, Indoor and outdoor efficacy testing of a broad-spectrum sunscreen against ultraviolet A radiation in psoralen-sensitized subjects, *J Am Acad Dermatol* (1987) **17**: 224–30.
12. Gange RW, Soparkar A, Matzinger E et al, Efficacy of a sunscreen containing butylmethoxydibenzoylmethane against ultraviolet A radiation in photosensitized subjects, *J Am Acad Dermatol* (1986) **15**: 494–9.
13. Kaidbey K, Gange RW, Comparison of methods for assessing photoprotection against ultraviolet A in vivo, *J Am Acad Dermatol* (1987) **16**: 346–53.

24
Microfine titanium dioxide: a new route to dermatological sun protection

E. Galley, D. Roberts and J. Ferguson
Boots Pharmaceuticals, Consumer Products Development, D98, 1 Thane Road, Nottingham NG2 3AA, UK

The solar ultraviolet (UV) electromagnetic spectrum covers wavelengths from 100 to 400 nm, and is conventionally subdivided into three energy bands: UVA, UVB and UVC. The UVA band covers wavelengths between 320 and 400 nm and is the lowest-energy band. UVB wavelengths are between 290 and 320 nm and are of higher energy than the UVA band. UVC wavelengths range from 100 to 290 nm and are the highest in energy. Terrestrial UV radiation comprises UVA and UVB only as UVC is absorbed by atmospheric ozone.

Excessive exposure to terrestrial UV radiation can cause skin damage. The conditions associated with the skin's exposure to UVB radiation are well documented.[1] These range from sunburn to actinic keratoses, elastosis and skin cancer. It is also documented that UVA can invoke cellular and connective tissue damage including photosensitization, photodermatoses and actinic skin aging.[2,3] Therefore, it is sensible to protect the skin from actinic damage by reducing its exposure to both UVB and UVA radiation. One way of achieving protection is to apply a sun cream.

Conventional sunscreen agents

A product developed to prevent actinic damage should fulfil three requirements: it should be safe, protect against UVA and UVB radiation and have good cosmetic acceptability. Cosmetic acceptability is dependent on good spreading properties, good skin feel, and the resultant product film being invisible on the skin. Failure to achieve this acceptability will result in poor patient compliance.

Most products currently used to protect the skin from UV radiation (UVR) are principally designed to prevent sunburning. They use organic sunfilters to absorb the UVR. These organic molecules have a number of limitations and can fail to meet the previously defined requirements of an actinic skin damage protective product in two ways. Firstly, organic sunfilters absorb light over relatively narrow wavebands. Figure 1 shows the opacity of a widely used sunfilter, 2-ethyl-hexyl-*p*-dimethylaminobenzoate, measured using a Phillips PU 8730 UV/VIS spectrophotometer. Efficient protection is afforded against the principal erythematous wavelengths; however, no protection is afforded above 340 nm. Consequently, subjects with long-wavelength UVA photosensitivity would receive no benefit from using products employing this molecule alone as the active sunfilter. The second limitation stems from the ability of these organic molecules to penetrate the skin. This has been shown to cause irritation, sensitization, and even photosensitization reactions in some individuals.[4]

Many dermatologists prefer products which rely on the pigment titanium dioxide to provide protection from actinic skin damage. Figure 2 shows the broad-spectrum protection offered by titanium dioxide. The efficiency is not as high as that of the organic sunfilters, but a degree of protection can be achieved when high concentrations of the pigment are included in formulations.

The safety profile of titanium dioxide is excellent. It has been used for 50 years in cosmetics, pharmaceuticals, paint, paper and food (food colour E171). It is an insoluble powder with little tendency to penetrate the skin. It is chemically and bio-

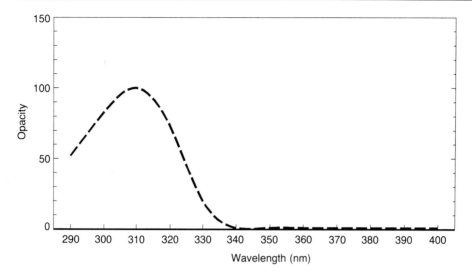

Figure 1

Opacity of 2-ethylhexyl-*p*-dimethylaminobenzoate.

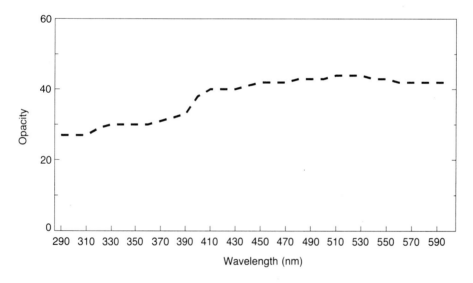

Figure 2

Opacity of pigmentary titanium dioxide.

logically inert and hence does not cause irritation or sensitization reactions. However, being a pigment, titanium dioxide has one serious limitation. Figure 2 shows that the compound has a fair opacity to UVR, but it has an even greater opacity to visible light (400–700 nm).

This results in products based on pigmentary titanium dioxide appearing very white when applied to the skin. The product is not cosmetically acceptable. The user looks like a white-faced clown and, consequently, patient compliance becomes a serious problem. If titanium dioxide is to be used to protect the skin from actinic damage, then ideally the opacity to UVR should be increased and, equally importantly, the skin whitening effect must be reduced.

Properties of microfine titanium dioxide

Since the time of Fresnel, almost 200 years ago, physicists have been proposing theories that define the relationship between opacity to electromagnetic radiation and pigment particle size and particle shape. These theories have been used to optimize the particle size and shape of pigmentary titanium dioxide in order to achieve maximum opacity to visible light (180–250 nm). It is also possible to apply the same theoretical considerations to select particles with reduced opacity to visible light and increased opacity to UVR.

The particle sizes with improved properties were found to be significantly smaller (10–100 nm) and more acicular than pigmentary titanium dioxide particles. They have become known as ultrafine or microfine titanium dioxide. Selecting these smaller particle sizes significantly alters the optical properties of titanium dioxide. Figure 3 shows a comparison between pigmentary titanium dioxide and microfine titanium dioxide. The microfine titanium dioxide has a higher opacity to UVR and a lower opacity to visible radiation than pigmentary titanium dioxide. When compared to the organic sunfilter 2-ethylhexyl-p-dimethylaminobenzoate (Figure 4), microfine titanium dioxide is found to have comparable UVB opacity but significantly higher UVA opacity. This suggests that products based on microfine titanium dioxide will have high efficiency and be cosmetically acceptable.

Chemical and physical analysis has been carried out on the microfine titanium dioxide. Chemical analysis shows that the changes in the optical properties do not result from changes in the 2:1 ratio of oxygen and titanium or from contamination by other elements. X-Ray crystallographic analysis shows that the fundamental crystal structure remains the same. Microfine titanium dioxide is identical, both chemically and physically, to pigmentary titanium dioxide.

Optimization of a product using microfine titanium dioxide

Studies were carried out to assess the effect of particle size variation on UVB, UVA and visible opacity. A series of particle sizes were selected with similar aspect ratios. Dispersions of the samples were prepared and opacity measurements determined using a Phillips spectrophotometer. Total UVB, UVA and visible light opacity was calculated by measuring the area under the opacity curve from 290 to 320 nm for UVB, 320 to 400 nm for UVA, and 400 to 700 nm for visible light. The

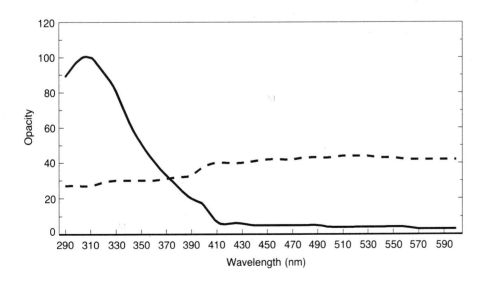

Figure 3

Comparison of the opacity of pigmentary (----------) and microfine (————) titanium dioxide.

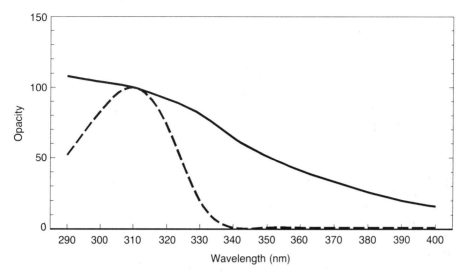

Figure 4

Comparison of the opacity of microfine titanium dioxide (────) and 2-ethylhexyl-*p*-dimethylaminobenzoate (--------).

relative opacity was then calculated by dividing the total opacity by the band width, i.e. for UVB

$$\text{Relative opacity} = \frac{\text{Total opacity}}{320 - 290} = \frac{\text{Total opacity}}{30}$$

Figure 5 shows a plot of one such evaluation. The particle size offering maximum relative UVB opacity is smaller than that offering maximum UVA opacity. This optimum particle size for UVA opacity also has significant visible light opacity and, consequently, may not be cosmetically acceptable. Therefore any particle size chosen must be a compromise between good UVA and UVB opacity and acceptable skin whitening due to visible light opacity.

We have found that such a compromise can be achieved by selecting a number of particle sizes and blending them. Such a blend has been formulated into a number of products which have been evalu-

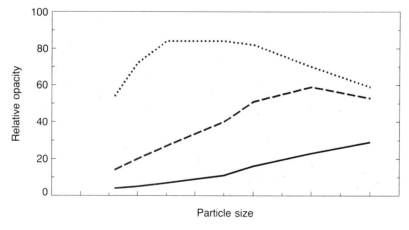

Figure 5

Comparison of relative opacity to visible (────), UVA (--------) and UVB (.......) radiation with changing particle size.

ated both in vitro and in vivo. The in vitro studies were carried out using a protocol derived from a method first described by Diffey and Robson.[5] This study was designed to assess the balance of UVB and UVA protection of the blended titanium dioxide based products and to compare these with other ethical sun protection products. Figure 6 shows the relative protection offered by a blended titanium dioxide based product with an in vivo sun protection factor (SPF) of 15 compared to two commonly prescribed SPF15 products (UK). The superior UVA protection of the blended titanium dioxide based product is readily apparent.

The in vivo clinical study was a comparative study on 11 patients with chronic actinic dermatitis. This study was designed to assess the level of UVA protection provided by the blended titanium dioxide based product with an SPF of 15 and to compare it with a leading UK prescribed SPF15 ethical sun protection product. Protection factors were estimated by inducing erythema with monochromatic light of 350 and 400 nm before and after product application. A summary of the results is depicted in Figure 7.[6]

The blended titanium dioxide product provided significantly higher protection at 350 nm ($p < 0.001$) and 400 nm ($p = 0.004$) than the most commonly prescribed sunscreen in the UK.

Cosmetic acceptability has been assessed subjectively and objectively. Spreading, rheology and skin feel have been assessed subjectively by a user panel. The skin colouring properties have been assessed both subjectively by user studies, and objectively using a Minolta chromameter to assess the whiteness of standard quantity applications (1 mg/cm) to skin, and to standard black Morest opacity cards. These assessments have shown blended particle size microfine titanium dioxide products do not significantly whiten the skin and that they are cosmetically acceptable for a wide range of skin types.

Conclusion

Products based on blended particle sizes of microfine titanium dioxide fulfil the requirements of a good sunscreen. Being based on titanium dioxide they have a good safety profile. They provide broad spectrum UVA and UVB protection and they are cosmetically acceptable. We can conclude that

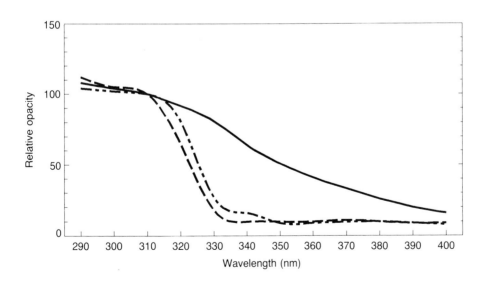

Figure 6

Comparison of the relative opacity of a product based on blended microfine titanium dioxide (———) and two prescribed ethical sun protection products (------- and – – – –) with the same declared SPF.

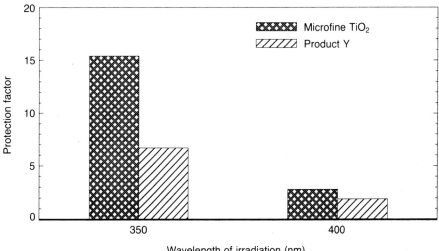

Figure 7

In vivo comparison of UVA protection of a blended titanium dioxide based product and a prescribed ethical sun protection product with the same declared SPF.

carefully selected particle size blends of microfine titanium dioxide are suitable for protecting normal and photosensitive skin from the adverse effects of the sun.

References

1. Hawke JLM, Parrish JA, Responses of normal skin to UV radiation. In: Regan JD, Parrish JA, (eds). *The science of photomedicine*, Plenum Press: New York, 1982, pp. 219–60.
2. Ferguson J, UVA: the neglected wavelengths? The importance of broad spectrum sun protection, *Soap Perf Cosmet* (1990) **63**: 47–52.
3. Sams WR, Sun induced aging. Clinical and laboratory observations in man, *Dermatol Clin* (1986) **4**: 509–16.
4. White IR, Photoallergens and photosensitivity: current problems. Presentation: The environmental threat to the skin, Cardiff, 14–17 April 1991.
5. Diffey BL, Robson J, A new substrate to measure sunscreen protection factors throughout the ultraviolet spectrum, *J Soc Cosmet Chem* (1989) **40**: 127–33.
6. Diffey BL, Farr PM, Sunscreen protection against UVB, UVA and blue light: an in vivo and in vitro comparison, *Br J Dermatol* (1991) **124**: 258–63.

25
Visual display units and facial rashes: fact or fiction?

Andrew J. Carmichael and Dafydd L. Roberts*

Department of Dermatology, University Hospital of Wales, Cardiff, UK, and *Department of Dermatology, Singleton Hospital, Swansea, UK

The explosion in information technology over the past decade has produced one very tangible change in the office environment — the visual display unit (VDU), sometimes also referred to as a visual display terminal. In the early 1980s a number of anecdotal reports appeared from Norway,[1,2] and the UK,[3] implicating VDUs in facial dermatoses. Subsequently, most of the literature on this putative association has emanated from Scandinavia. Whether this represents a genuine increased prevalence, or simply greater public awareness in Scandinavia, fuelled by one VDU case having been accepted by the Swedish National Insurance Board as an occupational disease,[4] is unresolved.[5]

With an ever-increasing proportion of office workers exposed to VDUs, we felt it important to establish whether there is evidence to support the suggestion that VDUs cause facial rashes, before 'magazine science' started to influence opinion in the offices of Britain. Our specific aim was to establish if VDU operators have an increased prevalence of facial complaints, within a population of office workers.

Method

Patients

The Driver Vehicle Licensing Agency (DVLA) for the UK is based in Swansea and has 3500 employees, the vast majority working in standard office conditions on one site. Preliminary enquiry suggested that approximately half the work-force spent a major part of their day (defined as an average of more than 2 h per day) working at VDUs and for the purpose of this survey these people were termed 'VDU operators'.

Questionnaire

In August 1990 a brief questionnaire entitled 'Skin problems in office workers' was distributed to all the employees at the DVLA. An introductory statement was deliberately vague, stating that 'The Dermatology Department in Singleton Hospital are carrying out a survey into skin problems and are inviting staff at the Agency to take part'. The confidential nature of the survey was emphasized and an outline of the results was promised, to be published in the house magazine 'Licence'. The questions fell under three headings: demographic details; occupational questions, focussing on the work environment; and skin complaints, with positive respondents asked to specify site, symptoms and appearance of affected skin. The questions were constructed to be answered with 'yes' or 'no' responses. Information on whether they were major VDU users was 'hidden' within the occupational questions, in an attempt to blind respondents to the principal aim of the study. Respondents were asked to complete the questionnaire within 1 month and return it to the on-site medical officer in an addressed envelope, which was provided.

Results

A total of 1102 questionnaires were completed, a response rate of approximately 40% of employees

Table 1 Profile of office workers in relation to VDU operator and facial skin complaint status.

	VDU operators (N = 655)		Non-VDU operators (N = 447)	
	Facial skin complaint	No facial complaint	Facial skin complaint	No facial complaint
Number	92 (14%)	563 (86%)	49 (11%)	398 (89%)
Mean age (years)	32.2	33.6	41.1	40.5
Mean period in post (years)	5.3	5.4	7.0	6.8
Female : male ratio	2.2 : 1	2.0 : 1	2.3 : 1	2.5 : 1

available to reply (allowing for sickness and annual leave). The respondents' mean age was 36.3 years, 759 (69%) were female, the mean period in their present post was 6 years, and 655 (59%) were VDU operators.

A total of 141 employees volunteered a facial complaint at the time of the survey, or within the previous 6 months, representing 12.8% of the respondents (Table 1). The 3.0% difference of skin complaints between VDU and non-VDU operators was not statistically significant ($\chi^2 = 2.27$, $P = 0.13$; 95% CI −0.8 to 7.0%).

The symptoms and appearance of those employees volunteering a facial skin complaint, classified according to VDU operator status, are summarized in Tables 2 and 3. No symptom or appearance was more frequently represented in the VDU operators in comparison with the control non-VDU operators.

Just 25 respondents admitted to using photocopying machines for more than 1 h per day, with three people (12%) volunteering a facial skin complaint, a similar proportion to the group as a whole.

Discussion

In a group of VDU operators we failed to demonstrate an association with facial skin complaints when compared with an on-site control population. No facial skin symptom or appearance discriminated VDU operators from non-VDU operators. There was no evidence for a specific 'VDU dermatosis'.

The low response rate is likely to have resulted in bias towards those with skin complaints, although we assume this would not have been selective with regard to VDU operator status, to alter interpretation of the data.

The nature of the facial dermatosis associated with VDUs has never been clearly defined. The original descriptions suggested a transient redness, sometimes with papules on the cheeks.[1-3] The facial rash in Rycroft and Calnan's four cases was only witnessed by the company's medical officer,

Table 2 Facial symptoms of office workers with a facial skin complaint

	Facial skin complaint	Itch	Burning	Pain
VDU operators (N = 655)	92	66	19	27
Non-VDU operators (N = 447)	49	32	12	12

Table 3 Facial appearance volunteered by office workers with a facial skin complaint.

	Facial skin complaint	Normal	Red	Dry	Greasy	Spots
VDU operators (N = 655)	92	37	45	52	31	46
Non-VDU operator (N = 447)	49	22	25	28	13	27

making the diagnosis uncertain.[3] Others have suggested that VDU exposure may provoke rosacea.[6,7] Whatever the facial dermatosis is, follow-up data indicate that the majority of cases improve within 8 months, without treatment and despite continued VDU exposure.[7]

The mechanism by which VDUs cause facial dermatoses has never been clearly elucidated. Both the X-ray emission and ultraviolet radiation of VDUs have been shown to be insignificant.[8] There have been suggestions that the electrostatic field associated with VDUs may result in deposition of irritants from the atmosphere, thereby predisposing to facial skin complaints.[9] Lower humidity would encourage this tendency and has been proposed as an explanation for the greater reporting of the problem in Scandinavia.[7] However, a provocation study found no relationship between the symptoms of patients and electrostatic or magnetic fields from VDUs.[10]

In addition to our survey, further evidence on the lack of a causal relationship between VDUs and facial rashes has recently been published. An epidemiological survey of 809 office employees from Sweden failed to demonstrate that objective facial skin signs were more common in workers exposed to VDUs.[11] Histopathological analysis of VDU exposed and non-exposed facial skin has shown no evidence of a difference.[12] It is interesting that the only parameter which Berg et al.[11] showed VDU exposure to influence, i.e. symptoms, is also the most subjective. It is certainly possible that the informed status of the Swedish VDU population led to bias on this count, explaining the disparity with our findings.

Conclusion

Facial dermatoses are a common problem[13] and exposure to VDUs has become well established as part of the office environment. It is not surprising that occasionally VDU exposure coincides with a facial dermatosis. We have failed to demonstrate an association between facial skin complaints and VDU usage. Equally, physical and histological examination of VDU exposed and non-exposed skin by others[11,12] has shown no evidence of an association.

Acknowledgements

We would like to thank the Personnel and Medical Departments at the Driver Vehicle Licensing Agency (DVLA) for their assistance. This study was supported by a grant from the West Unit, West Glamorgan Health Authority.

References

1 Nilsen A, Facial rash in visual display unit operators, *Contact Dermatitis* (1982) **8**: 25–8.
2 Tjonn HH, Report of facial rashes among VDU operators in Norway. In: Pearce BG, (ed.). *Health hazards of VDTs?* Wiley: Chichester, 1984, pp. 17–23.
3 Rycroft RJG, Calnan CD, Facial rashes among visual display unit operators. In: Pearce BG, (ed.). *Health hazards of VDTs?* Wiley: Chichester, 1984, pp. 13–15.
4 Lagerholm B, Bildskarmar och hudforandringar. Ingaende undersokningar motiverade. *Lakartidningen* (1986) **83**: 60–1.
5 Wahlberg JE, Liden C, Is the skin affected by work at visual display terminals? In: Taylor JS, (ed.). *Dermatologic clinics*, vol 6. *Occupational dermatoses*, W B Saunders Company: Philadelphia, 1988, pp. 81–5.
6 Liden C, Wahlberg JE, Does visual display terminal work provoke rosacea? *Contact Dermatitis* (1985) **13**: 235–41.
7 Berg M, Skin problems in workers using visual display terminals. A study of 201 patients, *Contact Dermatitis* (1988) **19**: 335–41.
8 Bergqvist UOV, Video display terminals and health. A technical and medical appraisal of the state of the art, *Scand J Work Environ Hlth* (1984) **10** (suppl 2): 1–87.
9 Cato Olsen W, Electric field enhanced aerosol exposure in visual display unit environments, Chr Michelsen Insititute, Department of Science and Technology, Bergen, April 1981: 1–40 (CMI 803604-1).
10 Swanbeck G, Bleeker T, Skin problems from visual display units: provocation of skin symptoms under experimental conditions, *Acta Dermatol Venereol (Stockh)* (1989) **69**: 46–51.
11 Berg M, Lidén S, Axelson O, Facial skin complaints and work at visual display units, An epidemiological study of office employees, *J Am Acad Dermatol* (1990) **22**, 621–5.
12 Berg M, Facial skin complaints and work at visual display units. Epidemiological, clinical and histopathological studies, *Acta Dermatol Venereol (Stockh)* (1989) (suppl 150): 1–40.
13 Berg M, Lidén S, An epidemiological study of rosacea, *Acta Dermatol Venereol (Stockh)* (1989) **69**: 419–23.

26
Skin complaints and visual display unit work: a psychophysiological approach

Mats Berg, Bengt B. Arnetz,* Sture Lidén, Peter Eneroth,† and Anders Kallner‡

Department of Dermatology, Karolinska Hospital, Stockholm, Sweden, *National Institute for Psychosocial Factors and Health, Stockholm, Sweden, †Research and Developmental Laboratory, Huddinge Hospital, and ‡Department of Clinical Chemistry, Karolinska Hospital, Stockholm, Sweden

Introduction

Since the autumn of 1985, many Swedish office employees have reported that skin problems are provoked by visual display unit (VDU) work. Most of the patients have had ordinary facial skin diseases[1,3] with pronounced subjective symptoms, but mild skin lesions. A large-scale epidemiological study[4] showed that subjective facial skin symptoms were more common among VDU-exposed workers, but objective skin signs and skin disease were as common in the non-exposed group. A study[5] using skin biopsies from the facial skin showed that there were no differences with regard to histopathological changes between VDU-exposed and non-VDU-exposed persons.[5] The only published provocation study found no relation between the symptoms of the patients and electrostatic or magnetic fields from the VDU.[6] The amount of ultraviolet or ionizing radiation emitted from the VDU screen is negligible.[7] There are on-going provocation studies not yet published, including other types of electrical field strengths, i.e. the electric AC fields, which are also emitted from VDUs. There is, however, no theoretical basis to support the hypothesis that these fields give rise to health hazards.[8]

A different school of thought has suggested that psychosocial stress may be an important factor in understanding VDU-associated skin problems. Despite the fact that information technology has radically changed the content of work as well as work organization, no controlled study has been carried out which has examined psychophysiological stress and skin complaints. The purpose of the present study was to evaluate the potential role of psychophysiological and organizational factors in the aetiology and clinical course of VDU-associated skin symptoms.

Materials and methods

In the present study, 50 persons exposed to VDUs were followed: half of them had subjective facial skin symptoms and the rest had no such skin complaints. The subjects were studied during a normal working day and during a day of leisure at their office. A comprehensive assessment of physiological, occupational and psychosocial factors was repeatedly performed throughout the 2 days of study. Blood and urine samples were collected four times a day during the two study days for the later determination of the levels of stress hormones (serum cortisol, prolactin, oestradiol, testosterone, thyroxin and growth hormone and urinary concentration of adrenalin and noradrenalin).

Results

The results show that the employees with skin complaints felt more stimulated in their work and had a higher decision latitude over work content and work organization compared to the control subjects. They reported, however, mental stress and eye complaints more frequently, and had significantly higher objectively registered itching frequency. They also had selective neuroendocrine activation during work but not during leisure, with changes in the stress hormones compared to the control subjects. There were no systematic differences between groups with regard to age and sex distribution, job functions, personality, socioeconomic factors, marital status, years of VDU work, alcohol or coffee consumption, or smoking habits. The pigmentation ability of the two groups was comparable.

Discussion

Our findings clearly show that employees with skin complaints suffer from more occupational stress compared to healthy controls working under similar objective conditions. This fact is reflected in higher stress hormone levels as well as subjective feelings of stress. Subjects with skin complaints also suffered from worse vision ergonomics and scratched themselves more frequently.

This study has shown that there are physiological differences in subjects with and without VDU-associated skin complaints. Since both groups were using VDUs to the same extent, our findings imply that there must be factors other than electromagnetic radiation contributing to the development of VDU-associated skin symptoms.

Based on our study we propose the following hypothesis: many employees working with computers suffer from occupational stress. This results in physiological changes characterized by elevated metabolism and increased dermal blood flow. This response may act as an unconditioned stimulus. The conditioning stimulus in this case would be the VDU work area. Once the conditioned response has been learned, the psychophysiological responses are elicited purely by the conditioned stimulus, i.e. the VDU. This model might help explain why people subsequently report symptoms in other electromagnetic environments.

The introduction of new technology has resulted in major changes in work content and work organization. These changes have in many cases resulted in a suboptimal organization with lack of performance feedback, discrepancy between mental capacity and goals of the worker and what is achievable by the software programs. The result of this discrepancy is a psychophysiological 'techno-stress'. We believe that further work in this area should include the psychosocial work environment and software ergonomic issues.

Our results show clearly that organizational factors and the psychosocial work environment[9] must be considered when VDU-associated skin problems are assessed in the workplace. Furthermore, for the persons with skin complaints, a conditioning mechanism[10] arising from a fear of health hazards is probably of importance.

In conclusion, the present study has shown physiological differences between persons with and without VDU-associated skin complaints. Corrective measures must entail many factors apart from merely installing 'low-emitting' VDUs. Tremendous financial resources have been misdirected to date without significantly improving the work environment of VDU workers suffering from skin complaints.

References

1 Berg M, Skin problems in workers using visual display terminals; a study of 201 patients, *Contact Dermat* (1988) **19**: 335–41.
2 Wahlberg JE, Lidén C, Is the skin affected by work at visual display terminals? *Dermatol Clinics* (1988) **6**: 81–5.
3 Lidén C, Contact allergy: a cause of facial dermatitis among visual display unit operators, *Am J Contact Dermat* (1990) **1**: 171–6.
4 Berg M, Lidén S, Axelson O, Skin complaints and work at visual display units; an epidemiological study of office employees, *J Am Acad Dermatol* (1990) **22**: 621–5.
5 Berg M, Hedblad M-A, Erhardt K, Facial skin complaints and work at visual display units; a histopathological study, *Acta Dermat (Stockh)* (1990) **70**: 216–20.
6 Swanbeck G, Bleeker T, Skin problems from visual display units, *Acta Dermato Venereol (Stockh)* (1989) **69**: 46–51.
7 Bergqvist U, Video display terminals and health: a technical and medical appraisal of the state of the art, *Scand J Work Environ Health* (1984) **10**: (suppl 2) 1–87.
8 Frankenhauser B, Video display terminals electromagnetic radiation and health. In: Knave B, Widebäck P-G, (eds). *Work with display units*, Elsevier: Amsterdam, 1987, pp. 81–4.
9 Arnetz B, Fjellner B, Eneroth P et al, Endocrine and dermatological concomitants of mental stress, *Acta Dermato (Stockh)* (1991) (suppl 156): 9–12.
10 MacQueen G, Marshall J, Perdue M et al, Pavlovian conditioning of rat mucosal mast cells to secrete mast cell protease II, *Science* (1989) **243**: 83–5.

27
A small solid state meter for measuring melanin pigmentation

Christopher Edwards and Robert Heggie
Department of Dermatology, University of Wales College of Medicine, Cardiff, UK

Introduction

Constitutive skin colour is an important parameter in both experimental and clinical medicine. Several skin disorders result in a diminution or even a complete loss of melanin, e.g. vitiligo. In other circumstances an increase in pigmentation can occur, for example in some scar tissue. Measurements of the amount of melanin present in the skin would help in the assessment of the severity of the disorder, and in monitoring the effects of therapy. Here non-invasive techniques of measurement are of particular use, for example in time-course studies, where exactly the same site can be measured repeatedly over time. It should also be remembered that pigmentary disorders are often presented for treatment because the patient feels disfigured. It is unlikely in these circumstances that the patient would be happy to agree to a biopsy, with accompanying scarring in the area of the disorder, just for a clinical measurement.

Dermatological photobiology deals with the effects of visible and ultraviolet radiation (UVR) on the skin. Normal short-term reactions to the UV portions of sunlight include stratum corneum thickening, erythema and increased melanin pigmentation. Methods of measurement of the amount of skin pigmentation have included the use of visual grading systems, and of filters, but instrumental measurement of one kind or another has become the method of choice. The construction of dose–response curves for the UVA spectrum for delayed pigmentation would be greatly facilitated by the use of objective linear measurements, if they were available.

Testing the efficacy of UVA sunscreens has recently been the subject of many studies. Since it is generally agreed that erythema of normal skin is not an appropriate end-point for UVA dose–response studies, many other methods have been proposed.[1-3] These include measuring erythema induced on psoralen-sensitized skin, and the assessment of both immediate and delayed pigmentation. Once again, a linear pigmentation measurement could be used to measure pigmentation as an end-point in UVA sunscreen studies.

The colour of skin as perceived by an observer is the result of many complex and interacting factors. Most important of these are the cutaneous pigments (the haemoglobins, melanin, carotenes and bilirubin), the stratum corneum (thickness and scaliness), the incident light, and the colour of the background. The perception of skin colour is greatly affected by the interpretation of the whole visual field by the brain, which produces differences in colour perception due to illumination and background colour as well as inter-individual variation in colour description and discrimination.

Clearly, visual methods of quantifying skin colour are to be avoided as far as possible. To this end, many measurements of skin colour have been attempted. These could be broadly categorized into two approaches. The first, called colorimetry, measures the overall colour of the skin using the tristimulus system.[4-6] This entails measuring three broad bandwidths of the visual spectrum and subsequently manipulating these tristimulus values according to a system which relates the three 'raw data' values to the colour perceptions and discriminations of a normal population. The determination of the exact mathematical manipulation of the measured values has been based on experiments conducted on surprisingly few subjects, and embodies the brain's response to colour in the final output variables. The whole philosophy is based on the quantification of colour as it would be seen by a human observer, and no separation of the contribution of individual (skin) pigments is possible.

The second approach, called reflectance photometry, relies on narrow-bandwidth measurements of the light diffusely scattered from within the skin. Different workers have chosen different numbers and wavelengths of measurements,[7-9] but all methods attempt to determine the slope of the melanin absorption spectrum with minimum interference from other skin pigments. The philosophy of the present study was to find a melanin index which is simply and only related to the amount of melanin pigment present.

The Cardiff melanin index meter

Previous reports have described instrumental designs which use the reflectance method to form melanin measurements, but these have been bulky, expensive and complicated, usually requiring a computer for control and/or calculation of the index. We describe here a very simple battery powered hand-held device which implements a two-wavelength melanin index. It is small and very simple to use, requiring only a 'set zero' adjustment and a 'read' button. A single number is presented which is related directly to the slope of the melanin absorption spectrum.

The meter consists of a hand-held probe and a small electronics control box (Figure 1). The probe contains a red and an infra-red emitting diode, a single photodiode receiver and drive and receive circuitry. The wavelengths chosen allow the slope of the melanin absorption band to be measured with minimum interference from the blood pigments (see Figure 2). The geometry of the light sources and the receiver is such that direct surface reflections 'miss' the receiver, thus maximizing the contribution to the received signal of the diffuse light re-emitted from the skin. The receiver is collimated to measure only the central 5 mm diameter of the approximately 12 mm diameter aperture of the probe (see Figure 3). Each light source is switched on and off (100% modulated) at independent, unsynchronized, frequencies. The receive

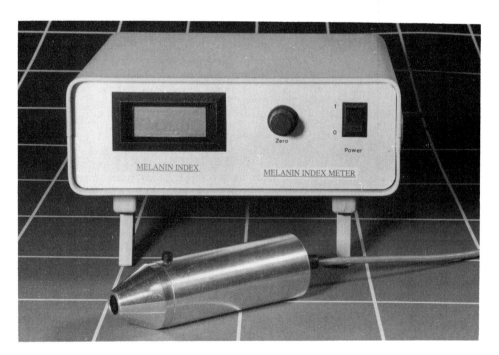

Figure 1

The Cardiff melanin index meter.

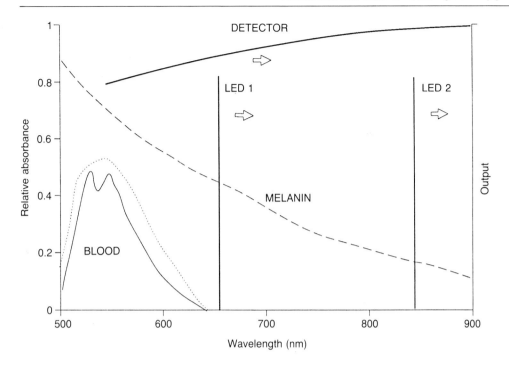

Figure 2

Approximate absorption spectra of cutaneous pigments and the output and receive response of the probe electro-optics. LED, light emitting diode.

signal is amplified and fed to two independent demodulators, each tuned to one of the driver modulation frequencies. These separate the red and the infra-red signals, and also reject any other signals not at the modulation frequencies, such as might arise from fluorescent lighting or from sunlight. The signals are then passed to a logarithmic ratio circuit, the (single) output of which is adjusted by a constant factor. This voltage is then presented as the melanin index. The logarithmic scale factor and the factor adjustment are designed to give a 0–200 range, which was chosen by experiment to give a reading of 25 to a very pale skin, and 150 to the darkest pigmented skin available. Thus a 0–200 range should encompass all skin types.

Evaluation

Preliminary evaluation of this meter was undertaken on a subject group with skin colour ranging from very pale Caucasian to very dark black. Two experiments were carried out to establish the range of values present in such a population, to relate these values to the Boston skin type, and to compare the meter measurements to an observer's judgment of skin colour.

The measurements were all made in the winter, in Cardiff, UK. No subjects had exposed their skin to sun or solarium light for the past 2 months. A melanin index measurement was made on the inner forearm of 25 subjects, who were assessed for their skin type according to the method of Fitzpatrick et al.[10] The results are summarized in Figure 4 and Table 1.

On 15 of these subjects, a further melanin index measurement was made on the outer forearm, avoiding hair. An independent observer, who was blind to this measurement, then arranged the subjects in a line with outer forearm skin colour changing from lightest to darkest from left to right. With the subjects thus arranged, it was felt that the eye was used to its best advantage, not to give an absolute measure of colour, but to rank adjacent

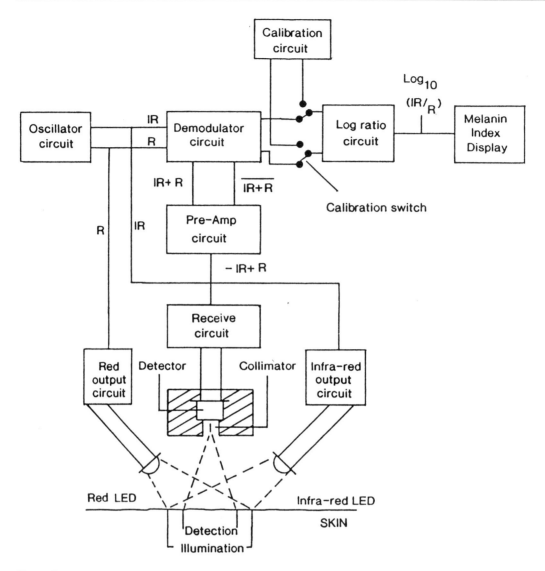

Figure 3

Schematic diagram of the melanin index meter.

forearms darker or lighter. The results of this experiment, shown in Figure 5, gave a Spearman's rank correlation coefficient of 0.88.

Conclusion

The results of the first experiment show that although the Boston skin type classification does not explicitly refer to skin pigmentation it nevertheless results in paler skinned individuals comprising the lower skin types. As experience tells us, the higher the skin type, the darker the skin. The great spread of values in each skin type group is witness to the fact that this is not a colour classification. The second experiment shows that the ranking of skin pigmentation by the meter is very close to that of an observer. Most of the differences between the two ranking results were on pairs of individuals who had very similar skin colour, and were very

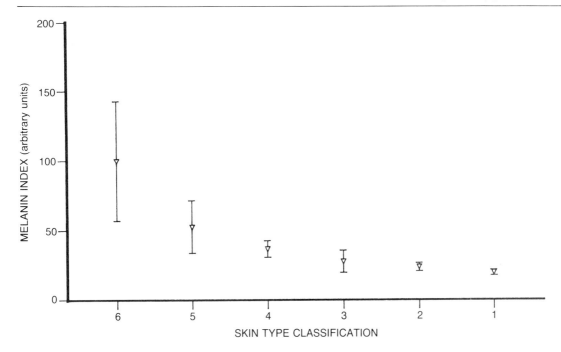

Figure 4

The melanin index (mean ±SD) of subjects grouped according to the sun reactivity classification of Fitzpatrick et al.[10]

Table 1 The melanin index measurements made on the inner forearm of 25 subjects.

Skin type	Melanin index (mean ±SD)
6	100 +/− 43
5	53 +/− 19
4	37 +/− 6
3	28 +/− 8
2	24 +/− 3
1	20 +/− 2

difficult to rank by eye. These individuals also gave very similar results when measured using the meter, and this led to the meter ranks of these two individuals being the opposite to the visual rank, so the disagreement between methods was probably not significant.

This meter is small, battery powered, hand held and extremely easy to use. It gives reproducible results which are in agreement with visual ranking, and it should be of considerable use in experimental and clinical photobiology.

References

1 Kaidbey K, Gange MD, Comparison of methods for assessing photoprotection against ultraviolet A in vivo, *J Am Acad Dermatol* (1987) **16**: 346–53.
2 Roelandts R, Sohrabvand N, Garmyn M, Evaluating the UVA protection of sunscreens, *J Am Acad Dermatol* (1989) **21**: 56–62.
3 Sayre RM, Agin PP, A method for the determination of UVA protection for normal skin, *J Am Acad Dermatol* (1990) **23**: 429–40.
4 Seitz JC, Whitmore CG, Measurement of erythema and

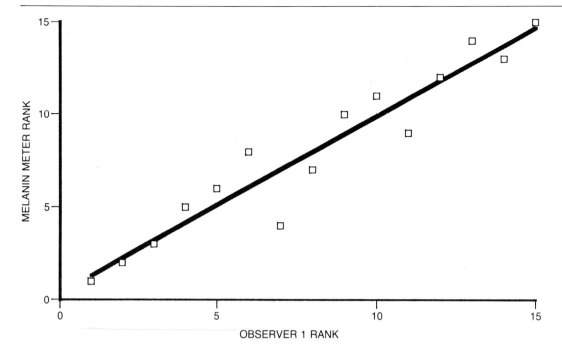

Figure 5

Comparison of the melanin index meter with a human observer for ranking the colour of inner forearm skin on 15 subjects of widely different degrees of pigmentation. Spearman's rank correlation coefficient = 0.88.

tanning responses in human skin using a tri-stimulus colourimeter, *Dermatologica* (1988) **177**: 70–5.
5 Herbin M, Venot A, Devaux JY et al, Color quantitation through image processing in dermatology, *IEE Trans Medical Imaging* (1990) **9**: 262–9.
6 Andreassi L, Casini L, Simoni S et al, Measurement of cutaneous colour and assessment of skin type, *Photodermatol Photoimmunol Photomed* (1990) **7**: 20–4.
7 Andersen PH, Bjerring P, Spectral reflectance of human skin in vivo, *Photodermatol Photoimmunol Photomed* (1990) **7**: 5–12.
8 Feather JW, Hajizadeh-Saffar M, Leslie G et al, A portable scanning reflectance spectrophotometer using visible wavelengths for the rapid measurement of skin pigments, *Phys Med Biol* (1989) **34**: 807–20.
9 Kollias N, Baqer BS, Spectroscopic characteristics of human melanin in vivo, *J Invest Dermatol* (1985) **85**: 38–42.
10 Fitzpatrick TB, Pathak MA, Parrish JA, Protection of human skin against the effects of the sunburn ultraviolet (290–320 nm). In: Fitzpatrick TB et al, (eds). *Sunlight and man—normal and abnormal photobiological responses*, University of Tokyo Press: Tokyo, 1974, p. 751.

28
Subacute cutaneous lupus erythematosus probably caused by occupationally acquired chronic ultraviolet radiation

Michael Buslau
Department of Dermatology, Johann Wolfgang Goethe-University, Theodor-Stern-Kai 7, D-6000, Frankfurt am Main, Germany

Introduction

There are limited data on skin effects caused by occupationally acquired chronic ultraviolet radiation (UVR). Furthermore, precise UVR threshold limits for preventing possible sequelae of occupationally acquired chronic UVR exposure are still lacking.[1] We report on a 59-year-old patient who worked from 1969 to 1990 checking aluminium coatings of lustre metal plates. Her place of work was lit by fluorescent lamps emitting unfiltered UVB and UVC rays. Since 1984 she has suffered from subacute cutaneous lupus erythematosus (SCLE). A few hours after starting work she regularly noticed pruritus and erythema on her face, forearms and hands. Her symptoms ameliorated during weekends and holidays. During the course of her disease her health worsened and she developed mild systemic signs of SCLE. Six medical and two technical experts' opinions were necessary to have her SCLE acknowledged as an occupational disease with a 40% degree of disability. To our knowledge this is the first case of occupationally acquired SCLE. This case raises the question of occupational trigger factors and their influence on autoimmune diseases and is also of importance because of the social aspects of occupational health hazards.

Case report

Case history

The female patient (born 1930) was completely healthy until the onset of subacute cutaneous lupus erythematosus (SCLE). Having completed her secondary education, she worked until 1969 on her parents' farm. At this time she had no problems with photosensitivity. From 1969 to 1990 she worked in a factory where her job was to take aluminium, steel and zinc cast press mouldings out of a galvanizing bath and to check the metal surface under bright artificial light. In 1983 the patient first noticed signs of increased photosensitivity. Within a few hours of starting work, the skin areas exposed to light (face, nape of the neck and forearms) began to itch and redden. These symptoms subsided when she was not working (e.g. evenings, weekends and holidays) but regularly returned upon recommencing work.

The patient presented at our department in 1984 on account of her symptoms and chronic discoid lupus erythematosus was diagnosed. At this point increased photosensitivity to UVB light was already documented and a possible occupational disease was considered. The ensuing clinical course, HLA antigens (B8 and DR3) and presence of Ro-antibodies in serum led to the diagnosis of SCLE. Transfer from her place of work was repeatedly advised, but was only undertaken in 1990. Only with intensive chloroquine therapy, intermittent glucocorticosteroid administration and subsequent use of UVR screening creams, could the patient resume working. However, these measures could not prevent a worsening of her clinical situation. Since 1989 the patient has shown bouts of depression and suicidal tendency and has complained of lethargy, tiredness and night sweats. Between 1984 and 1989 the patient was declared unfit on 11 occasions and had to be admitted twice to hospital for treatment.

Clinical picture

In 1989, at the last clinical assessment, the patient showed the following signs: centrofacial erythema with slight pityriasiform scaling but without infiltration and without scarring; multiple teleangiectasias on the face and neck; the scalp showed erythema with pityriasiform scaling; multiple small, sometimes excoriated and encrusted, spots were seen on the shoulders, both arms and extensor surfaces of the lower legs; fine-spotted de- and hyperpigmentation; the mediolateral aspects of the feet showed livedo reticularis; cuticle sclerosis and periungual erythema and atrophy; and erythema on the extensor sides of the fingers of both hands. Buccal mucous membranes were normal and no enlarged lymph nodes were found.

Laboratory data

Revelant pathological laboratory data (1989) are: BSR 100/125 mm (1984, 32/54 mm); BUN 34 g/l; immunoglobulin G (IgG) 2810 g/l; IgA 515 g/l; ANA 1:1280 (1984, 1:160); positive Ro- and La-antibodies; RNP antibodies; CRP; and RF. Urin: 50 erythrocytes/µl, protein 0.3 g/l. HLA: B8, B15, DR3, DR5 and DRw52.

Technical assessment

In 1986, an investigation of the radiation dosage at the patient's workplace was undertaken. Four different measuring points were chosen (in close proximity to the workbench: directly under the light close to the workbench, under a lamp on the conveyer belt and at 0.2 m above the workbench). The radiation spectrum in both the UV and visible regions, the light intensity, the UVA intensity and the effective UVB/C radiation were all measured. The results were compared with the UVR present in an office. In the subsequent report it was stated that:

> The patient's place of work is in a room measuring 36 × 36 m^2 enclosed at the top with a maximum height of 6 m. The roof windows are an extra 3.5 m high at their highest point. The light comes from a northerly direction. The fluorescent lights illuminating the room are 3.5 m above the floor and those illuminating the workbench are at a height of between 2.5–3.0 m. During cloudy weather, as when

these measurements were taken, most of the lighting is by uncovered artificial light sources, namely fluorescent lights (OSRAM type L58 W/25, universal white). The physical and biological data pertaining to the lights are given in Table 1.

The major part of the radiation intensity is in the visible range, wavelength >400 nm. In the UV range is a small line at 315 nm and a slightly larger line at 365 nm. There is a continuous background intensity with increasing wavelength from 320 and 420 nm (Figure 1). The illumination from different angles to the light source was between 65 and 520 Lux (office: 30–400 Lux) and between 510 and 820 Lux (office: 480–800 Lux). The UVA radiation was below the limit of detection (0.05 mW/cm^2). The effective UVB/C radiation was between 0.015 and 0.03 µW/cm^2 (office: 0.003–0.01 µW/cm^2).

After a total of six medical and two technical assessments, SCLE was recognized as an occupational disease with 40% of disability. Due to age, the patient took early retirement. She remains an out-patient and, after 5 months, no real clinical change in her symptoms has been seen, despite further chloroquine and glucocorticosteroid treatment.

Table 1 Technical and biological data of the OSRAM type L58 W/25, universal white, fluorescent tube.

UVR (mW/1000 lumen)	UVA	<0.001
	UVB	15.1
	UVC	92.4
Acute biological effects (h/1000 lux)	Conjuctivitis	1092
	Erythema	52
	Pigmentation	316

Discussion

UVR can be regarded as a potential environmental occupational skin hazard.[2] Skin lesions should be reckoned with under conditions of high actinic energy (acute UVR over-dosage). This is also the case in patients with normal UVR dosage but with drug- or disease-induced photosensitivity (chronic UVR effect).[3] In addition to the UV part of natural light, UVR emitted by artificial light, for example

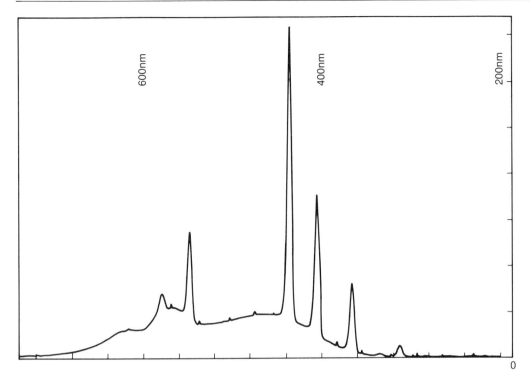

Figure 1

Occupationally acquired chronic UVR exposure: the radiation spectrum at 0.2 m above the patient's workbench.

fluorescent lamps, should be considered; hence the reports of exacerbation of rosacea, UVR-induced contact dermatitis and actinic reticuloid by fluorescent light. Whether fluorescent light can provoke a malignant melanoma remains a source of controversy.[4]

Employees at risk are those whose workbench is very close to the light source or those requiring very bright illumination. Increased UVR reflection from materials should also be taken into account. For example, aluminium welding produces a higher level of UVR than does steel welding.[5] Nebe and Lenz[6] have described the case of an arc welder with occupationally acquired CDLE and the subsequent healing of skin lesions on retraining as a mechanic. Wozniak[7] has described an arc welder in whom CDLE developed after 13 working years and whose CDLE was accepted as an occupationally acquired disease.

Many cumulative factors were present in our patient: the increased photosensitivity in cases of SCLE; the persistent 21-year exposure at work to UVB light from naked bright fluorescent mercury vapour lamps; the small distance between the source of illumination and the subject; and the reflection of UVR by the aluminium coatings. The fluorescent lamps at the patient's workplace produced UVB radiation together with a small amount of UVC. The radiation dosage, without accounting for that arising from reflection from the aluminium parts, was 10 times higher than that found in a normal office. Although the radiation dosage limits of the American Conference of Governmental Industrial Hygienists (ACGIH) were not exceeded in this case, it must be remembered that the ACGIH limits are based on acute UVR over-dosage and assume normal photosensitivity.

Carrie and Kühl[8] have proposed that a connection between occupation and lupus erythematosus may exist under the following conditions: (1) the condition must be linked to or originate from the exposed skin areas; (2) the case history must emphasize the effect of illumination; and (3) it should be possible to correlate the patient's occupation with the course or outbreak of the disease. Our patient fulfilled these criteria. The dependence of SCLE aggravation on her occupation was repeatedly documented. It is therefore all the more incomprehensible why six medical assessments were required before the patient could be removed from her place of work and her SCLE recognized as being occupationally acquired. At least three reasons for this can be proposed: (1) the triggering of such autoimmune skin diseases by environmental agents is, in terms of medical insurance and compensation, a relatively new field; (2) systematic checks on the possibly damaging effects of chronic UVR at work are lacking; and (3) there are as yet no compulsory limits governing cumulative UVR exposure at work.

Lehmann et al[9] have demonstrated that lupus erythematosus skin changes, particularly in patients with SCLE, can be induced experimentally by UVA and UVB exposure. At present it remains unclear whether an SCLE, under corresponding genetic predisposition, can be initially triggered by chronic UVR exposure at work. This would be of great importance in determining the amount of compensation to be awarded to workers. In the present case, in notifying the SCLE as an occupationally acquired disease, the possible effects of lupus erythematosus on organs other than the skin were not recognized as being occupationally acquired. It remains to be seen whether this situation requires revision.

References

1 Bergner Th, Przybilla B, UV exposure at the workplace. Determination of threshold limit values, *Hautarzt* (1990) **41**: 523–6.
2 Michailov P, Dogramadjev I, Berowa N, UV radiation as occupational environmental damage, *Berufsdermatosen* (1981) **29**: 5–8.
3 Nikolowski J. Schüle D, Pathogenesis and aggravation of occupational diseases caused by rays of different wave lengths, *Berufsdermatosen* (1975) **23**: 55–61.
4 Cohen R, Adams RM, Physical causes of occupational skin diseases: radiation. In: Adams RM, (ed). *Occupational skin disease*, 2nd edn, Saunders: Philadelphia, 1990, pp65–72.
5 Zenz C, Knight AL, Ultraviolet, microwave, laser, and infrared radiation. In: Zenz C, (ed). *Occupational Medicine*, Chicago: Year Book Medical Publishers, 1975, p564.
6 Nebe H, Lenz U, Untersuchungen über berufliche Noxen beim Lupus erythematodes. *Derm Mschr* (1971) **157**: 500–4.
7 Wozniak KD, Erythematodes chronicus discoides as an occupational disease, in an electric welder, *Berufsdermatosen* (1971) **19**: 187–96.
8 Carrié C, Kühl M, *Leitfaden der beruflichen Hautkrankheiten*, vol 2, George Thieme: Stuttgart, 1969.
9 Lehmann P, Hölzle E, Kind P et al, Experimental reproduction of skin lesions in lupus erythematosus by UVA and UVB radiation, *J Am Acad Dermatol* (1990) **22**: 181–7.

29
Seasonal influence on the occurrence of dry flaking facial skin

M. D. Cooper, H. Jardine and J. Ferguson
Consumer Products Development, Boots Pharmaceuticals, Nottingham, UK

There are many intrinsic factors that influence the outward appearance and function of the skin; likewise there are many extrinsic or environmental factors which either directly or indirectly have a physiological effect. It is generally accepted that dry skin conditions are more common during the winter months. Early studies attempted to attribute dryness and chapping of the skin to environmental factors, in particular relative humidity and absolute humidity, often using in vitro or animal models.[1] The aims of the present study were to monitor dry, flaking facial skin over a 14-month period, using simple subjective assessment techniques, and to determine any causative association with meteorological factors.

Subjects

A total of 55 female volunteers were accepted into the study (aged 18–58 years, average age 27 years) after exclusion for pregnancy and medical treatment for any abnormal skin condition. For various reasons, not all subjects attended every assessment. All subjects worked in an air-conditioned environment for approximately 7 h every day. They were allowed to use cosmetics and toiletries freely during the study, with the exception that no products were applied or used on the face on the morning of each assessment day. Use of topical medications available over the counter (such as anti-acne products) was not allowed on the test sites.

Methods

Skin type assessment

On attendance for assessment, each subject first had their forehead and whole left facial cheek skin types assessed by a trained assessor. The assessment scale uses standard visual descriptors (Table 1). Very few subjects demonstrated grades 1 or 5; later analyses were therefore simplified by combining skin types 1 and 2 to form a 'greasy' subgroup, and skin types 4 and 5 to produce a 'dry' subgroup.

Dry flaking skin assessment

Dry, flaking skin is most easily visualized by removal of the skin surface lipids after assessment of skin

Table 1 Skin type assessment scale.

Type 1	*Very greasy*: coarse texture, open pores, shiny patches, comedones and spots common
Type 2	*Slightly greasy*: open texture, occasional comedones/spots
Type 3	*Normal*: fairly open texture, occasional comedones and flake
Type 4	*Slightly dry*: fine texture, occasional flakes visible, some tightness
Type 5	*Very dry*: very fine texture, dull appearance, obvious flakes, tight.

type. This was achieved by adopting a standard swabbing technique using cotton wool and propan-2-ol, allowing the excess alcohol on the skin surface to evaporate before visual assessment.[2] The same trained assessor did every assessment in order to maintain continuity of scoring. The accuracy of this assessor's results was periodically checked by comparing these scores with those given by a second expert assessor.

Dry flaking skin was assessed every 4 to 5 weeks according to a novel assessment scale (Table 2). This scale was designed primarily to ease the visual burden of assessing multiple parameters, by examining three visual aspects of flaking skin separately: the grade (or size) of skin flakes, their density, and the area covered by the flakes. A flaking score was calculated for each assessed site by addition of scores for each of the three aspects. The scale of potential scores is, therefore, discontinuous and the data obtained were analysed using appropriate statistical techniques. It is reasonably well accepted that subjective assessment scales should not use any more than a five-point descriptor scale, because assessor proficiency diminishes as the number of assessment classes increases above this number. The composite scale used in the present study enables a more representative assessment of the condition than is possible using a single five-point assessment scale.

Table 2 Dry flaking skin subjective scoring scale.*

Flake size — scale 0 to 3
0 Dulled powdery appearance, no flakes visible
1 Very small but visible flakes
2 Intermediate sized flakes (at least two times size of 1)
3 Large flakes with obvious curling edges

Density of flakes — scale 0 to 3
0 No flakes, powdery only
1 Sparsely distributed flakes (size 1 to 3)
2 Non-uniform covering of flakes
3 Flakes in close proximity, with uniform covering of flaking area

Area of cover — scale 0 to 3
0 No flaking
1 Less than one-third of swabbed area flaking
2 One- to two-thirds of swabbed area flaking
3 Over two-thirds of swabbed area flaking

* Flaking score = sum of scores of flake size, density and area of cover. Possible scores: 0, 3, 4, 5, 6, 7, 8, 9.

Meteorological data

Temperature and wind speed data were obtained from the regional weather centre (height above mean sea level 117 m); relative humidity measurements were obtained locally using a wet and dry bulb whirling hygrometer. The highest and lowest temperatures reached each month were taken from the supplied data, and the mean cumulative wind speed was calculated by adding the daily mean wind speeds for each month.

Results and discussion

Meteorological effects on flaking levels

The average flaking scores are shown in the histogram in Figure 1. A periodic change during this study was clearly evident. Average scores were higher on the forehead regardless of season and, in comparison to cheek scores, were worse during the second winter of the study. The seasonal change in temperature (Figure 2) is as would be expected for a northern temperate zone. The direction of change in temperature is in direct opposition to the change in average flaking levels, suggesting that temperature may have some influence on the levels of dry flaking skin. Atmospheric humidity would also be expected to have some influence on the severity of the condition: relative humidity (RH) did not show a particular relationship with flaking levels in this study, although absolute humidity did (Table 3). The following expression was used to calculate absolute humidity (AH, in mg l^{-1}):

$$AH = \left(\frac{RH_T}{100} \times SVP_T\right)$$

where SVP is the saturated vapour pressure at temperature T (obtained from tables) and RH_T is the relative humidity at temperature T. Absolute humidity indicates the mass of water vapour present in a unit volume of the atmosphere, unlike relative humidity which is the ratio of the quantity of water vapour present in the atmosphere to the quantity which would saturate it at the existing temperature. So, the higher the temperature, the greater the water holding capacity of the atmosphere.

Average flaking scores for the forehead and cheek correlate negatively with both the highest

Seasonal influence on the occurrence of dry flaking facial skin 161

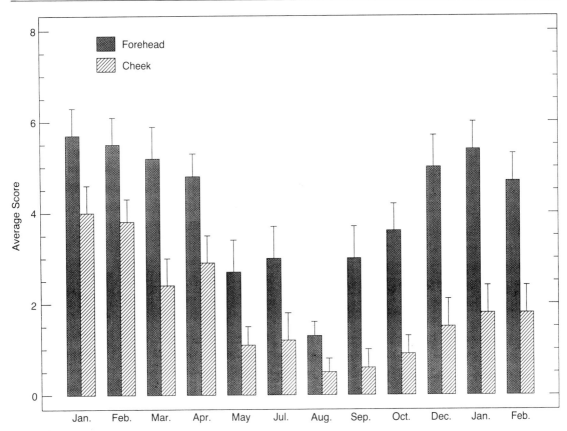

Figure 1

Monthly average flaking scores. Bars indicate ±2 standard errors of the mean. No data were obtained for June or November.

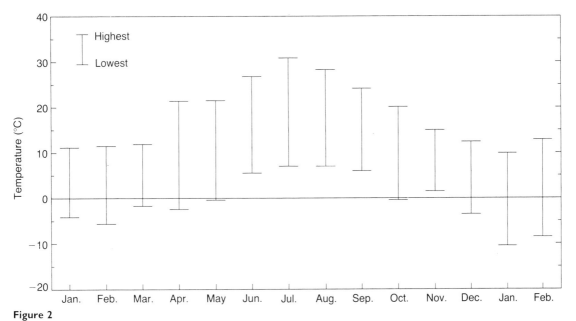

Figure 2

The highest and lowest temperatures recorded each month during the study.

and the lowest temperatures (Table 3), indicating that the lower the temperature, the higher the level of dry flaking skin (compare Figures 1 and 2). Although considered by some to be an important factor, relative humidity did not correlate significantly with the level of dry flaking skin in this study, but the relationship with absolute humidity (Figure 3) was significant ($r = 0.92$ forehead). This is in agreement with the early findings of Gaul and Underwood.[3] Both the moisture content of the atmosphere and the temperature of the surroundings appear to be specific environmental factors influencing the general condition of the epidermis.

The positive correlations obtained with mean cumulative wind speed (Table 3) suggest that we may have detected the effects of wind on the condition of the skin. Wind can alter the temperature gradient or water content gradient across the stratum corneum, resulting in an imbalance in condition between outer and deeper epidermal layers. The significance of the correlation obtained for the cheek could be the result of greater exposure of this area to the drying effects of wind.

Skin type and flaking

Examination of the seasonal data on dry flaking skin according to dry, normal or greasy skin types (Figure 4) shows that all forehead-skin types demonstrate a reduction in average scores during the summer (August). The pattern of change in cheek-skin types, however, is less straightforward, due perhaps to average flaking scores being much lower on this site (Figure 4). It is worth noting that the average flaking score for the group presenting a greasy-skin type on the forehead during the first winter (February) of the study (Figure 4), was higher than that obtained for the other two skin-type groups. This was also observed in the summer (August) for the forehead, and in May for the cheek.

Flaking score distribution

Sample distributions of flaking scores obtained during the different seasons in the study are presented in Figure 5. On the forehead the score distribution is skewed towards the high scores in winter (February), and towards the lower scores during summer (May and August), returning to a more normal distribution in December. A similar seasonal shift in score distribution was found for the cheek skin; this site shows a greater tendency towards a zero flaking score during August than did the forehead, and the February and December distributions are markedly negatively skewed. These selected distributions demonstrate the shift in score frequency according to season.

Many of the effects of climate changes are well known; changes in temperature and humidity in particular invoke biological thermoregulatory mechanisms and may alter sebaceous flow or composition. Exposure to ultraviolet radiation changes dramatically in quality and quantity according to season and perhaps even the seasonal change in daylight hours could have some direct or indirect effect. There are likely to be many more unknown natural and unnatural environmental influences on skin condition.

Whilst in this study we specifically considered the effects of the external environment, effects of the indoor environment, particularly in air-conditioned buildings, may well contribute to the overall condition of the skin. Alternate exposure to

Table 3 Correlation coefficients for average flaking scores against meteorological parameters.

	Temperature		Cumulative mean daily wind speed	Relative humidity	Absolute humidity
	Highest	Lowest			
Average forehead flaking score	−0.88*	−0.82*	+0.53	+0.39	−0.92*
Average cheek flaking score	−0.63*	−0.56*	+0.62*	+0.06	+0.60*

* Statistically significant ($p < 0.05$, Student's t-test).

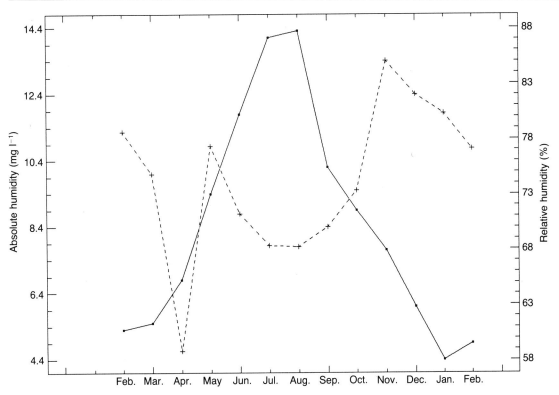

Figure 3

Relative humidity (----) and derived absolute humidity (——) data for 13 months of the study.

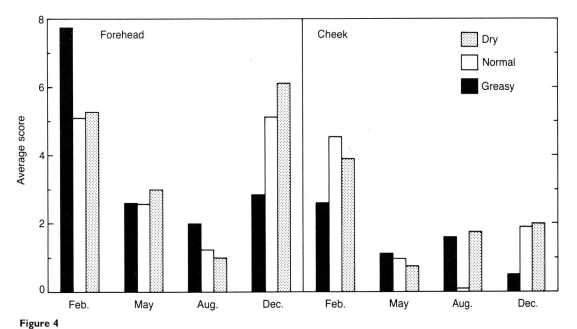

Figure 4

Average flaking scores calculated according to visually assessed skin type, for selected months showing seasonal changes (February, winter; May, spring; August, summer; December, autumn/winter).

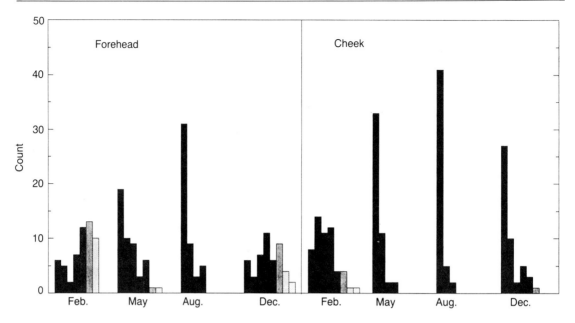

Figure 5

Flaking score distributions for selected months, showing seasonal changes. Bars are presented in ascending order of score (0, 3, 4, 5, 6, 7, 8, 9) from left to right in each distribution.

both 'controlled' indoor and 'uncontrolled' natural outdoor environments will undoubtedly put the skin under stress and affect its general condition, particularly if exposed to extremes of temperature and humidity. The dry, flaking skin condition studied here may, at least in part, result from such cyclical exposure.

This study demonstrates a seasonal change in the prevalence of a dry, flaking facial skin condition, and the incidence appears to be in part at least governed by environmental temperature and atmospheric moisture content.

References

1 Middleton JB, Allen BM, The influence of temperature and humidity on stratum corneum and its relation to skin chapping, *J Soc Cosmet Chem* (1974) **24**: 239–43.
2 Fairhurst E, Keyser AM, Forward GC, Investigations into the nature of 'dry' flaking skin, *12th IFSCC Congress, Paris* (1982) **3**: 147–51.
3 Gaul LE, Underwood GB, Clinical aspects of dry skin, *J Invest Dermatol* (1951) **18**: 9–12.

Part II: Chemical hazards in the environment

30
Xenobiotic metabolism in the skin

David R. Bickers and Hasan Mukhtar
Skin Diseases Research Center, Department of Dermatology, Case Western Reserve University, Cleveland, Ohio, USA

Introduction

The skin is a major interface between the body and the environment and functions as a portal of entry for certain types of xenobiotics, such as transdermally delivered drugs and selected toxic chemicals and physical agents. In the past the skin was considered to be a largely inert tissue with predominant barrier function, but in recent decades it has become clear that cutaneous tissue is a major contributor to and participant in the immunologic and inflammatory pathways important for homeostasis.

Cytochrome P450s

Humans exist in a potentially hostile environment replete with noxious, chemical and physical agents, and one system that has evolved to protect against the toxic effects of xenobiotics is known as the cytochrome P450 gene superfamily. This represents a large number of gene families that code for a limited number of isozymes which function to catalyse the oxidative metabolism of a diverse array of xenobiotics. One unusual aspect of the cytochrome P450 system is that, unlike classical enzyme substrate kinetics in which a single enzyme reacts with one or very few closely related substrates, cytochrome P450 dependent isozymes display a broad substrate specificity and yet, paradoxically, each is characterized by a high degree of substrate and product specificity.

Cytochrome P450s are, for the most part, located in the endoplasmic reticulum and are microsomal enzymes having as one major function the introduction of oxygen into substrates. This type of catalytic activity is characteristic of heme proteins such as cytochrome P450, as is the facilitation of electron transfer reactions that are vitally important for energy metabolism. In general, characteristic substrates for cytochrome P450 are highly lipophilic non-polar compounds that cannot be excreted efficiently in the urine. The cytochrome P450 catalysed introduction of oxygen into xenobiotics generally elicits two changes in these molecules, converting them into more polar water-soluble metabolites that are more readily excreted and which have little or no pharmacological activity. Thus, the cytochrome P450s provide an important defense mechanism for dealing with the various chemicals to which the body is exposed on a daily basis. In addition to xenobiotics, cytochrome P450s also catalyse the transformation of numerous endogenous compounds, including steroid hormones and lipids, and thus function as a mechanism for inactivating and enhancing the elimination of these biologically active substances.[1–5]

While the majority of the cytochrome P450s that have been identified to date are found in the liver, it is now known that virtually every tissue possesses variable types and amounts of these heme proteins, the distribution of which reflects a complex array of genetic and environmental influences.

Cytochrome P450 mediated metabolic activation

It is important to emphasize that while the cytochrome P450 system predominantly functions to convert pharmacologically or biologically active substrates into inactive metabolites, there are a number of situations where the opposite occurs in that inert precursors are converted into reactive metabolites capable of evoking certain kinds of toxic effects. This cytochrome P450 dependent metabolic activation pathway is implicated in the generation of reactive metabolites of certain types of environmental chemical carcinogens and this may be one decisive factor in determining an individual's risk of developing malignant neoplasms as a result of exposure to such chemicals.

In general then, there may be competing pathways within cells for the cytochrome P450 dependent metabolism of the inactivation and activation of xenobiotics. When inactivation predominates, the potential toxicity of substrates is decreased, whereas predominance of activation may predispose to certain kinds of toxicity.

Enzyme induction

Another interesting feature of the cytochrome P450 dependent enzyme system is the complex effects of various inherited and acquired influences on the expression of the genes that code for these isozymes. For example, the cytochrome P450s are generally inducible following exposure to certain kinds of chemical and physical influences. Thus, amplification of cytochrome P450 gene expression results in increased production of one or another isozyme that will, in turn, influence the rate of substrate turnover for that isozyme. On the other hand, cytochrome P450 isozyme expression may be inhibited by other factors so that the amount present at a given time in a target tissue will reflect an extraordinarily complex interplay of factors.

Cutaneous cytochrome P450

Over the past decade, our laboratory has been interested in characterizing cytochrome P450 isozyme expression in the skin. As a first approach to this problem it was necessary to develop innovative techniques for the preparation of microsomal suspensions from skin samples or from skin cells. Since the cutaneous compartment contains a number of structural proteins, among them keratins, collagens and elastins, which are highly resistant to mechanical disruption and solubilization, development of the ideal methodology for preparation of functional and intact microsomes has proven to be elusive. In general, skin microsomal protein is only 5–10% of that found in the liver, but the skin's strategic location as a portal of entry affords a unique opportunity for the metabolism of certain xenobiotics within the target tissue itself. This may be a particularly important influence on the role of cytochrome P450 in chemical carcinogenesis.

Measurement of cytochrome P450s

The name cytochrome P450 refers to the fact that these heme proteins absorb incident energy intensely around 450 nm under reducing conditions in the presence of carbon monoxide.[6-11] Thus, one standard approach to identifying cytochrome P450s is to measure them spectrally. Microsomes prepared from whole skin, from epidermis or from epidermal keratinocytes have all been shown to have spectrally detectable amounts of cytochrome P450 and, furthermore, treatment of animals or cultured cells with polycyclic aromatic hydrocarbon carcinogens such as benzo[a]pyrene (BP) results in increased amounts of cytochrome P450 in these preparations. Furthermore, the peak absorbance of the induced isozyme occurs near 448 nm and this 2 nm blue shift is characteristic of polyaromatic hydrocarbon carcinogen-inducible cytochrome P450 isozymes.

Purification of cutaneous cytochrome P450

The next challenge was to isolate and purify the induced cytochrome P450 isozyme and this was accomplished employing standard solubilization and chromatographic techniques that accomplished 40- to 50-fold purification of the enzyme P450 IAI in rodent epidermis. In vitro reconstitution experiments in which the purified isozyme was combined with a cytochrome P450 reductase and a lipid verified that substrates for cytochrome P450 IAI were metabolized by the purified heme protein.[12-16]

Immunophenotyping of cutaneous cytochrome P450s

Further characterization of the cytochrome P450 present in the skin was facilitated by the availability of monoclonal and polyclonal antibodies directed against various cytochrome P450 isozymes. One such monoclonal antibody known as 1-7-1 is directed against hepatic cytochrome P450 IA1 induced by treatment with carcinogens and another known as 2-66-3 is directed against cytochrome P450 IIB1 known to be induced by barbiturates. Using an enzyme-linked immunosorbent assay (ELISA) technique, the monoclonal antibodies were employed to characterize the nature of cytochrome P450 isozyme expression in rodent epidermis. Monoclonal antibody 2-66-3 reacted predominantly with microsomes prepared from untreated animals, whereas monoclonal antibody 1-7-1 reacted predominantly with microsomes prepared from carcinogen-treated animals.

These same antibodies were then used for immunoblot analysis of cytochrome P450 isozyme expression employing sodium dodecyl sulfate (SDS) polyacrylamide gel electrophoresis. Microsomes prepared from untreated and carcinogen-treated animals were shown to migrate in the gels to a position characteristic of cytochrome P450 isozymes and, furthermore, there were increased amounts of cytochrome P450 IA1 identified in these microsomes, indicating that carcinogen treatment enhanced the production of this isozyme in epidermal microsomes. In further studies, the same 1-7-1 antibody, as well as a polyclonal antibody prepared in our own laboratory directed against P-450 IA1, were each shown to bind to microsomes prepared from either the epidermis or the liver of neonatal rats.

The results were confirmed by employing the antibodies for immunophenotyping experiments in rodent skin using horseradish peroxidase staining. A single topical application of a carcinogenic chemical resulted in increased staining indicating enhanced expression of cytochrome P450 IA1. This first became apparent by 8 h and reached a maximum at 24 h before starting to decrease. The staining intensity was greatest in epidermal keratinocytes and in the sebaceous follicles of treated skin. These findings are consistent with the concept that epidermis and structures closely related to it are the predominant site of cytochrome P450 IA1 gene expression in mammalian epidermis.[17-24]

Cytochrome P450 gene expression in skin

While these observations concerning cytochrome P450 isozyme expression in skin were of interest, it seemed important to characterize the expression of the genes that encode for cytochrome P450 isozymes in the skin. Because of the low levels of cytochrome P450 in this tissue, it was necessary to employ more sensitive techniques to assess gene expression. The polymerase chain reaction (PCR) is a particularly useful approach since it is capable of accomplishing substantial amplification of genes expressed in a tissue. By employing oligomers that match the terminal nucleotides of the hepatic isozyme, it was possible to show that carcinogen treatment of rodent skin resulted in substantially increased expression of the cytochrome P450 IA1 gene message.[25,26] Furthermore, a time-course study verified that increased gene message was detectable as early as 6 h after treatment, reached a peak at 24 h, and by 36 h had started to decrease. Additional studies were conducted using human keratinocytes and these confirmed increased cytochrome P450 IA1 gene message following treatment with a carcinogenic chemical.

Chemical carcinogenesis and cutaneous cytochrome P450

What is the potential importance of these findings? One possible implication is the relationship of this type of gene expression to chemical carcinogenesis. The induction of cancer is a complex phenomenon that has been perhaps most carefully studied in the skin. Indeed, the first evidence implicating environmental exposure as a major factor in the development of human malignancy came from the observation of Sir Percival Pott, a London surgeon who, in 1775, drew attention to the unique susceptibility of chimney sweeps to scrotal skin cancer and proposed that this would be attributed to their chronic exposure to soot. This prescient finding anticipated by almost 150 years the studies of Japanese workers who, early in the 20th century, showed that repetitive application of crude coal tar to the ears of rabbits resulted in the development of malignant neoplasms. Subsequent studies showed that the cancer-causing components of coal tar were polycyclic aromatic hydrocarbons such as benzo[a]pyrene and that these hydrocarbons were metabolized by cytochrome P450 dependent microsomal enzymes.

Studies in rodent epidermis, in cultured human keratinocytes and in organ cultures of human skin have verified the cytochrome P450 dependent metabolism of benzo[a]pyrene.[27-9] This is an example of a metabolic activation process in which oxygen is initially introduced into the hydrocarbon at the 7,8-position to form benzo[a]pyrene 7,8-

oxide. This epoxide is in turn a substrate for a non cytochrome P450 dependent enzyme known as epoxide hydrolase which cleaves the epoxide residue to yield the 7,8-dihydrodiol of benzy[a]pyrene. This diol is then a substrate for cytochrome P450 IA1 which inserts another oxygen at the 9,10-position to yield diastereomers of benzo[a]pyrene-7,8-diol-9,10-epoxide. One of these diol-epoxide isomers can bind to DNA and may thereby initiate the neoplastic process in skin cells.

Carcinogenesis is a complex multi-step process which includes initiation, promotion and malignant conversion. Cytochrome P450 dependent metabolic activation has been implicated in both initiation and conversion, but appears to play a particularly important role in the initiation process, for example, perhaps by evoking oncogene expression. Further studies are needed to define the role of cytochrome P450 mediated metabolic activation in the various stages of carcinogenesis.

Anticarcinogenesis

One novel approach to diminishing the cytochrome P450 dependent metabolic activation process that is crucial for tumor initiation by polycyclic aromatic hydrocarbons is to identify non-toxic inhibitors of this catalytic activity which might be expected to reduce the risk of cancer induction. Indeed, our studies have shown that naturally occurring polyphenolic compounds that occur in fruits and vegetables, and which include ellagitannins such as ellagic acid and tannic acid, are powerful inhibitors of cytochrome P450 dependent catalytic activity and of enzyme enhanced binding of chemical carcinogens to DNA. Pre-treatment of rodents with topically applied ellagitannins or administration of small amounts in the drinking water substantially diminish the incidence of malignant squamous cell carcinoma that develop in animals treated with polycyclic aromatic hydrocarbon carcinogens. Similar results have been achieved with epicatechins which are present in green tea, suggesting that it may be possible to diminish the risk of certain types of human malignancy using this approach.

Conclusions

The skin is a remarkably active tissue from a metabolic perspective. Our studies have shown that the cutaneous compartment expresses multiple genes of the cytochrome P450 superfamily and that one of these, cytochrome P450 IA1, may play an important role in the susceptibility of the skin to chemical carcinogenesis. Our studies re-emphasize that even small amounts of certain enzymes in target tissues at portals of entry to the body may have a decisive influence over the risk of certain kinds of toxic responses. Furthermore, metabolic responses in the skin may provide important clues to cytochrome P450 isozyme distribution that could be employed as one approach to assessing an individual's risk for certain kinds of environmentally induced neoplasms or other toxic responses. Furthermore, the ability to introduce genes into cells suggests that it may be possible to introduce genes programmed to detoxify certain kinds of environmental responses.

References

1 Mukhtar H, Khan WA, Cutaneous cytochrome P-450, *Drug Metab Rev* (1989) **20**: 657–73.
2 Kappus H, Drug metabolism in the skin. In: Greaves MW, Shuster S, (eds). *Pharmacology of the skin*, vol II, Springer-Verlag, New York, 1989, pp. 123–64.
3 Bickers DR, Drugs, carcinogen and steroid hormone metabolism in the skin. In: Goldsmith LA, (ed.). *Biochemistry and physiology of the skin*, Oxford University Press: New York, 1991, in press.
4 Kao J, Carver MP, Cutaneous metabolism of xenobiotics, *Drug Metab Rev* (1990) **22**: 363–410.
5 Bronaugh RL, Stewart RF, Storm JE, Extent of cutaneous metabolism during percutaneous absorption of xenobiotics, *Toxicol Appl Pharmacol* (1989) **99**: 534–43.
6 Conney AH, Induction of microsomal enzymes by foreign chemicals and carcinogenesis by polycyclic aromatic hydrocarbons: GHA Clowes Memorial Lecture, *Cancer Res* (1982) **42**: 4875–917.
7 Omura T, Sato R, The carbon monoxide-binding pigment of liver microsomes, I. Evidence for its hemoprotein nature, *J Biol Chem* (1964) **239**: 2370–8.
8 Ryan DE, Levin W, Purification and characterization of hepatic microsomal cytochrome P-450, *Pharmacol Ther* (1989) **45**: 153–239.
9 Levin W, The 1988 Bernard B. Brodie Award lecture. Functional diversity of hepatic cytochrome P-450, *Drug Metab Dispos* (1990) **18**: 824–30.
10 Nebert DW, Nelson DR, Coon MJ, et al, The P450 superfamily: update on new sequences, gene mapping, and recommended nomenclature, *DNA Cell Biol* (1991) **10**: 1–14.
11 Jakoby WB, Ziegler DM, The enzymes of detoxification, *J Biol Chem* (1990) **265**: 20715–8.
12 Khan WA, Das M, Stick S, Javed S et al, Induction of

epidermal NAD(P)H : quinone reductase by chemical carcinogens: a possible mechanism for the detoxification, *Biochem Biophys Res Commun* (1987) **146**: 126–33.

13 Pohl RJ, Philpot RM, Fouts JR, Cytochrome P-450 content and mixed-function oxidase activity in microsomes isolated from mouse skin, *Drug Metab Dispos* (1976) **4**: 442–50.

14 Bickers DR, Dutta-Choudhury T, Mukhtar H, Epidermis: a site of drug metabolism in neonatal rat skin. Studies on cytochrome P-450 content and mixed-function oxidase and epoxide hydrolase activity, *Mol Pharmacol* (1982) **21**: 239–47.

15 Alvares AP, Bickers DR, Kappas A, Polychlorinated biphenyls: a new type of inducer of cytochrome P-448 in the liver, *Proc Natl Acad Sci USA* (1973) **70**: 1321–5.

16 Mukhtar H, Raza H, Bickers DR, Purification of β-naphthoflavone inducible neonatal rat epidermal cytochrome P-450, *FASEB J* (1990) **4**: A600 (abstract).

17 Khan WA, Park SS, Gelboin HV et al, Monoclonal antibodies directed characterization of epidermal and hepatic cytochrome P-450 isozymes induced by skin application of therapeutic crude coal tar, *J Invest Dermatol* (1989) **93**: 40–5.

18 Ichikawa T, Hayashi S, Nosiro M et al, Purification and characterization of cytochrome P-450 induced by benz[a]anthracene in mouse skin microsomes, *Cancer Res* (1989) **49**: 806–9.

19 Mukhtar H, Das M, Steele JD et al, HPLC separation of multiple isozymes of epidermal cytochrome P-450 in neonatal Sprague-Dawley rats, *Clin Res* (1986) **34**: 991A (abstract).

20 Thomas PE, Bandiera S, Reik LM et al, Polyclonal and monoclonal antibodies as probes of rat hepatic cytochrome P-450 isozymes, *Fed Proc* (1987) **46**: 2563–6.

21 Gelboin HV, Friedman FK, Monoclonal antibodies for studies of xenobiotic and endobiotic metabolism, *Biochem Pharmacol* (1985) **34**: 2225–7.

22 Guengerich FP, Turvy CG, Comparison of levels of several human microsomal cytochrome P-450 enzymes and epoxide hydrolase in normal and disease states using immunochemical analysis of surgical liver samples, *J Pharmacol Exp Ther* (1991) **256**: 1189–94.

23 Khan WA, Park SS, Gelboin HV et al, Epidermal cytochrome P-450: immunochemical characterization of isoform induced by topical application of 3-methylcholanthrene to neonatal rats, *J Pharmacol Exp Ther* (1989) **249**: 921–7.

24 Whitter TB, Guengerich FP, Baron J, Effects of topical application of 3-methylcholanthrene on xenobiotic metabolizing enzymes in rat skin, *Fed Proc* (1985) **44**: 1115 (abstract).

25 Batula N, Sagara J, Gelboin HV, Expression of P_1-450 and P_3-450 DNA coding sequences as enzymatically active cytochromes P-450 in mammalian cells, *Proc Natl Acad Sci USA* (1987) **84**: 4073–7.

26 Mukhtar H, Khan IU, Haqqi TM et al, Polymerase chain reaction based detection of cytochrome P450 gene families in mammalian epidermis, *J Invest Dermatol* (1991) **96**: 581.

27 Finnen MJ, Herdman ML, Shuster S, Distribution and sub-cellular localization of drug metabolizing enzymes in the skin, *Br J Dermatol* (1985) **113**: 713–21.

28 Das M, Bickers DR, Mukhtar H, Epidermis: the major site of cutaneous benzo(a)pyrene and benzo(a)pryene 7,8-diol metabolism in neonatal Balb/C mice, *Drug Metab Dispos* (1986) **14**: 637–42.

29 Moloney SJ, Fromson JM, Bridges JW, Cytochrome P-450 dependent deethylase activity in rat and hairless mouse skin microsomes, *Biochem Pharmacol* (1982) **31**: 4011–8.

31
Cutaneous hazards associated with the use of cosmetics

Anton C. de Groot
Department of Dermatology, Carolus Hospital, 5200 BD 's-Hertogenbosch, The Netherlands

Introduction

A cosmetic product is any substance or preparation intended for placing in contact with the various external parts of the human body (epidermis, hair, lips and external genital organs) or with the teeth and the mucous membranes of the oral cavity with a view to cleaning them, perfuming them or protecting them, to keep them in good condition, change their appearance and/or correct body odours (Directive 76/768/EEC, 6th Amendment, 1991).

Cosmetics have been used for millennia to embellish the physical, mental, and spiritual well-being of mankind. These products are used with one or more of the following purposes: for the daily care and hygiene of the body (soap, shampoo, toothpaste, moisturizing and cleansing cream); to enhance attractiveness (make-up, hair colour, permanent wave, setting and styling gel, and nail lacquer); to obtain a pleasant smell (deodorant, perfume, aftershave, and mouthfreshener); for protection (sunbathing products); and for the masking of skin defects, e.g. vitiligo and port wine stains.

It has been shown that cosmetics can bring substantial psychological benefit. Nevertheless, side-effects of cosmetic products do occur. They can be classified as follows: irritation (objective and/or subjective), contact allergy, photosensitivity, contact urticaria (immediate contact reactions), acne/folliculitis, colour changes of the skin and appendages, miscellaneous local side-effects, and systemic side-effects.[1] This chapter deals with some aspects of irritation and contact allergy arising from cosmetic products.

Frequency and nature of side-effects

Relative to their widespread use, serious adverse reactions from cosmetic products are rare. Nevertheless, side-effects from cosmetics and toiletries are by no means rare. Their frequency and nature has been investigated both in patients consulting the dermatologist and in the general population.

General population

A total of 1609 individuals (838 men, 771 women, aged 33–64 years, average age 47.5 years) were asked the following question: 'Have you experienced side-effects of cosmetics or toiletries in the preceding 5 years?'. It was explained that everyday products such as soap, shampoo and toothpaste were to be included, and that mild reactions such as itching and dryness of the skin also were to be reported.[2]

Of the 1609 subjects interviewed, 196 (12.2%) claimed to have suffered from side-effects. The percentage in women was 16% and that in men 9%. The most frequently reported subjective symptom was itching, following by a feeling of dryness, burning of the skin and prickling sensations. Twenty-three subjects (12%) had no visible skin changes. The others described a variety of skin eruptions. The products that were blamed for the adverse reactions are summarized in Table 1.

Women ascribed most reactions to soap, facial cream, deodorant, shampoo and eye shadow. Among men soap also ranked first, followed by aftershave, deodorant and shower foam. Even

Table 1 Cosmetics to which side-effects were attributed

Women (N = 124)			Men (N = 72)		
Cosmetic	Number	%	Cosmetic	Number	%
Soap	51	41	Soap	35	49
Facial cream	41	33	Aftershave	16	22
Deodorant	31	25	Deodorant	14	19
Shampoo	20	16	Shower foam	9	12
Eye shadow	14	11	Massage oil	2	3
Bath/shower foam	9	7	Wife's hair lacquer	2	3
Facial make-up	8	6	Shaving soap	1	1
Perfumes	8	6			
Mascara	5	4			
Depilatory cream	3	2			

though most reactions were described as mild, and over 60% of the patients could solve the problem by stopping the use of the suspected products and using a different brand instead, 62 patients (32%) consulted the family physician for the cosmetic-related problems. Twenty-seven patients had been referred to the dermatologist. Twenty of them were patch-tested, but in no case was any cosmetic allergy proven. This, together with the type of complaints reported, suggested that irritation was the major cause of reactions to the cosmetics.[2] Atopic individuals were over-represented in the population claiming side-effects, and it was concluded that atopics are at higher risk of developing irritant reactions to cosmetics.[2] Both conclusions were confirmed in a subsequent study.[3]

A total of 982 regular clients of beauticians were interviewed on cosmetic-related side-effects experienced in the preceding 5 years. Of these clients, 254 (26%) claimed to have had such reactions. Of these, 150 were patch tested with the European standard series and a cosmetic screening series of 15 known cosmetic allergens. Only a few patients had positive patch-test reactions to cosmetic allergens: colophony, 1 (1%); wool alcohols, 3 (2%); balsam of Peru, 1 (1%); formaldehyde, 2 (1%); fragrance mix, 3 (2%); and Kathon CG, 3 (2%). The diagnosis of cosmetic allergy was judged to be 'proven' in three cases (2%), and 'possible' in seven individuals (5%). Thus, in only 10 (7%) out of 150 patients with side-effects from cosmetics and toiletries was contact allergy to these products considered to be the cause. The majority of reactions were due to irritation from personal cleanliness products such as soaps, shampoos, bath foams and deodorants.

This study also showed that irritant effects of cosmetics may worsen pre-existing dermatoses such as seborrhoeic dermatitis, acne and rosacea. As in the previous study,[2] it was demonstrated that an atopic diathesis predisposes to cosmetic-related irritant side-effects.[3]

Patients consulting the dermatologist

In dermatological practice, allergy to cosmetic products has been diagnosed in 0.6% of all referrals and in approximately 5.5% of all patients patch-tested for suspected allergic contact dermatitis.[4] This percentage appears to be increasing: of 576 patients tested in 1987–88, 57 (10%) were allergic to cosmetic products.[5] No figures on side-effects other than contact allergic reactions have been published.

Products causing cosmetic allergy and responsible allergens

A total of 119 patients (102 (86%) women, 17 (14%) men) with proven cosmetic-related contact allergy were investigated in a prospective study.[4] The diagnosis was usually made on the basis of a positive patch-test to a cosmetic product. Sometimes, patch-tests with cosmetics were negative, but use tests or repeated open application tests (ROATs) proved the existence of cosmetic allergy.

More than half of all reactions were caused by skin-care products (N = 67, 56%). Next were nail cosmetics (N = 16, 13%), followed by perfumes

($N = 10, 8\%$), hair cosmetics ($N = 7, 6\%$), deodorants ($N = 6, 5\%$) and lip cosmetics ($N = 5, 4\%$).

In order to identify the allergens, 81 patients (68%) were tested with all ingredients of the suspected cosmetic products, 38 (32%) with one or more allergens known to be present in the cosmetics used. All were tested with the European standard series. In this series most reactions were observed to the fragrance mix ($N = 31$, 26%), followed by balsam of Peru ($N = 12$, 10%), formaldehyde ($N = 10$, 8%), wool alcohols ($N = 6$, 5%), quaternium-15 ($N = 5$, 4%) and colophony ($N = 5$, 4%). Ingredient patch-testing revealed a total of 53 cosmetic allergens (Table 2).

The most frequent contact allergen was Kathon CG, which gave a reaction in 33 patients (28%). Second was toluene sulphonamide/formaldehyde resin which caused allergy in 15 patients (13%), followed by oleamidopropyl dimethylamine (13 patients, 11%). Of the classes, preservatives were the most important category implicated with 47 reactions (32%). Fragrances followed with 39 reactions (27%), and emulsifiers with 21 reactions (14%).

Ingredient labelling in the European Community

Dermatologists often see patients with contact dermatitis caused or worsened by cosmetic products. Adequate diagnosis, treatment, and advice are possible only if the offending ingredients can be identified. European Community regulations do not require cosmetic manufacturers to list all ingredients on their products; only about 30 groups of chemicals must be declared on the label. As an almost invariable consequence, little information is provided on the product or package label. Dermatologists, therefore, often have to contact the manufacturers of the cosmetics used by their patients, which usually takes time and sometimes results in undesirable delays in diagnosis or no diagnosis at all. After the allergens responsible for the dermatitis have been identified, patients need advice on which products to avoid and on those that can be used without risking a recurrence of dermatitis. Currently, this is virtually impossible. The solution to the problem is simple: all ingredients of cosmetics and toiletries must be listed on the products or the package label, or both.[5]

The working party European Community Affairs of the European Society of Contact Dermatitis have demonstrated[5] that ingredient labelling would be of great benefit to dermatologists (who could identify the causative allergens); to patients with allergies to cosmetics and to those sensitized to ingredients used in cosmetic products (who could continue using cosmetics without the risk of allergic dermatitis due to cosmetics); and to cosmetic science and the cosmetic industry (which would be provided with data to make its products safer).

The percentage of the general population that is allergic to cosmetics or cosmetic ingredients has been roughly estimated as 2–3% of adults. Consequently, a significant part of the population would benefit from ingredient labelling of cosmetics. The cosmetic industry would suffer no major long-term disadvantages from ingredient labelling, and slight inconveniences could readily be overcome.

Table 2 Classes of causative ingredients ($N = 147$) in 119 patients with cosmetic allergy

		No. of patients
Preservatives		47 (32%)
Kathon CG	33	
Diazolidinyl urea	3	
Quaternium-15	3	
Imidazolidinyl urea	2	
Propylparaben	2	
Other	4	
Fragrances		39 (27%)
Unspecified	15	
Specified	24	
Eugenol	4	
Hydroxycitronellal	4	
Cinnamic alcohol	2	
Citronellol	2	
Geraniol	2	
Isoeugenol	2	
Other	8	
Emulsifiers		21 (14%)
Oleamidopropyl dimethylamine	13	
Cocamidopropyl betaine	3	
Cocamide DEA	2	
Lauramide DEA	1	
Other	2	
Toluenesulphonamide/formaldehyde resin		15 (10%)
Lanolin (derivatives)		4 (3%)
Acetylated lanolin	1	
Eucerit	1	
Lanolin	1	
Lanolin oil	1	
Miscellaneous		21 (14%)

Intensive and repeated consultations have been undertaken with the chairman and the members of the European Commission, members of the Europarliament, consumer organizations and the cosmetic industry. Press conferences and radio/television interviews have been held in various countries. These efforts to convince the legislative authorities of the usefulness and necessity of cosmetic ingredient labelling appear to have been successful.

On 5 February 1991, The Commission of the European Communities published its proposal for a Council Directive amending for the sixth time Directive 76/768/EEC on the approximation of the laws of the Member States relating to cosmetic products. The following point was added to article 6 which states what must be mentioned on the product and the package:

> A list of ingredients in descending order of weight at the time they are added. This list shall be preceded by an appropriate indication including the word 'ingredients'. Where this is impossible for practical reasons, the ingredients must appear on an enclosed leaflet, with either abbreviated information on the container and the packaging or the symbol given in Annex VIII referring the consumer to the ingredients specified. Perfume and aromatic compositions and their raw materials shall be referred to by the word 'perfume'. Ingredients of a concentration of less than 1% may be listed in any order after those of a concentration of more than 1%. Colouring agents may be listed in any order after the other ingredients.

The ingredients may be expressed in a language easily understood by the consumer. To this end, the Commission shall adopt a common ingredients nomenclature.

Member States must take all necessary measures to ensure that from 1 January 1997 neither manufacturers nor importers established within the Community place on the market products which fail to comply with the provisions of the Directive; after 31 December 1997 such products cannot be sold or disposed of to the ultimate consumer.

Roughly, the situation, if indeed adopted, will be the same as in the USA. It will be important for the European Society of Contact Dermatitis to continue conferring with the Commission to achieve optimal conditions.

References

1 Groot AC de, Adverse reactions to cosmetics, Dissertation, University of Groningen, The Netherlands, 1988.
2 Groot AC de, Nater JP, van der Lende R et al, Adverse effects of cosmetics and toiletries: a retrospective study in the general population, *Int J Cosm Sci* (1987) **9**: 255–9
3 Groot AC de, Beverdam ECA, Tjong Ayong C et al, The role of contact allergy in the spectrum of adverse effects caused by cosmetics and toiletries, *Contact Dermatit* (1988) **19**: 195–201.
4 Groot AC de, Bruynzeel DP, Bos JD et al, The allergens in cosmetics, *Arch Dermatol* (1988) **124**: 1525–9.
5 Groot AC de, Labelling cosmetics with their ingredients, *Br Med J* (1990) **300**: 1636–8.

32
Occupational plant dermatitis

R. J. G. Rycroft
St John's Dermatology Centre, St Thomas's Hospital, London SE1 7EH, UK

Even in industrialized agriculture, plants remain a more frequent cause of occupational skin disease than chemicals.[1] Forestry, horticulture and floristry are similarly afflicted. Contact dermatitis accounts for the overwhelming majority of cases, there being an unusual predominance of allergic over irritant contact dermatitis, at least in horticulture and floristry.[2]

The major scourges of outdoor workers of all kinds are poison oak and poison ivy sensitization in areas such as the western USA,[3] and Compositae (Asteraceae) sensitization in many other areas such as the midwestern USA, southern Australia, India and Europe.[4] *Frullania*,[5] a liverwort, and *Cladonia*,[6] a lichen, are additional causes of serious occupational disability among foresters. Airborne contact dermatitis occurs in all these occupational dermatoses.

Among horticulturalists and florists there is a second group of major causes: tulips, alstroemeria, daffodils and, to a lesser extent, primula. 'Tulip fingers' occurs mainly in those who handle the bulbs, but alstroemeria dermatitis occurs mainly from handling the flowers. Both are allergic. 'Daffodil itch' or 'lily rash' is endemic among those who cut, bunch and pack daffodils: this is mainly an irritant contact dermatitis, although sensitization can also occur.[7] Primula allergy is probably more of a domestic than an occupational problem.[8]

Plants of the Anacardiaceae other than poison oak and poison ivy sensitize mango pickers (*Mangifera indica*); operatives processing cashew nuts, cashew-nut shell oil or its industrial products, such as varnishes (*Anacardium occidentale*),[9] oriental lacquer craftsmen (*Rhus verniciflua*),[10] and woodworkers (Rengas wood).[11]

Other common allergic causes include *Codiaeum variegatum* (confusingly also known as 'croton' but to be distinguished from *Croton*, which is highly irritant), recently reported in a florist's delivery driver,[12] colophony in Pinaceae,[13] and garlic, onion, chives and leeks (Alliaceae).[14]

Other common irritant causes include *Dieffenbachia*,[15] *Opuntia* (sabra dermatitis),[16] chicory,[17] and many of the Cruciferae (Brassicaceae)[18] and Euphorbiaceae.[19]

The staple cereal crops oats and barley can cause both irritant and allergic contact dermatitis.[20] Tobacco more commonly causes irritation, rarer cases of sensitization mainly occurring in cigarette and cigar factories.[21]

The Rutaceae[22] and Apiaceae (Umbelliferae)[23] are well known for causing phytophotodermatitis, examples being rue and giant hogweed, respectively. Phototoxicity among celery (Apiaceae) harvesters occurs particularly when it is fungally (or sometimes bacterially) infected.[24] String trimming of weeds puts gardeners at risk from plants such as cow parsley (Apiaceae).[25]

Contact urticaria, irritant or allergic, occurs from a wide variety of plants and plant products encountered occupationally, including lettuce, potato, citrus fruits and strawberries.[26] Protein contact dermatitis from type I allergies to fruits and vegetables occurs in food handlers.[27]

Accurate diagnosis depends on careful history taking as well as appropriate investigation. Patch, prick, scratch, scratch-chamber, open and rub tests may be required.[28] A workplace visit may be needed to detect a plant previously missed.

A change of occupation can often be avoided if the cause can be identified accurately enough, but may be indicated in isolated allergic contact dermatitis or for sensitive-skinned individuals in wet work.

Prevention depends upon pre-employment examination to exclude at least those with previous histories of severe childhood eczema, particularly if with hand involvement, occupational hygiene, truly protective gloves,[29] and rational use of skin-care products.[30] Hyposensitization, although theoretically possible, is too critical a procedure to be recommended routinely.

References

1 O'Malley M, Thun M, Morrison J et al, Surveillance of occupational skin disease using the supplementary data system, *Amer J Ind Med* (1988) **13**: 291–9.
2 Fregert S, Occupational dermatitis in a 10-year material, *Contact Dermat* (1975) **1**: 96–107.
3 Epstein WL, Poison oak and poison ivy dermatitis as an occupational problem, *Cutis* (1974) **13**: 544–8.
4 Diepgen TL, Häberle M, Bäurle G, Fallstricke in der Berufsdermatologie: das aerogene Kontaktekzene auf Pflanzen (Pitfalls in occupational dermatology: airborne contact dermatitis) *Dermat Beruf Umwelt* (1989) **37** 23–5.
5 Mitchell JC, Industrial aspects of 112 cases of allergic contact dermatitis from *Frullania* in British Columbia during a 10-year period, *Contact Dermat* (1981) **7**: 268–9.
6 Salo H, Hannuksela M, Hausen B, Lichen picker's dermatitis (*Cladonia alpestris* (L.) Rab.), *Contact Dermat* (1981) **7**: 9–13.
7 Gude M, Hausen BM, Heitsch H et al, An investigation of the irritant and allergenic properties of daffodils (*Narcissus pseudonarcissus* L., Amaryllidaceae). *Contact Dermat* (1988) **19**: 1–10.
8 Ingber A, Menné T, Primin standard patch testing: 5 years experience, *Contact Dermat* (1990) **23**: 15–19.
9 Reginella RF, Fairfield JC, Marks JG, Hyposensitization to poison ivy after working in a cashew nut shell oil processing factory, *Contact Dermat* (1989) **20**: 274–9.
10 Kawai K, Nakagawa M, Kawai K et al, Hyposensitization to urushiol among Japanese lacquer craftsmen, *Contact Dermat* (1991) **24**: 146–7.
11 Goh CL, Occupational allergic contact dermatitis from Rengas wood, *Contact Dermat* (1988) **18**: 300.
12 Cleenewerck M-B, Martin P, Occupational contact dermatitis due to *Codiaeum variegatum* L., *Chrysanthemum indicum* L., *Chrysanthemum x hortorum* and *Frullania dilatata* L. In: Frosch PJ, Dooms-Goossens A, Lachapelle J-M, et al, (eds). *Current topics in contact dermatitis*, Springer-Verlag: Berlin, 1989, pp. 149–57.
13 Lovell CR, Dannaker CJ, White IR, Dermatitis from X *Cupressocyparis leylandii* and concomitant sensitivity to colophony, *Contact Dermat* (1985) **13**: 344–5.
14 Lautier R, Wendt V, Kontaktallergie auf Alliaceae. Fallbeschreibung und Literaturübersicht (Contact allergy to *Alliaceae*. Case report and literature study), *Dermat Beruf Umwelt* (1985) **33**: 213–5.
15 Ippen I, Wereta-Kubek M, Rose U, Haut- und Schleimhautreaktionen durch Zimmerpflanzen der Gattung Dieffenbachia (Skin and mucous membrane reactions from house plants of the species *Dieffenbachia*), *Dermat Beruf Umwelt* (1986) **34**: 93–101.
16 Banerjee K, A case report of sabra dermatitis, *Ind J Dermatol* (1977) **22**: 159–62.
17 Rycroft RJG, Lovell CR, Harries PG et al, Occupational irritant contact dermatitis from chicory, *Boll Dermatol Allergol Profess* (1987) **2**: 77–82.
18 Van Ketel WG, Bruynzeel DP, Contact dermatitis due to plants in Amsterdam, *Boll Dermatol Allergol Profess* (1987) **2**: 132–8.
19 Urishibata O, Kase K, Irritant contact dermatitis from *Euphorbia marginata*, *Contact Dermat* (1991) **24**: 155–6.
20 Cronin E, Contact dermatitis from barley dust, *Contact Dermat* (1979) **5**: 196.
21 Rycroft RJG, Smith NP, Stok ET et al, Investigation of suspected contact sensitivity to tobacco in cigarette and cigar factory employees, *Contact Dermat* (1981) **7**: 32–8.
22 Ena P, Camarda I, Phytophotodermatitis from *Ruta corsica*, *Contact Dermat* (1990) **22**: 63.
23 Goitre M, Roncarolo G, Bedello PG et al, Occupational phytophotodermatitis from *Heracleum mantegazzianum*: isolation of furocoumarins, *Boll Dermatol Allergol Profess* (1987) **2**: 177–84.
24 Ashwood Smith MJ, Ceska O, Chaudhury SK, Mechanism of photosensitivity reactions of diseased celery, *Br Med J* (1985) **290**: 1249.
25 Oakley AMM, Ive FA, Harrison MA, String trimmer's dermatitis, *J Soc Occup Med* (1986) **36**: 143–4.
26 Grattan CEH, Harman RRM, Contact urticaria to strawberry, *Contact Dermat* (1985) **13**: 191–2.
27 Cronin E, Dermatitis in food handlers. In: Cullen JP, Dahl MV, Golitz LE et al, (eds). *Advances in dermatology*, vol 4, Year Book: Chicago, 1989, pp. 113–23.
28 Hannuksela M, Tests for immediate hypersensitivity. In: Maibach HI (ed.). *Occupational and industrial dermatology*, 2nd Edn, Year Book: Chicago, 1987, pp. 168–78.
29 Marks JG, Allergic contact dermatitis to *Alstroemeria*, *Arch Dermatol* (1988) **124**: 914–6.
30 Thiboutot DM, Hamory BH, Marks JG, Dermatoses in floral shop workers, *J Am Acad Dermatol* (1990) **22**: 54–8.

33
Xenobiotic experimentation: predicting percutaneous penetration

Jonathan Hadgraft and Keith R. Brain
The Welsh School of Pharmacy, University of Wales, P.O. Box 13, Cardiff CF1 3XF, UK

It has been known for many years that substances applied to the skin can penetrate sufficiently to produce systemic effects. In the case of pesticides and industrial chemicals it is important to know the rate of penetration in order to assess the possible toxic effects of inadvertent contact with the material. The most relevant data for assessing the risks from topical exposure to xenobiotics are obtained from in vivo human studies. Conducting human in vivo studies on toxic materials raises serious ethical considerations, particularly until a full toxicity file has been established. In addition, deconvoluting in vivo topical data requires knowledge of the clearance kinetics of the parent compound and its metabolites. This is normally obtained following intravenous administration. Due to the potentially toxic nature of pesticides the amounts that can be administered by the intravenous route have to be very small. This leads to considerable analytical difficulties and it is often necessary to administer the compound in radiolabelled form. Additional ethical problems are then encountered, together with the problem of verification of the integrity of the radiolabelled species.

Current regulatory requirements for registration of pesticides necessitate extensive in vivo experimentation on animals, but the relevance of the results from these is debatable. There are clear structural differences in the relative numbers of hair follicles, epidermal thickness, etc. Recently, the significance of skin lipids has been demonstrated and there are considerable differences in both the content and composition of these between man and experimental animals. Clearance kinetics and metabolism will also differ. It has not been possible to identify a simple correction factor which can be used to correct the permeability coefficient for humans. Rank orders of permeabilities have been produced for certain compounds, but these can be altered by the presence of surfactants and other formulation recipients.

Determining the potential for skin penetration of a new compound

There is increasing interest from all regulatory authorities and industry in the development of in vitro methods of permeation assessment, and their validation by comparison with in vivo determinations. Accessing sufficient quantities of human skin for large scale in vitro penetration studies is difficult and in vitro studies using animal tissues can be misleading or incorrect because of the interspecific variability described above. As a result of our involvement in the in vitro assessment of skin permeation of both pesticides and therapeutic agents, it has become apparent that an estimation of the expected flux of a compound is beneficial in determining the experimental design, particularly with regard to the choice of analytical technique.

Model synthetic membranes have been evaluated as an alternative in vitro method. A number of different lipid-impregnated membranes have been investigated,[1] particularly tetradecane and isopropylmyristate, and some correlations have been found. Further extensive validation is required but it is possible that more suitable model lipids may be identified, such as dipropyleneglycolpelargonate.[2] However, it must be appreciated that the lipids actually present in the intercellular channels of the stratum corneum are complex and form ordered bilayer structures. Any future developments must therefore consider this structuring, which can be altered by the presence of formulation components or the diffusing agent itself. The modelling approach has the attractions that it is not subject to the biological variation found with real tissues, and that it allows the physical chemistry of the transfer process to be probed. When the physicochemical determinants of transfer have been identified it should be possible to construct mathematical models which will predict the absorption profile of a permeant based on simple physicochemical parameters. Our initial attempts to produce mathematical models of skin absorption[3] have shown promise and are discussed below.

Mathematical models

In the simplest terms, the skin can be regarded as a bilaminate structure composed of an outer layer, the stratum corneum, which provides the rate-limiting barrier to the ingress of most compounds. Underlying this is the living viable epidermis which is a significant barrier for extremely lipophilic xenobiotics. The stratum corneum is largely lipophilic in nature whereas the underlying tissue is aqueous; therefore any model must consider the partitioning of the permeant between these layers. The most rigorous approach is to examine the permeation process by considering solutions to Fick's laws of diffusion with appropriate boundary conditions. Due to the complex nature of the skin and the slow transfer properties within it, the solutions require that the non-steady-state kinetics are examined. The solutions to these equations are complex and can only be achieved in the most basic of cases. They have been considered for an interpretation of the diffusion of some esters of nicotinic acid[4] and have been useful in determining that for these compounds the route of transfer is via the intercellular channels that surround the keratinocytes.

The knowledge of the route of penetration has been very useful in interpreting the mechanisms by which permeants cross the barrier function of the skin and how their physicochemical properties influence the absorption rate. Studies using visualization techniques have confirmed the importance of the intercellular route[5] and considerable efforts have been made to identify and quantify the complex array of skin lipids that are located in the channels. The interaction of the permeants and formulation components with the structured lipids will be important in controlling the rate of absorption and any mechanisms by which this can be predicted will be crucial in a complete model of percutaneous penetration. Due to the mathematical problems of identifying unique solutions to Fick's laws of diffusion, more simplistic kinetic approximations have been examined which appear to be useful in predicting absorption rates. The kinetic model retains physicochemical relevance by approximating the different diffusion and partition steps by a series of consecutive and competitive first-order processes. The elements of the model together with a schematic representation of the skin are shown in Figure 1. The various rate constants have the following significance.

The constant k_1 describes diffusion through the stratum corneum, it can be related to the absolute diffusion coefficient within the stratum corneum, D_{SC}, and the diffusional pathlength l_{SC} by the equation

$$k_1 = D_{SC}/l_{SC}^2$$

It should be remembered that the diffusional pathlength is not simply the thickness of the stratum corneum but the tortuous route through the intercellular channels which can be some 15 times the thickness.[4] Following the analysis of the skin penetration of a range of compounds it has been suggested[3] that k_1 can be approximated from the molecular weight (M) of the diffusant by the equation

$$k_1 \text{ (per hour)} = 0.911 \, M^{-1/3}$$

The relationship is crudely based on the fact that the diffusion coefficient is related to the molecular size of the permeant and a cube-root dependency has been found to be adequate for molecules with molecular weights less than 750 D. Further verification of this relationship is required and it will also be necessary to determine whether or not the skin has a molecular weight cut-off for diffusion. It is also possible to examine the way in which penetration enhancers affect the rate of penetration. The constant k_1 will be increased by those such as Azone® and oleic acid which are known to disrupt the structured lipids in the stratum corneum. At the moment there are insufficient data to predict the exact manner in which k_1 will be affected but in the optimization of formulation design it is useful to consider what influence any formulation components may have on the absorption rate.[6] For example, non-ionic surfactants incorporated into the formulation may act as penetration enhancers; the magnitude of effect will vary depending on the

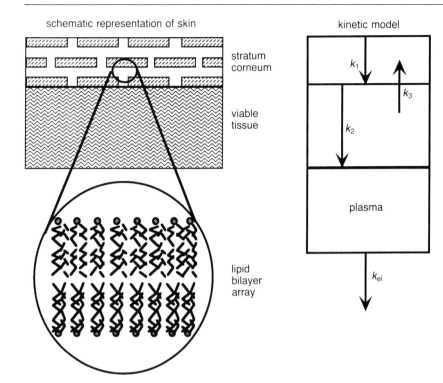

Figure 1

A diagrammatic representation of skin and the associated kinetic model.

physicochemical properties of the penetrant. The more lipophilic the diffusant, the less significant the presence of the type of enhancer that affects the lipid disordering in the stratum corneum. The relative magnitudes of effect can be predicted using the kinetic model. Differences in skin permeability are found at different anatomic sites on the body, these can also be taken into consideration by varying k_1.

The constant k_2 describes the further diffusion of the drug through the viable epidermis, a region which for diffusional purposes resembles an aqueous protein gel. A similar molecular-weight-dependent equation has been identified:

$$k_2 \text{(per hour)} = 14.4\, M^{-1/3}$$

It is well established that lipophilic materials form reservoirs in the stratum corneum and in the model the partitioning behaviour between the stratum corneum and the viable tissue needs to be taken into account and be able to predict reservoir formation. In the kinetic model this is achieved by the competitive rate constant k_3. The ratio k_3/k_2 should provide the partition coefficient of the permeant between the stratum corneum and the viable tissue. The larger the partition coefficient the larger k_3 and the more the material will accumulate in the stratum corneum. An empirical relationship between k_3, k_2 and the octanol pH 7.4 partition coefficient, K_{oct}, has been demonstrated.[3]

$$k_3/k_2 = K_{oct}/5$$

Once the permeant has reached the base of the viable tissue it encounters the microvasculature and rapid uptake and distribution in the systemic circulation occurs. If the volume of distribution (V_d) and elimination rate constant (k_{el}) from the plasma are known, the output from the body (k_{out}) is equal to the product of the two, i.e. $V_d k_{el}$. If the input through the skin (k_{in}) can be predicted from the kinetic model it is then possible to estimate both the amount of xenobiotic absorbed and the associated plasma concentration (C_p). The latter quantity is obtained by equating the input and output functions.

$$k_{in} = C_p k_{out}$$

Before the input can finally be estimated one additional consideration must be addressed. The permeant will have a finite solubility in the skin lipids and a constraint has to be built into the model to allow for the fact that the skin lipids can be saturated with the permeant. The solubility constraint can be estimated by two approaches. The better of the two[7] requires a knowledge of the solubility of the material in octanol [S_{oct}, g/l]. If this is known, the maximum amount of material that can accumulate (per square centimetre) in the skin [sc] is given by:

$$\log [sc] = 1.31 \log[oct] - 0.13$$

If the octanol solubility is unknown another way of estimating [sc] is using the melting point (m.p., °K) since thermodynamic considerations predict that solubilities are related to melting points.[7] The equation that can be used is:

$$\log [sc] = 1.91 \,(10^3/\text{m.p.}) - 2.956$$

Data analysis of a range of diverse compounds[8] using these solubility constraints and the kinetic model for percutaneous penetration described above show that the former method of calculating skin solubility gives a more reliable result. However, the octanol solubilities of the permeants under investigation are not always available whereas the melting points usually are. For compounds that are liquid at room temperature the solubility in the skin lipids is not thought to be a limitation and materials such as nitroglycerin and nicotine which are liquids at ambient temperatures and which are neither excessively polar nor lipophilic permeate the skin rapidly.

Some penetration enhancers (e.g. propylene glycol and N-methylpyrrolidone) act by increasing the solubility of the penetrant in the stratum corneum, these effects can also be estimated using the modelling approach by simple scaling of the allowable solubility in the stratum corneum.

With the in-built solubility limitation and a linear combination of the rate constants k_1, k_2 and k_3, the easiest way to obtain solutions to the kinetic model is to use numerical methods. STELLA software (High Performance Systems Inc.) used on the Apple Macintosh computer provides an ideal computer-based environment for building the basic model shown in Figure 1 and entering the different rate constants.

It is also possible to add features to the model to allow for such processes as metabolism and evaporation from the site prior to absorption. Although these different loss processes have been considered mathematically, there are currently insufficient data to provide good estimates of the precise rate constants involved.[9]

Repeat dosing to the same site can be considered. The effects will be highly dependent on the physicochemical nature of the permeant. It is also easy to model an additional barrier on to the skin surface, as would be encountered when an operative was wearing protective clothing. The effects of the additional barrier can be assessed and the influence of a xenobiotic which forms a reservoir in the clothing after repeated use predicted.

The utility of the model can be considered by application to some drugs which are currently delivered via the transdermal route and for which both physicochemical and pharmocokinetic parameters are available in the literature. The β-blocking agent bupranolol has been investigated for transdermal delivery and plasma levels determined.[10] Using the kinetic model above and the relevant physicochemical and pharmacokinetic parameters it is possible to estimate the plasma levels that should be attained. Figure 2 shows a comparison of the predicted and experimentally determined levels. The correlation is good and the figure also demonstrates the feasibility of describing repeated-dose applications.

Many pesticides have low melting points but are very lipophilic materials. The low melting point and high partition coefficient will mean that they will partition favourably into the stratum corneum but partitioning into the deeper viable tissue will be very slow and it will take a long time to establish maximum flux. Figure 3 shows the plasma-time profile for a theoretical material with a molecular weight of 250 D, log P of 3.0 and a melting point of 100°C. It is assumed that 25 mg is applied over an area of 25 cm^2 and the pharmacokinetics are such that the volume of distribution and elimination half-life are 100 l and 3 h, respectively. Formulation effects can be examined; for example, the figure also shows the effect of a formulation component which increases the solubility in the stratum corneum by a factor of 10 and also promotes partition into the viable tissue by a factor of 10.

Very polar materials tend to have high melting points and will not partition into the lipids of the stratum corneum. Their fluxes will also be slow. Figure 3 also shows the profile that would be seen for a penetrant with log $P = -2$ and a melting point of 300°C.

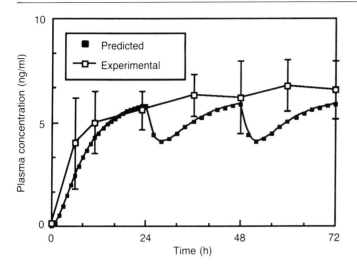

Figure 2

A comparison between the predicted and experimentally determined plasma levels of bupranolol after repeated transdermal delivery.

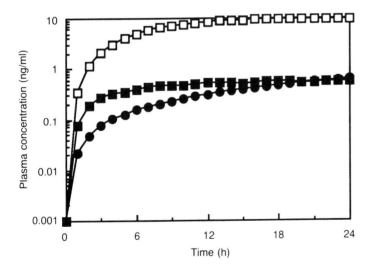

Figure 3

The theoretical profiles of three xenobiotics which have a molecular weight of 250 D, a clearance half-life of 3 h and a volume of distribution of 100 l. A total of 25 mg is applied over a surface area of 25 cm^2. (■) log P = 3.0, melting point = 100°C. (□) The same compound but a formulation component has increased its solubility in the stratum corneum by a factor of 10 and reduced its partitioning between the stratum corneum and the viable tissue by a similar factor. (●) log P = −2, melting point = 300°C.

Conclusions

Mathematical models are useful in predicting the expected fluxes of xenobiotics. This may be particularly useful when ethical considerations preclude in vivo studies. They are useful in assessing the amounts of materials that will penetrate in an in vitro experiment which is essential for determining the appropriate choice of receptor phase and analytical technique. In any modelling it is important, prior to an in vivo human experiment, to confirm the prediction using an in vitro evaluation using excised human skin. The utility of this can be demonstrated in the development of a transdermal delivery system for the administration of the antidepressant Rolipram.[11] Initial mathematical modelling showed that therapeutic levels of 4 ng/ml could be achieved. This was confirmed using an in vitro excised human skin study. A volunteer study was then conducted and the experimentally determined plasma levels were 2 ng/ml, within a factor of 2 of the predictions. Combinations of the appropriate mathematical model and carefully designed in vitro experiments should allow risk assessments of xenobiotics which can be regarded with some confidence.

References

1. Hadgraft J, Ridout G, Development of model membranes for percutaneous absorption measurements. II. Dipalmitoyl phosphatidyl choline, linoleic acid and tetradecane, *Int J Pharmaceut* (1988) **42**: 97–104.
2. Leahy DE, DeMeere ALJ, Wait AR et al, A general description of water–oil partitioning rates using the rotating diffusion cell, *Int J Pharmaceut* (1989) **50**: 117–32.
3. Hadgraft J, Brain KR, Predicting pesticide percutaneous penetration, *Pestic Sci* (1990) **30**: 81–9.
4. Albery WJ, Hadgraft J, Percutaneous absorption: in vivo experiments, *J Pharm Pharmacol* (1979) **31**: 140–7.
5. Elias PM, Epidermal lipids, membranes, and keratinisation, *Int J Dermatol* (1981) **20**: 1–19.
6. Guy RH, Hadgraft J, Physicochemical aspects of percutaneous penetration and its enhancement, *Pharm Res* (1988) **5**: 753–8.
7. Hadgraft J, Cordes G, Wolff M, Prediction of the transdermal delivery of β-blockers. In: Rietbrock N, (ed). *Die Haut als Transportorgan für Arzneistoffe*, Steinkopff-Verlag: Darmstadt, 1990, pp. 133–43.
8. Kasting GB, Smith RL, Cooper ER, Effect of lipid solubility and molecular size on percutaneous absorption. In: Shroot B, Shaefer H, (eds). *Skin pharmacokinetics*, Karger: Basel, 1987, pp. 138–53.
9. Hadgraft J, Guy RH, A theoretical description of the effects of volatility and substantivity on percutaneous absorption, *Int J Pharmaceut* (1984) **18**: 139–48.
10. Green PG, Hadgraft J, Wolff M, Physicochemical aspects of the transdermal delivery of bupranolol, *Int J Pharmaceut* (1989) **55**: 265–9.
11. Hadgraft J, Hill S, Hümpel M et al, Investigations on the percutaneous absorption of the antidepressant Rolipram in vitro and in vivo, *Pharm Res* (1990) **7**: 1307–12.

34
Chemical irritation and predisposing environmental stress (cold wind and hard water)

W. E. Parish
Unilever Research & Engineering, Colworth Laboratory, Colworth House, Sharnbrook, Bedford MK44 ILQ, UK

Introduction

The macroscopic effects of moderate or severe irritants are obvious, but necrosis masks many of the biomolecular changes. The more challenging problems in research on inflammation are the changes in mild irritation, the generation of cytokines, and interaction of receptors and ligands with regulation of epidermal hyperplasia and differentiation, and leukocyte infiltration. The changes in mild irritation are also more relevant to repeated natural environmental insults that change the susceptibility of individuals to irritation by substances that are normally well tolerated.

The skin is a very effective barrier to many potentially irritant substances. It is capable of selective absorption, and of metabolizing susceptible substances. It constantly renews itself and is quick to repair damage to its integrity. Though some insults may have a persistent effect, the constant state of adaptation usually results in a new steady state.

A change in environmental exposure resulting in persistent mild irritation is followed by adaptation and a new steady state as the skin becomes tolerant or hardened. What has been insufficiently studied are the anecdotal histories such as that of an individual who becomes tolerant after a new exposure to mild irritation on a factory assembly line, or to an applied product, e.g. an aftershave lotion, may be no longer tolerant to the previous factory operation or product. This is analogous to a soft hand exposed to friction and, after the immediate physical irritation, becomes calloused although when the occupation ceases the hand becomes soft again and susceptible to further friction.

Epidermal responses to environmental and chemical irritants

The essential features of mild irritation, as resulting from adverse evironmental exposure, are summarized in Figure 1. The main defects, decrease of the lipid barrier and increased transepidermal water loss, are associated with desquamation, loss of surface corneal elasticity and, eventually, surface cracks. Repair is associated with lipid synthesis, proliferation of basal keratinocytes with transient hyperkeratosis until a new steady state is achieved. Repeated insults that do not resolve, initiate an autoinflammatory cycle and may also predispose to irritation from previously tolerated substances.

Individual features of inflammation are not only defects in the integrity of skin function, but are also triggers stimulating repair. Transepidermal water loss (TEWL) is a good example of a defect resulting from exposure to irritants that is also a stimulus to repair. The epidermis synthesizes ceramide lipids which are deposited as lamellar bilayers in the stratum corneum to form the barrier controlling water loss. Damage to this barrier results in loss of water. The amount and rate of loss of water is the stimulus to increased synthesis of lipid by keratinocytes until the barrier is repaired, after which the lipid synthesis returns to the normal rate (Figure 2).[1]

The hyperproliferation of mildly irritated or healing epidermis is another example of a feedback regulating control. Recently it has been reported that the glycosphingolipids and ceramides of the lipid barrier undergo some degradation releasing sphingosine. Sphingosine inhibits protein kinase C

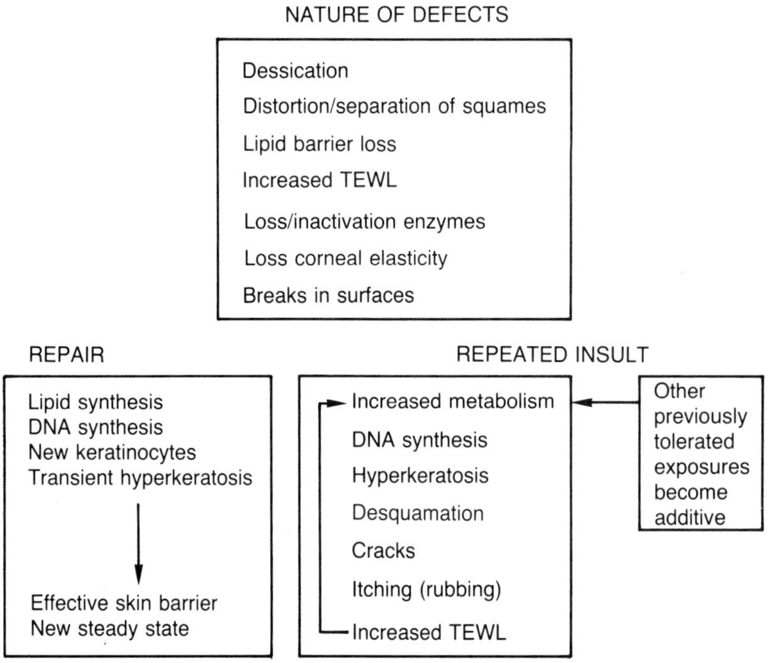

NATURE OF DEFECTS
Dessication
Distortion/separation of squames
Lipid barrier loss
Increased TEWL
Loss/inactivation enzymes
Loss corneal elasticity
Breaks in surfaces
REPAIR
Lipid synthesis
DNA synthesis
New keratinocytes
Transient hyperkeratosis
Effective skin barrier
New steady state
REPEATED INSULT
Increased metabolism
DNA synthesis
Hyperkeratosis
Desquamation
Cracks
Itching (rubbing)
Increased TEWL
Other previously tolerated exposures become additive

Figure 1

The sequence of changes seen in mild environmental damage.

WATER LOSS (TEWL)
STIMULUS
CERAMIDE LAYER
INCREASED LIPID SYNTHESIS REPAIR OF BARRIER

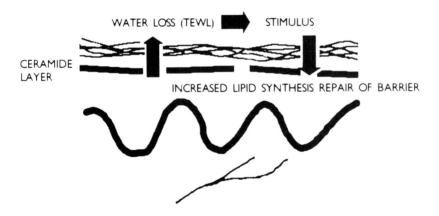

Figure 2

Diagrammatic representation of transepidermal water loss becoming the stimulus to increased lipid synthesis and repair of the barrier. Based on data from Grubauer et al.[1]

which has an essential role in cell proliferation and DNA synthesis. The sphingosine released controls proliferation by the basal cells.[2] It is probable that, during a period of regeneration and repair to the lipid layer, the degradation of lipids and the release of sphingosine are reduced, thus removing the feedback control of proliferation, resulting in increased basal cell mitoses (Figure 3).

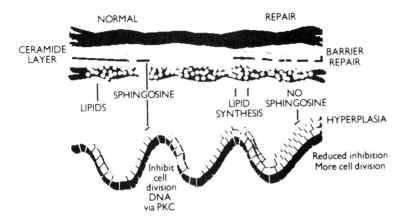

Figure 3

Diagrammatic representation of regulatory feedback control of basal cell proliferation by sphingosine released by degradation of the lipid barrier layer. It is possible that one of the contributory changes leading to increased proliferation by the basal cells after mild irritation is cessation of sphingosine release while the lipid barrier is being repaired. Based on data from Wertz and Downing.[2]

Although the macroscopic changes of inflammation induced by different irritants appear very similar, critical studies on human volunteers exposed to several irritants showed significant differences in epidermal response: sodium lauryl sulphate induced parakeratosis and spongiosis, nonanoic acid induced dyskeratosis with cytoplasmic condensation, and propylene glycol induced basket weave corneum and slight spongiosis. Although benzalkonium and croton oil both induced spongiosis, the nature of the overall changes differed.[3] In tests on human skin in vitro, histological differences between the effects of acid, alkali and clostridial toxin were not so clear cut. Rodent epidermis, being only two or three cells deep, is not a suitable material for such tests. However, there are distinct differences in the amounts of epidermal enzymes released after in vitro topical application of acid, alkali or bacterial toxins, and in the histochemical changes that occur.[4,5] Thus irritants vary in their early effects on the epidermis and in the endogenous substances released, although the macroscopic changes they cause appear very similar.

Much of the degeneration and necrosis observed as secondary or tertiary events following exposure to irritants is due to leucocyte infiltration and activated substances in plasma. Leucocytes, particularly neutrophils, infiltrate the damaged skin and release enzymes which accelerate necrosis and cleave the damaged tissue from normal tissue, facilitating rapid healing. Without the leucocyte infiltration and vascular response there may be little evidence of epidermal damage. The effects of mild irritants applied to living mice for 4 h, with the skin being taken for histological examination at 24 h, were compared with the changes seen in the skin of mice which were killed just before application of the same substance for 4 h, and the carcase maintained at body temperature for 24 h. The in vivo test showed leucocyte infiltration, erythema and destruction of the keratinocytes made susceptible by chemical treatment, whereas the epidermis of mice treated with the irritant after death showed some hydropic degeneration and a few dead cells.[5] This strongly indicates that the role of neutrophils includes inducing much of the epidermal necrosis. In further tests in which mild irritants (1% sodium hydroxide (NaOH), or 3% sodium lauryl sulphate (SLS) or 100% ethanol) were applied to the skin of freshly killed rabbits for 4 h, no consistent changes were seen in samples taken immediately or after 24 h in skin stained for succinic dehydrogenase, acid phosphatase, glucose-β-phosphatase and ATPase, although changes were observed in skin from rabbits treated in vivo, provided that there was leucocyte infiltration.[6] The test provided evidence of variable responses to different irritants in that histochemical reaction products were missing after treatment with one irritant (SLS) but increased by another (NaOH).

Effects of cold dry wind

Opportunity was taken to examine the skin of hands exposed for 3 h to a cold dry wind with a chill factor estimated to be about 20. On day 4 to 5 the hands were macroscopically rough and appeared dry and erythematous. Tape-strip preparations were examined by confocal laser microscopy, and histochemically by staining for lipid (oil red O), acid phosphatase, non-specific esterase and lysozyme. Silicone impressions were examined for roughness using scanning electron microscopy and profilometry. Elasticity was examined by means of a caliper pinch test in which the surface of the skin was raised and time taken for it to retract was measured. Elasticity of the corneum was measured by raising it on the point of a needle. Comparison of the observations made on day 4 to 5 after exposure and on day 18 to 19 (Table 1) showed that exposure resulted in a surface accumulation of dry sheets of corneum, with a significantly roughened surface (Figure 4). Surface lipid as seen in oil red O preparations, acid phosphatase and non-specific esterase was reduced. The values for the two enzymes at 18 to 19 days tended to be greater than seen on other occasions in preparations from the same subject, but no quantitative analysis was done.

The physical irritant effects of short exposure to a severe cold dry wind may be summarized as follows. The stratum corneum showed dessication, desquamation, degeneration/fragmentation, roughness and fine fissures, loss of enzymes, decreased lipid content, and decreased elasticity. The effect on keratinocytes was probably reduced metabolism followed by a rebound metabolic burst, and transient impedence of lipid formation. The dermis showed reduced elasticity, and reduced blood supply during chilling followed by a rebound erythema.

The deterioration of the corneal squames, formation of fine fissures, and decrease in the lipid and enzymes, would favour increased susceptibility to other physical or chemical irritants. No tests were made to assess increased susceptibility resulting from this environmental physical irritation, although the hands were exposed to normal domestic practices without any observed adverse effects.

Hard water as a potential environmental irritant

Water is another potential environmental irritant hazard. Hands are frequently exposed to water, and effects sometimes attributed to detergents and other chemicals may be due to or exacerbated by water, with or without cold winds. Water varies much in quality, and poor condition of skin and hair in some individuals is attributed to hard water. Preliminary tests were made with the objective of preparing a detailed protocol for examining the effects of hard water on skin, particularly on hands.

Tests were done using hard water containing 605 mg/l total solids and 150 mg/l calcium (osmotic pressure was 13 to 14 m.osmol) and spring water containing 30 mg/l calcium. The test was done over 14 days with exposure of one hand to the hard water and the other hand to the soft water for 7 days; the hands were then alternated for 7 days. There was no exposure of the hands to soap or detergents, and exposure to water other than that used for the test was reduced to a minimum, with plastic disposable gloves being used for dirty tasks, bathing and showering. Exposure of the hands to the test water was about 80 min each day (either 80 min or 40 + 40 min) and equal for each hand.

Table 1 Effects of exposure to cold dry wind for 3 h.

Examination	Results	
	Day 4 to 5	Day 18 to 19
Image analysis of tape strips by confocal laser microscopy	Dessicated sheets of corneum. Some fragmented	Flatter, more single cells. Intact
Scanning electron microscopy of silicone impressions	Rough, desquamated scales	Regular pattern, smoother

Elasticity
  Prick test
  Raised corneum on point of needle
	Elevation slowly decreased	Normal response in 2 seconds

Histochemistry*
  Lipid
  Acid phosphatase
  Non-specific esterase
  Lysozyme
	0
	+/0
	+/0
	+
		++
		+++
		+++
		+

* 0, nil or irregular small amounts; + to +++, increasing intensity and regularity of staining.

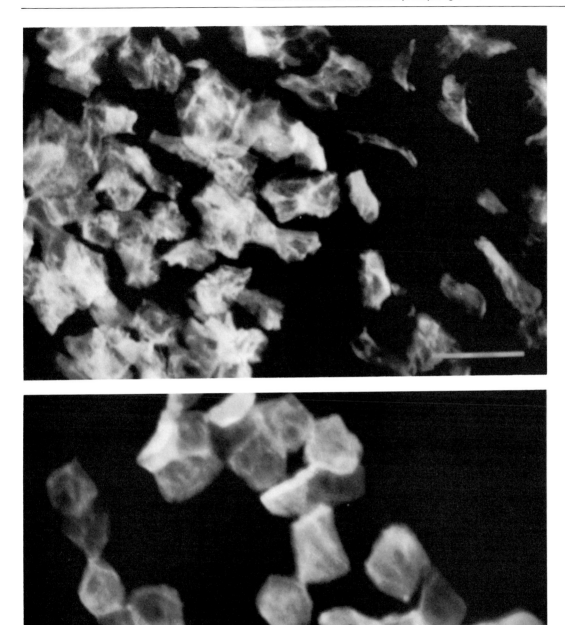

Figure 4

(a) Corneal squames examined by means of the confocal laser microscope 4 days after exposure to cold dry wind. (Chill factor approximately 20.) Scale bar is 50 μm. (b) Corneal squames during restitution of the stratum corneum. Well formed single cells of regular shape, or in small sheets conjoined edge-to-edge.

The volume of water used was 2 l at room temperature.

Hands were examined for TEWL using a Servomed evaporimeter. Three readings were made at each site before other sampling procedures were carried out. There was some variation between the replicate readings because it is difficult to examine a flat surface not traversed by a tendon or vein. Lipid concentrations were determined from five consecutive tape strips, and from tape giving low background readings which were extracted, and examined using high performance thin layer liquid chromatography (HPTLC). Samples were examined for total fatty acids, ceramide and cholesterol. Tape strips of the stratum corneum were also examined for acid phosphatase by histochemical staining and for morphology by using the confocal laser microscope. Silicone impressions were examined for roughness by means of profilometry.

The results obtained (Table 2) show that on each occasion the hand exposed to hard water showed increased TEWL, reduced lipid content, and a slight increase in acid phosphatase. Although the hand exposed to hard water appeared to have a scaly surface there was no evidence of increased roughness by profilometry and only slight changes were detected using the confocal microscope.

A separate examination of the surface corneal squames by X-ray probe analysis revealed a 10-fold greater deposition of calcium on the hard-water exposed hand compared to the soft-water exposed one.

A repeat experiment of 1 month duration in which exposure to hard and distilled water was compared did not result in such clear-cut results, although the analyses are not complete.

It is difficult to make a long-term examination of the surface change of hands as they are continually exposed to the environment and to friction. The surface is uneven which does not facilitate TEWL measurements or sampling of the stratum corneum, particularly by silicone impression. The cross-over technique of alternate exposure of the left and right hands does not remove all the limitations, although it should control the effects of the greater use of the dominant hand.

The cause of the adverse effect is still to be determined. The hard water used was not toxic in that, after membrane filtration and its use as the diluent for culture medium, it supported growth of fibroblasts as well as, or slightly better than, medium prepared with distilled water. Water itself has some adverse effect after prolonged exposure. It is possible that soluble calcium may penetrate the stratum corneum and impede normal differentiation of corneocytes and lipid synthesis in the stratum granulosum. Low concentrations of calcium stimulate the growth of primary cultures of keratinocytes; increasing calcium concentrations decrease colony formation.[7] There is an optimal concentration of calcium for regulating epidermal differentiation in vitro, including expression of the granular cell layer products filaggrin and cornified envelope precursor; increasing the amount of calcium decreases differentiation.[8] Calcium also has a regulatory activity in interepidermal cell binding[9] and is believed to be necessary for the binding of lamellar bodies to the granular cell layer membranes and, therefore, to the formation of the bilayer lipid water barrier.

If there is sufficient soluble calcium in hard water to penetrate the skin, there are several processes in the outer epidermis that are susceptible to calcium imbalance which can result in dysfunction and, possibly, greater susceptibility to irritants.

Predictive tests for identifying and classifying irritants

It is required by the European Economic Community (EEC), the US Food and Drug Administration (USFDA) and other authorities that all new substances are examined for their potential as irritants. In the EEC, irritant or corrosive substances must be labelled with a risk phrase according to the severity of risk. The standard procedure for classifying the potential of substances to induce irritation or corrosion is the 4 h topical application under an occlusive patch; the

Table 2 Comparison of the effects of hard and soft water over 7 days exposure (cross-over left and right hands, total 14 days, preliminary results).

Test	Calcium concentration (mg/l)	
	(soft water)	(hard water)
TEWL	−	+
Lipid concentrations	+	−
Acid phosphatase stratum corneum	−	(+)
Profilometry	−	−
Confocal laser microscopy	−	(+)

−, decreased; (+), slightly increased; +, increased.

albino rabbit being the preferred species. The much greater susceptibility of the rabbit to irritation (Table 3) and the exaggerated, i.e. not representative in practice, conditions of the 4 h application, have led to much criticism that the procedure and classification is not relevant to man. This is a misconception. The tests are designed to identify hazard, i.e. the potential of a substance to induce a particular biological effect.[10] The relevance, or risk for man is a separate consideration. The judgement of risk is not based solely on the potency of the substance to induce hazard, but also on the known activity of similar substances, the concentration, physical state, and the route and frequency of exposure. Identification of hazard is based on the most discriminating test; hence the requirement by regulatory authorities for the 4 h test in rabbits.

Classification is subject to the strict conduct of the protocol, but there are several variables which have a profound influence: (1) species of test animal; (2) method of preparation of the skin; (3) phase of hair cycle; (4) physical state of the test substance; (5) nature of the occlusive patch; and (6) criteria used to assess the reaction.[11] Moreover, there are variations in the protocols required by different regulatory authorities (Table 4) and these also influence classification. Nevertheless, when critically and conscientiously done, the rabbit irritation test detects the irritant hazard potential of substances, and enables comparisons between substances to be made. Labelling for hazard rather than for risk to man, and the substitution of in vitro techniques for in vivo tests are different issues.

In vitro tests for identifying irritants

Several in vitro tests using different end-points of cell damage have been proposed as alternatives to

Table 3 Comparison of the susceptibility of rabbit and man to irritants (10% sodium lauryl sulphate by occlusive patch for 2 h).*

Erythema	Exposure time (h)		
	1	24	48
Response of the majority			
Rabbit ($n = 6$)	Very slight	Moderate	Moderate/severe
Man ($n = 31$)	None	None	None
Number showing greatest effect			
Rabbit ($n = 6$)	Very slight (6)	Severe (2)	Severe (2)
Man ($n = 31$)	Moderate (3)	Moderate (3)	Moderate (1)

+ From Parish and Holland.[11]

Table 4 Predictive irritation tests: variations in official test methods.*

	EEC and OECD	EPA	AFNOR France	Official France
Product	Chemicals	Pesticides	Chemicals	Cosmetics
No. of animals	At least 3	At least 6	6	6
Skin-site state	Intact	Intact	Intact and abraded	Intact and abraded
Exposure	4 h	4 h	4 h	24 h
Dressing	Semi-occlusive	Semi-occlusive	Occlusive	Occlusive

* EEC, European Economic Community; OECD, Organization for European Corporation and Development; EPA, Environment Protection Agency (USA); AFNOR, Association Française de Normalisation.

the use of live animals for predicting irritant properties of substances, although most have been applied to surfactant-induced damage to the eye. No simple in vitro test can reproduce the many features that occur during an inflammatory response in a complex organ like skin. Nevertheless, some of the events of direct toxic damage to epithelium can be reproduced in culture, although the subsequent changes arising from the leucocyte infiltration which induce the macroscopic signs of irritation are lacking. The in vitro target tissues are single cell cultures, usually as monolayers, and usually fibroblasts, keratinocytes or corneal (eye), organ preparations of skin as taken from the body or cultured. Recently, reconstructed skin, known as living skin equivalents, has been used.

Organ preparations, particularly keratome slices of skin, are effective in detecting corrosive and irritant substances but have limitations. In the EEC classification, corrosion, which to a pathologist designates as immediate destruction of tissue, refers to a full depth skin necrosis after 3 min or 3 min to 4 h exposure in a rabbit test. Corrosion can be detected in vitro using several techniques, one of the most reliable being the fall of electrical resistance across the treated skin slice which distinguishes corrosive chemicals from those inducing irritation or other minor damage.[12,13]

Keratome preparations of human skin may also be used to detect irritant properties of substances applied to the corneal surface. Among the criteria used to assess damage are the release of enzymes (acid phosphatase, neutral protease and lactate dehydrogenase), histology and histochemistry, and the use of isotope-labelled lysine and isoleucine.[4,5] The results (Table 5) show that the technique reliably detects irritants, particularly weak irritants, but it is not possible to rank different irritants for their potency. There are other drawbacks, e.g. the availability of surgical samples of skin, the differences in response of some samples, and the handling of potentially infected material.

An alternative is to use cultures of differentiated epidermis grown on collagen–fibroblast rafts, known as living skin equivalents.[14,15] It has been shown that, using benzoyl peroxide as a test substance, it is possible to assess damage by histology and generation of lipoxygenase products from skin equivalents pretreated with tritiated arachidonic acid.[16] Theoretically, the skin equivalent is a good approximation of skin in vivo, but the value of its application to detect irritants may be exaggerated. In our experience using 3-[4,5-dimethylthiazol-2-yl]-2,5-diphenyltetrazolium bromide (MTT) as an end-point of irritation potential as judged by inhibition of metabolism, the contribution to the test result from the keratinocytes may not be significantly more than that arising from the fibroblasts.

Further development and refinement of in vitro tests for identifying irritants is essential, but sufficient experience has already been gained to substitute in vitro for in vivo tests. Major difficulties lie in the selection of the techniques gaining general approval and validation to satisfy regulatory authorities.

Table 5 Results from in vitro skin tests, using epidermal keratome preparations, related to irritation and corrosivity occurring in vivo.*

Test substances	Degree of severity of change†		
	Ensyme release‡	Histology histochemistry‡	Isotope utilization§
Weak irritants	++	+	+++ (I)
Moderate irritants			
Alkalis	+	W	++ (D)
Acids	++	+	ND
Bacterial toxins	+	++	+ (I)
Corrosive chemicals	0	0 to ++	0

* From Parish.[4]
† 0, No change detected; W, weak response; I, increase; D, decrease; ND, not done.
‡ Results from 24 h exposure.
§ Increase or decrease (compared to control) in use of [^{14}C]lysine and [^{14}C]isoleucine after 4 h exposure to the chemical or injection of a bacterial toxin.

References

1. Grubauer G, Elias PM, Feingold KR, Transepidermal water loss: the signal for recovery of barrier structure and function, *J Lipid Res* (1989) **30**: 323–33.
2. Wertz PW, Downing DT, Free sphingosine in human epidermis, *J Invest Dermatol* (1990) **94**: 159–61.
3. Willis CM, Stephens CJM, Wilkinson JD, Epidermal damage induced by irritants in man: a light and electron microscopic study, *J Invest Dermatol* (1989) **93**: 659–99.
4. Parish WE, Relevance of in vitro tests to in vivo acute skin inflammation: potential in vitro applications of skin keratome slices, neutrophils, fibroblasts, mast cells and macrophages, *Food Chem Toxicol* (1985) **23**: 275–85.
5. Parish WE, Evaluation of in vitro predictive tests for irritation and allergic sensitization, *Food Chem Toxicol* (1986) **24**: 481–94.

6 Parish WE, Inflammatory mediators applied to in vitro toxicology: studies on mediator release and two-cell systems, *Toxic in vitro* (1990) **4**: 231–41.
7 Dykes PJ, Jenner LA, Marks R, The effect of calcium on the initiation and growth of human epidermal cells, *Arch Dermatol Res* (1982) **273**: 225–31.
8 Yuspa SH, Kilkenny AE, Steinert PM et al, Expression of murine epidermal differentiation markers is tightly regulated by restricted extracellular calcium concentrations in vitro, *J Cell Biol* (1989) **109**: 1207–17.
9 Patel H, Marcelo C, Voorhees JJ et al, In vitro alterations of epidermal cell adhesion induced by temperature, substrate and cations, *J Invest Dermatol* (1981) **76**: 474–9.
10 EEC Council Directive, 88/379/EEC On laws, regulations and administrative provisions relating to the classification, packaging and labelling of dangerous substances, *Off J Eur Commun* (15 October 1988) **L259**: 10.
11 Parish WE, Holland GH, Experience on the conduct and interpretation of tests for skin irritancy. In: *Classification of chemicals as skin irritants*, European Chemical Industry Ecology and Toxicology Centre: Brussels, 1987, pp68–108.
12 Oliver GJA, Pemberton MA, The identification of corrosive agents for human skin in vitro, *Food Chem Toxicol* (1986) **24**: 513–5.
13 Oliver GJA, Pemberton MA, Rhodes C, An in vitro skin corrosivity test — modification and validation, *Food Chem Toxicol* (1986) **24**: 507–12.
14 Bell E, Ehrlich HP, Buttle DJ et al, Living tissue formed in vitro and accepted as skin-equivalent tissue of full thickness, *Science* (1981) **211**: 1051–4.
15 Regnier M, Arselineau D, Lenoir MC, Human epidermis reconstructed on dermal substrates in vitro: an alternative to animals in skin pharmacology, *Skin Pharmacol* (1990) **3**: 70–85.
16 Dykes PJ, Edwards MJ, O'Donovan MR et al, In vitro reconstitution of human skin: the use of skin equivalents as potential indicators of cutaneous toxicity, *Toxic in vitro* (1991) **5**: 1–8.

35
Immunotoxicity of heavy metal compounds

Hans-Christian Schuppe, Peter Kind, Clive Stringer* and Ernst Gleichmann*

Department of Dermatology, Heinrich-Heine-University, Moorenstr. 5, D-4000 Düsseldorf 1, Germany, and *Division of Immunology, Medical Institute of Environmental Hygiene at the Heinrich-Heine-University, Auf'm Hennekamp 50, D-4000 Düsseldorf 1, Germany

There is growing awareness that the immune system may be a sensitive target for a wide variety of chemicals, including occupational and environmental pollutants, food contaminants, drugs, and their metabolites.[1,2] In this respect, heavy metal compounds have attracted considerable attention.[2,3] Experimental animal studies and observations in humans indicate that the immunotoxic properties of heavy metal compounds are heterogeneous: direct immunosuppressive effects resulting in increased susceptibility to infectious agents or neoplasia have to be distinguished from metal-induced hyper-reactivity which may lead to autoimmunity and/or allergy.[2] However, the pathogenic mechanisms triggering these reactions, e.g. the precise mechanism of sensitization, are unknown. The overview presented here focuses on the immunostimulatory effects inducible by mercury, gold and platinum compounds. With reference to insights from clinical medicine, mouse models were established to investigate the genetic, cellular and chemical/molecular requirements for the induction of immunopathological reactions to mercury, gold and platinum compounds.

Clinical immunopathology of mercury, gold and platinum compounds

Mercury

Inorganic and organic mercury compounds play an important role as occupational and environmental pollutants; in addition, some of them have been used as drugs, and others are still ingredients in preservatives, disinfectants and ointments.[4-6] For the general population the dominating exposure to mercury arises from dental amalgams.[4] Apart from dose-dependent neurotoxic and nephrotoxic effects, mercury compounds can induce a variety of immunopathological alterations in man (Table 1). Mercury compounds are well-known contact sensitizers.[5,6] However, positive patch-test results to mercurials, including preservatives such as merthiolate, are more common than is clinically manifest contact dermatitis.[6] Furthermore, chronic exposure to mercury may lead to nephrotic syndrome due to a membranous glomerulonephritis with granular immunoglobulin G (IgG) deposits in the mesangium and at the glomerular basement membrane.[7] In chronically exposed workers circulating immune complexes and anti-laminin autoantibodies have also been described.[4]

Gold

Compounds containing gold in the Au(I) state, such as disodium aurothiomalate (Na$_2$AuTM), are widely used for the treatment of rheumatoid arthritis. However, the pharmacological mechanism of these slow-acting drugs as well as the reason for an unusually high frequency of immunological side-effects are unknown.[8] After several months of treatment, adverse immune reactions necessitate discontinuation of therapy in up to one-third of patients.[9] Based on a classification developed from studies of murine graft-versus-host (GVH) disease,[10] the adverse reactions to Au(I) drugs may be divided into stimulatory and hypoplastic immunopathological alterations (Table 1). Immunopoten-

Table 1 Survey of immunopathological reactions inducible by mercury, gold and platinum compounds in humans.*

	Compounds†	Clinical manifestations
Mercury	$HgCl_2$, CH_3HgCl, merbromin, merthiolate, amalgam	Contact dermatitis. Membranous glomerulonephritis with mesangial and glomerular basement membrane deposits of IgG. Circulating immune complexes, anti-laminin autoantibodies
Gold	Disodium aurothiomalate (Na_2AuTM), aurothioglucose, auranofin	Lichenoid dermatitis, stomatitis, immune complex glomerulonephritis, alveolitis, eosinophilia, increased serum IgE, formation of antinuclear autoantibodies, thrombocytopaenia, granulocytopaenia, aplastic anaemia
	$AuCl$, $AuCl_3$, $NaAuCl_4$, $KAu(CN)_2$	Contact dermatitis
Platinum	$Na_2[PtCl_6]$, $(NH_4)_2[PtCl_6]$, $(NH_4)_2[PtCl_4]$; cis-$[Pt(NH_3)_2Cl_2]$‡	Rhinitis, conjunctivitis, asthma, urticaria; anaphylactic shock. Contact dermatitis (?)

* See text for references.
† Selected examples.
‡ Anaphylactic reactions.

tiating effects include (lichenoid) dermatitis, stomatitis, eosinophilia and, occurring at lower frequency, immune complex glomerulonephritis, alveolitis, lymphadenopathy, hyper-γ-globulinaemia with increased serum IgE levels and formation of antinuclear autoantibodies (ANA); hypoplastic effects may result in hypo-γ-globulinaemia and aplastic anaemia.[9] Human leucocyte antigens (HLA) B8 and DR3, as well as the non-HLA-linked status of slow sulphoxidation, increase the risk of developing these immune reactions upon exposure to Au(I) drugs.[8] Apart from exanthematous eruptions induced by antirheumatic Au(I) compounds, contact sensitization to both Au(I) and Au(III) salts has been described, sometimes with persistent dermatitis-like or granulomatous patch-test reactions[5] (Table 1).

Platinum

The potent sensitizing properties of certain complex salts of platinum are well documented in workers involved in platinum refining processes[11-14] (Table 1). Up to 50% of exposed persons may develop symptoms of immediate-type allergy such as conjunctivitis, rhinitis, bronchial asthma, or urticaria.[11] Other cutaneous symptoms including pruritus and dermatitis are not well characterized.[5,11] Total serum IgE levels may be elevated.[12-14] The diagnosis of platinum related occupational disease can be confirmed by means of the skin-prick test or by bronchoprovocation eliciting immediate-type reactions to minute doses (10^{-2} to 10^{-8} mol/l) of hexa- and tetra-chloroplatinate complexes $[Pt(IV)Cl_6]^{2-}$ or $[Pt(II)Cl_4]^{2-}$.[12,14] In contrast to these hazardous but highly specific in vivo tests, attempts to demonstrate platinum specific serum IgE or IgG antibodies in radioallergosorbent tests (RAST) remained inconclusive.[14] Moreover, it has been shown that platinum salts can elicit a non-specific histamine release from human basophils, even in the absence of free proteins.[14] Drug-induced anaphylaxis was observed after intravenous administration of the antineoplastic agent cis-dichlorodiaminine platinum.[15]

Murine models for analysing the immunotoxicity of mercury, gold and platinum compounds

Assessment of immunotoxicity by systemic exposure

Comparable to routine toxicology, the assessment of the immunopathological alterations induced by heavy metal compounds is based on long-term systemic exposure of experimental animals, e.g. rodents.[1] In order to evaluate accurate dose–response relationships, parenteral exposure routes (subcutaneous, intramuscular and intraperitoneal) represent a reasonable approach. However, the probable or known route of exposure in humans (inhalation, oral and epicutaneous) must also be considered. Apart from the route of application, the frequency and duration of treatment, the pharmacokinetics, the chemical properties of the compound, and the age, sex, and genetic status of the host are critical parameters. Screening for immunopathological changes includes haematological tests, the histology of lymphoid organs, antibody production, quantification of lymphocyte subpopulations, proliferative and cytotoxic T cell responses, macrophage function, and natural killer cell activities. The data presented here focus on immunoglobulin production, especially autoantibody formation and IgE dysregulation. Delayed-type hypersensitivity (DTH) reactions are demonstrated by means of an ear-swelling test following short-term skin sensitization.

Local lymph node reactivity: the popliteal lymph node assay

The popliteal lymph node (PLN) assay, originally developed for quantifying local GVH reactions,[16] has proved to be a simple and predictive test system for characterizing the immunogenicity, mainly T-cell-sensitizing potential, of low molecular weight chemicals including drugs, metal compounds and non-metal contact allergens.[2,3,17] In the direct PLN assay using mice or rats, the test compound is administered subcutaneously without adjuvant into one hind footpad. The contralateral footpad is not injected or is treated with the solvent only, thus serving as an intra-individual control. Within a few days after injection, an ensuing immune reaction can be assessed by removing and weighing both PLNs. In addition, cell counts, [^{3}H]thymidine incorporation into the PLN, and flow cytometry can be performed. The results are expressed as a PLN index comparing the measured parameter(s) from the injected side with those of the control side. With most chemicals tested (including heavy metal compounds) peak PLN reactions occur between days 4 and 10. Maximum PLN weight indices rarely exceed a level of 10 in the mouse.

When the primary PLN enlargement has subsided (usually after 4–6 weeks), the specificity of the PLN reaction can be demonstrated by an enhanced secondary PLN response to a suboptimal dose of the priming, but not unrelated chemical, injected into the pretreated hind footpad.

In order to demonstrate sensitization of T lymphocytes from animals exposed systemically, an adoptive transfer PLN assay has been established. Spleen or lymph node cells (or isolated T cell populations) from donor mice are inoculated into one hind footpad of syngeneic recipients and re-stimulated with a suboptimal dose of the priming agent.

Another local lymph node assay is the auricular lymph node assay in mice.[18] This test was designed to detect the contact sensitizing potential of chemicals applied topically on the dorsal ear.

Mercury

The various immunopathological effects inducible by $HgCl_2$ were first studied in the rat.[19] Similar observations can be made in the mouse[20–22] (Table 2), a species that offers a number of advantages concerning immunological and genetic characterization. On repeated administration of subtoxic doses of $HgCl_2$ (0.5 mg/kg three times per week), susceptible mouse strains, such as A.SW or B10.S (both carrying the H-2^s haplotype), develop an autoimmune disorder within a few weeks. In contrast to saline treated control animals, $HgCl_2$ treated H-2^s mice exhibited antinuclear autoantibodies (ANA) with persistently high titres of antinucleolar autoantibodies (ANolA) and immune-complex glomerulonephritis.[21] $HgCl_2$ induced ANolA primarily react with fibrillarin, a protein associated with the small nucleolar RNA U3.[23] ANolA with the same specificity can be detected in sera obtained from scleroderma patients.

Apart from autoantibody formation, mercury responsive mice show a dramatic increase in total serum IgE levels which peak 2 weeks after the first injection and rapidly decline by week 4.[22,24] Compared to pretreatment levels or saline-treated

Table 2 Survey of the immunopathological reactions inducible by mercury, gold and platinum compounds in in-bred mouse strains.*

	$HgCl_2$	Na_2AuTM†	$Na_2[PtCl_6]$
Chronic systemic exposure‡			
Increase in total serum			
IgE	+	+	(+)
IgG1	+	+	−
IgM	−	+	−
Autoantibody formation			
ANA§	+	+	(+)
ANolA§	+	+	−
anti-GBM//	+	ND	ND
Immune complex glomerulonephritis	+	+	ND
H-2 haplotype encoding			
Responsiveness	$H-2^s > H-2^b$	$H-2^s > H-2^b$	$H-2^b$
Non-responsiveness	$H-2^d$	$H-2^d$	$H-2^d$
Dermal exposure			
Contact sensitivity (DTH)	+	ND	ND
H-2 haplotype encoding			
Responsiveness	$H-2^d > H-2^b$		
Non-responsiveness	$H-2^s$		
*Local lymph node reactivity***		Au(I)††	Au(III)‡‡
Primary PLN response	+	−	+	+
Secondary PLN response	+	−	+	+
Adoptive secondary PLN response§§	+	−	+	+
Responsiveness of athymic nude mice	−	−	−	−

* See text for references.
ND, not determined.
† Disodium aurothiomalate.
‡ $HgCl_2$: 0.5 mg/kg three times weekly subcutaneously. Na_2AuTM: 22.5 mg/kg weekly intramuscularly. $Na_2[PtCl_6]$: 20–100 μg/kg three times weekly s.c.
§ Antinuclear autoantibodies (ANA); antinucleolar autoantibodies (ANolA).
// Anti-glomerular basement membrane antibodies.
** Determined by means of the popliteal lymph node (PLN) assay.
†† Na_2AuTM and AuCl.
‡‡ $AuCl_3$ and $HAuCl_4$.
§§ Transfer of splenic T cells from chronically treated syngeneic mice.

animals, Hg-treated A.SW mice develop a 160-fold increase in IgE. A significant increase is found in IgG1 and IgG2A levels, which persist, unlike IgE, during further treatment.[24] IgM levels remain unaltered.

Susceptibility to these mercury induced immunopathological changes is genetically controlled[19,21,22] (Table 2). In rats and mice, both major histocompatibility (MHC) class II loci as well as unknown non-MHC loci determine responsiveness. In contrast to mercury susceptible strains (A.SW and B10.S) carrying the H-2^s haplotype, H-2^d mice (BALB/c, DBA/2 and B10.D2) are non-responders or low-responders for ANA/ANolA and hyper-IgE induction. H-2^b mice (C57BL/6) are intermediately susceptible. Inside the MHC, it is the A locus that determines responsiveness for mercury induced ANolA formation.[21] In the presence of a susceptibility allele at A, such as A^s, co-expression of H-2E decreases susceptibility.

There are several lines of evidence indicating that T cells play a central role in the development of mercury induced immunopathological effects. Congenitally athymic rats and mice fail to react to mercury compounds.[19,25] In euthymic rats of a responder strain (Brown–Norway), $HgCl_2$ preferentially activated CD4$^+$ T cells, and these cells were capable of transferring the autoimmune disorder to syngeneic recipients.[26] Furthermore, hyper-IgE and hyper-IgG1 induction as well as an increased expression of MHC class II molecules on B cells[27] of responder mice indicate that interleukin-4 (IL-4) producing T helper (T_H) cells could initiate polyclonal B cell activation. Evidence for the importance of IL-4 arises from experiments in which mercury exposed responder mice (H-2^s)

were treated simultaneously with anti-mouse IL-4 monoclonal antibody.[24] Anti-IL-4 treatment completely abrogated the mercury induced increase in serum IgE and partially inhibited the increase in IgG1 but not IgG2A. Concerning the IgG subclass distribution among mercury induced ANolA, titres of IgG1 ANolA were significantly reduced while those of IgG2a, IgG2b, and IgG3 are increased.[24]

These data suggest that systemic exposure to $HgCl_2$ might impair the balance of cytokines produced by T_H cells in responsive animals. In the mouse, long-term $CD4^+$ T-cell clones can be functionally subdivided according to their lymphokine profile.[28] T_H1 cells synthesize predominantly IL-2 and IFNg, and promote DTH reactions; T_H2 cells provide B-cell help and enhance IgE production via IL-4, IL-5, IL-6 and IL-10 which can antagonize T_H1 activity. There is growing evidence that the functional T_H1/T_H2 dichotomy also plays an important role in the modulation of immune responses in vivo.[28,29] Applying the T_H1/T_H2 concept to the $HgCl_2$ model, it is conceivable that, in $H-2^s$ mice, $HgCl_2$ preferentially activates the T_H2 subset. The non-responder state of $H-2^d$ mice concerning autoimmunity and IgE dysregulation might be due to a lack of mercury induced T_H2 activation.

The concept of a T_H1/T_H2 imbalance induced by $HgCl_2$ is also supported by experiments investigating contact sensitization to $HgCl_2$[30] (Table 2). Five days after repeated epicutaneous application of $HgCl_2$ (0.1% in acetone) on the flanks, an ear-swelling reaction can be elicited by ear challenge (0.05% $HgCl_2$ in acetone/olive oil). DBA/2 and B10.D2 (both $H-2^d$) mice but not B10.S ($H-2^s$) mice are able to mount a DTH reaction to $HgCl_2$ peaking with a maximal increase in ear thickness of 10–14% (controls <3%) on day 4 after challenge. Histologically, the reaction is paralleled by dermal infiltration of mainly polymorphonuclear cells. These results demonstrate that $H-2^d$ mice are not generally unresponsive to $HgCl_2$. In contrast to $H-2^s$ mice, the T_H1 subset might be preferentially activated by mercury in $H-2^d$ mice.

Gold

At least some of the immunological side-effects seen in man also develop in susceptible mouse strains treated with weekly intramuscular injections of Na_2AuTM (22.5 mg/kg)[8] (Table 2). A.SW or B10.S mice carrying the $H-2^s$ haplotype are susceptible to the development of an autoimmune disorder resembling that inducible by $HgCl_2$. Within 10 weeks of treatment, ANA and ANolA can be detected in sera of all mice, with ANolA titres up to 1 : 2560. In addition, Na_2AuTM induces hyper-γ-globulinaemia with gradually increasing serum levels of total IgE, IgG and IgM in the same animals. As intermediate responders, about 70% of C57BL/6 ($H-2^b$) mice were ANA positive. Kidneys from Na_2AuTM treated C57BL/6 mice show prominent mesangial and vascular IgG deposits. DBA/2 ($H-2^d$) mice as well as Na_2TM treated control animals fail to mount any reaction.

In contrast to the potent immunostimulatory properties of chronically administered Na_2AuTM, this Au(I) compound and Na_2TM fail to induce primary PLN responses when tested in various mouse strains[8] (Table 2). However, Au(III) salts, such as $AuCl_3$ and $HAuCl_4$, can induce strong primary PLN reactions, which are dose dependent and T-cell dependent. Secondary PLN responses upon local challenge indicate specificity. However, when Au(III) is reduced to Au(I) by addition of Na_2TM or methionine prior to administration, immunogenicity is significantly decreased. Thus, the oxidation state of gold (Au(III) versus Au(I)) plays a major role in its T-cell immunogenicity, suggesting that the Au(I) of Na_2AuTM must be oxidized to Au(III) before T cells are sensitized and adverse immunological reactions develop. The hypothesis is supported by results obtained with the adoptive transfer PLN assay. Splenic T cells from mice chronically treated with Na_2AuTM elicit a significant secondary PLN response to Au(III), but not Au(I) upon challenge in untreated syngeneic recipients. A probable site for in vivo oxidation of Au(I) compounds is the macrophages.[8]

Platinum

Although some immunopathological alterations inducible by complex platinum salts have been studied in rats,[31] the precise mechanism of sensitization is still unclear. The mouse PLN assay allows demonstration of the immunogenicity of platinum compounds (Table 2). $Na_2[PtCl_6]$ and $(NH_4)_2[PtCl_6]$ induce dose-dependent primary PLN responses in the nanomolar range.[32] In C57BL/6 mice, peak reactions occur around day 6 following injection of 90–180 nmol per animal. PLN reactivity to hexachloroplatinates proves to be T-cell dependent as athymic nude mice fail to mount any response. Differences between various immunocompetent strains of mice reveal that platinum induced PLN responses are genetically controlled. Furthermore,

$[PtCl_6]^{2-}$ primed mice generate a marked secondary response, suggesting antigen specificity. Immunogenicity of platinum in mice is not confined to hexachloroplatinates but other compounds such as the antineoplastic agent cis-dichlorodiaminine platinum can induce comparable PLN reactions.

Preliminary data on mice chronically treated with $Na_2[PtCl_6]$ (20–100 μg/kg three times weekly subcutaneously) indicate that platinum salts can induce ANA with a homogenous staining pattern in up to one-third of C57BL/6 mice but not B10.S mice.[33] Comparable to rat experiments, additional monthly intraperitoneal injections of a classical adjuvant such as $Al(OH)_3$ enhance total serum IgE levels (Table 2).

Conclusions

The immunotoxic properties of mercury, gold and platinum salts include a variety of immunostimulatory effects in both man and experimental animals. Apart from allergic reactions such as contact dermatitis (mercury and gold), or bronchial asthma (platinum), these metal compounds give rise to autoimmune disorders. In murine models, the spectrum of metal-induced immunopathological effects resembles GVH disease, suggesting that T_H cells play a dominant role in their development. In fact, T-cell-deficient, congenitally athymic mice fail to mount local or systemic immune reactions to mercury, gold or platinum compounds. Hyper-Ig (IgE) induction and autoantibody formation in susceptible mouse strains indicate that IL-4 producing T_H2 cells can initiate polyclonal B-cell activation during systemic exposure to heavy-metal compounds. However, the same compound, e.g. $HgCl_2$, may elicit T_H1-mediated DTH reactions. A metal-induced imbalance of T_H1/T_H2 functions, namely the profile of lymphokines preferentially produced, might determine the type of immunopathological alterations that ensue. The type of T_H response is closely linked to MHC class II alleles governing susceptibility to mercury, gold and platinum induced immune reactions.

The precise epitope recognized by the T cells and the mechanisms which give rise to the T cell–B cell interactions are unknown. The protein binding capacity of heavy-metal compounds might affect membrane proteins, intracellular proteins or processing of proteins within immunocompetent cells. One of the hypotheses to be considered is a metal-induced modification of MHC class II molecules and/or self-peptides at the cell surface of B cells and accessory cells creating foreign epitopes. On the other hand, the metal salts could alter T cell receptor functions or amplify T cell–B cell adhesion via other membrane proteins.

A simple method for revealing the T-cell-sensitizing potential of metal compounds in vivo is the PLN assay. Primary PLN responses proved to be dose dependent and specific. The striking difference in T cell immunogenicity found between Au(I) and Au(III) salts demonstrates that, in addition to the original chemical and physical properties of the compound tested, the long-term fate of the compound after incorporation is of critical importance. The concept that immunogenic metabolites are generated within immunocompetent cells, for example oxidation of Au(I) in macrophages, should be generally considered.

Although extrapolation is difficult, insights from murine models should improve the assessment of immunotoxicological risks associated with the exposure to heavy-metal compounds in man. Further studies are necesssary to develop reliable assays characterizing metal-induced activation of murine and human T cells and their lymphokine profiles in vitro.

Acknowledgements

Parts of this work were supported by the programme on Environment and Allergy, Grant No. 07ALL050, from the Federal Ministry of Research and Technology (BMFT), Bonn, Germany and a grant from Degussa AG, Hanau, Germany.

References

1. Dean JH, Thurmond LM, Immunotoxicology: an overview, *Toxicol Pathol* (1987) 15: 265–71.
2. Gleichmann E, Kimber I, Purchase IFH, Immunotoxicology: suppressive and stimulatory effects of drugs and environmental chemicals on the immune system, *Arch Toxicol* (1989) 63: 257–73.
3. Gleichmann E, Kind P, Schuppe H-C et al, Tests predicting sensitization to chemicals and their metabolites, with special reference to heavy metals. In: Dayan AD, Hertel RF, Heseltine E et al, (eds). *Immunotoxicity of metals and immunotoxicology*, Plenum Press: New York, 1990, pp139–51.
4. Friberg L, Eneström S, Inorganic mercury. In: Dayan AD, Hertel RF, Heseltine E et al, (eds). *Immunotoxicity of metals and immunotoxicology*, Plenum Press: New York, 1990, pp163–73.
5. Cronin E, *Contact dermatitis*, Churchill Livingstone: Edinburgh, 1980.

6. Wekkeli M, Hippmann G, Rosenkranz AR et al, Mercury as contact allergen, *Contact Dermatit* (1990) **22**: 295–6.
7. Fillastre JP, Mery JP, Druet P, Drug-induced glomerulonephritis. In: Solez K, Whelton A, (eds). *Acute renal failure*, Marcel Dekker: New York, 1985, pp389–407.
8. Schuhmann D, Kubicka-Muranyi M, Mirtschewa J et al, Adverse immune reactions to gold. I. Chronic treatment with an Au(I) drug sensitizes mouse T cells not to Au(I), but to Au(III) and induces autoantibody formation, *J Immunol* (1990) **145**: 2132–9.
9. Sambrook PN, Browne LD, Champion D et al, Terminations of treatment with gold sodium thiomalate in rheumatoid arthritis, *J Rheumatol* (1982) **9**: 932–4.
10. Gleichmann E, Pals ST, Rolink AG et al, Graft-versus-host reactions (GVHR): clues to the etiopathology of a spectrum of immunological diseases, *Immunol Today* (1984) **5**: 324–32.
11. Roberts HE, Platinosis. A five year study of the effects of soluble platinum salts on employees in a platinum laboratory and refinery, *Arch Ind Hyg* (1951) **4**: 549–59.
12. Biagini RE, Bernstein IL, Gallagher JS et al, The diversity of reaginic immune responses to platinum and palladium metallic salts, *J Allergy Clin Immunol* (1985) **76**: 794–802.
13. Murdoch RD, Pepys J, Hughes EG, IgE antibody responses to platinum group metal salts. A large scale refinery survey, *Br J Ind Med* (1986) **43**: 37–43.
14. Merget R, Schultze-Werninghaus G, Muthorst T et al, Asthma due to the complex salts of platinum — a cross-sectional survey of workers in a platinum refinery, *Clin Allergy* (1988) **18**: 569–80.
15. Khan A, Hill JM, Grater W et al, Atopic hypersensitivity to cis-dichlorodiaminine-platinum and other platinum complexes, *Cancer Res* (1975) **35**: 2766–70.
16. Ford WL, Burr W, Simonsen M, A lymph node weight assay for graft-versus-host activity of rat lymphoid cells, *Transplantation* (1970) **10**: 258–66.
17. Kammüller ME, Thomas C, De Bakker JM et al, The popliteal lymph node assay in mice to screen for the immune disregulating potential of chemicals — a preliminary study, *Int J Immunopharmacol* (1989) **11**: 293–300.
18. Kimber I, Weisenberger C, A murine local lymph node assay in mice for the identification of contact allergens: assay development and results of an initial validation study, *Arch Toxicol* (1989) **63**: 274–82.
19. Pelletier L, Tournade H, Druet P, Immunologically mediated manifestations of metals. In: Dayan AD, Hertel RF, Heseltine E et al, (eds). *Immunotoxicity of metals and immunotoxicology*, Plenum Press: New York, 1990, pp163–73.
20. Hultman P, Eneström S, Murine mercury-induced immune-complex disease: effect of cyclophosphamide treatment and importance of T cells, *Br J Exp Pathol* (1989) **70**: 227–36.
21. Mirtscheva J, Pfeiffer C, De Bruijn JA et al, Immunological alterations inducible by mercury compounds. III. H-2A acts as an immune response and H-2E as an immune 'suppression' locus for $HgCl_2$-induced antinucleolar autoantibodies, *Eur J Immunol* (1989) **19**: 2257–61.
22. Pietsch P, Vohr H-W, Degitz K et al, Immunological alterations inducible by mercury compounds. II. $HgCl_2$ and gold sodium thiomalate enhance serum IgE and IgG concentrations in susceptible mouse strains, *Int Arch Allergy Appl Immunol* (1989) **90**: 47–53.
23. Reuter R, Tessars G, Vohr H-W et al, Mercuric chloride induces autoantibodies against U3 small nuclear ribonucleoprotein in susceptible mice, *Proc Natl Acad Sci USA* (1989) **86**: 237–41.
24. Ochel M, Vohr H-W, Pfeiffer C et al, Il-4 is required for the IgE and IgG1 increase and IgG1 autoantibody formation in mice treated with mercuric chloride, *J Immunol* (1991) **146**: 3006–11.
25. Stiller-Winkler R, Radaskiewicz T, Gleichmann E, Immunopathological signs in mice treated with mercury compounds. I. Identification by the popliteal lymph node assay of responder and non-responder strains, *Int J Immunopharmacol* (1988) **4**: 475–84.
26. Pelletier L, Pasquier R, Rossert J et al, Autoreactive T cells in mercury-induced autoimmunity. Ability to induce the autoimmune disease, *J Immunol* (1988) **140**: 750–4.
27. van Vliet E, Thissen D, Gleichmann E, Mercuric chloride induces mouse T cells to produce interleukin-4 in vitro, *Immunobiology* (1990) **181**: 161–2.
28. Mosmann TR, Coffman RL, Two types of mouse helper T cell clones, *Adv Immunol* (1989) **7**: 111–47.
29. Locksley RM, Scott P, Helper T-cell subsets in mouse leishmaniasis: induction, expansion and effector function, *Immunol Today* (1991) **12**: A58–61.
30. Stringer C, Kind P, Gleichmann E, Contact sensitivity to $HgCl_2$ in mice, *Immunobiology* (1990) **181**: 238–9.
31. Murdoch RD, Pepys J, Enhancement of antibody production by mercury and platinum group metal halide salts. Kinetics of total and ovalbumin-specific IgE synthesis, *Int Arch Allergy Appl Immunol* (1986) **80**: 405–11.
32. Schuppe H-C, Haas-Raida D, Kulig J et al, T-cell-dependent popliteal lymph node reactions in mice inducible by platinum compounds, (1991) (submitted).
33. Schuppe H-C, Haas-Raida D, Kulig J et al, Platinum compounds induce pathological immune reactions in mice, *Immunobiology* (1990) **181**: 238.

36
Human skin response to irritants: the effect of UVA and UVB radiation on the skin barrier

Percy Lehmann, Erhard Hölzle, Bodo Melnik and Gerd Plewig
Department of Dermatology, Hautklinik, Heinrich-Heine-University, Moorenstrasse 5, 4 Düsseldorf 1, Germany

Introduction

By choosing appropriate chemicals ('irritants'), concentrations and certain modes of application, it is possible to induce most of the typical skin lesions known to dermatology on normal skin. Thus, irritation models exist for the study of skin reactivity under various conditions, e.g. in young and aged, in winter and summer, and in healthy and diseased skin.[1,2] Previous studies have shown that skin reactivity to different primary irritants is increased during cold dry winter seasons compared to hot humid summer months.[3]

Epidermal thickening and melanogenesis are protective mechanisms induced by solar irradiation to prevent further actinic damage. There is also evidence that UVB, PUVA, and to a lesser extent UVA can exert a local and also a systemic immunosuppressive effect.[4,5] However, experimental studies on the influence of UV irradiation on skin irritability are scant.[6]

As the protective effect of the skin against environmental agents is mainly exerted by the stratum corneum, we investigated the structure and lipid composition of the horny layer in correlation with skin reactivity towards primary irritants under the modulating influence of UVA and UVB irradiation. In each experimental model the influence of UVA and UVB on the skin barrier and barrier functions was examined separately.

Materials and methods

Irritation models

Two test areas on the back of 30 volunteers (aged 18–31 years) were irradiated with UVA and UVB thrice weekly for three successive weeks. Altogether, 9×100 J/cm^2 UVA and 9×1.5 minimal erythema dose (MED) UVB were applied.

For the UVA irradiation a high intensity metal halide radiator (UVASUN 3000, Mutzhas, Munich, Germany) was used, which emits radiation in the range 330–460 nm.[7] The UVB irradiation was performed with a UV 800 unit lamp equipped with fluorescent bulbs (285–350 nm; Philips TL 20W/12, Waldmann, Villingen/Schwenningen).

After the third week, skin reactivity to primary irritants was evaluated using the following irritation tests on normal, UVA and UVB irradiated skin.

Alkali resistance test

The time required to induce 10 tiny erosions by application of 0.1 N NaOH under the constant pressure of a glass block ($3.5 \times 2 \times 1.5$ cm) was measured.

Dimethylsulphoxide test

Wheals were induced by a 5-min exposure to 100, 95 and 90% dimethylsulphoxide (DMSO). The DMSO solution was applied using a plastic block (15 × 3 × 0.5 cm) in which holes (8 mm in diameter) had been drilled. Skin reaction was evaluted on a 1+ to 4+ scale.

Sodium lauryl sulphate test

After a 24-h application of 1, 2 and 3% sodium lauryl sulphate (SLS) in Duhring chambers, skin irriation was evaluated on a 1+ to 4+ scale.[1,6]

Stratum corneum thickness

In a second series of experiments, biopsies were taken and processed for electron microscopic evaluation of the stratum corneum according to a modification of the method described by Holbrook and Odland.[8] Two days after the third irradiation ($n = 4$) and 2 days after completion of the irradiation series ($n = 10$) 4-mm biopsies were taken from test sites and untreated skin, fixed in 2% glutaraldehyde and 1% osmium tetroxide and embedded in epoxy resin (Epon 812) for electron microscopic evaluation. In order to assure preservation of full thickness stratum corneum, the biopsy was positioned by the aid of two teflon rings between two dialysis membranes for fixation, dehydration and embedding (Figure 1).

Stratum corneum lipids

To investigate further the UVR modulation of the skin barrier stratum corneum lipids were extracted in vivo with ethanol/diethyl ether and quantified after high performance thin layer chromatography. A thorough description of the lipid extraction, thin layer chromatography, and quantification of the lipids has been given elsewhere.[9,10] As we were interested in the deeper stratum corneum barrier lipids, the upper horny cell layers were removed by two strippings with adhesive tape before lipid extraction.

Statistical analysis

From the individual data a mean, standard variation, variance, and standard error of the mean was calculated. The data were tested using an *F*-test for homogeneous distribution. In case of homogeneity a paired Student's *t*-test was used, otherwise a Wilcoxon *U* test was used.

Results

Irritation models

The alkali resistance time was significantly longer in the pre-irradiated areas compared to untreated skin ($P \leq 0.001$). In non-irradiated skin, the time

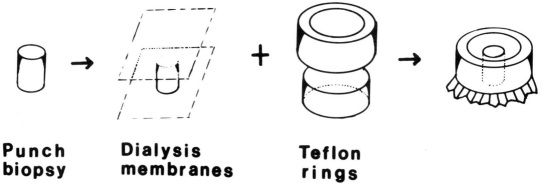

Figure 1

Technique to ensure preservation of full thickness stratum corneum during the processing of tissue for electron microscopy.

taken to induce 10 tiny erosions was 10.10 min (sd ± 2.78), in UVA-irradiated skin 12.58 min (sd ± 3.39) and in UVB-irradiated skin 17.40 min (sd ± 3.28) (Figure 2). The difference between UVA- and UVB-irradiated skin was also significant ($P \leq 0.001$).

The reactivity to DMSO was lowered by pre-irradiation at all concentrations tested. Again, UVB was more effective than UVA (Figure 3). The differences were significant between non-irradiated and pre-irradiated test areas as well as between UVA- and UVB-irradiated skin.

Pre-irradiation also rendered the skin more resistant to SLS at all concentrations used (Figure 4). The differences were significant between normal skin compared to pre-irradiated skin but

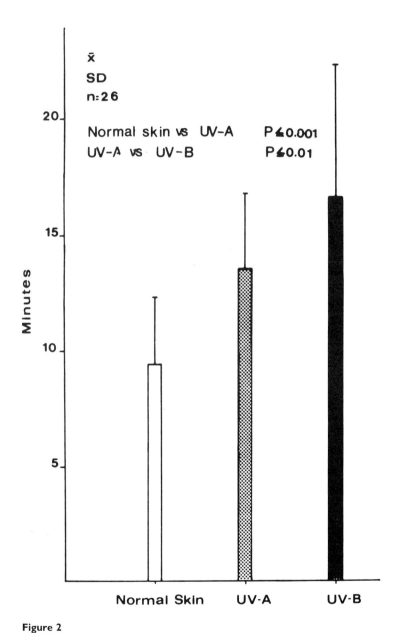

Figure 2

Prolonged alkali resistance time on pre-irradiated test areas compared to normal skin.

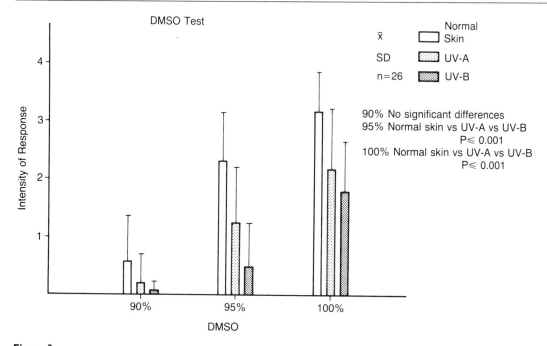

Figure 3

Skin reactivity to DMSO is reduced in the irradiated areas.
UVB is more effective than UVA.

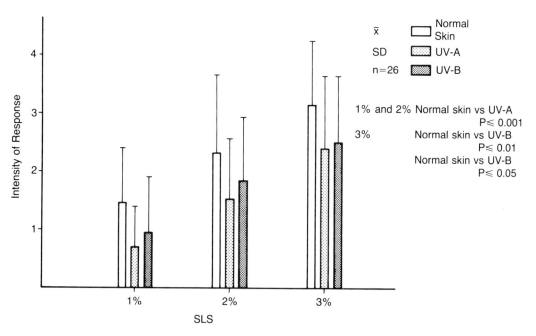

Figure 4

Reduced skin reactivity to SLS in pre-irradiated areas. There is no significant difference between UVA and UVB irradiation.

not between UVA- and UVB-irradiated areas. Thus, in all three irritation models UVA and UVB irradiated areas were more resistant to damage than normal skin. It appeared that the barrier function after UV irradiation was improved. In the majority of experiments UVB irradiation provided a higher degree of protection than UVA irradiation.

Stratum corneum thickness

In non-irradiated skin the mean number of horny cell layers was 16.6. (sd ± 4.4), in UVA-irradiated skin the mean value was 16.8 (sd ± 5.3) and in UVB irradiated areas it was 22.6 (sd ± 4.2). After three irradiations the mean value in the UVA treated sites was 15.8 (sd ± 1.9) and in the UVB-irradiated skin it was 20.9 (sd ± 4.6) (Figure 5). Thus, UVB irradiation led to a significant increase of horny cell layers, which was detectable after as soon as 1 week, whereas UVA did not alter the thickness of the stratum corneum significantly.

Stratum corneum lipids

UVB and, to some extent, UVA exposure resulted in an increase in the amount of all stratum corneum lipids (Table 1). These lipis were ceramides, free sterols, free fatty acids, triglycerides, cholesterol/wax esters, squalene and alkanes. The distribution of the different lipid classes and the quantitative changes following UV irradiation is shown in Figure 6. There was a significant increase in the fractions of alkanes, squalene, triglycerides and free fatty acids after UVA and after UVB treatment.

Table I Effect of UVA and UVB on the total amount of extracted lipid ($n = 20$).

	Extracted lipid ($\mu g/cm^2$)	sem
Before irradiation	43.5	5.0
After UVA irradiation	79.7	11.7*
After UVB irradiation	87.1	11.6*

*$P < 0.01$.

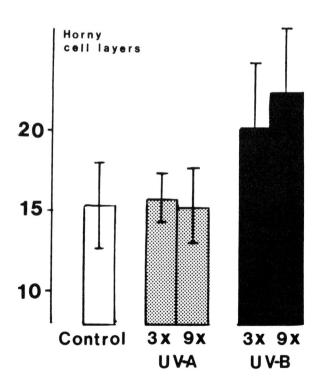

Figure 5

Number of horny cell layers counted on normal skin and after three or nine irradiations with UVA or UVB, respectively.

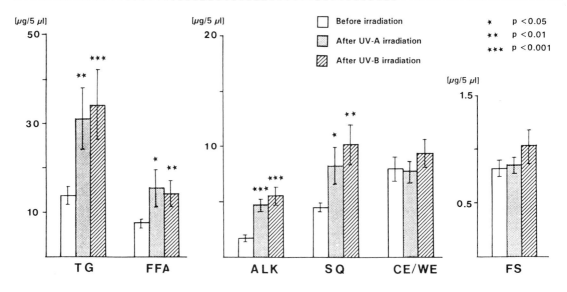

Figure 6

Effect of UVA and UVB on the composition of stratum corneum lipids ($x \pm$ sem). TG, triglycerides; FFA, free fatty acids; ALK, alkanes; SQ, squalene; CE/WE, cholesterol esters/wax esters; FS, free sterols.

Ten subfractions in the ceramide region were separated. An increase in the amount of extracted ceramides after UVA and UVB irradiation was detected in 9 out of 10 subfractions (Figure 7). Two fractions (7a and 7b) were only detectable after UVA or UVB irradiation.

Discussion

Although UV radiation is used to treat dermatoses with impaired barrier function, e.g. atopic dermatitis, the underlying mechanisms for the treatment effects are unknown. To clarify this subject functional (skin reactivity), ultrastructural and lipid biochemistry studies were performed on UV-irradiated skin.

It was demonstrated that UVB as well as UVA irradiation rendered the skin more resistant to primary irritants. This may explain the higher skin irritability seen during the winter months compared to the summer season[3] and the beneficial effects of therapeutic UV irradiation in some dermatoses.

There may be several ways in which UV irradiation can improve barrier function. The induction of a 'Lichtschwiele' (light barrier) after UVB irradiation probably accounts partly for the barrier improvement. However, after UVA irradiation no change in the horny cell layer count was detectable, despite improvement in barrier function. The increase in stratum corneum lipids, which was detected after UVA and UVB irradiation, explains the demonstrated effects of pre-irradiation on the skin reactivity against primary irritants.

Ceramides and acylceramides are believed to be the essential lipid constituents which are functionally and structurally responsible for the maintenance of the epidermal permeability barrier.[11] The beneficial effects of UV irradiation on barrier properties thus may be explained on a morphological basis for UVB (induction of a 'Lichtschwiele') but also by UV-induced biochemical modifications of the stratum corneum lipids after UVB and UVA irradiation. It is possible that impaired barrier function of atopic dry skin might be improved by UV-mediated normalization of diminished stratum corneum ceramides in atopic skin.[12]

References

1   Frosch P, *Hautirritation und empfindliche Haut (Skin irritation and sensitive skin)*, Grosse Scripta 7, Grosse: Berlin, 1985.

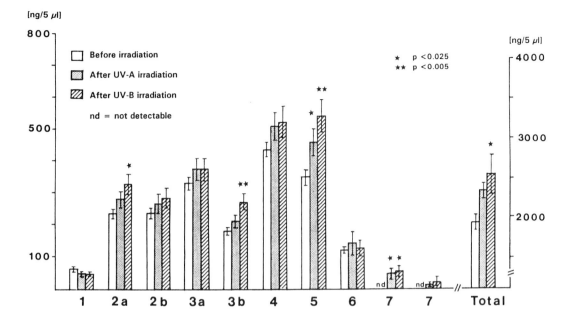

Figure 7

Increase in stratum corneum ceramides after UV irradiation ($x \pm$ sem). Ceramides are depicted in decreasing order of polarity, ceramide 1 being the most polar.

2 Lehmann P, Photodiagnostische Testverfahren. Experimentelle Untersuchungen zur UV-Gewöhnung der Haut, provokative Testverfahren bei Lichtdermatosen und im tierexperimentellen Modell, Habilitationsschrift (Photodiagnostic test procedures. Investigations on skin adaptation to UV-injury, provocative UV-testing in photodermatoses and in animal models), 1989, Heinrich-Heine-Universität, Düsseldorf.

3 Agner T, Serup J, Seasonal variations of skin resistance to irritants, *Br J Dermatol* (1989) **121**: 323–8.

4 Kripke ML, Photoimmunology: the first decade. In: Hönigsmann H, Stingl G, (eds). *Current problems in dermatology 15: Therapeutic photomedicine*, Karger: Basel, 1986, pp164–75.

5 Kripke ML, Morison WL, Modulation of immune function by UV radiation, *J Invest Dermatol* (1985) **85**: 62s–6s.

6 Lehmann P, Helbig S, Hölzle E et al, Bestrahlung mit UV-A oder UV-B wirkt protektiv gegenüber Irritantien (Irradiation with UVA or UVB is protective against primary irritants), *Zentralbl Hautkr* (1988) **154**: 686–92.

7 Mutzhas MF, Hölzle E, Hofmann C et al, A new apparatus with high radiation energy between 330–460 nm: physical description and dermatological applications, *J Invest Dermatol* (1981) **76**: 42–7.

8 Holbrook KA, Odland GF, Regional differences in the thickness (cell layers) of the human stratum corneum: an ultrastructural analysis, *J Invest Dermatol* (1974) **62**: 415–22.

9 Melnik BC, Hollmann J, Erler E et al, Microanalytical screening of all major stratum corneum lipids by sequential high-performance-thin-layer-chromatography, *J Invest Dermatol* (1989) **92**: 231–4.

10 Wefers H, Melnik BC, Flür M et al, Influence of UV-irradiation on the composition of human stratum corneum lipids, *J Invest Dermatol* (1991) **96**: 959–62.

11 Elias P, Epidermal lipids, barrier function and desquamation, *J Invest Dermatol* (1983) **80**: 44s–9s.

12 Melnik B, Hollmann J, Plewig G, Decreased stratum corneum ceramides in atopic individuals — a pathobiochemical factor in xerosis?, *Br J Dermatol* (1988) **119**: 547–8.

37
Sodium lauryl sulphate penetration through human skin

Bo Forslind, Axel Emilson and Magnus Lindberg*
EDRG, Department of Medical Biophysics, Karolinska Institute, Stockholm, and *Department of Occupational Dermatology, University Hospital, Uppsala, Sweden

Introduction

The main skin barrier function is assigned to the stratum corneum of the epidermis. The structure of stratum corneum has been described by Elias[1] in terms of a two-compartment model, 'the brick and mortar model', which visualizes the corneocytes as the bricks and intercellular lipids as the mortar. This model implies that the barrier for water and water-soluble substances is localized to the intercellular lipid bilamellar layers.

The intercellular spaces between corneocytes are filled with stacked multiples of lipid bilayers.[1–3] The function of the stratum corneum barrier will depend on several factors, including the composition and mass of the lipid, the fluidity of the lipids as well as the hydration of the stratum corneum. If the lipids are in a crystalline phase, i.e. below the characteristic transition temperature, they will be maximally close-packed and allowed minimal mobility, which will make passage even for small molecules like water difficult. On the other hand, in the fluid crystalline state, the lipid mobility in the bilayer plane as well as the permeability through the bilayers will increase with rising temperature.

The fact that the permeability of lipid bilayers is more or less directly related to the fluidity of the constituent lipids means that the permeability will be influenced by the length and the saturation of the fatty acyl carbon chains. The multiple lipid bilayers of the stratum corneum barrier are composed of long fatty acid chains.[4] Available data suggest that the thermal transition of the stratum corneum lipids from the close-packed crystalline state to a more fluid crystalline state occurs within the temperature range of 38–40°C,[5] i.e. at temperatures well above normal skin temperature.[6]

Detergents are known to interact with biological membranes and the effect may be an increased permeability. The mechanism is most probably due to the interaction with the intercellular lipid bilayers, inducing increasing disorder in the packing of the lipids.[7] In addition, detergents may cause a decrease in the transition temperature for the layer as a whole.[8]

The aim of our present, ongoing study is to investigate the influence of temperature on the penetration of detergents, notably sodium lauryl sulphate (SLS). This, the most commonly used detergent to induce skin irritation, is studied in relation to its penetration through human skin in an in vitro system. The influence of temperature was our main concern, and only the physical aspects of the barrier function were considered.

In order to evaluate the effect on the transition temperature by SLS itself, penetration experiments with a lower SLS-detergent concentration were performed.

Materials and methods

Materials

SLS labelled with ^{35}S, initial specific activity 1mCi, was obtained from Amersham International. Unlabelled SLS was obtained from KEBO, Stockholm.

Full-thickness human skin was obtained at plastic reconstruction surgery of the female breast region.

The skin was either used fresh from the operating theatre or frozen at −28°C for various periods of time before the experiments were started.

A horizontal static diffusion cell model was used for the penetration studies. The area of skin exposed to solutes was 1.33 cm², and the volume of each chamber was 60 ml. As only the physical properties of the skin barrier were considered, we used distilled water as the vehicle in order to avoid the protein extracting capacity of physiological salt solutions.

At the end of the experiment, the radioactivity of the substance in the donor and recipient chambers was determined by liquid scintillation counting (Packard liquid spectrometer system, model 2425, Packard Inc.) using Biofluor (NEN Research) scintillation fluid.

Diffusion cell studies

The skin was freed from subcutaneous fat tissue, cut into small pieces (approximately 1.5 cm × 1.5 cm) and mounted in the diffusion cell with the epidermal side of the skin towards the donor chamber.

Two different donor solutions were used: (i) 2% SLS with added [^{35}S]SLS, $N = 18$; frozen <1 month, $N = 11$; frozen ≥1 month, $n = 7$; (ii) 0.5% SLS with [^{35}S]SLS added, $N = 15$; frozen <1 month, $n = 5$; 10 fresh samples.

The recipient solution initially contained only distilled water. Each experiment set was run at ambient temperature (22°C) and with thermostatic control at 40°C and 60°C, for 18 h.

Scintillation procedure

Three samples (2 ml) were taken from the recipient chamber of each temperature set. In addition, 2 ml of the donor solution was sampled. The samples were dried in heat chambers overnight and after complete evaporation of the solutions, 4 ml Biofluor scintillation fluid was added and the sealed vessels were continuously agitated for 48 h. Subsequently the radioactivity was determined by means of scintillation counting. An average value was calculated for each temperature and the value for the 22°C experiment was set as 100% to which the data at 40°C and 60°C were related.

Table 1 Penetration of 2% SLS at 40°C and 60°C (related to 22°C as 100%)

Sample	22°C	N	40°C	N	60°C	N
All skin	100	18	273	18	641	16
Fresh skin	100	11	327	11	829	11
Frozen skin	100	7	188	7	227	5

Data analysis

Statistical analysis was done using Student's t-test.

Results

Experiments with 2% SLS

The penetration of [^{35}S]SLS at temperatures above ambient was significantly increased ($P < 0.05$) as compared to baseline penetration at ambient temperature (22°C).

When considering the possible difference between the pre-history of our samples, i.e. non-frozen versus frozen, the data indicate that some differences in penetration occur. Thus the increase in penetration related to temperature is not as prominent in the samples which had been frozen for >1 month. Statistical evaluation of the differences shown between the frozen and non-frozen samples is not feasible at present as the number of samples in each subgroup was too small for such an analysis to be made (Table I)(Figure 1).

Experiments with 0.5% SLS

The penetration of [^{35}S]SLS at 40°C was only slightly increased compared to baseline. At 60°C, penetration was conspicuous in comparison to the 20°C data. It is notable that the increase in penetration is related to temperature in a non-linear fashion in the temperature range 20–60°C (Figure 2).

Discussion

The results obtained support a tentative model for the organization of the stratum corneum lipids where the transition from a crystalline phase to a fluid crystalline phase occurs just below 40°C. The

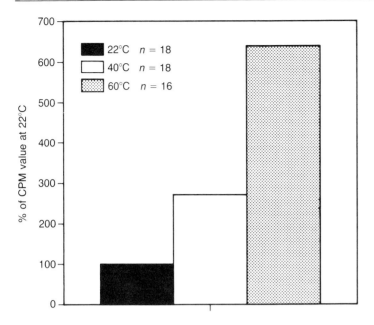

Figure 1

Penetration of [^{35}S]SLS (2.0% SLS) through human skin.

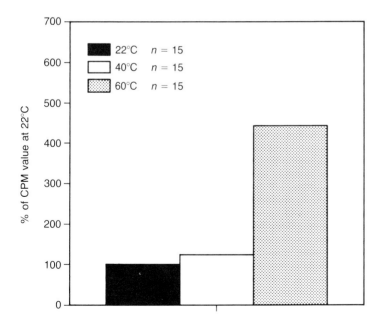

Figure 2

Penetration of [^{35}S]SLS (0.5% SLS) through human skin.

conspicuous increase in SLS and nickel permeability at 40°C compared to 22°C is in accordance with the concept that at temperatures above the transition temperature, i.e. in the fluid crystalline phase, the membrane units are less densely packed than below the transition temperature. This will consequently result in a higher permeability for water and other compounds at 40°C compared to conditions prevailing at ambient temperature. At 60°C the membranes are expected to show a still higher degree of disorder, which may even approach a chaotic state. Hence the barrier function should drop to a minimum, as the data obtained indicate.

The answer to the question why skin samples that were frozen for >1 month showed slightly different properties compared to the fresh skin samples should probably be sought in the quantitative changes in the membranes related to their content of proteins, proteolipids and glycolipids. It is well known that frozen pure lipid preparations return to their original bilamellar structural organization on thawing. Configuration changes in the quaternary, tertiary and secondary structure of the said components probably perturb the bilamellar organization to a certain extent upon freezing and thawing. Thus, fresh samples are probably more representative of the in vivo situation than previously frozen ones.

The 0.5% SLS experiments resulting in a minor increase of penetration of [^{35}S]SLS at 40°C compared to 22°C can be explained in terms of 'trapping' of the detergent in the intercellular lipid bilayers. Since the absolute amount of SLS is smaller with this lower detergent concentration, the trapping will be more conspicuous than is the case with 2.0% SLS.

Acknowledgements

This study was generously supported by Sterisol AB, the funds of the Karolinska Institute and Edvard Welander foundation (B.F. and M.L.) and the Anders Otto Swärds foundation (A.E.).

References

1 Elias PM, Epidermal lipids, barrier function and desquamation, *J Invest Dermatol* (1983) **80**: 44–9.
2 Landmann L, Epidermal permeability barrier: transformation of lamellar granule disks into intercellular sheets by a membrane fusion process, *J Invest Dermatol* (1986) **87**: 202–9.
3 Swartzendruber DC, Wertz PW, Kitko DJ et al, Molecular models of the intercellular lipid lamellae in mammalian stratum corneum, *J Invest Dermatol* (1989) **92**: 251–7.
4 Gray GM, White RJ, Glycosphingolipids and ceramides in human and in pig epidermis, *J Invest Dermatol* (1978) **70**: 336–41.
5 Refeld SJ, Plachy WZ, Williams ML et al, Calorimetric and electron spin resonance examination of lipid transitions in human stratum corneum: molecular basis for normal cohesion and abnormal desquamation in recessive x-linked ichthyosis, *J Invest Dermatol* (1988) **91**: 494–505.
6 Tanaka T, Sakanashi T, Kaneko N et al, Spin labeling study on membrane fluidity of epidermal cell (cow snout epidermis), *J Invest Dermatol* (1986) **87**: 745–7.
7 Golden GM, Guzek DB, Kennedy AH et al, Stratum corneum lipid phase transitions and water barrier properties, *Biochemistry* (1987) **21**: 2382–8.
8 Inoue T, Iwanage T, Fukushima K et al, Interaction of surfactants with bilayer of negatively charged lipid: effect on gel-to-liquid crystalline phase transition of dilauroylphosphatidic acid vesicle membrane, *Chem Phys Lipids* (1988) **48**: 189–96.

38
Do transition metals in household and personal products play a role in allergic contact dermatitis?

D. A. Basketter, E. G. Barnes and C. F. Allenby*

*Environmental Safety Laboratory, Unilever Research, Sharnbrook, MK44 1LQ, UK, and *Lister Hospital, Stevenage, Herts, UK*

Introduction

The transition metals nickel, cobalt and chromium are a major cause of allergic contact dermatitis (ACD).[1] Concern is expressed periodically that traces of nickel, cobalt or chromium in household and/or personal products may contribute to the incidence of ACD, especially that expressed as hand eczema in housepersons.[2-5] The refractory nature of hand eczema and its association particularly with nickel allergy is well known.[6] Nevertheless, whilst not always easy to interpret, epidemiological data do indicate that there is little or no relationship between the overall incidence of ACD to the transition metals and trace levels in household or personal products.[7] To investigate this issue further, we assessed whether trace levels of the three named metals could elicit allergic skin reactions in previously sensitized individuals and considered factors affecting the threshold of sensitivity.

Materials and methods

Nickel sulphate (99.999%) and cobalt chloride (99.999%, 2 ppm nickel by analysis) were obtained from Aldrich (Gillingham, UK). Potassium dichromate (Analar grade), sodium dodecyl sulphate (SDS) (99%) and ethylene diamine tetraacetic acid (Analar grade) were obtained from BDH (Poole, UK).

Panels of subjects allergic to either nickel, cobalt or chromium, as judged by positive patch test and/or clinical history, were recruited. Ethical approval was obtained for each of the studies.

Dilutions of the metal salts were applied to both normal and surfactant treated skin of the back and forearm. Patches were applied in Finn chambers on Scanpor tape (Epitest, Oy) in the standard way either to the back or to the forearm for 48 h and read according to the International Contact Dermatitis Research Group (ICDRG) scale.

Metal analyses on products and on patch-test materials were carried out by atomic absorption or plasma emission spectrophotometry.

Results

The dose response to challenge with nickel in a panel of 20 nickel allergic subjects is shown in Table 1. On normal back or forearm skin, only a minority reacted to 10 ppm. None responded at the 1 ppm level. However, sensitivity was enhanced on forearm skin pretreated by immersion in SDS,[8] such that two subjects reacted weakly but positively to 0.5 ppm.

In a small panel of cobalt allergic subjects (Table 2), none reacted to a concentration of less than 1000 ppm cobalt on normal back skin. The threshold was significantly reduced to between 1 and 10 ppm by pretreatment of the test site with SDS for 24 h.[9]

Table 3 presents the data for a group of chromium allergic subjects. Whilst 2 of 14 subjects reacted to a concentration of approximately 9 ppm chromium, none reacted to 0.09 ppm. Although the study did not include pretreatment of skin sites with SDS, patch tests with fabric washing powder at up to 1% (equivalent to 0.16 ppm chromium) failed to elicit any reproducible positive reactions.[10]

Table 1 Nickel dose response (panel size 20).

	Nickel concentration (ppm)			
	10	5	1	0.5
Back skin	3	1	0	ND
Forearm skin	3	3	0	ND
SDS treated forearm skin	12	6	3	2

ND, not done.

Table 2 Cobalt dose response (panel size 6).

	Cobalt concentration (ppm)				
	10 000	1000	100	10	1
Back skin	6	1	0	0	0
SDS treated back skin	ND	6	5	3	0

ND, not done.

Table 3 Chromium dose response (panel size 14 or 7).

	Chromium concentration (ppm)				
	1770	885	88.5	8.9	0.09
Back skin	14	11	2*	2	0*

* Panel size 7.

Table 4 Effect of EDTA on allergic reactions to nickel, cobalt and chromium.

	Without EDTA	With EDTA*
Nickel	10	5
Cobalt	6	1
Chromium	11	9

* Approximately equimolar EDTA except for chromium with a three-fold molar excess.

In some circumstances it is possible to chelate the transition metals to reduce their effective concentration. To model this, reactions were assessed in the presence and absence of EDTA (Table 4). EDTA was very effective at reducing the frequency of responses to nickel and cobalt, but not to chromium.

Since allergy to the transition metals discussed in this paper is common, and subjects can react to quite low levels, it is important to ensure that trace contamination of household and personal products is acceptably low. Table 5 summarizes the analytical data on nickel, cobalt and chromium trace contamination of 325 products from 15 European countries. Maximum levels found were rarely in excess of 1 ppm, and were commonly below the limit of detection for the product matrix.

Discussion

There is concern that trace contamination of products by the transition metals nickel, cobalt and chromium can give rise to eczema in subjects with an existing allergy.[2–5] Whilst household products such as detergents and bleaches have been implicated in the past,[3,11,12] there are also occasions when personal products have been found to be responsible.[13–15] Thus, although the important and substantial sources of metal contact are well known (jewellery, cement, etc.; see Burrows[16] for a review), it is important to identify the levels in other consumer products and relate these to individual susceptibility, particularly in damaged skin.

Analysis of a wide range of Unilever products from 15 European countries, with rare exceptions, showed levels of nickel, cobalt and chromium to be <1 ppm. The clinical studies described[8–10] have shown that under 'worst case' conditions of 48 h occluded application onto surfactant damaged skin, the minimum eliciting concentration for these metals is generally in the range 1–10 ppm.

On the basis of these data we consider that, if the three metals are kept to these very low levels, then the risk of transition metal dermatitis via contact with household or personal products, even in very sensitive individuals, is extremely low.

References

1 Fowler JF, Allergic contact dermatitis to metals, *Am J Contact Dermatit* (1990) **1**: 212–23.
2 Nava C, Campiglio R, Caravelli G et al, I sali di chromo e nichel come causa di dermatite allergica da contatto con detergenti (Chrome and nickel salts as a cause of allergic contact dermatitis from detergents), *Med Lav* (1987) **78**: 405–12.
3 Vilaplana J, Grimalt F, Romaguera C et al, Cobalt content of household cleaning products, *Contact Dermatit* (1987) **16**: 139–41.

Table 5 Analysis of the nickel, chromium and cobalt content of products from 15 European countries.

	Concentration detected (ppm)*								
	Nickel			Cobalt			Chromium		
	Mean	Min.	Max.	Mean	Min.	Max.	Mean	Min.	Max.
4 toothpastes	<1	—	<1	<1	—	<1	1	<1	1.2
11 hand creams	<1	—	<1	<1	—	<1	<1	—	<1
6 shampoos	<1	—	<1	<1	—	<1	<1	—	<1
3 conditioners	<1	—	<1	<1	—	<1	<1	—	<1
1 hair dye	<1	—	<1	<1	—	<1	<1	—	<1
4 roll on deodorants	<1	—	<1	<1	—	<1	<1	—	<1
3 stick deodorants	<1	—	<1	<1	—	<1	<1	—	<1
1 facial wash	<1	—	<1	<1	—	<1	1.1	—	1.1
1 liquid soap	<1	—	<1	<1	—	<1	<1	—	<1
1 nail varnish	<1	—	<1	<1	—	<1	<1	—	<1
1 lipstick	<1	—	<1	<1	—	<1	<1	—	<1
6 aerosol deodorants	<1	—	<1	<1	—	<1	<1	—	<1
213 fabric washing powders	<1.0	<0.2	16.0†	<0.22	<0.1	0.6	<1.2	<0.1	5.8†
39 dish washing liquids	<0.25	<0.2	0.8	<0.24	<0.1	0.25	<0.36	<0.2	1.4
19 fabric washing liquids	<0.29	<0.15	0.8	<0.22	<0.1	0.25	<0.28	<0.2	0.5
2 fabric softeners	<0.2	—	<0.2	<0.25	—	<0.25	<0.2	—	<0.2
2 bleaches	<0.2	—	<0.2	<0.25	—	<0.25	0.7	0.6	0.8
8 hard surface cleaners	<0.24	<0.13	0.3	<0.25	—	<0.25	0.52	0.4	0.8

* Values are the mean, minimum (min.) and maximum (max.) in parts per million.
† High values found in 1987, now reduced to mean 1.0 ppm nickel and 1.2 ppm chromium.

4   Angelini G, Vena GA, Allergia da contatto al nichel. Considerazioni su vecchie e nuove acquisizioni (Contact allergy to nickel. A consideration of old and new sources), Boll Dermatol Allergol Profess (1989) 4: 5–29.
5   Kokelj F, Nedoclan G, Daris F et al, Nichel e cromo nei detergenti da toilette (Nickel and chrome in detergents and toiletries), Boll Dermatol Allergol Profess (1989) 4: 31–7.
6   Wilkinson DS, Wilkinson JD, Nickel allergy and hand eczema. In: Maibach HI, Menne T, (eds). Nickel and the skin: immunology and toxicology, CRC Press, Boca Raton, FL, 1989, p. 133.
7   Kaestner W, Metallspuren in Waschmitteln und allergiehaeufigkeit — gibt es erkenntnisse ueber einenursaechlichen zusammenhang? (Traces of metals in detergents and the incidence of allergy — is there a correlation between these?) Seifen-Oele-Fette-Wacshe (1988) 149: 213, 269.
8   Basketter DA, Allenby CF, A model to simulate the effect of detergent on skin and evaluate any resulting effect on contact allergic reactions, Contact Dermatit (1990) 23: 291.
9   Allenby CF, Basketter DA, Minimum eliciting patch test concentrations of cobalt, Contact Dermatit (1989) 20: 185–90.
10 Allenby CF, Goodwin BFJ, Influence of detergent washing powders on minimal eliciting patch test concentrations of nickel and chromium, Contact Dermatit (1983) 9: 491–9.
11 Malten KE, Schutter K, van Senden KG et al, Nickel sensitization and detergents, Acta Dermat Venereol (Stockh) (1969) 49: 10–13.
12 Garcia-Perez A, Martin-Pascual A, Sanchez-Misiego A, Chrome content in bleaches and detergents: its relationship to hand dermatitis in women, Acta Dermatol (1973) 53: 353–8.
13 Kasahara N, Nakayama H, Cosmetic dermatitis and metal sensitization, Hifubuyo-Shinryo (1990) 12: 247–50.
14 Van Ketel WG, Liem DH, Eyelid dermatitis from nickel contaminated cosmetics, Contact Dermatit (1981) 7: 217.
15 Goh CL, Ng SK, Kwok SF, Allergic contact dermatitis from nickel in eyeshadow, Contact Dermatit (1989) 20: 380–1.
16 Burrows D, Mischievous metals — chromate, cobalt, nickel and mercury, Clin Exp Dermatol (1989) 14: 266–72.

39
The effect of area of application on the intensity of response to a cutaneous irritant

Peter J. Dykes, Stephanie Hill and Ronald Marks
Department of Dermatology, UWCM, Cardiff CF4 4XN, UK

Introduction

The use of predictive patch testing for the determination of irritancy potential is widespread. Both animal and human models are used in an attempt to predict the behaviour of a material when in general use. Several factors are involved in the development of a cutaneous irritant response. For example, the nature of the irritant and the time it spends in contact with the skin are important. The concentration of an irritant can also be crucial in the development of irritancy, as can environmental factors such as relative humidity and temperature. Variables such as body site and age can also be relevant. There is, however, little information concerning any effect of varying the area of application on the intensity of the cutaneous response. With predictive animal irritancy testing there seems to be no general agreement and the size of patch varies from 100 to 2500 mm^2 according to the protocol being followed.[1] With human studies the original observation of Kligman and Wooding seems to hold sway.[2] That is, above the minimum of 50 mm^2 the size of patch has no influence on the results.

In the light of recent reports concerning the effect of area of application on the development of sensitization reactions,[3,4] we decided to reinvestigate the effect of area of application on the cutaneous irritant response. This has been assessed in human subjects using both subjective and objective methods of assessment following application of aqueous solutions of sodium lauryl sulphate.

Materials and methods

Study population

Twenty volunteer subjects (14 male and 6 female; mean age 38.2 years) were recruited for the study. All subjects were normal, healthy volunteer subjects to whom the nature of the study had been explained and, after full explanation, had signed a witnessed, informed consent form. Ethical approval for the study was obtained from the Joint Ethics Committee of the South Glamorgan Area Health Authority and University of Wales College of Medicine prior to commencement. The test site was the volar aspect of the forearm.

Determination of minimal irritant dose

Each subject was tested for sensitivity to aqueous sodium lauryl sulphate (SLS). Increasing concentrations of SLS, up to 2%, were applied under occlusion. After 24 h occlusion, the patches were removed and the sites left untreated. The degree of erythema was then assessed at 48 h and the minimal irritant dose (MID) defined as that concentration which produced a moderate, uniform erythema.

Data presented here has been accepted for publication in the British Journal of Dermatology

Application of sodium lauryl sulphate solutions

Applications of each individual's MID were made under occlusion for 24 h using 9, 25, 100, 225 and 400 mm² squares of filter paper soaked in the appropriate SLS solution. In other words, a constant dose per unit area was applied. At 25 h (1 h after removal) and 48 h, the sites were assessed for erythema, capillary blood flow and oedema.

Assessment of cutaneous irritancy

The methods of assessing cutaneous irritancy were as follows.

(a) Sites were scored for erythema using an arbitrary 0–4 scale.
(b) Sites were assessed subjectively for erythema using a 100 mm visual analogue scale (VAS).
(c) Erythema was measured objectively using a solid-state erythema meter.[5] The meter used was an adaptation of the design originally described by Diffey et al.[6]
(d) Cutaneous blood flow was measured using a laser Doppler blood flow meter (Periflux, Perimed, Sweden).
(e) Oedema was assessed using pulsed A-scan ultrasound.[7]

Statistical analysis

The data were analysed on a within-subject basis using the Friedman non-parametric two-way analysis of variance. If a significant difference was found ($P < 0.05$) further comparisons were made between pairs of treatments (i.e. 9 versus 25 mm², 25 versus 100 mm², etc.) using a Wilcoxon test. All procedures were carried out using a Unistat IV statistical package (Unistat Ltd, P.O. Box 383, Highgate, London) on an Olivetti PCS286 personal computer.

Results

The results of arbitrary scale scores at 25 and 48 h are presented as means and standard deviations in Figure 1. An increase in the mean score was noted at 25 mm² with a further increase at 100 mm². There was little change at 225 mm² but a further smaller increase at 400 mm². This finding was confirmed by the statistical analysis which showed significant differences between 9 and 25 mm² and between 25 and 100 mm² (25 and 48 h) and between 225 and 400 mm² (48 h only). The results of the VAS scores for erythema showed a similar pattern to the arbitrary scores (Figure 2), with statistically significant increases in scores up to a plateau at about 100 mm².

The results for the objective measurements of erythema, capillary blood flow and oedema are presented in Figures 3, 4 and 5, respectively. All show a similar type of curve to the subjective forms of assessment.

Discussion

Sodium lauryl sulphate has been used extensively by investigators as a model of cutaneous irritancy and its dose response and age and site variations are well documented.[8–10] In the present study the response to SLS was characterized in terms of erythema, alteration of capillary blood flow and induction of oedema. Using a constant dose per unit area this study has clearly shown an increase in the intensity of the cutaneous irritant reaction with area of contact of irritant. The two subjective visual scoring systems showed an increase in perceived intensity with area up to 100 mm². That this was not an optical illusion created by the differences in size was demonstrated by the erythema index values which gave almost identically shaped curves. Changes in capillary blood flow and the increase in skin thickness (oedema) also indicated variation in response with area.

The significance of the shape of the curve obtained in this experiment is not clear. The drop off at small areas may be related to lateral diffusion of SLS in the stratum corneum. This would lead to reduced levels of irritant in the papillary dermis. As the area increased this effect would rapidly disappear. An alternative hypothesis is that some kind of recruitment of capillaries occurs when larger areas are tested. That is, when only a small number of capillaries are involved, diffusion of inflammatory mediators is rapid. With increasing numbers involved the mediator concentration rises and intensifies the reaction by 'autocrine' stimulation or by stimulating adjacent capillaries. Once beyond a certain level, the capillaries are maximally stimulated and a plateau is reached.

The importance of these findings with regard to predictive patch testing in human subjects is clear. A minimum area of 100 mm² is necessary to deter-

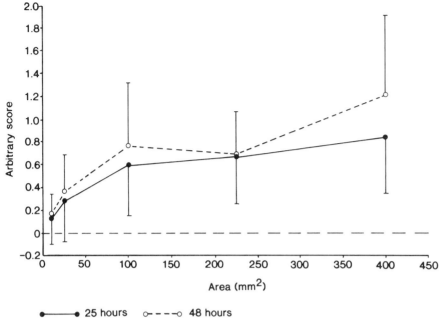

Figure 1

The effect of increasing area on erythema as assessed by an arbitrary scoring system. Results are expressed as mean score ± standard deviation. The following pairs of differences were statistically significant ($P < 0.05$, Wilcoxon): 25 h, 9 versus 25 mm^2, 25 versus 100 mm^2; 48 h, 9 versus 25 mm^2, 25 versus 100 mm^2, 225 versus 400 mm^2.

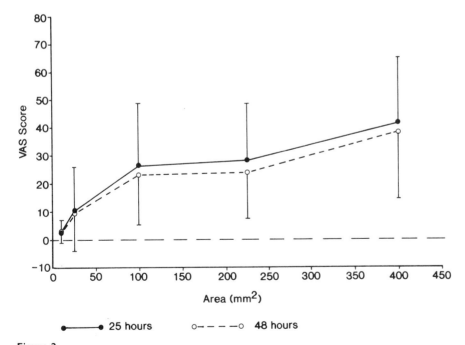

Figure 2

The effect of increasing area on erythema as assessed using a visual analogue scale (VAS) system. Results are expressed as mean VAS score ± standard deviation. The following pairs of differences were statistically significant ($P < 0.05$, Wilcoxon): 25 h, 9 versus 25 mm^2, 25 versus 100 mm^2, 225 versus 400 mm^2; 48 h, 9 versus 25 mm^2, 25 versus 100 mm^2, 225 versus 400 mm^2.

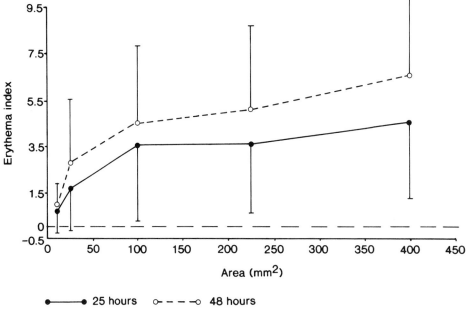

Figure 3

The effect of increasing area on erythema as assessed using an erythema meter. Results are expressed as mean erythema index ± standard deviation. The following pairs of differences were statistically significant ($P < 0.05$, Wilcoxon): 25 h, 9 versus 25 mm^2, 25 versus 100 mm^2; 48 h, 9 versus 25 mm^2, 25 versus 100 mm^2, 225 versus 400 mm^2.

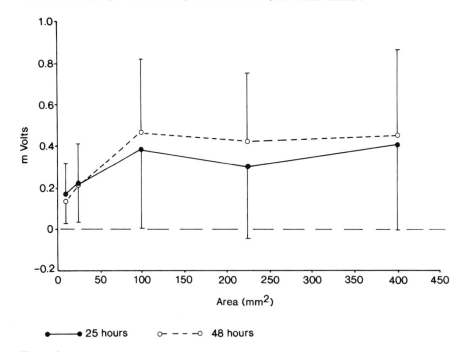

Figure 4

The effect of increasing area on capillary blood flow as assessed by a laser Doppler device. Results (in millivolts) are expressed as mean ± standard deviation. The following pairs of differences were statistically significant ($P = 0.05$, Wilcoxon): 25 h, 25 versus 100 mm^2; 48 h, 25 versus 100 mm^2.

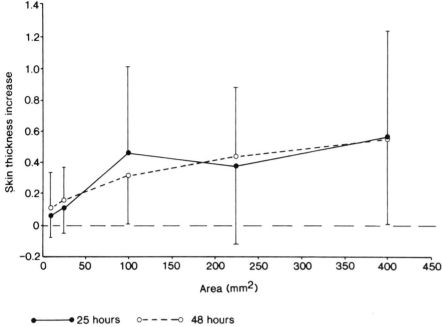

Figure 5

The effect of increasing area on cutaneous oedema as assessed by A scan ultrasound. Results (in microseconds) are expressed as mean ± standard deviation. The following pairs of differences were statistically significant ($P < 0.05$, Wilcoxon): 25 h, 9 versus 25 mm^2, 25 versus 100 mm^2, 225 versus 400 mm^2; 48 h, 25 versus 100 mm^2.

mine the irritant potential of a material. Smaller areas of application may well lead to false-negative results. These results may well be of significance in the development of industrial dermatitis. In addition to the concentration of irritant, the area of contact may be critical in the development of subsequent reactions.

References

1. Roper SS, Dermatotoxicology: animal irritancy testing. In: Rietscher RL, Spencer TS, (eds). *Methods for cutaneous investigation*, Marcel Dekker: New York, 1990, pp. 19–46.
2. Kligman AM, Wooding WM, A method for the measurement and evaluation of irritants on human skin, *J Invest Dermatol* (1967) **49**: 78–94.
3. White SI, Friedmann PS, Moss C et al, The effects of altering area of application and dose per unit area on sensitization to DNCB, *Br J Dermatol* (1986) **115**: 663–8.
4. Rees JL, Friedman PS, Matthews JNS, The influence of area of application on sensitization to dinitrochlorobenzene, *Br J Dermatol* (1990) **122**: 29–31.
5. Pearse AD, Edwards C, Hill S et al, Portable erythema meter and its application to use in human skin, *Int J Cosmetic Sci* (1990) **12**: 63–70.
6. Diffey BL, Oliver RJ, Farr PM, A portable instrument for quantifying erythema induced by ultraviolet irradiation, *Br J Dermatol* (1984) **111**: 663–72.
7. Tan CY, Statham B, Marks R et al, Skin thickness measurement by pulsed ultrasound: its reproducibility, validation and variability, *Br J Dermatol* (1982) **106**: 657–67.
8. Bruynzeel DP, van Ketel WG, Scheper RJ et al, Delayed time course of irritation by sodium lauryl sulphate: observation on threshold reactions, *Contact Dermatit* (1982) **8**: 236–9.
9. Wilhelm KP, Surber C, Maibach HI, Quantification of sodium lauryl sulphate irritant dermatitis in man. Comparison of four techniques: skin colour reflectance, transepidermal water loss, laser Doppler flow measurement and visual scores, *Arch Dermatol Res* (1989) **281**: 293–5.
10. Agner T, Serup J, Sodium lauryl sulphate for irritant patch testing — a dose response study using bioengineering methods for determination of skin irritation, *J Invest Dermatol* (1990) **95**: 543–7.

40
Contact dermatitis to paraphenylenediamine in hairdressers

Baldassarre Santucci, Gian Carlo Fuga, Carlo Cannistraci, Walter Marmo, Antonio Cristaudo and Mauro Picardo
Dermatological Institute Ospedale S. Gallicano, Via di S. Gallicano 25 a, 00153 Rome, Italy

Dermatitis of the hands among hairdressers has been fully described by several authors.[1-4] According to Cronin, '... there are two patterns of contact dermatitis: one, eczema of the fingers (EF), occurs in apprentices and trained hairdressers, especially those with an atopic background. The prognosis is bad and the more affected workers are likely to change their job. The second type is characterized by dry irritant skin over the metacarpophalangeal joints (MCPJ), and occurs in younger apprentices, doing many shampoos each day. The changes resemble those of winter chapping and are always greatest over the metacarpophalangeal joint. Atopy is not a factor in these patients and the prognosis is better. Patients require gloves and emollients and they can continue hairdressing'.[4] However, in our opinion MCPJ depends on many factors and may represent an interim state, and is not always curable within a few days of ceasing to work with shampoos. The aim of the present work was to investigate how the clinical differences in the two patterns may be explained using non-invasive methods.

Materials and methods

Twelve young hairdressers (6 men and 6 women, aged 15–19 years) were included. Six of these had EF and six had MCPJ. None had a personal or familial atopic background. They had been shampooing frequently and tinting each day, without gloves, from 1–36 months (Table 1). All subjects were patch tested using substances from the Inter-

Table 1 Summary of the clinical patterns of the examined subjects.

Subject No	Age (years)	Sex	Length of work (months)	Onset of symptoms	Pattern of dermatitis	Patch-test response	No. of shampoos per day	No. of tints per day
1	17	F	1	10 days	MCPJ	—	30	—
2	17	F	12	5 months	MCPJ	—	9	5
3	19	M	12	6 months	MCPJ	—	14	4
4	18	F	12	6 months	MCPJ	Ni	12	6
5	15	F	1	15 days	MCPJ	—	12	4
6	17	M	2	1 month	MCPJ	Ni	15	4
7	19	F	36	6 months	EF	PPD + PTD	10	4
8	15	F	8	2 months	EF	PPD + Ni	10	4
9	16	M	24	8 months	EF	PPD + PTD	10	6
10	19	F	36	9 months	EF	PPD + Ni	10	4
11	16	F	24	6 months	EF	PPD + PAP	8	6
12	17	F	24	2 months	EF	PPD	8	2

MCPJ, metacarpophalangeal joint dermatitis; EF, eczema of the fingers; Ni, nickel; PPD, *p*-phenylenediamine, PTD, *p*-toluylendiamine; PAP, *p*-aminophenol.

national Contact Dermatitis Research Group (ICDRG) standard series (Trolab) and the following substances relevant to hairdressing: pyrogallol 1%, p-toluylendiamine (PTD) 1%, o-nitro-p-phenylendiamine 1%, resorcinol 1%, ammonium persulphate 1%, ammonium thioglycollate 2%, p-aminophenol (PAP) 1%, all in petrolatum (Firma, Florence). Using Finn chambers on Scanpor, the tests were read at 48 and 72 h according to the ICDRG scale. After 15 days both the stained and the apparently healthy skin of the dorsa of the hands was examined using computerized capillaroscopy, reflected digitized optical densitometry and reflected optical microscopy.

Cronin[4] has compared the changes found in MCPJ with the effects of winter chapping.[5] In the present study, subjects with winter chapping who gave negative responses to patch tests were studied as controls.

Capillaroscopic observation was carried out using a reflected light microscope (Zeiss OMPI 1-F), with a fixed lens (f:50), magnification changer (0,4,0,6,1), enlargement of the tube (f: 2 = 160) and the interface for the camera (2×). The capillaroscopic image, filmed with a charge coupled device (CCD) camera, was displayed on a high definition colour monitor and then recorded with a 3/4 in. video recorder. The video signal coming from the camera or video recorder, after decoding from phase alternative time (PAL) to red-green-blue (RGB), was run through a computer which, appropriately configured, digitizes and visualizes the signal on a high-definition monitor. The system was suitably calibrated such that any magnification of the microscopic field corresponded to a precise metric value for the pixel of the digitized image. The computer elaborated a grid which, overlapping the digitized image being examined, determined the diameter and length of the capillaries with micrometric precision. In particular, to measure the diameter, the software enabled us to determine the distance between two diametrically opposite points on each side of the vessels, on the basis of purely orthogonal geometry or on the basis of a quantitative and qualitative analysis of the colour.

The erythema and the colour of the skin was evaluated by means of optical reflected densitometry.[6,7] A light reflected densitometer (X-Rite 404) was used. A graphic representation of the colour surveyed by the densitometer was made using a 386 personal computer with mathematical co-processor. The graphic card, capable of representing 32 760 colours, was connected to a high-resolution monitor with persistent phosphor and to a Ratmek photographic apparatus. The values obtained from the densitometer were inserted into the computer which computed them automatically into cyan – magenta – yellow (CMY), RGB, hue luminescence saturation (HLS) or hue saturation visual (HSV) systems[7] and reproduced the colour under examination on the monitor. The quantification of erythema index (EI) was obtained by subtracting the logarithm to the base 10 of the inverse reflectance (R) of the red light from that of the green light and then using the scale of complementary colours:

$$EI = \log R_{magenta} - \log R_{cyan}$$

The difference between the EI of damaged skin and EI of the apparently healthy skin represents the gradient of erythema (GE). Digitized optical reflected microscopy was carried out using the capillaroscopic apparatus described above.

In order to microscopically determine the depth of pigment deposits, the most superficial corneal layers of the diseased skin examined were stripped with adhesive tape.

Statistical analysis

Student's t-test was used to evaluate the difference in the number of pervious capillaries per square millimetre between EF and MCPJ and in the GE of the two groups.

Students' t-test for paired data was used to evaluate the difference of the EI values between EF and healthy skin and between MCPJ and healthy skin.

Results

The patch test responses to the ICDRG standard series and to the substances relevant to hairdressing are shown in Table 1.

Capillaroscopic observations

In normal skin of the dorsa of the hands, the mean number of pervious capillaries per square millimetre was 25. These values were within the range of mean values found by us in normal subjects (25 ± 1.7 per square millimetre). For subjects with EF and MCPJ the mean values were 37.7 and 32, respectively (Tables 2 and 3; $t = 2.46$; $p < 0.05$).

Table 2 Erythema index (EI), number of pervious capillaries (per square millimetre) and gradient of erythema (GE) found in the examined subjects.

	EI	No. of capillaries	GE
Healthy skin	0.11	25	
Eczema of fingers	0.16	37.7	1.5
Metacarpophalangeal joint	0.14	32	1.27
Winter chapping	0.17	38.1	1.54

Table 3 Statistical evaluation of the differences found in the subjects examined.

		t	p
EI	EF/HS	2.85	<0.01
	MCPJ/HS	2.60	<0.05
No. of capillaries	EF/MPCJ	2.46	<0.05
GE	EF/MPCJ	3.20	<0.01

EI, erythema index; GE, gradient of erythema; EF, eczema of the fingers; MCPJ, metacarpophalangeal joint dermatitis; HS, healthy skin.

Computerized optical reflected densitometry

The mean EI values found in healthy skin, EF and MCPJ were 0.11, 0.16 and 0.14, respectively (Table 2, t (EF/healthy skin) = 2.85, $p < 0.01$; Table 3, t (MCPJ/healthy skin) = 2.60, $p < 0.05$).

The mean GE values found in EF and MCPJ were 1.5 and 1.27, respectively (Tables 2 and 3; $t = 3.20$, $p < 0.01$).

Optical reflected microscopy

In both EF and MCPJ, deposits of brownish linear or granular pigment in the upper epidermis which were more evidence in MCPJ were observed (Figures 1 and 2). The microscopic observation carried out after adhesive tape stripping revealed that pigment deposits were in the deepest corneal layers in EF (Figure 3).

For the subjects with winter chapping the following data were found: mean EI 0.17, mean GE 1.54, mean number of pervious capillaries 38.1 (Table 2). No deposits of pigment were observed (Figure 4).

Discussion

The two patterns of hand dermatitis seen in all subjects were the same as those described by Cronin.[4] In the present study MCPJ seemed to arise earlier than EF and was found in subjects doing more shampooing than tinting. These subjects gave negative responses to patch testing with substances relevant to hairdressing. The two positive responses to nickel found in the subjects affected by MCPJ (Table 1) seemed to be more linked to the wearing of metal objects than to hairdressing. Positive responses to at least one of the tested substances related to hairdressing were found only in subjects with EF and in all of the EF subjects. These subjects had also been hairdressing for longer and had been shampooing relatively less than tinting (Table 1). The diseased skin appeared more coloured than the normal skin in both patterns. A statistically significant difference between the colours of EF and MCPJ, and between each of them and the apparently healthy skin examined, was found (Table 3).

The hyperchromatic areas, more evident on the joints in MCPJ, were microscopically filled with linear or granular amounts of brownish pigment. These substances were probably pigment polymers of partly oxidized aromatic compounds, mainly p-phenylenediamine (PPD), which is widely used in Italy for tinting. The deposits were sometimes present in the upper epidermis, disappearing with adhesive tape stripping; sometimes, particularly in EF, they were present at deeper levels. The amount of pigment was less in EF (Figure 3) and this could be due both to the greater amount of inflammation and to greater capillary dilatation. The amount of pigment present seems to depend more on the type of the work done than on the length of time spent at work (Table 1).

In MCPJ there seemed to be a positive relationship between the quantity and depth of the pigment and the involvement of capillaries: the deeper the pigment deposit the greater the capillary involvement.

The hands of the subjects with winter chapping did not show any pigment but only a variable degree of capillary involvement (Figure 4).

More numerous and open capillaries were found on the hands of subjects with EF (Figure 3) and the difference from subjects with MCPJ was statistically significant (Table 3). The healthy skin in both types of disorder did not show any pigment or capillary involvement.

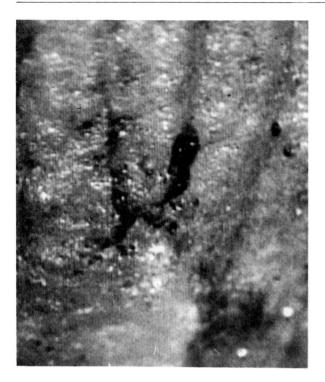

Figure 1

Deposits of brownish granular pigment in the upper epidermis in MCPJ.

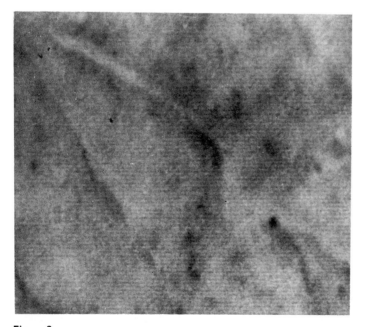

Figure 2

Moderate deposits of pigment after adhesive tape stripping in MCPJ. Limited involvement of capillaries.

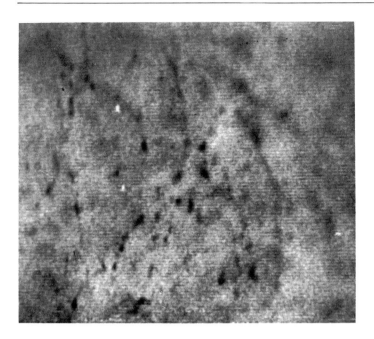

Figure 3

Deep deposits of pigment and numerous enlarged capillaries in EF.

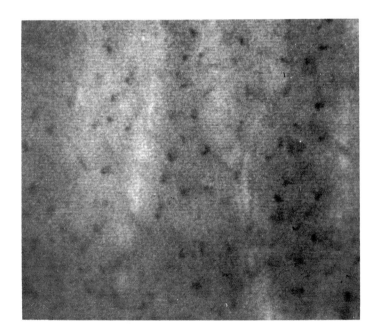

Figure 4

Strong degree of capillary involvement without any pigment in winter chapping.

The colour of the diseased areas seems to depend on both the amount of pigment and the number of capillaries involved. These changes cannot only be ascribed to the degreasing effect of repeated shampooing as the normal skin on the hands was exposed to the same shampoos and did not show any staining. Shampoos are probably damaging because, apart from lowering barrier function, they removed fresh tinting, facilitating the penetration of dangerous partly oxidized PPD. The presence of this foreign substance may have other dangerous effects. It is worth stressing two points: (1) the quantity of deposited substances may interfere with the reducing events and the scavenger capability of the skin[8] which are individual characteristics. The greater the amount the stronger the possibility of depleting reducing protective substances. (2) Depending on the concentration applied, PPD is known to produce a toxic effect on cultured human keratinocytes partly due to oxygen radicals and the generation of oxidation products. These phenomena may induce the release of lipo-oxygenase substrates leading to inflammatory reactions.[9]

In conclusion, in our opinion, the changes found in the hands of the hairdressers studied originated from the repeated use and penetration of PPD. The deposited PPD with concomitant capillary involvement and the experimental findings seem to suggest that MCPJ may be an interim state. The prognosis is dependent on many factors: to continue hairdressing may be a risk and a few days of rest may not be sufficient to eliminate PPD. Wearing gloves should be compulsory for all workers. Because most refuse to wear gloves for various reasons, the only way to prevent this problem is to remove PPD from the market.

References

1 Marks R, Cronin E, Hand eczema in hairdressers, *Aust J Dermatol* (1977) **18**: 123–6.
2 Wilkinson DS, Hambly EM, Prognosis of hand eczema in hairdressing apprentices, *Contact Dermatit* (1978) **4**: 63.
3 Cronin E, Kullavanijaya P, Hand dermatitis in hairdressers, *Acta Dermat (Stockh)* (1979) (suppl 85): 47–50.
4 Cronin E, Dermatitis of the hands in beauticians. In: Maibach HI, (ed). *Occupational and industrial dermatology*, 2nd edn, Year Book Medical Publishers Inc.: Chicago, 1987, pp. 267–70.
5 Fuga GC, Spina C, Di Palma A et al, Microcirculation. Usefulness of information in capillaroscopy, *Proc 6th Conf Med Inform*, Medinfo 89, Singapore, 11–15 December 1989.
6 Leonard F, Kalis B, Demange L, Mesure quantitative de l'érythème cutanée par photodensitometrie, *Nouv Dermatol* (1987) (suppl VI): 245–7.
7 Fuga GC, Spina C, Cavallotti C et al, Computerized reflected optical densitometry. Research on the colour of the skin. Lecture notes in medical informatics, *Proc Med Informatic Europe 90*, Glasgow, 20–23 August 1990.
8 Schmidt RJ, Khan L, Chung LY, Are free radicals and not quinones the haptenic species derived from urushiols and other contact allergenic mono- and dihydric alkylbenzenes? The significance of NADH, glutathione, and redox cycling in the skin, *Arch Dermatol Res* (1990) **282**: 56–64.
9 Picardo M, Cannistraci C, De Luca C et al, Effect of *para* group substances on human keratinocytes in culture, *Contact Dermatit* (1990) **23**: 236.

41
Euxyl K 400: a new allergen in cosmetic products

Antonella Tosti, Liliana Guerra and Federico Bardazzi
Istituto di Clinica Dermatologica dell'Università, Via Massarenti 1, 40138 Bologna, Italy

Euxyl K 400 is a new preservative system for cosmetics and toiletries, first introduced on the European market in 1985 and used in Italy since 1987. Its active ingredient is a synergistic mixture of 2-phenoxyethanol and 1,2-dibromo-2,4-dicyanobutan. It is supplied by the manufacturer (Schülke & Mayr, Hamburg) as a solution containing 20% of 1,2-dibromo-2,4-dicyanobutan in 2-phenoxyethanol. Over the last 2 years, we have included Euxyl K 400 in our standard patch-test series.

Materials and methods

From September 1988 to March 1991, 2540 consecutive patients affected by contact dermatitis were patch tested with Euxyl K 400 2.5% in petrolatum, using Finn Chambers on Scanpor tape and reading at 2, 3 and 4 days.

A positive reaction to Euxyl K 400 was found in 29 patients (1.14%). Doubtful reactions were always verified by retesting and by observing the change in the reactions over 1 week. No cases of active sensitization were detected.

The source of Euxyl K 400 sensitization was traced in 11 patients who had been using one or more cosmetic products containing this preservative system. Of the 29 patients, 15 agreed to undergo additional tests: (a) patch tests with Euxyl K 400 0.5% in petrolatum; (b) patch tests with phenoxyethanol 5% in petrolatum; (c) a provocative use test in which the patients were asked to apply a generic skin-care lotion preserved with Euxyl K 400 0.1% to the right antecubital fossa, a similar lotion preserved with methyl and propyl paraben 0.2% and diazolidinylurea 0.2% to the left antecubital fossa, twice daily for 2 weeks; and (d) six patients were also patch tested with serial dilutions (2%, 1.5%, 1% and 0.5%) of Euxyl K 400 in petrolatum and ethanol, and with Euxyl K 400 0.5% in water.

All results were assessed using the ICDRG grading scale.

Results

Euxyl K 400 0.5% in petrolatum gave a strong positive reaction (+--/++-/++-) in five patients, and a slight positive reaction (+--/+--/+--) in three patients. Two patients positively reacted to phenoxyethanol 5% in petrolatum (+--/++-/++-). Five patients reacted to the provocative use test with the lotion containing Euxyl K 400, developing an itching dermatitis in the right antecubital fossa after 5–7 days. All six patients tested with the serial dilutions of Euxyl K 400 reacted to each of the concentrations of Euxyl K 400 in petrolatum and ethanol, except for Euxyl K 400 0.5% in ethanol. All these patients also showed a positive reaction to Euxyl K 400 0.5% in water. This indicates that Euxyl K 400 0.5% in water is adequate for detecting sensitization to the preservative.

In 6 of the 15 patients the source of Euxyl K 400 sensitization was traced: three patients were using leave-on products preserved with Euxyl K 400, and two patients were sensitized by rinse-off products containing Euxyl K 400. In one patient, who reacted to phenoxyethanol 5% in petrolatum, the source of sensitization was detected in several leave-on and rinse-off products containing phenoxyethanol.

In the last few years numerous manufacturers have started using Euxyl K 400 as an alternative to other antimicrobials. Enquiries of the major Italian manufacturers revealed that, since 1989, Euxyl K 400 has been added to numerous cosmetic formulations. Phenoxyethanol unassociated with 1,2-dibromo-2,4-dicyanobutan is also used extensively in the cosmetics industry.

Contact dermatitis from Euxyl K 400 has occasionally been described in the literature.[1,2] We have previously reported that sensitization to this preservative is not rare in Italy.[3]

We believe that Euxyl K 400 should be added to the cosmetic patch-test tray. Since the frequency of sensitization to any allergen is strongly related to actual exposure, sensitization to Euxyl K 400 may possibly become more common when this preservative system becomes a widely used ingredient of cosmetic formulations.

References

1 Senff H, Exner M, Gortz J et al, Allergic contact dermatitis from Euxyl K 400, *Contact Dermatit* (1989) **20**: 381–2.
2 de Groot AC, Weyland JW, Contact allergy to methyldibromoglutaronitrile in the cosmetics preservative Euxyl K 400, *Am J Contact Dermatit* (1991) **2**: 31–2.
3 Tosti A, Guerra L, Bardazzi F et al, Euxyl K 400: a new sensitizer in cosmetics, *Contact Dermatit* (1991) **24**: in press.

42
The skin equivalent as a genotoxicity model

M. J. Edwards, P. J. Dykes, V. Merrett and R. Marks
Department of Dermatology, University of Wales College of Medicine, Heath Park, Cardiff CF4 4XN, UK

Introduction

Many chemical mutagens share a common property in that they require metabolic activation by cellular enzymes. The cytochrome P450 enzyme system has been shown to activate polycyclic aromatic hydrocarbons (PAHs) by forming highly reactive electrophilic intermediates which react with nucleophilic centres in cellular DNA. This process is thought to be one of the initial steps in the process of chemical carcinogenesis.[1,2]

In many short-term in vitro mutagenicity tests the target cells are either bacterial or rodent with metabolic activation being provided by cell free tissue extracts (S9). The need for metabolic activation suggests that human cells process carcinogens in different ways to bacteria or other mammalian species. Even within the same organism the various cell types differ in their ability to absorb, activate and repair DNA lesions.[3] The skin equivalent provides the opportunity of reassembling some of the cellular components of human skin into a differentiating and functional tissue which may be used as a realistic in vitro model for chemical risk assessment.

In view of the wealth of information available on the mechanism by which benzo[a]pyrene (B[a]P) exerts its mutagenic effect, it was used in this study to assess the suitability of the skin equivalent as a genotoxicity model. The carcinogenicity of B[a]P is associated with its ability to bind to cellular DNA following metabolic activation by cytochrome P450. This enzyme system metabolizes B[a]P to a number of products among which the bay region diol epoxide has been shown to bind to the exocyclic 2-amino group of guanine.[4] The (+)− (7R)- trans-anti-B[a]P-7,8-dihydrodiol-9,10-epoxide: deoxyguanosine ((7R)-trans-anti-BPDE-deoxyguanosine) adduct formed within the cellular DNA following exposure to B[a]P has been associated with the mutagenic activity of this PAH.[5]

Methods and materials

Materials

Benzo[a]pyrene, snake venom phosphodiesterase, alkaline phosphatase, proteinase K, ribonuclease A, DNase I cholera toxin, transferrin and triiodothyronine were obtained from the Sigma Chemical Company. [G-^{3}H]B[a]P (specific activity 50–80 Ci/mmol) was obtained from Amersham UK. Redistilled high purity phenol was obtained from ICN Biomedicals Ltd, UK. The materials used in the culture of keratinocytes were purchased from sources described previously.[6] Bond elute C18 reverse-phase cartridges and the high performance liquid chromatography (HPLC) system were obtained from Jones Chromatography, Hengoed, UK. The HPLC system consisted of a Milton Roy CM 4000 multiple solvent delivery system, a variable wavelength spectromonitor 3100 and a JCL 6000 data-acquisition system.

HPLC analysis of B[a]P adducts

The B[a]P : deoxyribonucleoside adducts were analysed by reverse-phase HPLC on a Spherisorb ODS

I (25 × 0.46 cm: 5 μm) reverse-phase column. The column was eluted with methanol : water (40 : 60) for 35 min at a flow rate of I ml/min, then for 45 min with methanol : water (55 : 45). Fractions (1 ml) were collected and the radioactivity measured in each fraction by liquid scintillation counting. Structural assignments of the individual adducts were based on comparison with published data.[7,8]

Results

Figures 1–3 illustrate typical HPLC profiles of the DNA adducts isolated from skin equivalent, human skin explants and mouse skin explants which had been treated with [^{3}H]-B[a]P for 24 or 48 h. The principal DNA adduct isolated from these tissues was (+)-(7R)-trans-anti-BPDE-2N-deoxyguanosine (peak 4). Four minor DNA adducts were also detected in the DNA digests from skin equivalents and human skin explants. By comparison with published data,[7,8] the following structural assignments were given to the minor B[a]P : DNA adducts. In order of elution from the HPLC column, peak 3 was designated (−)-(7S)-trans-anti-BPDE-2N-deoxyguanosine; peak 5 was syn-BPDE-2N-deoxyguanosine. Both peaks I and 2 were DNA adducts formed by the reaction of B[a]P with deoxycytosine.

Profiles of DNA adducts isolated from mouse skin explants which had been exposed to [^{3}H]-B[a]P for 24 to 48 h at 37°C were qualitatively very similar to the DNA adducts extracted from skin equivalents and human skin explants. In addition to the four minor DNA adducts extracted from skin equivalents and human skin explants, a single late-eluting B[a]P adduct peak (peak 6) was detected in mouse skin explants (Figure 3). By comparison with published data,[7,8] this B[a]P adduct was assigned the structure B[a]P-6N-deoxyadenosine.

Quantitative differences were observed between the tissues when the data was expressed in terms of the amount of extractable DNA. Higher levels of [^{3}H]-B[a]P adducts were detected in the DNA from skin equivalents when compared with human or mouse skin explants. Table I illustrates the peak ratio of each adduct extracted from the three tissues after a 24-h exposure to [^{3}H]-B[a]P. The data show that the minor B[a]P adduct peak ratios relative to (+)-(7R)-trans-anti-BPDE-deoxyguanosine (peak 4) were very similar to both skin equivalents and human skin explants. The mouse skin explants displayed one major difference when the peak ratios were compared with skin equivalents or human skin explants. Relatively large amounts of the minor DNA: 6N-deoxyadenosine adducts were detected in mouse skin explants.

Table I Ratio of the minor B[a]P induced DNA adducts formed in skin equivalents and human and mouse skin explants relative to the major B[a]P induced DNA adduct (+)-trans-anti-BPDE-deoxyguanosine.

B[a]P adduct	Peak ratio		
	Mouse	Human skin	Skin equivalents
1	0.315	0.272	0.277
2	0.350	0.337	0.364
3	0.475	0.429	0.417
4	1.00	1.00	1.00
5	0.145	0.235	0.280
6	0.250	0.045	0.001

Tissues exposed to [^{3}H]Benzo[a]pyrene for 24 h at 37°C. Peak ratios were calculated relative to peak 4, (+)-(7R)-trans-anti-BPDE-deoxyguanosine.

Conclusion

The metabolic activation of B[a]P has been compared in skin equivalents and mouse and human skin explants. Qualitative analysis of the DNA adducts formed in these tissues by reverse-phase HPLC has provided an effective method for the comparison of their genotoxic potential.

The detection of B[a]P : DNA adducts in the epidermis of the three tissues under study demonstrated that they are capable of activating B[a]P to genotoxic metabolites. Quantitative analysis of the data showed that the skin equivalent contained the largest number of DNA adducts per unit of extractable DNA. This may be due to the permeability of skin equivalent to B[a]P when compared with skin explants. Alternatively, the skin equivalent may contain higher levels of B[a]P metabolizing enzymes. Mammalian skin contains an inducible cytochrome P450 enzyme system which contributes to the activation of PAHs. It is possible that the culture conditions under which the skin equivalents were grown may in part cause the induction of PAH activating enzymes.

The close similarity in peak ratios between skin equivalents and human skin explants provides good evidence that the skin equivalent is a valid in vitro model of human skin. The skin equivalent model has a number of advantages over other in vitro risk-assessment methods. The skin equivalent cannot

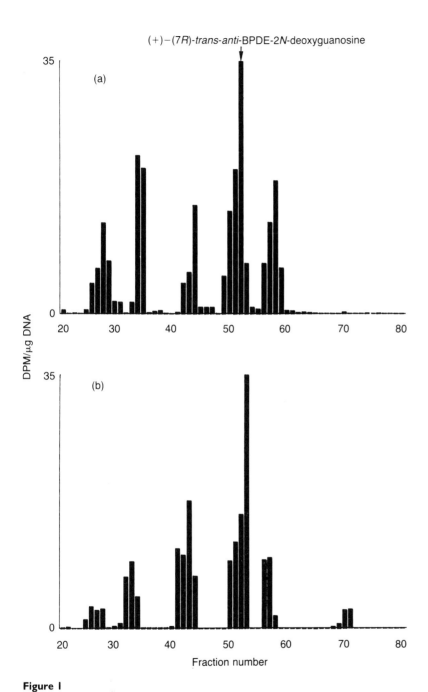

Figure 1

HPLC profile of the [^{3}H]-B[a]P : DNA adducts extracted from skin equivalents (a) exposed to [^{3}H]-B[a]P for 24 h at 37°C or (b) exposed to [^{3}H]-B[a]P for 48 h at 37°C. The arrow indicates the position of (+)-(7R)-*trans-anti*-BPDE-deoxyguanosine.

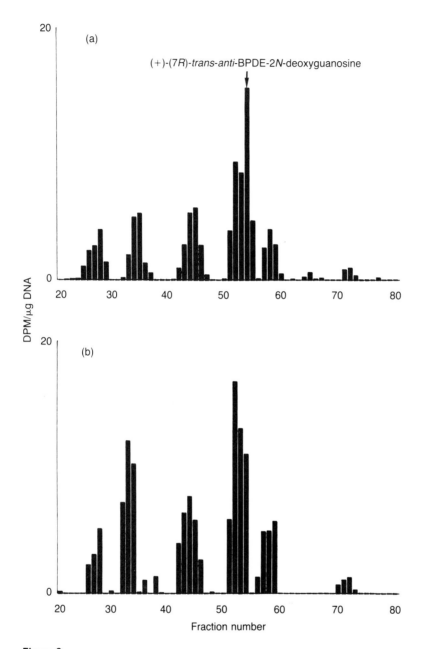

Figure 2

HPLC profile of the [^{3}H]-B[a]P : DNA adducts extracted from human skin explants (a) exposed to [^{3}H]-B[a]P for 24 h at 37°C or (b) exposed to [^{3}H]-B[a]P for 48 h at 37°C. The arrow indicates the position of (+)-(7R)-*trans-anti*-BPDE-deoxyguanosine.

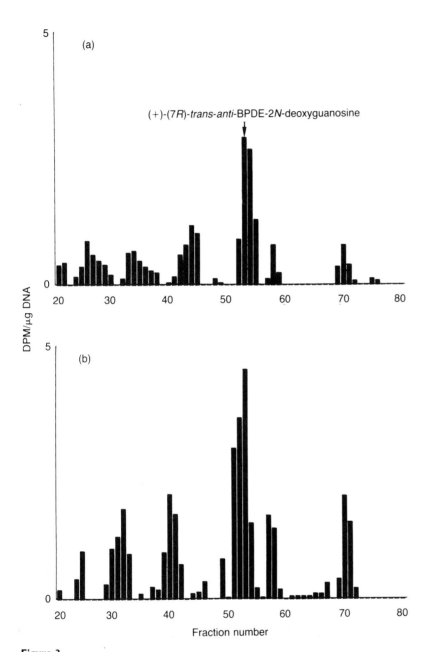

Figure 3

HPLC profile of the [^{3}H]-B[a]P : DNA adducts extracted from mouse skin explants (a) exposed to [^{3}H]-B[a]P for 24 h at 37°C or (b) exposed to [^{3}H]-B[a]P for 48 h at 37°C. The arrow indicates the position of (+)-(7R)-*trans-anti*-BPDE-deoxyguanosine.

represent the complete in vivo situation as human skin contains a wide range of cell types. However, the model does contain a multilayered structure with stratum corneum and differentiating epithelium. The model also has the advantage of being potentially useful for detecting genotoxic compounds present in topical dermatological formulations and for modelling the potential risk arising from materials in the industrial workplace.

References

1 Miller JA, Carcinogenesis by chemicals: an overview, *Cancer Res* (1970) **30**: 559–76.
2 Wright AS, The role of metabolism in chemical mutagenesis and chemical carcinogenesis, *Mutation Res* (1980) **75**: 215–41.
3 Kouri RE, Lubet RA, McKinney CE et al, Aryl hydrocarbon hydroxylase activity 'of mouse and humans', *Environ Sci Res* (1983) **29**: 179–97.
4 Osborne MR, Beland FA, Harvey RG et al, The reaction of 7,8-dihydroxy-9,10-epoxy-7,8,9,10-tetrahydro-benzo[α]pyrene with DNA, *Int J Cancer* (1976) **18**: 362–8.
5 DiGiovanni J, Decina PC, Prichett WP et al, Formation and disappearance of benzo[a]pyrene:DNA adducts in mouse epidermis, *Carcinogenesis* (1985) **6**: 741–7.
6 Dykes PJ, Edwards MJ, O'Donovan MR et al, In vitro reconstruction of human skin: the use of skin equivalents as potential indicators of cutaneous toxicity, *Toxic in vitro* (1991) **5**: 1–8.
7 Weston A, Grover PL, Sims P, Metabolic activation of benzo[α]pyrene in human skin maintained in short term organ culture, *Chem–Biol Interact* (1983) **45**: 359–71.
8 Huckle KR, Smith RJ, Weston WP et al, Comparison of hydrocarbon : DNA adducts formed in mouse skin *in vitro* and in organ culture *in vitro* following treatment with benzo[a]pyrene, *Carcinogenesis* (1986) **7**: 965–70.

43
Some new and alternative approaches to skin irritation testing

D. Jírová, Ž. Nikolová, S. Fiker and H. Jančí

Institute of Hygiene and Epidemiology, Department of Environmental Health, Šrobárova 48, 100 42 Prague 10, Czechoslovakia

Introduction

The spectrum of topical agents with a potentially negative effect on skin or mucosal surfaces is relatively broad. For their safe use it is essential to assess the early signs of local disease that might eventually lead to the development of more serious problems after repeated and intensified contact.

Until recently, procedures used for predicting irritant effects of topical agents employed the classical method elaborated by Draize. This test continues to attract criticism because of its unsatisfactory reliability and the growing costs of the test, as well as for ethical reasons.

One of the available alternatives to tackle this problem appears to be the use of in vitro tissue-culture techniques. This standard testing system makes it possible to use the cells of several species and to compare them with the response of human cells.[1-3]

Aims of the study

The aims of the present study were; (i) to select in vitro tissue-culture methods suitable for detecting early cellular lesions after a low-level exposure to chemicals; (ii) to verify the suitability of these methods for assessing the irritant effects of the selected topical agents; (iii) to compare the test results obtained with the in vitro techniques used with classical techniques in vivo; and (iv) to apply in vitro tests for estimating the degree of toxicity in a broader group of topical agents.

Materials and methods

For comparative studies the chemical substances included surface active agents and preservatives which come in regular contact with human skin or mucous membranes (Table 1). The degree of toxicity was estimated in a broader group of shampoos and toothpastes.

The in vivo responses in albino rabbits were established according to French standards for chemical toxicity testing.[4] Skin irritation was also evaluated in a group of human volunteers.[5]

For in vitro tests human peripheral blood mononuclear cells and rabbit splenocytes were used as cellular test substrates. Attention was focussed on the viability of these cells, their general growth characteristics and their metabolic and functional activities.

The substances were added in increasing concentrations to the tissue-culture medium. The maximum non-toxic concentration was established for each substance and test.

The in vitro techniques included a test of vitality of human peripheral blood lymphocytes,[6] a test of the activity of lactic dehydrogenase in human peripheral blood lymphocyte culture,[6] the responsiveness to phytohemagglutinin (PHA) stimulation in human peripheral blood culture[7] and the migration activity of splenocytes derived from rabbit spleen fragments.[8]

The human lymphocytes were prepared from peripheral venous blood (30 IU heparin/ml). Lymphocytes were isolated on Ficoll-Hypaque gradient, washed in minimal essential medium (MEM) three times and adjusted to a concentration of 4×10^6

Table 1 Substances tested in comparative studies

Formaldehyde HCHO (39.1% active substrate)	Preservative	Lachema, ČSFR
Kathon CG (structures: 5-chloro-2-methyl-4-isothiazolin-3-one and 2-methyl-4-isothiazolin-3-one) (1.5% active substrate)	Preservative	Rohm and Haas Comp., France
Sodium lauryl sulphate $CH_3(CH_2)_{11}$–O–SO_3–Na (pure substrate)	Surface active agent (anion active)	Lachema, ČSFR
Aminoxide Ws35 R–CO–NH–CH_2–CH_2–N(CH_3)(CH_3)–O (pure substrate)	Surface active agent (non-ionic)	Th. Goldschmidt AG, BRD
Aminookis R–N(CH_3)(CH_3)–O (30% active substrate)	Surface active agent (non-ionic)	Nipkem BLR

cells/ml in MEM with 10% fetal calf serum (FCS), and 1 ml aliquots were placed in closed plastic test tubes and then centrifuged at 200 g. The supernatant was removed and 1 ml of the substance being tested in the appropriate concentration was added. Controls contained cells in cultivation medium only. The cultures were incubated for 24 h at 37°C.

The vitality (V) of cells was determined by means of the Trypan blue stain, before the culture was established and after 24 h of cultivation; measurements were the average of observations made in triplicate. The results are presented as the index of vitality, the ratio between the vitality found in experimental cultures and that found in control cultures at the end of cultivation.

The supernatant of the peripheral lymphocyte culture was tested for lactate dehydrogenase (LDH) activity (L) after 24 h of cultivation employing spectrophotometric procedures. The results are presented as an index of LDH activity.

Human peripheral venous blood (30 IU heparin/ml) diluted 1:20 in MEM with 5% FCS, was cultivated in the presence of PHA (40 μg/ml) and the substance tested for responsiveness to (PHA) stimulation (P) at 37°C and in 5% CO_2 for 76 h (Dynatech plates 8 × 12 wells, flat bottom, volume of culture 0.2 ml). For the next 14 h [^{3}H]thymidine (60 kBq in 7 μl) was added to each well. At the end of cultivation the cultures were harvested and the [^{3}H]thymidine incorporation measured. The results are presented as the stimulation index (P).

The migration activity of splenocytes derived from rabbit spleen fragments was determined as follows. Aseptically excised rabbit (*Chinchila*) spleen was cut on a sterile paraffin plate into pieces about 1 mm in diameter. These fragments were washed in MEM. Increasing concentrations of the substance in MEM with 10% FCS were pipetted in volumes of 0.15 ml into wells (Dynatech plates 8 × 12, flat bottom). Each concentration was placed into four wells, one fragment was transferred into each well. Controls contained fragments in cultivation medium only. After 24 h of cultivation at 37°C and in 5% CO_2, the migration zones of the spleen cells were measured. The results are presented as the migration index (M), the ratio between the experimental migration zone to the control zone.

Statistical evaluations comprised the correlations between the concentrations of the substances and the values obtained. The significance of the correlations was tested at the 5% significance level. By means of linear regression the borderline concentration, relevant to the highest non-toxic concentration, for each individual, substance and method was determined.

Results

The results of the tests in vivo suggest that rabbit skin has a higher sensitivity than does human skin. We failed to confirm regular higher reactivity of the scarified in contrast to non-scarified skin. The results are documented in the case of formaldehyde (Figure 1), sodium lauryl sulphate (Figure 2) and Kathon CG (Figure 3). Similar results were obtained with Aminoxide Ws35 and Aminookis.

Responses to the test substances with both in vivo and in vitro tests were analogous, they were dose dependent and of non-specific toxicity. The results in the case of formaldehyde are shown in Figure 4. Similar results were obtained with other substances. Toxic effects for the different substances were reached at different concentrations depending on the biological character of the substance concerned. Figure 5 shows the highest non-toxic concentrations for in vivo and in vitro tests for substances tested in the comparative study.

To estimate the degree of toxicity in a broader group of topical agents, we used the rabbit splenocyte migration activity test. According to the highest non-toxic concentration we can well document the effect of various products in a group of shampoos (Table 2).

The splenocyte migration activity method was also effective in routine tests of some toothpastes. The highest non-toxic concentration correlates with the content of tenzide expressed as sodium lauryl sulphate or Etoxon (Table 3).

Discussion

The practical value of tests in vitro is the rapid availability of data on the character of test substance effects, defined conditions of testing in

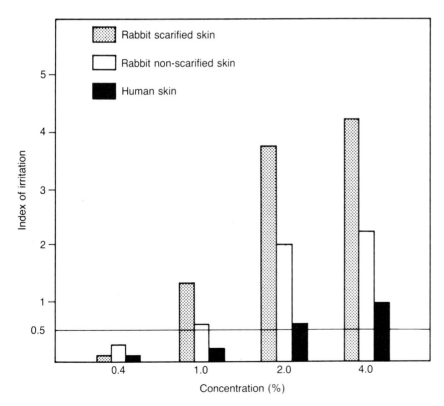

Figure 1

In vivo primary skin irritation of formaldehyde.

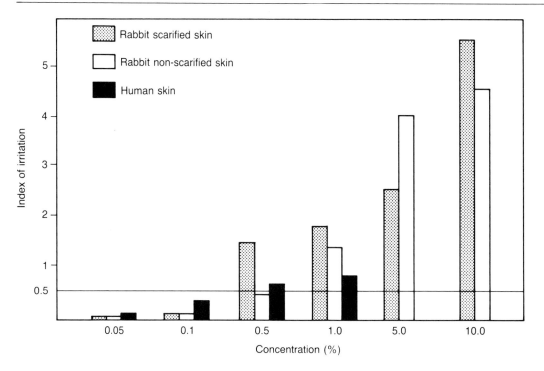

Figure 2

In vivo primary skin irritation of sodium lauryl sulphate.

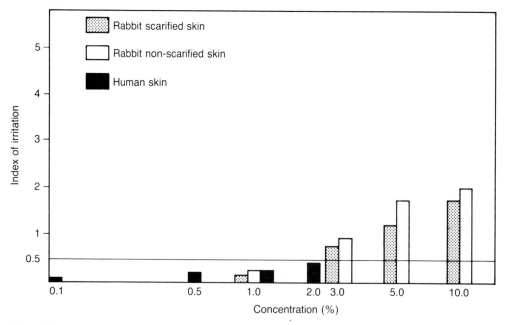

Figure 3

In vivo primary skin irritation of Kathon CG.

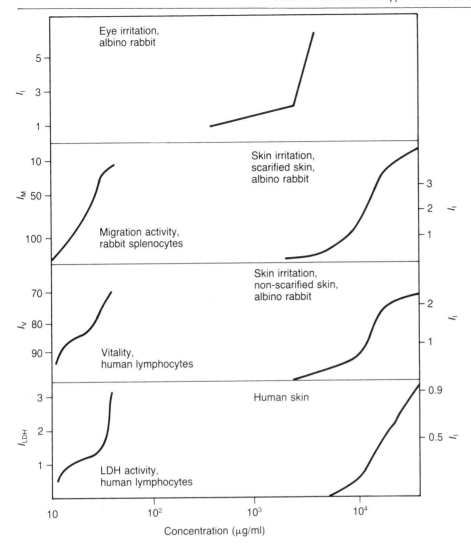

Figure 4

Responses to in vivo and in vitro tests with formaldehyde.

the tissue culture, accuracy and objectivity of the test results, low cost, standardization and reliability. This mode of testing provides important complementary information on the biological properties of the substances examined in vivo. It is considered to have the potential to become a practical method of testing in routine practice.[1,2,5,8,9,11]

Various cell types, including haemapoietic cells, peritoneal exudate macrophages, keratinocytes, splenocytes, liver cells and tumour cells, e.g. leukaemic cells, HeLa cells and T lymphoblastoid cells, have advantages at times.[3] In our study the human peripheral lymphocytes and rabbit splenocytes were used as the cellular substrate for tests in vitro. The reasons for using these cells were their easy accessibility, high sensitivity and the wide variety of pathophysiological changes that may be detected and influenced. Another reason is their analogy to a certain type of skin cell in some features, e.g. membrane markers, and their regular occurrence in the cellular infiltrate of both the irritant and allergic skin response.[10]

Responses to the test substance were dose dependent and showed non-specific toxicity. The in vitro methods were found to correlate well with the in vivo methods. They were more sensitive than in vivo techniques and could easily distinguish

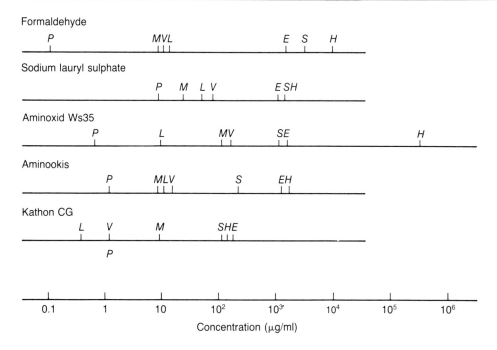

Figure 5

The highest non-toxic concentration of various substances as determined in vitro and in vivo. P, PHA stimulation test (human peripheral blood); M, migration activity (rabbit splenocytes); V, vitality (human peripheral lymphocytes); L, LDH activity (human peripheral lymphocytes); E, eye irritation (white rabbits); S, skin irritation (white rabbits); H, skin irritation (humans).

Table 2 Screening test — migration activity of rabbit splenocytes

Group of shampoos	Non-toxic concentration (μg/ml)
Derma tonic Kinder Schaumbad Shampoo mit Kamille, Gnann, Germany	600
Palmolive Baby Shampoo, Colgate, Austria	
Matchroom Conditioning Shampoo, Coty, UK	
Wella Balsam Shampoo for Normal Hair, Wella, Germany	
Old Spice Shampoo for Men, Shulton, UK	
Laginella Krauter Duft Shampoo, Gnann, Germany	500
XZ Shampoo Mildes, Berner, Finland	400
Poly Kur Balsam Shampoo, Henkel, Austria	400
XZ Shampoo Weinzen Heim Ol, Berner, Finland	250
Mild Shampoo, Catzy, Poland	
Siten Shampoo, Costas Minas, Cyprus	200
Phileas Gel Shampooing/Douche, Nina Ricci, France	
Shamtu Weissdorn Shampoo gegen, Shuppen, Blendax, Germany	150
Siten Shampoo Citron, Costas Minas, Cyprus	100
Head Shoulders Shampoo, Pro-Quality, Canada	Toxic
Crisan Shampoo Activ — Kur gegen Shuppen	Toxic

Table 3 Screening test — migration activity of rabbit splenocytes

Group of toothpastes	Non-toxic concentration (μg/ml)	Expressed as	
		SLS	Etoxon
Bis acidentol Deni denta Nhu'ṅgoc (Vietnam)	1000	1.88	2.36
Fytodent Azu Extradent Fluorodent (Finland) Macleans (UK)	2500	1.58	1.92
Elmex for children Perlička for children New Macleans (UK)	5000	0.65	0.61
Sotenal 2	10 000	0.27	0.26
Carlotherm	50 000		

SLS, sodium lauryl sulphate.

the particular effect of the substance under test. As is evident from Figures 4 and 5, the PHA stimulation test in the whole-blood culture is highly effective in the assessment of low-toxicity agents. The viability test and the test of LDH activity in human lymphocyte culture is well suited to establishing cell membrane integrity. The method of rabbit splenocyte migration activity turned out to be quite suitable for screening purposes (Tables 2 and 3).

Conclusions

The in vitro methods described here are very sensitive and useful for routine screening. They represent an ethical alternative approach to screening for irritation. Subsequent tests in vivo can then be performed on a limited number of experimental animals and human volunteers. The effects of new chemical substances should be evaluated using as many tests as possible.

The suggested series of in vitro tests can provide extended information on the mechanism controlling the action of the substances under test. This is of most importance in establishing adequate criteria for the safe application of substances in practice.

References

1 Goldemberg RL, In vitro toxicity testing, Drug Cosmet Ind (1985) 136: 24–96.
2 Wilcox DK. Bruner LH, In vitro alternatives for ocular safety testing — an outline of assays and possible future developments, ATLA — alternatives Lab Animals (1990) 18: 117–28.
3 Stringer DA, Skin irritation, ECETOC Monograph No. 15, Brussels, 1990.
4 Norme Française Homologuée NF-T 03-263, April 1982; Norme Française Homologuée NF-T 03-264, April 1982.
5 Nilson GE, Otto V, Assessment of skin irritancy in man by laser doppler flowmetry, Cont Dermatol (1982) 6: 401–6.
6 Jírová D, Fiker S, Teisinger J, In vitro tests for detecting toxic effects of dermotrophic substances, Rev Inst Pasteur Lyon (1986) 19: 233–44.
7 Horký J, Manifestation of radiation injury of human lymphocytes using PHA mitogenic stimulation in different culture systems, Physiol Bohemoslov (1986) 35: 497–512.
8 Švejcar J, Johanovský J, Pekárek J, In vitro technique of cell migration from the spleen and/or artificial fragments. In: Bloom BR, Glade PR, (eds). In vitro methods in cell-mediated immunity, Academic Press: London, 1971, p. 263.
9 Loden M, The simultaneous penetration of water and sodium lauryl sulfate through isolated human skin, J Soc Cosmet Chem (1990) 41: 227–33.
10 Green I, Immunological identification and function of dermal and epidermal cells, Br J Dermatol (1984) 3s (suppl 27): 1–10.
11 Muller C, Animal test alternatives: Rockefeller, John Hopkins utilize separate routes, Drug Cosmet Ind (1985) 136: 36–42.

44
Cutaneous manifestations of tetrachlorodibenzo-*p*-dioxin in children and adolescents

Ruggero Caputo
1st Department of Dermatology, University of Milan, Milan, Italy

After an accident in a chemical plant in Seveso, Italy, on 10 July 1976, 2,3,7,8-tetrachlorodibenzo-*p*-dioxin (TCDD) spread over a populated area. The event was exceptional because children were also affected and because the contamination took place not only through direct exposure but also through inhalation and the ingestion of contaminated foods, especially fruits and vegetables.

Dermatological manifestations were recognized as early lesions and late or acneform lesions. The early lesions appeared within a few hours or a few days after the accident and were ascribed to direct cutaneous exposure to the toxic cloud or to the contaminated soil.

Of 1660 people examined in the period from 20 to 40 days after the accident, 447 showed irritative cutaneous lesions. The main clinical features were erythema and oedema of exposed areas, vesiculo-bullous and necrotic lesions on the palms, and papulonodular lesions on the trunk and arms.

The acneform lesions (chloracne) appeared some 30–60 days after the accident and were considered to result both from direct exposure to TCDD and to the inhalation or intake of contaminated foods.

Chloracne was demonstrated in 44 subjects, 28 of whom had suffered from early lesions. Most of the patients were children aged 2–10 years or adolescents. The eruption (Figure 1) was characterized by comedo-like and cystic lesions; the malar region was the most frequently affected, while the centrofacial region was constantly and inexplicably spared, as has been reported in other chloracne cases.[1]

Severe manifestations were detected in only eight children, all of whom had shown early lesions. These subjects had follicular hyperkeratosis associated with comedones on the limbs. In three children granuloma annulare- or erythema elevatum diutinum-like lesions occurred on the palms, and two sisters had comedones and cysts of the axillae. The yearly follow-up of chloracne subjects revealed a progressive attenuation of signs and

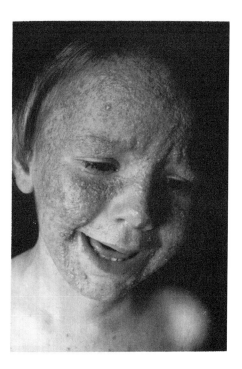

Figure 1

A severe case of chloracne with sparing of the centrofacial region.

symptoms, and the onset of atrophic-cicatricial lesions about 1 year after the accident in 36 patients. The degree of scarring varied from pitting, as in atrophoderma vermiculatum, to extensive scarring in the most severe cases.

In conclusion, the dermatological findings in the years following this accident demonstrated the following points. (i) Chloracne is the most reliable and typical sign of poisoning by TCDD. (ii) Chloracne, especially in prepubertal children, is the most sensitive indicator of environmental pollution. (iii) Chloracne has a predilection for children and adolescents. (iv) Chloracne is more severe in subjects who experience early, irritative lesions, and the severity of clinical signs is related to the degree of topical TCDD exposure and, probably, to TCDD inhalation and ingestion. (v) To our knowledge[2] none of the patients who suffered from chloracne subsequently developed systemic lesions or important laboratory abnormalities. (vi) Atrophic scars are the only sequelae of the accident.

References

1 Tindall JP, Chloracne and chloracnegens, *J Am Acad Dermatol* (1985) **13**: 539–58.
2 Moccarelli P, Marocchi A, Brambilla P, Clinical laboratory manifestations of exposure to dioxin in children. A six-year study of the effects of an environmental disaster near Seveso, Italy, *J Am Med Assoc* (1986) **256**: 2687–95.

45
Systemic toxicity in man secondary to percutaneous absorption*

Susanne Freeman and Howard I. Maibach
University of California Hospital, San Francisco, CA 94143-0989, USA

Human skin is exposed to chemicals from birth to death. Although not generally appreciated, some chemicals are more toxic, at least in animals, topically than orally. Furthermore, many compounds are absorbed to a greater degree from the skin than orally and, on whole body exposure produces systemic absorption of grams of material. This chapter focuses on the limited epidemiological data, depending largely on case reports.

Factors affecting absorption

Many drugs for topical use on the skin and mucous membranes are capable of producing systemic side-effects the occurrence and severity of which depend largely on factors that affect the absorption of topically applied drugs.

The integrity of the barrier

The stratum corneum layer of the epidermis is the skin's main barrier to transepidermal absorption. Follicular orifices and sweat gland ducts may provide additional pathways for absorption. Anything which alters the structure or function of the stratum corneum will affect epidermal absorption. The integrity of this barrier, with resultant increase in percutaneous absorption, is reduced by any inflammatory process of the skin, such as any form of dermatitis or psoriasis. Similarly, removal of the stratum corneum by stripping or damage by alkalis, acids, etc., will increase percutaneous absorption.

* Updated with permission from Haddad L and Winchester J, Clinical Management and Drug Overdose, 2nd ed., W. B. Saunders, Philadelphia, 1990.

The physico-chemical properties of the substance

Absorption decreases with increasing molecular size. It is affected by the relative water/lipid solubility of the drug and the relative solubility of the drug in its vehicle compared with its solubility in the stratum corneum.

Occlusion

The penetration of topical drugs may be increased by the use of an occlusive covering, by a factor of 10 or more. This is because of increased water retention in the stratum corneum, increased blood flow, increased temperature, and increased surface area after prolonged occlusion (skin wrinkling).

The vehicle containing the drug

The greater the affinity of a vehicle for the drug it contains, the less the percutaneous absorption of the drug. The physical properties of vehicles, especially the degree of occlusion they produce, affect percutaneous absorption, as discussed above (e.g. greases). Structural or chemical damage to the barrier layer can be caused by the vehicle used; vehicles such as dimethyl sulphoxide cause greatly increased percutaneous absorption. In general, higher concentration of the drug in its vehicle enhances penetration.

Site of application

Regional differences in permeability of skin largely depend on the thickness of the intact stratum. According to the findings of a study by Feldmann and Maibach[1] the highest total absorption of hydrocortisone is that from the scrotum, followed (in decreasing order) by absorption from the forehead, scalp, back, forearms, palms and plantar surfaces.

Age

The greatest toxicological response to topical administration has been seen in the infant. The preterm infant does not have intact barrier function and hence is more susceptible to systemic toxocity from topically applied drugs.[2,3]

A normal full-term infant probably has a fully developed stratum corneum with complete barrier function.[4] Yet, according to Wester et al,[5] topical application of the same amount of a compound to both the adult and the newborn child results in a 2.7-fold greater systemic availability in the newborn. This is because the ratio of surface area to body weight in the newborn is three times that in the adult. Therefore, given an equal area of application of a drug to the skin of the newborn and adults, the proportion absorbed per kilogram of body weight is much more in the infant.

Temperature

Increased skin temperature usually enhances penetration.

Metabolism

Like the liver, the skin is capable of metabolizing drugs and foreign substances. It contains many of the enzyme systems of the liver, and its metabolizing potential has been estimated to be about 2% of that of the liver.[6]

Systemic side-effects caused by topically applied drugs and cosmetics

Topically applied drugs and cosmetics can cause allergic or irritant contact dermatitis. However, this type of side-effect, usually limited to the skin, is outside the scope of the present article. The reader is referred to the textbooks by Cronin[7] and Fisher[8] for references to contact dermatitis. Systemic side-effects from topically applied chemicals can sometimes result from either a toxic (irritant) reaction or a hypersensitivity reaction. The latter can be an anaphylactic type of reaction which is the extreme manifestation of the contact urticaria syndrome.[9] Many topical drugs and cosmetics have reportedly caused anaphylactic reactions.

While anaphylactic reactions to topical medicaments are uncommon, their potentially serious nature warrants attention. However, reports of toxic (as distinct from allergic) reactions to applied drugs and cosmetics are more numerous and include many medicaments which have been used safely for many years, but which can be toxic under specific circumstances.

Antibiotics

Chloramphenicol

Oral administration of chloramphenicol may lead to aplastic anaemia.[10] A case of marrow aplasia with a fatal outcome after topical application of chloramphenicol in eye ointment has been described by Abrams et al.[11] There have been three earlier reports of bone marrow aplasia after the use of chloramphenicol containing eye drops.

Clindamycin

Topical clindamycin is widely used in the treatment of acne vulgaris. It is estimated that 4–5% of clindamycin hydrochloride is absorbed systemically.[12] The degree of absorption largely depends on the vehicle, ranging from 0.13% (acetone) to 13.92% (DMSO).[13] Several cases of topical clindamycin associated diarrhoea have been reported.[14–16]

Pseudomembranous colitis is a well-recognized side-effect of systemic administration of clindamycin. A case of pseudomembranous colitis after topical administration has been reported.[17] It was concluded that all patients receiving topical clindamycin should be warned to discontinue therapy and consult their physician if intestinal symptoms occur.

Gentamicin

Ototoxicity is a well-known hazard of systemic gentamicin administration. However, topical application to large thermal injuries of the skin has similarly caused ototoxic effects, ranging from mild to severe hearing loss, with an associated decrease in vestibular function.[18] In the two patients described, the measured serum levels of gentamicin were 1.0–3.0 μg/ml and 3.3–4.3 μg/ml, respectively. Drake[19] described a woman who developed tinnitus each time she treated her paronychia with 0.1% gentamicin sulfate cream. Use of gentamicin ear drops may also be associated with ototoxic reactions.[20]

Neomycin

Just as ototoxicity is a well-known hazard of parenteral neomycin administration, so has deafness been reported after almost any form of local treatment, including treatment of skin infections and burns,[21–23] application as an aerosol for inhalation, instillation into cavities,[24] irrigation of large wounds,[25] and use of neomycin containing eardrops.[26] Kellerhals[27] has reported 13 cases of inner-ear damage in which the use of eardrops containing neomycin and polymycin were incriminated. All cases had perforated tympanic membranes and Kellerhals concluded that these drops (and also those containing chloromycetin, colistin and polymycin) should not be used in such cases for periods longer than 10 days.

Antihistamines

Diphenylpyraline hydrochloride

Diphenylpyraline hydrochloride has been used topically in Germany for the treatment of eczematous and other itching dermatoses. Symptomatic psychosis has been observed in 12 patients, nine of whom were children. The amount of active drug applied ranged from 225 to 1350 mg. The first symptoms of intoxication were psychomotor restlessness in all cases, usually within 24 h. Other symptoms included disorientation, and optic and acoustic hallucinations. All symptoms disappeared 4 days after discontinuation of the topical medication.[28]

Promethazine

Bloch and Beysovec[29] have reported a 16-month-old male weighing 11.5 kg who was treated with 2% promethazine cream for generalized eczema. After approximately 15–20 g of the cream had been applied, the child fell asleep. He woke a few hours later with abnormal behavior, loss of balance, inability to focus, irritability, drowsiness and failure to recognize his mother. One day later all symptoms had spontaneously disappeared. A diagnosis of promethazine toxicity through percutaneous absorption was made. Known symptoms of promethazine toxicity include disorientation, hallucinations, hyperactivity, convulsions and coma.

Antimicrobial agents

Boric acid

The toxicity of this mildly bacteriostatic substance is described by Done.[30] Undoubtedly the use of borates should be abandoned because of their limited therapeutic value and high toxicity. In recent times few cases of borate intoxication have been reported, probably due to its decreasing use.

Castellani's solution

Castellani's solution (or paint) is an old medicament mainly used for the local treatment of fungal skin infections. It contains boric acid (5.0), fuchsin (5.0), resorcinol (100.0), water (705.0), phenol (40.0; 90%), acetone (50.0), and spirit (100.0).

Lundell and Nordman[31] have reported a case in which two applications of Castellani's solution severely poisoned a 6-week-old boy who became cyanotic with 41% methemoglobin. The authors state that this case demonstrates that the application of Castellani's solution to napkin eruptions and other areas where absorption is rapid, may cause serious complications.

Another case report[32] states that hours after the application of Castellani's paint to the entire body surface except the face of a 6-week-old infant for severe seborrheic eczema, the child became drowsy and had shallow breathing. The authors state that phenol was detected in the urine of four out of 16 children treated with Castellani's paint.

Hexachlorophene

Since 1961 hexachlorophene[33] has been used extensively in hospital nurseries, mainly for reducing the incidence of staphylococcal infections among the newborn. In addition, it has been an ingredient of many medical preparations, cosmetics and other consumer goods.

Hexachlorophene readily penetrates damaged skin and its absorption through intact skin has also been demonstrated.[34–36]

In 1972 in France, as a result of the accidental addition of 6.3% of hexachlorophene to batches of baby talcum powder, 204 babies fell ill and 36 died from respiratory arrest.[37,38] This report was followed by animal experiments with hexachlorophene confirming that the drug is neurotoxic.

Consequently, in 1972 the US Food and Drug Administration (USFDA) banned the use of hexachlorophene to prescription use only, or as a surgical scrub and hand wash for health-care personnel. Hexachlorophene was excluded from cosmetics except as a preservative in levels not exceeding 0.1%.

Because of the high absorption through damaged skin and its proven neurotoxicity, hexachlorophene is contraindicated for the treatment of burns or application to otherwise damaged skin. Premature infants are also at risk. The safety of hexachlorophene for routine bathing of babies is still controversial. Plueckhahn et al[39] and Hopkins[40] have reviewed the benefits and risks of hexachlorophene.

4-Homosulfanilamide

4-Homosulfanilamide (sulfamylon acetate; 4-H-S) is a topical sulfonamide which was used for the treatment of large burns. It has nowadays been largely replaced by silver sulfadiazine. Sulfamylon is a carbonic anhydrase inhibitor and has been found to cause hyperchloremic metabolic acidosis in patients with extensive burns treated with its topical application, caused by percutaneous absorptions of the drug.[41,42] Reversible pulmonary complications[43] and methemoglobinuria[44] have also been reported.

Iodine and povidone iodine

Povidone iodine (betadine) is a water-soluble iodine complex which retains the broad-range microbiocidal activity of iodine without the undesirable effects of iodine tincture. However, toxicity still occurs from povidone iodine absorbed percutaneously, mainly when it is used on large areas of burnt skin or on neonates.[45]

Phenol

Phenol (carbolic acid) is no longer widely used as a skin antiseptic, but in dilutions of 0.5–2.0% it is sometimes prescribed as an antipruritic in topical medicaments and is used for phenol face peels.

It has been shown that as much as 25% of phenol is absorbed from 2 ml of a solution of 2.5 g phenol/litre water applied to the skin of the forearm and left on for 60 min.[46] The toxic dose for adults has been estimated to be 8–15 g.

Phenol induced ochronosis has been reported[47] in patients who for many years treated leg ulcers with wet dressings containing phenol.

There have been several case reports of fatal reactions to percutaneously absorbed phenol. One was caused by accidental spillage of phenol,[48] one due to treatment of burns with a phenol containing preparation,[49] and another due to the application of phenol to wounds.[50] A 1-day-old child died after application of 2% phenol to the umbilicus.[51]

Several cases of sudden death or intra- or post-operative complications have been reported after phenol face peels.[52] Major cardiac arrhythmias were noted[53] in 10 out of 43 patients during phenol face peels. However, this item is rather controversial and some authors feel that when the procedure is done over more than than 1 h, and when the dose applied is carefully monitored, phenol face peels are safe.[54,55] Poisoning due to phenol ingestion is described by Haddam.[56]

Resorcinol

Resorcinol is used for its keratolytic properties in the treatment of acne vulgaris. It is also a constituent of the antifungal Castellani's solution. Formerly, leg ulcers were treated with external applications of resorcinol containing applications.

Resorcinol can penetrate human skin. It has an anti-thyroid activity similar to that of methylthiouracil, although it is chemically unrelated to any of the known groups of antithyroid drugs. Consequently, several cases of myxoedema caused by percutaneous absorption of resorcinol, especially from ulcerated surfaces, have been described.[57,58]

Methemoglobinemia in children, caused by absorption of resorcinol applied to wounds, has been reported.[59,60] Cunningham[61] reported a case in which an ointment containing 12.5% resorcinol applied to the nappy area of an infant produced cyanosis, hemolytic anaemia and hemoglobinemia. The author found seven reported cases in the literature of acute poisoning in babies as a consequence of topical resorcinol application, in some instances to limited areas; five fatalities were recorded.

A case of severe poisoning of a 6-week-old infant due to two applications of Castellani's paint has been described.[62]

Although the use of resorcinol in young children and for leg ulcers should be avoided, topical resorcinol, when used for acne vulgaris, appears to be safe.[63]

Silver sulfadiazine

Sulfadiazine silver cream is widely used for the topical treatment of burns. Intended primarily for the control of pseudomonas infections, this bactericidal agent acts on the cell membranes and cell walls of a variety of Gram-positive and Gram-negative bacteria, as well as on yeasts. Its relative freedom from appreciable side-effects has contributed to its popularity.

Absorption of sulfonamide from burns to 17–46% body area treated with sulfadiazine silver showed that 20–25% of the daily topical dose could be accounted for as conjugated sulfonamide. Unconjugated drug represented from 35–95% of the total output. Total plasma, sulfonamide concentration did not exceed 10 μg/ml.[64]

There has been one report of nephrotic syndrome following topical therapy.[65] Several authors have reported leukopenia during treatment with silver sulfadiazine.[66–68] Current evidence suggests a causal relationship between silver sulfadiazine and leukopenia, although the mechanism of this reaction is unknown. Examination of bone marrow aspirates show hyperplasia with no evidence of maturation arrest. The drug presumably affects the white blood cells peripherally.[68] The sulfadiazine induced leukopenia is at its nadir within 2–4 days of the start of therapy. The leucocyte count returns to normal levels within 2–3 days and recovery is not affected by continuation of therapy. The erythrocyte count is not affected.

Triclocarban

Triclocarban (trichlorocarbanilide, TCC) is a bacteriostatic agent which has been used as an antimicrobial in toilet soap since 1956. The percutaneous absorption of TCC has been studied by Scharpf et al[69] who showed that, after a simple shower employing a whole-body lather with approximately 6 g of soap containing 2% TCC, about 0.23% of the applied dose of TCC was recovered in feces afer 6 days, and 0.16% of the dose in the urine afer 2 days. At all sampling times, blood levels of radioactivity were below the detection limit of 10 ppb. There have been several reports[70, 71] of methemoglobinemia presumably induced by topical TCC in neonates.

Arsenic

The toxicity of ingested or inhaled arsenic has been described by Robertson.[72] Fowler's solution, which was for a long time used orally in the treatment of psoriasis, contained arsenic. Arsenical keratoses and malignancies are well recognized long-term reactions to this.

Carmustine

Topical carmustine (BCNU) has been used for the treatment of mycosis fungoides, lymphomatoid papulosis and parapsorias en plaques. Percutaneous absorption of BCNU has been demonstrated in man. Zackheim et al (to be published) treated 91 patients with mycosis fungoides and related disorders with topical BCNU. Mild to moderate reversible bone marrow depression occurred in three patients. Their data suggest that hematological toxicity arises primarily from the shorter intensive schedules; the prolonged use of up to 100 mg/week appears to be safe. Although an occasional mild elevation in the blood urea nitrogen or serum glutamic oxaloacetic transaminase (SGOT) was noted in patients treated with courses exceeding 600 mg, no such changes were seen with lower doses. In the study by Zackheim et al, there were no apparent long-term harmful effects on the hematopoietic system or internal organs.

Camphor

Camphor is a pleasant-smelling cyclic ketone of the hydroaromatic terpene group. When rubbed on the skin, camphor is a rubefacient but, if not virorously applied, produces a feeling of coolness. It is an ingredient of a large number of over-the-counter remedies (with a camphor content of 1–20%), taken especially for symptomatic relief of chest congestion and muscle aches, but its effectiveness is rather dubious.

Camphor is readily absorbed from all sites of administration, including topical application to the skin.

The compound is classified as a class IV chemical, i.e. a very toxic substance. Hundreds of cases of intoxication have been reported, usually after accidental ingestion in chidren.

Cosmetic and other agents

Henna dye and p-phenylenediamine

The use of a henna dye is traditional in Islamic communities. The dye is used on nails, skin and hair by married ladies and, traditionally, also by the major participants in marriage cermonies, when the bridegroom and best man also apply henna to their hands.

Henna consists of the dried leaves of *Lawsonia alba* (family Lythraceae), a shrub which is cultivated in North Africa, India and Sri Lanka. The coloring matter, lawsone, is a hydroxynaphthoquinone and this is associated with fats, resin and henna tanin in the leaf. Dyeing hair or skin with powdered henna is a somewhat lengthy procedure and in order to speed up this process, Sudanese ladies mix a 'black powder' with henna; this accelerates the fixing process of the dye to a matter of minutes. This 'black powder' is paraphenylenediamine. The combination of henna and 'black powder' is particularly toxic and over 20 cases of such toxicity, some fatal, have been noted in Khartoum alone in a 2-year period. Initial symptoms are those of angioneurotic edema with massive edema of the face, lips, glottis, pharynx, neck and bronchi. These occur within hours of the application of the dye-mix to the skin. The symptoms may then progress on the second day to anuria and acute renal failure with death occurring on the third day. Dialysis has helped some patients, but others have died from renal tubular necrosis.[73] Whether this toxicity is due to *p*-phenylenediamine per se (probably grossly impure) or whether its toxicity is potentiated in its combination with henna powder is unknown. Systemic administration of the 'black powder' leads to similar symptoms, and several deaths due to ingestion with suicidal intent have been reported.[74]

Diethyltoluamide

Diethyltoluamide has been used as an insect repellent since 1957. Although diethyltoluamide has an overall low incidence of tonic effects, prolonged use in children has been discouraged because of reports of toxic encephalopathy.[75,76] In one case the bedding, nightclothes and skin of a 3½-year-old girl were sprayed daily for 2 weeks with a total of 180 ml of 15% diethyltoluamide. Shaking and crying spells, slurred speech and confusion developed. Improvement occurred after vigorous medical treatment including anticonvulsants. In another report, one of two children displaying signs of severe tonic encephalopathy died after prolonged hospitalization. At autopsy, edema of the brain and congestion of the meninges was found.

Dimethyl sulfoxide

The toxicology of topical dimethyl sulfoxide (DMSO) has been investigated by Kligman.[77] In this study, 9 ml of 90% DMSO was applied twice daily to the entire trunk of 20 healthy volunteers for 3 weeks. The following laboratory tests were done: complete blood count, urinalysis, blood sedimentation rate, SGOT, BUN and fasting blood sugar determinations. At the end of the study, all laboratory values had remained normal. Except for the appearance of cutaneous signs as erythema, scaling, contact urticaria, stinging and burning sensations, the drug was tolerated well by all but two individuals, who developed systemic symptoms. In one, a toxic reaction developed on day 12 which was characterized by a diffuse erythematous and scaling rash accompanied by severe abdominal cramps; the other had a similar rash and complained of nausea, chills and chest pains. These signs, however, abated in spite of continued administration of the drug.

To investigate possible side-effects of chronic exposure to DMSO another 20 volunteers were painted with 9 ml of 90% DMSO applied to the entire trunk, once daily for a period of 26 weeks. Neither clinical nor laboratory investigations showed adverse effects of the drug. However, most subjects did experience the well-known DMSO induced disagreeable oyster-like breath odour, to which they eventually became insensitive. One fatality due to a hypersensitivity reaction has been reported.[78]

Dinitrochlorobenzene

Dinitrochlorobenzene (DNCB), a potent contact allergen, has been used with some success for the treatment of recalcitrant alopecia areata. Today, however, its use has been discouraged because suspicion has been aroused that DNCB may be mutagenic. Another drawback for its use is its ability to potentiate epicutaneous sensitization to non-related allergens.[79] DNCB is absorbed in substantial amounts through the skin, and about 50% of the applied dose is ultimately recoverable in the urine.[80]

A possible systemic reaction to DNCB has been reported:[81] a 25-year-old man was treated with 0.1% DNCB in an absorbent ointment base for alopecia areata after prior sensitization. After 2 months of daily application the patient experienced generalized urticaria, pruritus and dyspepsia. Discontinuation of drug led to cessation of all symptoms, which recurred after reintroduction of DNCB therapy.

Ethyl alcohol

Twenty-eight children with alcohol intoxication from percutaneous absorption have been described by Gimenez et al[82] from Buenos Aires, Argentina. Apparently, in that area it is (or was) a popular procedure to apply alcohol soaked cloths to the abdomen of babies as a home remedy for the treatment of disturbances of the gastrointestinal tract such as cramps, pain, vomiting and diarrhoea, or because of crying, excitability and irritability. The children were of both sexes and ranged in age from 33 months to 1 year (mean 12 months, 27 days). Alcohol soaked cloths had been applied on the babies' abdomen under rubber pants, and the number of applications varied from one to three; it was estimated that each application contained approximately 40 cm^3 ethanol. Medical consultation took place from 1 to 23 h after application. Alcoholic breath and abdominal erythema were valuable clues to the diagnosis.

All 28 children showed some degree of central nervous system depression, 24 showed miosis, 15 hypoglycaemia, five convulsions, five respiratory depression and two died. Eleven children had blood alcohol levels of 0.6–1.49 g%. Of the two who died, one was autopsied: the findings were consistent with ethyl alcohol intoxication.

More recently, a case of acute ethanol intoxication in a preterm infant of 1800 g due to local application of alcohol soaked compresses on the legs as a treatment for puncture hematomas has been reported.[83]

Topically applied ethanol in tar gel[84] and beer containing shampoo has caused antabuse effects in patients on disulfiram therapy for alcoholism, through percutaneous absorption.

Fumaric acid monethyl ester

The effect of systemically and/or topically administered fumaric acid monoethyl ester (ethyl fumarate) on psoriasis has been studied by Dubiel and Happle[85] in six patients. Two patients who had been treated with locally applied ointments, consisting of 3% or 5% ethyl fumarate in petrolatum, developed symptoms of renal intoxication.

Local anaesthetics

Benzocaine

Methemoglobinemia has been reported following the topical application of benzocaine to both skin and mucous membranes.[86-90] However, this is an uncommon occurrence;[91] most cases occurred in infants.

Lidocaine

Lidocaine hydrochloride is widely used for both topical and local injection anesthesia. When the drug is applied to mucous membranes, blood levels simulate those resulting from intravenous injection.[92] Serum lidocaine concentrations higher than 6 μg/ml are associated with toxicity.[93] The signs are those of central nervous system stimulation followed by depression and later inhibition of cardiovascular function. Systemic toxicity from viscous lidocaine applied to the oral cavity in two children has been described.[94,95] In one, the mother had been applying lidocaine hydrochloride 2% solution to the infant's gums with her finger 5–6 times daily for 1 week; the child experienced two generalized seizures within 1 h. Urine examined using thin layer chromatography revealed a large amount of lidocaine, and a blood level of 10 μg/ml was determined.[95] The other child had a seizure after having received 227.8 mg/kg oral viscous lidocaine for stomatitis herpetica over a 24-h period. In this case, however, ingestion and resorption from the gastrointestinal tract may have contributed to the clinical picture. It has been suggested that for pediatric patients viscous lidocaine should be applied with an oral swab to individual lesions, thus limiting buccal absorption by decreasing the surface area exposed to lidocaine.[94]

Mercurials

The toxicology of mercury has been comprehensively described by Aronow.[96] With a few exceptions, the use of mercury in medicine is considered to be outdated. However, attention should be paid to the possibility of mercurial poisoning even nowadays, as mercury may still be present in many drugs, and in many countries even in over-the-counter remedies, often without mention on the label.

Although there are considerable differences between various mercurials regarding the rate of absorption through the skin, all mercurial preparations are a potential hazard and may cause intoxication. Metallic mercury is readily absorbed through intact skin; absorption of ammoniated mercury chloride in psoriatic patients has been demonstrated by Bork et al.[97]

Young[98] examined 70 psoriatic patients treated with an ointment containing ammoniated mercury before, during and after treatment. Symptoms and signs of mercurial poisoning could be detected in 33 patients.

Nephrotic syndrome has been reported in a 24-year-old man using an ammoniated mercury containing ointment for psoriasis.[99,100] Nephrotic syndrome due to topical mercury was also reported by Lyons et al.[101]

There have been two case reports[102,103] of children who died following the treatment of an omphalocele with merbromin (an organic mercurial antiseptic).

In view of the risks of both systemic side-effects and contact allergic reactions to mercurials, there seems to be no justification for the continuing use of these drugs in dermatological therapy.

Monobenzone

Monobenzone (monobenzyl ether of hydroquinone) is used topically by patients with extensive vitiligo to depigment their remaining normally pigmented skin. A patient who had been applying the drug for 1 year had an anterior linear deposition of pigment on both corneas. In 11 additional patients with vitiligo who were using monobenzone, acquired conjuctival melanosis occurred in two patients and pingueculae in three.[104]

2-Napththol

2-Naphthol (β-naphthol) is used in peeling pastes for the treatment of acne and between 5% and 10% of a cutaneous dose has been recovered from the urine.[105,106] The extensive application of 2-napththol ointments has been responsible for systemic side-effects, including vomiting and death.[107,108]

Hemels[106] concluded that 2-naphthol containing pastes should be applied for short periods of time and to a limited area not exceeding 150 cm^2.

Insecticides

Lindane is the γ isomer of benzene hexachloride and is widely used in the treatment of scabies and pediculosis, usually in a 1% lotion which is applied to the entire body and left on for 24 h (in the case of scabies). The percutaneous absorption of the drug has been studied.[109–111] The general toxicology has been described by Haddad.[112]

Intoxication from excessive topical therapeutic application of lindane has been documented.[113–115] The issue of possible toxic reactions to a single therapeutic application of lindane, notably central nervous system toxicity, has not yet been settled.[116–119] Most authors seem to agree that the benefits to be derived from the use of lindane as a scabicide and pediculicide outweigh the risks involved.[120–123] The risk of toxicity appears minimal when lindane is used properly according to directions. Solomon et al,[120] in their review of lindane toxicity, provide dosing recommendations.

Malathion

The detailed toxicology of malathion has been described by Haddad.[124] Malathion is used in the treatment of lice, a single application of 0.5% in a solution being customary. Used in this way, it is generally safe.

Ramu et al[125] have reported on four children with intoxication following hair washing with a solution containing 50% malathion in xylene for the purpose of louse control. Malathion is also a weak but definite skin sensitizer.[126]

Podophyllum

The toxicity of podophyllum has been described by Haddad[127] and by Cassidy et al.[128] Although there have been a significant number of case reports describing serious neurologic illness or death following the application of podophyllum, these are generally related to its use in widespread lesions. Podophyllum (20%) in tincture of benzoin is still indicated by isolated venereal warts.[129] Its use is contraindicated in pregnancy. Following application it should be washed off after a specific period of time.

Salicylic acid

The general toxicology of salicylates has been described by Proudfoot,[130] including its absorption through the skin. Salicylic acid is widely used in dermatology as a topical application for its keratolytic properties. Cases of salicylate poisoning after topical use of salicylic acid have been reported on several occasions. Taylor and Halprin[131] used 6% salicylic acid in a gel base under plastic suit occlusion in adults with extensive psoriasis. During their 5-day study, serum salicylates never exceeded 5 mg/100 ml and no patient developed toxicity. However, toxicity was noted by von Weis and Lever[132] who found serum salicylate levels ranging from 46 to 64 mg/100 ml. Salicylic acid therapy for extensive lesions may be especially dangerous for children. An unpublished review[133] revealed 13 deaths associated with the widespread use of salicylic acid preparations, and all but three occurred in children. This compound should not be used on large areas (more than 25%) of the skin of a child.[133]

In 1952, Young[98] collected eight fatal cases of salicylate poisoning with symptoms of vomiting, tinnitus, stupor, Cheyne–Stokes respiration and nuchal rigidity.

Von Weis and Lever[132] reported on three adults with extensive psoriasis who were treated with an ointment containing 3% or 6% salicylic acid six times daily. Between days 2 and 4, symptoms of salicylism developed in all three patients. The levels of salicylic acid in the serum ranged from 46 to 64 mg/100 ml. Within 1 day after discontinuation of the ointment, the symptoms had largely disappeared. The serum salicylic acid in the serum decreased to zero within a few days.

The same authors also recorded 13 deaths resulting from intoxication with salicylic acid following the application of salicylic ointment to the skin, reported in the literature up to 1964, and several non-fatal intoxications. The 13 deaths included three patients with psoriasis, five cases of scabies, three of dermatitis, one of lupus vulgaris and one of congenital ichthyosiform erythroderma. Ten of the fatal cases occurred in children, three of them being under 3 years of age.

The most dramatic account in the literature is that of two plantation workers in Bougainville, in the Solomon Islands, who were painted twice a day with an alcoholic solution of 20% salicylic acid to tinea imbricata involving about 50% of the body. The victims were comatose within 6 hours and dead within 28 h.[134]

Wechselberg[135] reported on a 3-month-old baby with scaly erythroderma treated in hospital with 1% salicylic acid in soft paraffin. After 10 days, the child began to vomit and lose weight. Later hyperpnea developed and an increasing somnolence. When the treatment was stopped, the child recovered rapidly.

Recently, a case of salicylic acid intoxication leading to coma in an adult patient with psoriasis, who had been treated with 20% salicylic acid in petrolatum, has been described.[136]

Selenium sulfide

Ransone et al[137] have reported a case of systemic selenium toxicity in a woman who had been shampooing her hair two or three times weekly for 8 months with selenium sulfide suspension.

Silver nitrate

Ternberg and Luce[138] observed fatal methemoglobinemia in a 3-year-old girl suffering from burns involving 82% of the body surface who was treated with silver nitrate solution.

Another complication of the use of silver nitrate in the treatment of large burns is electrolyte disturbance, especially in children. Due to the hypotonicity of the silver nitrate dressings, hyponatremia, hypokalemia and hyperchloremia may develop.[139,140] Also, loss of other water soluble minerals and vitamins may occur. Post-mortem examinations of patients treated with silver nitrate have revealed that silver has been deposited in internal organs showing that absorption of silver from topical preparation does occur.[141] It should be mentioned that the excessive use of silver containing drugs has led to local and systemic argyria[141] and to renal damage involving the glomeruli with proteinuria.[142]

Steroids

Corticosteroids

It has been amply documented that topically applied glucocorticosteroids are absorbed through the skin.[143] Systemic absorption in quantities sufficient to replace endogenous production is not uncommon. However, iatrogenic Cushing's syndrome resulting from the use of topical steroids is rare. Pascher[144] has summarized the relevant data of 12 cases.

Systemic side-effects of topical corticosteroids occur more frequently in children than adults[145] and in patients with liver disease because of retarded degradation of the drug.[146] The two main causes of systemic side-effects are hypercorticism leading to an iatrogenic Cushing's syndrome and suppression of the hypothalamic–pituitary–adrenal axis.[147]

It is not easy to provide data on 'safe' uses of topical corticosteroids but, as for the potent corticosteroid clobetasol-17-propionate, 0.05% is the dose recommended to be limited to 45 g per week.[148]

Sex hormones

Estrogens. Topical application of estrogen containing preparations may lead to resorption of these hormones and systemic estrogenic effects. Beas et al[149] have reported on seven children with pseudoprecocious puberty due to an ointment containing estrogens. The common factor found in every patient was the use of the same ointment for the treatment or prevention of ammoniacal dermatitis for a period of 2–18 months with 2–10 daily applications. Endocrinological and radiological studies excluded other possible causes of sexual precocity. The most important clinical signs were: intense pigmentation of mammillary areola, linea alba of the abdomen and the genitals, mammary enlargement and the presence of pubic hair. Three female patients also had vaginal discharge and bleeding. Estrogenic contamination of the ointment was suspected and confirmed by a biological test of the vaginal opening of castrated female guinea-pigs. After discontinuation of the incriminated topical drug, all symptomatology progressively disappeared in every patient.

Pseudoprecocious puberty has also been observed in young girls after contact with hair lotions and other substances containing estrogens.[150–152] Such contact has led to gynecomastia in young boys.[153,154] Gynecomastia in a 70-year-old man from exposure to 0.01% dienestrol cream used by his wife for atrophic vaginitis and as a lubricant before intercourse has been reported.[155]

Estrogen cream for the treatment of baldness has also caused gynecomastia, which was persistent in the reported case.[156] In adult males both oral and topical administration of estrogens may result first in pigmentation of the areola and then in gynecomastia.[157,158]

Tars

Coal tar

A case of methemoglobinemia in an infant following the 5-day application of an ointment containing 2.5% crude coal tar and 5% benzocaine to about half the body surface has been reported.[159]

Dithranol

Dithranol has been used since 1916 for the treatment of psoriasis. Although it causes irritant dermatitis and discoloration of the skin, its use is generally considered to be devoid of systemic side-effects.

Comment

In this chapter we have summarized the literature citations and the basic aspects of percutaneous penetration. The purpose of this chapter is to alert the reader to the potential for systemic toxicity from topical exposure. Demonstrating causality (rather than association) requires careful documentation. Combining knowledge of the inherent molecular and animal toxicology, cutaneous penetration, and metabolism with the adverse human reaction literature permits a more precise determination of causality. With each of the examples presented here, the original citations combined with the further documentation noted below should permit more discriminate causality judgements.

The above data focus the need for controlled studies on the toxicity of chemicals with skin exposure. Recent texts emphasizing current approaches and technology are those by Marzulli and Maibach[160] and Bronaugh and Maibach.[142,161]

Acknowledgement

We have drawn heavily upon the useful studies of J. P. Nater and A. C. de Groot in Chapter 16 of *Unwanted Effects of Cosmetics and Drugs Used in Dermatology*, 2nd edn, Elsevier, Amsterdam, 1985.

References

1. Feldmann RJ, Maibach HI, Regional variation in percutaneous penetration of 14C cortesol in man, *J Invest Dermatol* (1967) **48**: 181.
2. Nachman RL, Esterly NB, Increased skin permeability in pre-term infants, *J Pediatr* (1971) **89**: 628–32.
3. Greaves SJ, Ferry DJ, McQueen EJ, Serial hexachlorophene blood levels in the premature infant, *NZ Med J* (1975) **81**: 334–6.
4. Rasmussen JE, Percutaneous absorption in children. In: Dobson RL, (ed.). *1979 year book of dermatology*, Chicago: Year Book Medical, 1979, pp15–38.
5. Wester RC, Noonan PK, Cole MP et al, Percutaneous absorption of testosterone in the newborn rhesus monkey: comparison to the adult, *Pediatr Res* (1977) **11**: 737–9.
6. Pannatier A, Jenner B, Testa B et al, The skin as a drug-metabolizing organ, *Drug Metab Rev* (1978) **8**: 319–43.
7. Cronin E, *Contact dermatitis*, Churchill Livingstone: Edinburgh, 1980.
8. Fisher AE, *Contact dermatitis*, 3rd edn, Lea and Febiger: Philadelphia, 1986.
9. Von Krogh G, Maibach HI, The contact curticaria syndrome. In: Marzulli FN, Maibach HI, (eds). *Dermatotoxicology*, 3rd edn, Hemisphere Publishing Corp: Washington, 1987, chap 15, p341.
10. Wilson AJ, Mielke CH, Haematological consequences of poisoning. In: Haddad LM, Winchester JF, (eds). *Poisoning and drug overdose*, W. B. Saunders: Philadelphia, PA, 1983, chap 96, p893.
11. Abrams SM, Degnan TJ, Vinciguerra V, Marrow aplasia following topical application of chloramphenicol eye ointment. *Arch Intern Med* (1980) **140**: 576.
12. Barya M, Goldstein JA, Kane A et al, Systemic absorption of clindamycin hydrochloride after topical application, *J Am Acad Dermatol* (1982) **7**: 208.
13. Franz TJ, On the bioavailability of topical formulations of clindamycin hydrochloride, *J Am Acad Dermatol* (1983) **9**: 66.
14. Stoughton RB, Topical antibiotics for acne vulgaris: current usage, *Arch Dermatol* (1979) **115**: 486.
15. Voron DA, Systemic absorption of topical clindamycin, *Arch Dermatol* (1978) **114**: 798.
16. Becker LE, Bergstresser PR, Whiting DA et al, Topical clindamycin therapy for acne vulgaris: a cooperative clinical study, *Arch Dermatol* (1981) **117**: 482.
17. Milstone EB, McDonald AJ, Scholhamer CF, Pseudomembranous colitis after topical application of clindamycin, *Arch Dermatol* (1981) **117**: 154.
18. Dayal VS, Smith EL, McCain WG, Cochlear and vestibular gentamycin toxicity: a clinical study of systemic and topical usage, *Arch Otolaryng* (1974) **100**: 338.
19. Drake TE, Reaction of gentamycin sulfate cream, *Arch Dermatol* (1974) **110**: 638.
20. Mittelman H, Ototoxicity of 'ototopical' antibiotics: past, present, and future, *Trans Am Acad Ophthal Otolaryng* (1972) **76**: 1432.

21 Friedmann I, Aerosols containing neomycin, *Lancet* (1977) **i**: 1662.
22 Anonymous, Warning on aerosols containing neomycin, *Lancet* (1977) **i**: 1115.
23 Bamford MFM, Jones LF, Deafness and biochemical imbalance after burns treatment with topical antibiotics in young children, *Arch Dis Childhood* (1978) **53**: 326.
24 Masur H, Whelton PK, Whelton A, Neomycin toxocity revisited, *Arch Surg* (1976) **3**: 822.
25 Kelly DR, Nilo EN, Berggren RB, Deafness after topical neomycin wound irrigation, *New Engl J Med* (1969) **280**: 1338.
26 Goffinet M, A propos de la toxicite cliniquement presumable de certaintes gouttes otiques, *Acta Oto-Rhino-Laryng Belg* (1977) **31**: 585.
27 Kellerhals B, Horschaden durch ototoxische Ohrtropfen. Ergebnisse einer Umfrage, *HNO (Berl)* (1978) **26**: 49.
28 Cammann R, Hennecke H, Beier R, Symptomatische Psychosen nach Kolton-Gelee-Applikation, *Psychiat Neurol Med Psychol* (1971) **23**: 426.
29 Bloch R, Beysovec L, Promethazine toxicity through percutaneous absorption, *Contin Practice* (1982) **9**: 28.
30 Done AK, Borates. In: Haddad LM, Winchester JF, (eds). *Clinical management of poisoning and drug overdose*, W. B. Saunders: Philadelphia, PA, 1983, pp929.
31 Lundell E, Norman R, A case of infantile poisoning by topical application of Castellani's solution, *Ann Clin Res* (1973) **5**: 404.
32 Rogers SCF, Burrows D, Neill D, Percutaneous absorption of phenol and methylalcohol in magenta paint B.P.C., *Br J Dermatol* (1978) **98**: 559.
33 Haddad LM, Miscellany. In: Haddad LM, Winchester JF, (eds). *Clinical management of poisoning and drug overdose*, W. B. Saunders: Philadelphia, PA, 1983, chap 101, p929.
34 Tyrala EE, Hillman LS, Hillman RE et al, Clinical pharmacology of hexachlorophene in newborn infants, *J Pediatr* (1977) **91**: 481.
35 Curley A, Hawk RE, Kimbrough RD et al, Dermal absorption of hexachlorophane in infants, *Lancet* (1971) **ii**: 296.
36 Alder VD, Burman D, Coroner-Beryl D et al, Absorption of hexachlorophene from infant's skin, *Lancet* (1972) **ii**: 384.
37 Pines WI, Hexachlorophane: why FDA concluded that hexachlorophene was too potent and too dangerous to be used as it once was?, *FDA Consumer* (1972) **6**: 24.
38 Anonymous, Hexachlorophene today, *Lancet* (1982) **i**: 500 (editorial).
39 Plueckhahn VC, Ballard BA, Banis JM et al, Hexachlorophene preparations in infant antiseptic skin care: benefit, risks and the future, *Med J Aust* (1978) **2**: 555.
40 Hopkins J, Hexachlorophene: more bad news than good, *Food Cosm Toxicol* (1979) **17**: 410.
41 Otten H, Plempel M, Antibiotika und Chemotherapeutika in Einzeldar-stellungen. Chemotherapeutika mit breitem Wirkungsbereich. Sulfon-amide. In: Otten H, Plempel M, Seigenthaler G, (eds). *Antibiotika-Fibel*, Thieme-Verlag: Stuttgart, 1975, pp110–45.
42 Leibman PR, Kennelly MM, Hirsch EF, Hypercarbia and acidosis associated with carbonic anhydrase inhibition: a hazard of topical mafenide acetate use in renal failure, *Burns* (1982) **8**: 395.
43 Albert Th A, Lewis NS, Warpeha RL, Late pulmonary complications with use of mafenide acetate, *J Burn Care Rehab* (1982) **3**: 375.
44 Ohlgisser M, Adler MN, Ben-Dov B et al, Methemoglobinaemia induced by mafenide acetate in children. A report of two cases, *Br J Anaesth* (1978) **50**: 299.
45 Mofenson HC, Caraccio TR, Greensher J, Iodine. In: Haddad LM, Winchester JF, (eds). *Poisoning and drug overdose*, Chapter 66. W. B. Saunders: Philadelphia, PA, 1983, chap 66, p697.
46 Baranowski-Dutkiewicz B, Skin absorption of phenol from aqueous solutions in men, *Int Arch Occup Environ Hlth* (1981) **49**: 99.
47 Cullison D, Abele DC, O'Quinn JL, Localized exogenous ochronosis. Report of a case and review of the literature, *J Am Acad Dermatol* (1983) **8**: 882.
48 Johnstone RT, *Occupational medicine and industrial hygiene*, CV Mosby: St Louis, MO, 1948, p216.
49 Cronin RD, Brauer RO, Death due to phenol contained in Foille^R, *J Am Med Assoc* (1949) **139**: 777.
50 Diechmann WB, Local and systemic effects following skin contact with phenol — a review of the literature, *J Ind Hyg* (1949) **31**: 146.
51 Von Hinkel GK, Kitzel HW, Phenolvergiftungen bei Neugeborenen durch kutane Resorption, *Dtsch Gesunh-Wes* (1968) **23**: 240.
52 Del Pizzo A, Tanski EL, Chemical face peeling — malignant therapy for benign disease?, *Plast Reconstr Surg* (1980) **66**: 121 (editorial).
53 Truppman ES, Ellerby JD, Major electrocardiographic changes during chemical face peeling, *Plast Reconstr Surg* (1979) **63**: 44.
54 *Tromovitch TA, Safety of chemical face peels, J Am Acad Dermatol (1982) 7: 137 (letter).*
55 Baker TJ, The voice of polite dissent, *Plat Reconstr Surg* (1979) **63**: 262.
56 Haddam LM, Phenol, dinotrophenol and pentachlorophene. In: Haddad LM, Winchester JF, (eds). *Poisoning and drug overdose*, W. B. Saunders: Philadelphia, PA, 1983, chap 87, p810.
57 Berthezene F, Fournier M, Bernier E et al, L'Hypothyroidie induite par la resorcine, *Lyon Med* (1973) **230**: 319.
58 Thomas AE, Gisburn MA, Exogenous ochronosis and myxoedema from resorcinol, *Br J Dermatol* (1961) **73**: 378.
59 Flandin C, Rabeau H, Ukrainczyk M, Intolerance à la resorcine, Test cutane, *Soc Derm Syph* (1953) **12**: 1804.
60 Murray MC, An analysis of sixty cases of drug poisoning, *Arch Pediatr* (1926) **43**: 193.
61 Cunningham AA, Resorcin poisoning, *Arch Dis Childhood* (1956) **31**: 173.
62 Lundell E, Nordman R, A case of infantile poisoning by topical application of Castellani's solution, *Ann Clin Res*

(1973) 5: 404.
63 Yeung D, Kanto S, Nacht S et al, Percutaneous absorption, blood levels and urinary excretion of resorcinol applied topically in humans, *Int J Dermatol* (1983) **22**: 321.
64 Gabriolove JL, Luria M, Persistent gynecomastia resulting from scalp inunction of estradiol: a model for persistent gynecomastia, *Arch Dermatol* (1978) **114**: 1672.
65 Owens CH, Yarborough DR, Brackett NR, Nephrotic syndrome following topically applied sulfadiazine therapy, *Arch Intern Med* (1974) **134**: 332.
66 Chan CK, Jarrett F, Moylan JA, Acute leukopenia as an allergic reaction to silver sulfadiazine in burn patients, *J Trauma* (1976) **16**: 395.
67 Jarrett F, Ellerbe S, Demling R, Acute leukopenia during topical burn therapy with silver sulfadiazine, *Am J Surg* (1978) **135**: 818.
68 Fraser GL, Beaulieu JT, Leukopenia secondary to sulfadiazine silver, *J Am Med Assoc* (1979) **241**: 1928.
69 Scharpf LG, Hill ID, Maibach HI, Percutaneous penetration and disposition of tricarban in man, *Arch Environ Hlth* (1975) **30**: 7.
70 Fisch RO, Berglund EB, Bridge AG et al, On triclocarban and methemoglobinemia. Quoted in Marzulli F and Maibach HI, *Dermatotoxicology*, 3rd ed. Hemisphere Press: Washington, 1985.
71 Ponte C, Richard J, Bonte C et al, Methemoglobinemies chez le nouveau-nie. Discussion du role etiologique du trichlorcarbanilide, *Ann Pediatr* (1974) **21**: 359.
72 Robertson WO, Arsenic and other heavy metals. In: Haddad LM, Winchester JF, (eds). *Clinical management of poisoning and drug overdose*, W. B. Saunders: Philadelphia, PA, 1983, chap 59, p656.
73 D'Arcy PF, Fatalities with the use of a henna daye, *Pharm Int* (1982) **3**: 217.
74 El-Ansary EH, Ahmed MEK, Clague HW, Systemic toxicity of *para*-phenylenediamine, *Lancet* (1983) **i**: 1341.
75 Grybowksy J, Weinstein D, Ordway N, Toxic encephalopathy apparently related to the use of an insect repellent, *N Engl J Med* (1961) **264**: 289.
76 Zadicoff C, Toxic encephalopathy associated with use of insect repellent, *J Pediatr* (1979) **95**: 140.
77 Kligman, AM, Dimethyl sulfoxide — Part 2, *J Am Med Assoc* (1965) **193**: 151.
78 Bennett CC, Dimethyl sulfoxide, *J Am Med Assoc* (1980) **244**: 2768.
79 De Groot AC, Nater JP, Bleumink K et al, Does DNCB therapy potentiate epicutaneous sensitization to non-related contact allergens? *Clin Exp Dermatol* (1981) **6**: 139.
80 Feldman RJ, Maibach HI, Absorption of some organic compounds through the skin in man, *J Invest Dermatol* (1970) **54**: 399.
81 McDaniel DH, Blatchley DM, Welton WA, Adverse systemic reaction to dinitrochlorobenzene, *Arch Dermatol* (1982) **118**: 371 (letter).
82 Gimenez ER, Vallejo NE, Roy E et al, Percutaneous alcohol intoxication, *Clin Toxicol* (1968) **1**: 39.
83 Castot A, Garnier R, Lanfranchi E et al, Effets systematiques indesirables des medicaments appliquels sur la peau chez l'enfant. *Therapie* (1980) **35**: 423.
84 Ellis CN, Mitchell AJ, Beardsley GR Jr, Tar gel interaction with disulfiram, *Arch Dermatol* (1979) **115**: 1367.
85 Dubiel W, Happle R, Behandlungsversuch mit Fumarsaure monoathylester bei Psoriasis vulgaris, *Z Haut-u Geschlkr* (1972) **47**: 545.
86 Haggerty RJ, Blue baby due to methemoglobinemia, *N Engl J Med* (1962) **267**: 13303.
87 Meynadier J, Peyron J-L, Resorption transcutanée des medicaments, *Rev Pract (Paris)* (1982) **32**: 41.
88 Steinberg JB, Zepernick RGL, Methemoglobinemia during anesthesia, *J Pediatr* (1962) **61**: 885.
89 Adriani J, Zepernick R, Summary of methemoglobinemia: study of child receiving benzocaine, OTC, vol 060150, (letter).
90 Olson ML, McEvoy GK, Methemoglobinemia induced by local anesthetics, *Am J Hosp Pharm* (1981) **38**: 89.
91 American Medical Association, *AMA Drug Evaluations*, 3rd edn, Publishing Sciences Group: Littleton, MA, 1977, p269.
92 Adriani J, Zepernick R, Clinical effectiveness of drugs used for topical anesthesia, *J Am Med Assoc* (1964) **118**: 711.
93 Seldon R, Sasahara AA, Central nervous system toxicity induced by lidocaine, *J Am Med Assoc* (1967) **202**: 908.
94 Giard MJ, Uden DL, Whitelock DJ, Seizures induced by oral viscous lidocaine, *Clin Pharm* (1983) **2**: 110.
95 Mofenson HC, Caraccio TR, Miller H et al, Lidocaine toxicity from topical mucosal application, *Clin Pediatr* (1983) **22**: 190.
96 Aronow R, Mercury. In: Haddad LM, Winchester JF, (eds). *Clinical management of poisoning and drug overdose*, W. B. Saunders: Philadelphia, PA, 1983, chap 56, p637.
97 Bork K. Morsches B, Holzmann H, Zum Problem der Quecksilber-Resorption aus weisser Prazipatatsalbe, *Arch Dermatol Forsch* (1973) **248**: 37.
98 Young E, Ammoniated mercury poisoning, *Br J Dermatol* (1960) **72**: 449.
99 Silverberg DS, McCall JT, Hunt JC, Nephrotic syndrome with use of ammoniated mercury, *Arch Intern Med* (1967) **120**: 581.
100 Turk JL, Baker H, Nephrotic syndrome due to ammoniated mercury, *Br J Dermatol* (1968) **80**: 623.
101 Lyons TJ, Christer CN, Larsen FS, Ammoniated mercury ointment and the nephrotic syndrome, *Minnes Med* (1975) **58**: 383.
102 Stanley-Brown EG, Frank JE, Mercury poisoning from application to omphalocele. *J Am Med Assoc* (1971) **216**: 2144 (letter).
103 Clark JA, Kasselberg AG, Glick AD et al, Mercury poisoning from merbromin (Mercurochrome^R) therapy of omphalocele, *Clin Pediatr (Philad)* (1982) **21**: 445.
104 Hedges TR III, Kenyon KR, Hanninen LA et al, Corneal and conjuctival effects of monobenzone in patients with vitiligo, *Arch Ophthalmol* (1983) **101**: 64.
105 Harkness RA, Beveridge GW, Isolation of 2-naphtol from urine after its application to skin, *Nature (London)* (1966) **211**: 413.

106　Hemels HGWM, Percutaneous absorption and distribution of 2-naphtol in man, *Br J Dermatol* (1972) **87**: 614.
107　Osol A, Farrar GE Jr, *The dispensatory of the United States of America*, 24th edn, Lippincott: Philadelphia, PA, 1947.
108　*Merck Index*, 9th edn, Merck and Co: Rahway, NJ, 1976, p291.
109　Feldmann RJ, Maibach HI, Percutaneous penetration of some pesticides and herbicides in man, *Toxicol Appl Pharmacol* (1974) **28**: 126.
110　Ginsburg CM, Lowry W, Reisch JS, Absorption of lindane (gamma benzene hexachloride) in infants and children, *J Pediatr* (1977) **91**: 998.
111　Hosler J, Tschanz C, Higuite C et al, Topical application of lindanecream (Kwell) and antipyrine metabolism, *J Invest Dermatol* (1980) **74**: 51.
112　Haddad LM, The carbamate, organochlorine and botanical insecticides; insect repellents. In: Haddad LM, Winchester JF, (eds). *The clinical management of poisoning and drug overdose*, W. B. Saunders: Philadelphia, PA, 1983, chap 68, p711.
113　Lee B, Groth P, Scabies: transcutaneous poisoning during treatment, *Pediatrics* (1977) **59**: 643.
114　Telch J, Jarvis DA, Acute intoxication with lindane (gamma benzene hexachloride), *Can Med Assoc J* (1982) **126**: 662.
115　Davies JE, Dedhia HV, Morgade C et al, Lindane poisonings, *Arch Dermatol* (1983) **119**: 142.
116　USFDA, Gamma benzene hexachloride (Kwell) and other products alert, *FDA Drug Bull* (1976) **6**: 28.
117　Lee B, Groth P, Scabies: transcutaneous poisoning during treatment, *Pediatrics* (1977) **59**: 643.
118　Matsuoka LY, Convulsions following application of gamma benzene hexachloride, *J Am Acad Dermatol* (1981) **5**: 98.
119　Pramanik AK, Hansen RC, Transcutaneous gamma benzene hexachloride absorption and toxicity in infants and children, *Arch Dermatol* (1979) **115**: 1224.
120　Solomon LM, Fahrner L, West DP, Gamma benzene hexachloride toxicity. A review, *Arch Dermatol* (1977) **113**: 353.
121　Shacter B, Treatment of scabies and pediculosis with lindane preparations: an evaluation, *J Am Acad Dermatol* (1981) **5**: 517.
122　Rasmussen JE, The problem of lindane, *J Am Acad Dermatol* (1981) **5**: 507.
123　Kramer MS, Hutchinson TA, Rudnick SA et al, Operational criteria for adverse drug reactions in evaluating suspected toxicity of a popular scabicide, *Clin Pharmacol Ther* (1980) **27**: 149.
124　Haddad LM, The organophosphate insecticides. In: Haddad LM, Winchester JF, (eds). *The clinical management of poisoning and drug overdose*, W. B. Saunders: Philadelphia, PA, 1983, chap 67, p704.
125　Ramu A, Slonim EA, Egal F, Hyperglycemia in acute malathion poisoning, *Isr J Med Sci* (1973) **9**: 631.
126　Milby TH, Epstein WL, Allergic sensitivity to malathion, *Arch Environ Hlth* (1964) **9**: 434.
127　Haddad LM, Miscellany. In: Haddad LM, Winchester JF, (eds). *The clinical management of poisoning and drug overdose*, W. B. Saunders: Philadelphia, PA, 1983, chap 107, p965.
128　Cassidy DE, Drewry J, Fanning JP, Podophyllum toxicity: a report of a fatal case and a review of the literature, *J Toxic Clin Toxicol* (1982) **19**: 35.
129　Chamberlain MJ, Reynolds AL, Yeoman WB, Toxic effect of podophyllum application in pregnancy, *Br J Med* (1972) **3**: 391.
130　Proudfoot AT, Salicylates and salicylamide. In: Haddad LM, Winchester JF, (eds). *The clinical management of poisoning and drug overdose*, W. B. Saunders: Philadelphia, PA, 1983, chap 50, p575.
131　Taylor JR, Halprin K, Percutaneous absorption of salicylic acid, *Arch Dermatol* (1975) **106**: 740.
132　Von Weiss JF, Lever WF, Percutaneous salicylic acid intoxication in psoriasis, *Arch Dermatol* (1964) **90**: 614.
133　United States Department of Health, Education and Welfare, Food and Drug Administration, OTC Antimicrobial II Advisory Panel. Quoted by Rasmussen JE, Percutaneous absorption in children. In: Dobson RL, (ed.). *Year Book of Dermatology*, Year Book Medical Publishers: Chicago, IL, 1979, p28.
134　Lindsey CP, Two cases of fatal salicylate poisoning after topical application of an antifungal solution, *Med J Aust* (1968) **1**: 353.
135　Wechselberg K, Salizylsaure-Vergiftung durch perkutane Resorption 1%-iger Salizylvaseline, *Anasth Prax* (1969) **4**: 103.
136　Treguer G, Le Bihan G, Colignier M et al, Intoxication salicylée par application locale de vaseline salicylée à 20% chez un psoriasique, *Nouv Presse Med* (1980) **9**: 192.
137　Ransone JW, Scott NM, Knoblock EC, Selenium sulfide intoxication, *N Engl J Med* (1973) **9**: 631.
138　Ternberg JL, Luce E, Methemoglobinemia: a complication of the silver nitrate treatment of burns, *Surgery* (1968) **63**: 328.
139　Anonymous, Burns and silver nitrate, *J Am Med Assoc* (1965) **193**: 230 (editorial).
140　Connely DM, Silver nitrate — ideal burn wound therapy?, *NY J Med* (1970) **70**: 1642.
141　Bader KF, Organ deposition of silver following silver nitrate therapy of burns, *Plast Reconstr Surg* (1966) **37**: 550.
142　Bronaugh R, Maibach H, *Percutaneous absorption*, 2nd edn, Marcel Dekker: New York, 1990.
143　Feldmann RJ, Maibach HI, Penetration of ^{14}C hydrocortisone through normal skin, *Arch Dermatol* (1965) **91**: 661.
144　Pascher F, Systemic reactions to topically applied drugs, *Int J Dermatol* (1978) **17**: 768.
145　Feiwell M, James VHT, Barnett ES, Effect of potent topical steroids on plasma-cortisol levels of infants and children with eczema, *Lancet* (1969) **i**: 485.
146　Burton TT, Cunliffe WJ, Holti G et al, Complications of topical corticosteroid therapy in patients with liver dis-

ease. *Br J Dermatol* (1974) **9** (suppl 10): 22.

147 May PH, Stern EJ, Ryter RJ et al, Cushing syndrome from percutaneous absorption of triamcinolone cream, *Arch Intern Med* (1976) **136**: 612.

148 Van der Harst LCA, Smeenk G, Burger PM et al, Waardebepaling en risicoschatting van de uitwendige behandeling met clobetasol-17-propionaat (Dermovate), *Ned T Geneesk* (1978) **122**: 219.

149 Beas F, Vargas L, Spada RP et al, Pseudoprecocious puberty in infants caused by a dermal ointment containing estrogens, *J Pediatr* (1969) **75**: 127.

150 Bertaggia A, A case of precocious puberty in a girl following the use of an estrogen preparation on the skin, *Pediatria (Napoli)* (1968) **76**: 579.

151 Landolt R. Murset G, Vorzeitige Pubertatsmerkmale als Folge unbeabsichtigter Ostrogenverabreichung, *Schweiz Med Wschr* (1968) **98**: 638.

152 Ramos AS, Bower BF, Pseudosexual precocity due to cosmetics ingestion, *J Am Med Assoc* (1969) **207**: 369.

153 Stoppelman MRH, Van Valkenburg RA, Pigmentaties en gynecomastie ten gevolge van het gebruik van stilboestrol bevattend haarewater bij kinderen, *Ned T Geneesk* (1955) **99**: 3925.

154 Edidin DV, Levitsky LL, Prepubertal gynecomastia associated with estrogen-containing hair cream, *Am J Dis Child* (1982) **136**: 587.

155 DiRaimondo CV, Roach AC, Meador CK, Gynecomastia from exposure to vaginal estrogen cream, *N Engl J Med* (1980) **302**: 1089 (letter).

156 Gabrilove JL, Luria M, Persistent gynecomastia resulting from scalp inunction of estradiol: a model of persistent gynecomastia, *Arch Dermatol* (1978) **114**: 1672.

157 Bazex A, Salvader R, Dupre A et al, Gynecomastie et hyperpigmentation areolaire apres oestrogenotherapie locale antiseborrheque, *Bull Soc Franc Dermatol Syph* (1967) **74**: 466.

158 Goebel M, Mamillenhypertrophie mit Pigmentierung nach lokaler Oestrogentherapie im Kindesalter, *Hautarzt* (1969) **20**: 521.

159 Goluboff N, MacFadyen DJ, Methemoglobinemia in an infant, *J Pediatr* (1955) **47**: 222.

160 Marzulli F, Maibach H, *Dermatotoxicology*, 4th edn, Hemisphere Press: Washington, 1991.

161 Bronaugh R, Maibach H, *Percutaneous penetration in vitro*, CRC Press, Boca Ratan Fl., 1991.

46
Ivy Shield: a new barrier cream for the prevention of poison ivy dermatitis

Dédée F. Murrell* and Elise A. Olsen

Division of Dermatology, Department of Medicine, Duke University Medical Center, Durham, NC 27710, USA, and *Department of Dermatology, University of North Carolina at Chapel Hill, Chapel Hill, NC 27514, USA

Introduction

Poison ivy/oak (Rhus) dermatitis frequently and sometimes severely afflicts individuals active in the outdoors[1]. Efforts to prevent Rhus dermatitis have focused on desensitization, the application of detoxicants, early washing of the exposed skin, and application of barrier creams. The side effects of desensitization (pruritis ani and erythematous nodules) have limited its application as a means of preventing Rhus dermatitis[2]. Two agents which chemically inactivate Rhus oleoresin have been tested.[3,4] Both detoxicating agents were only effective if mixed with the Rhus extract prior to skin contact.

Early removal of the Rhus extract, even within 5 min, has been unsuccessful as a means of preventing dermatitis.[5] Even a minute dose of antigen in contact for only a few minutes may trigger an immune response in sensitive individuals. Moreover, during outdoor activities, washing the exposed areas immediately after contact with the Rhus plants is impractical and often impossible.

The main advantage of a barrier cream in the prevention of Rhus dermatitis is that the preparation can be applied in anticipation of exposure. Barrier creams tested thus far have included chloroamide,[4] white petrolatum,[6] ferric chloride ointment,[6] sodium perborate,[6,7] kaolin, bentonite, silicone, organoclay (Ivyguard),[8] and linoleic acid dimers (Stokogard).[9] Of all these, only organoclay and linoleic acid dimers have shown some promise. Ivy Shield (Interpro, Haverhill, MA, USA) is a barrier cream that has been successfully used in industry to prevent irritant contact dermatitis and it was of interest to investigate whether it might also be of benefit in preventing allergic contact dermatitis in the form of Rhus dermatitis.

This study evaluated the efficacy of Ivy Shield alone and Ivy Shield with kaolin in the prevention of experimentally-induced Rhus dermatitis. Kaolin has been used previously as a barrier cream.[8]

Methods

Caucasian subjects between 18 and 45 years of age, in good health and with a positive patch test to Rhus extract (1 : 100) were included in the study. Rhus extract (Hollister-Stier, Spokane, WA, USA) was applied for 4 h to patients' upper arms and the area was evaluated at 72 h for erythema, induration and vesiculation. A positive test score was ≥ 3 out of a possible total of 9. Women of child-bearing potential were excluded if pregnant, breast feeding, or not using reliable methods of contraception. Subjects who had applied topical steroids to the forearms within 2 weeks or who had taken systemic immunosuppressants within 1 month of study entry, those with a history of diabetes mellitus or autoimmune disorders, or those with any dermatitis on their upper extremities were also excluded. All subjects participating in the study gave written informed consent. The study conformed to a randomized controlled double-blind design. The procedures were approved by the Investigational Review Board at Duke University Medical Center.

Procedure

If forearm hair was dense, subjects' forearms were first shaved. The forearms were then washed with Hibiclens (ICI Pharmaceuticals, Wilmington, DE, USA) and water and three 4×4 cm target areas marked on each forearm. A randomized schema, taking into account distal to proximal location on either forearm, was computer generated for Ivy Shield A and Ivy Shield B (with kaolin) and a control. Ivy Shield A and Ivy Shield B were applied to one of three target areas on each forearm by a study nurse uninvolved in the efficacy analysis. One target area on each forearm remained untreated as a control (C). Ivy Shield was rubbed in for 60 s and allowed to dry for 20 min. Closed patch tests were then applied to each site. A 1:50 commercial preparation of Rhus extract freshly diluted to 1:100 in 95% alcohol was then applied in 0.02-ml aliquots onto 8 mm filter paper discs (Epitest Ltd, Oy, Finland). The discs were then placed in the center of each target area, covered with a Finn chamber (Allerderm Labs, Mill Valley, CA, USA) and held in place with 2.5 cm Dermcal tape (Johnson & Johnson, New Brunswick, NJ, USA). After 4 h the patches were removed and the arms thoroughly washed with Hibiclens and water.

Assessment

Subjects returned on days 2, 3, 4 and 7 for assessment by a single experienced observer (D.F.M.) who was blinded to the application process. Erythema, induration and vesiculation were each graded on a scale of 0 to 3 with 0.5 increments where: 0 = no reaction; 1 = mild reaction; 2 = moderate reaction; and 3 = severe reaction. The total of each of these parameters on a given day represented the global severity score. Subjects were given Atarax (Hydroxyzine) 10 mg p.o. (Roenig Division, Pfizer, New York, NY, USA) if they developed severe pruritus. After their final assessment on day 7, subjects were also given Temovate (Clobetasol proprionate) ointment 0.5% (Glaxo Inc., Research Triangle Park, NC, USA) to apply twice a day for 2 weeks to any residual dermatitis.

Statistical methods

The data were analysed using the Wilcoxon signed rank test. Repeated-measures analysis of variance confirmed that patient, site, and arm made no difference to the data interpretation.

Results

Twenty healthy Caucasian volunteers (11 men, 9 women), ranging in age from 19 to 43 years (mean 28.5 years) entered the study. The mean degree of global dermatitis on a scale of 0 to 9, where 9 is the most severe, in unprotected areas (control sites) was 2.5 (± 0.2), 3.4 (± 0.3), 3.9 (± 0.3), and 3.3 (± 0.3) on the second, third, fourth and seventh day after exposure to Rhus extract, respectively. The severity of Rhus dermatitis peaked in the majority of control areas on day 4 of assessment and on day 7 in the areas treated with Ivy Shield A and Ivy Shield B.

There was an average reduction in mean global severity of dermatitis of 35% ($P \leq 0.05$) for areas treated with Ivy Shield A and 30% ($P \leq 0.05$) for Ivy Shield B compared to control values (Figure 1). The mean peak global severity score was reduced by 38% ($P \leq 0.05$) for Ivy Shield A and 34% ($P \leq 0.05$) for Ivy Shield B compared to control values. There was no statistically significant difference in the prevention of Rhus dermatitis afforded by Ivy Shield with kaolin (Ivy Shield B) compared with Ivy Shield alone (Ivy Shield A).

Rhus dermatitis was completely prevented by Ivy Shield A and B in only one of the 20 subjects. Each forearm provided three direct comparisons: Ivy Shield A vs. control, Ivy Shield B vs. control and Ivy Shield A vs. Ivy Shield B. For any one of these three direct comparisons, there were two for each of the 20 subjects or 40 per day of assessment. Hence, over four assessments there should have been 160 direct comparisons of two differently protected areas. One subject failed to attend his last assessment, leaving 158 of the latter comparisons. The severity of dermatitis pretreated with Ivy Shield A was diminished in 113/158 (71%, $P \leq 0.05$), equivalent in 13/158 (8%) comparisons, and more severe than control areas in 33/158 (21%) comparisons. The corresponding figures for areas treated with Ivy Shield B compared to control areas were 116/158 (73%, $P \leq 0.05$), 26/158 (16%) equal to control, and 26/158 (16%) worse than control.

The subjects were arbitrarily further divided into those with moderately severe dermatitis (peak individual global severity score ≥ 5) and those with mild dermatitis (peak individual global severity

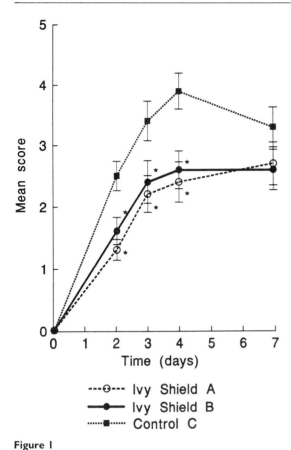

Figure 1

The relationship between mean global severity score (range 0 to 9) and time (days) for Ivy Shield A, Ivy Shield B vs. control (C).

score ≤5). The 6 subjects with moderately severe dermatitis and the 14 subjects with mild dermatitis had mean peak global severity scores of 6.2 and 2.7, respectively (in their control sites). Both Ivy Shield A and Ivy Shield B reduced the mean peak global score in subjects with severe dermatitis by 28%. In contrast, the mean peak global dermatitis score in subjects with mild dermatitis was reduced by 52% and 45% by Ivy Shields A and B, respectively.

Discussion

Ivy Shield is a novel type of barrier cream containing TEA stearate, Stearamide MEA, Ethoxydiglycol, acetic acid and water. The preparation relies on adherence to the skin, rather than absorption, to prevent contact of the Rhus antigen with the skin. Ivy Shield (A) was field-tested in 1987.[10] Thirty-two Rhus-sensitive forestry workers reported their subjective experience of using Ivy Shield (A) each work day over an average of 4 weeks. A reduction in the severity and frequency of Rhus dermatitis was experienced by 28/32 (88%) subjects. Ivy Shield has also been shown to be an equivalent or more protective barrier than kaolin, silicone or bentonite in 9/10, 7/8 and 9/11 direct comparisons, respectively, in open patch tests of threshold concentrations of Rhus extract as tested in seven subjects by Epstein.[10]

This study presents supporting evidence for the efficacy of Ivy Shield in moderating Rhus dermatitis. Ivy Shield with and without kaolin reduced the severity of an experimentally-induced Rhus dermatitis. The target areas of forearm skin pretreated with Ivy Shield A and Ivy Shield B had less severe dermatitis than control sites in 71% and 73% of 158 direct comparisons, respectively. Both Ivy Shield A and B reduced the mean global dermatitis score and the mean peak global dermatitis score. The reduction in the mean peak global score was proportionately greater in those subjects with mild dermatitis compared with those subjects with moderately severe dermatitis. The presence of kaolin afforded no additional protection over Ivy Shield alone.

Ivy Shield completely prevented Rhus dermatitis in 1/20 patients. This inability to prevent dermatitis completely in this model may be due to the severity of dermatitis created by the model. Our system thus provides a more rigorous screen for barrier efficacy and simulates a heavy exposure of Rhus antigen. In contrast previous investigators of barrier creams have used threshold concentration of Rhus extract,[4,8,9] and/or used open patch tests rather than closed patch tests.[8]

As Ivy Shield was efficacious in this rigorous system, it may prove to be a useful agent for workers chronically exposed to Poison ivy/oak. More work needs to be done to compare the efficacy of Ivy Shield with linoleic acid dimers (Stokogard) and organoclay (Ivygard) in this system. However, it is encouraging that Ivy Shield did demonstrate significant barrier properties against allergic contact dermatitis due to poison ivy and it would be interesting to tests its efficacy in other areas of dermatology.

Acknowledgements

We gratefully acknowledge the assistance of Elizabeth A. Turney, B.S.P.H., and Gary Koch, Ph.D., at the Department of Biostatistics, University of North Carolina at Chapel Hill. This study was supported in part by a grant from Interpro Inc., Haverhill, MA, USA.

References

1. Orchard S, Barrier creams, *Dermatol Clin* (1984) **2**: 619–29.
2. Epstein WL, Byers VS, Baer H, Induction of persistent tolerance to urushiol in humans, *J Allergy Clin Immunol* (1981) **68**: 20–5.
3. Sizer IW, Prokesch CE, The destruction by tyrosinase of the irritant principles of poison ivy and related toxicants, *J Pharm Exp* (1945) **84**: 363–74.
4. Thurmon FM, Ottenstein B, Bessman MJ, Chemical and biological tests with the toxic substance of poison ivy (urushiol) and its absorption by amberlite exchange resins, *J Invest Dermatol* (1955) **25**: 9–20.
5. Shelmire BS, Contact dermatitis from weeds: patch testing with their oleoresin, *J Am Med Assoc* (1939) **113**: 1085–90.
6. Howell JB, Evaluation of measures for prevention of ivy dermatitis, *Arch Dermatol Syph* (1943) **48**: 373–8.
7. Schwartz L, Warren LH, Goldman FH, Protective ointment for the prevention of poison ivy dermatitis, *Pub Hlth Rep* (1940) **55**: 1327–33.
8. Epstein WL, Topical prevention of poison ivy/oak dermatitis, *Arch Dermatol* (1989) **125**: 499–501.
9. Orchard S, Fellman JH, Storrs FJ, Poison ivy/oak dermatitis. Use of polyamine salts of a linoleic acid dimer for topical prophylaxis, *Arch Dermatol* (1986) **122**: 783–9.
10. US Department of Argiculture, *Technol and Dev News* (1988) **Jul.–Aug.**: 2.

47
Can health hazard associated with chemical contamination of the skin be predicted from simple in vitro experiments?

C. Surber,†§ K.-P. Wilhelm,†‡ H. I. Maibach† and R. H. Guy*

School of Medicine and School of Pharmacy, Departments of Dermatology, Pharmacy and Pharmaceutical Chemistry,* University of California,*† San Francisco, USA, University of Lübeck,‡ Germany, University of Basel,§ Switzerland

Introduction

Risk assessment following dermal exposure to toxic occupational and evironmental chemicals is a complex problem. An accurate evaluation of the potential hazard requires a sensible estimate of the amount of material that has entered the body by permeation across the skin. This determination requires that we have knowledge of the rate-limiting barrier in percutaneous absorption, and the key physicochemical determinants that control molecular flux through the skin.[1,2] This literature establishes that the outermost layer of skin, the stratum corneum (SC), is typically the major barrier to percutaneous penetration. Furthermore, previous research has shown that a chemical's partition coefficient (PC) between, for example, a lipophilic solvent, such as octanol, and water can, under certain circumstances, be used as a relative indicator of inherent skin permeability.[3] These empirical estimates, however, ignore the heterogeneous structural complexity of the SC and at best provide only qualitative predictions.

In this investigation, our aim was to validate simple procedures to quantify chemical partitioning between the SC (and/or other skin layers) and a vehicle (i.e. the medium, such as water or an organic solvent, in which the chemical is presented to the skin surface). We hypothesize that the distribution parameters derived from such a study will be more predictive in risk assessment. The experiments reported here examine the effect of several variables (chemical concentration, equilibration time, SC preparation technique, and SC source and vehicle) on the SC/vehicle partitioning phenomenon.

Materials and methods

Skin preparation

Dermotomed human skin (0.5 mm, Dermatom Mod. B; Padgett, Kansas City, MO, USA) was obtained from cadavers at autopsy. The skin samples were stored for up to a maximum of 3 days in phosphate buffered saline at 4°C prior to isolation of the SC. 'Sunburn' SC samples were taken from the forehead of one individual and were used without further treatment. Full-thickness rhesus monkey skin was provided by the California Primate Research Center, University of California, Davis. Subcutaneous fat was carefully removed and the full-thickness skin was then treated as indicated below. Hairless guinea-pig SC was prepared from full-thickness skin removed after killing the animal (Charles River Inc., Wilmington, MA, USA).

One of the following three techniques was used to separate epidermis from dermis: (1) the skin specimen was submerged in a 20 mM EDTA solution of 15 mM sodium phosphate (pH 7.2) in normal saline for 5 h at 37°C (EDTA treatment); (2) the tissue was submerged in phosphate buffered saline (pH 7.2) for 45 s at 50°C (heat treatment in water); or (3) the tissue was sandwiched in aluminum foil, which was pressed on a slide warmer for 45 s at 50°C (heat treatment on metal). After these treatments, the SC/epidermis layer was peeled from the dermis with dissection forceps. The thin sheets of SC/epidermis were then placed dermal side down on a filter paper soaked with 0.0001% trypsin (pH 8.2) for 24 h at 25°C. After digestion of the epidermal layer the SC was gently rinsed and then dried at 37°C in an incubator. Dry SC was stored in a desiccator.

Delipidization was done as follows. Dry, pre-weighed SC samples were placed in a glass beaker containing 50 cm^3 2:1 chloroform/methanol and were gently agitated for 24 h at 25°C. The delipidized SC samples were then removed, rinsed twice with fresh chloroform/methanol, and dried. Lipid content was determined by the change in weight of the SC after solvent extraction.

Partition coefficient determination

Partitioning experiments used one of four membrane phases (full-thickness skin, dermis alone, SC + epidermis or SC) and either water or isopropylmyristate (IPM) as the vehicle phase. Chemical partitioning between the skin sample and the vehicle was determined by measuring the disappearance of ^{14}C radiolabeled solute from the vehicle and the concomitant increase of radioisotope in the skin sample. The skin/vehicle partition coefficient was defined as PC = C_s/C_v, where C_s is the solute concentration in 1000 mg skin and C_v is the concentration in 1000 mg vehicle. In a typical experiment, 500 µl of the vehicle solution and an accurately weighed, dry skin sample (3–8 mg) were placed in a screw-cap borosilicate glass vial, which was capped with a teflon septum. The vial contents were equilibrated, with gentle occasional agitation, for various time intervals at 25°C. The skin sample was then removed, gently blotted on filter paper, and immediately dissolved in Soluene-350 (Packard Instrument Co., Inc., Dowers Grove, IL, USA). An aliquot of the vehicle (300–400 µl) was removed from the vial. Concentrations of radiolabeled compound in the vehicle and in the dissolved skin sample were then determined by liquid scintillation counting (Tri Carb 1500; Packard Instrument Co., Inc., Dowers Grove, IL, USA). All experiments were performed in quintuplicate.

Compounds

The phenols were obtained from Moravek Biochemicals Inc., Brea, CA, USA. The compounds used were [ring-^{14}C] 4-acetaminophenol (AC), 4-cyanophenol (CY), 4-iodophenol (I) and 4-pentyloxyphenol (PO); ^{14}C polychlorinated biphenyls (54%) (PCB), 1,1,1-trichloro-2,2-bis(p-chlorophenyl)ethane (DDT), atrazine (AT) and benzo[a]pyrene (B[a]P) were from Amersham Inc., The Netherlands. Radiochemical purity was determined by thin layer chromatography (TLC) and was found to be ≥ 98% for all compounds.

Results and discussion

The objective of the study was to assess the rigor of simple, in vitro experimental procedures for determining the skin vehicle partition coefficients (PC) of potentially toxic chemicals. As the PC is a key parameter in percutaneous absorption, a simple means of evaluating this quantity should significantly improve quantitative risk assessment following dermal exposure. Although a variety of skin/vehicle PC measurements have been made previously,[3-7] the results presented here, using chemicals spanning a wide range of physicochemical properties, constitute a unique and in-depth examination of the variables that can influence skin/vehicle partitioning.

Figure 1 shows the effect of equilibration time on the SC/water partitioning of the four phenols studied. The experiments indicating an incubation time of 0 h actually involved contact between SC and the aqueous phenol solution for approximately 3 min. The lipophilic phenols (I and PO) appeared to reach equilibrium within 6 h; the PCs of AC and CY, however, continued to increase with increasing contact time. While a long equilibration period is desirable when measuring liquid–liquid two-phase partitioning, care must be exercised when a biological membrane constitutes one of the phases. This is because prolonged contact between membrane and solvent (i.e. the other phase in the partitioning system) may alter the inherent properties of tissue and hence the degree to which it can take up a distributing solute. For example, the data in Figure 1 may suggest that the behaviour of AC and CY is due to an increasing level of SC hydration and concomitant uptake of bulk water and solute dissolved therein. From the standpoint of risk assessment, monitoring the partitioning process as a function of time is clearly sensible as most actual exposures are unlikely to proceed to equilibrium state. The kinetics of partitioning, therefore, are valuable addenda to the thermodynamic information.

The effect of varying the initial aqueous phase drug concentration (C_i) on the SC/water PC of the four phenols is presented in Table 1. As expected, the PC values tend to decrease with increasing C_i. For example, artifacts due to adsorption will be reduced as C_i is raised and the PC will be expected

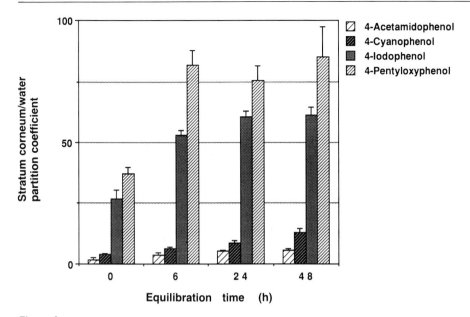

Figure 1

Stratum corneum/water partition coefficients (mean ± SD; $N = 5$) of four phenols determined as a function of equilibration time.

Table 1 Effect of initial aqueous phase chemical concentration (C_i, µg/cm³) on SC/water partitioning.*

Acetamidophenol		Cyanophenol		Iodophenol		Pentyloxyphenol	
C_i	PC	C_i	PC	C_i	PC	C_i	PC
0.05	6.1 ± 0.4	0.05	11 ± 2.6	0.07	74 ± 6.7	0.11	90 ± 14
0.53	4.6 ± 0.7	0.43	8.5 ± 2.6	0.72	54 ± 4.7	1.01	79 ± 14
5.25	5.8 ± 0.2	4.32	6.1 ± 0.5	7.11	47 ± 3.1	11.30	79 ± 5.5

* The SC was obtained from the thigh of a 32-year-old male Caucasian. The SC was separated by the 'heat treatment in water' procedure described in the text. The equilibration time was 24 h. Values are means ± SD, $N = 5$.

to attain a limiting value. Again, with respect to dermal exposure, the usefulness of examining the 'vehicle' concentration of the contacting chemical is self-evident when, for example, a body burden calculation is required.

The data in Table 2 demonstrate how delipidization of SC affects the SC/water PCs of AC and PO, which represent hydrophilic and lipophilic phenols. While delipidization leads to a significant ($P \leq 0.05$, Student's t-test for paired data) increase in the PC of AC for both SC sources, a small, but not consistently significant, *decrease* in PO partition coefficient was observed. The measurement of a PC using 'damaged' SC is a useful exercise if

Table 2 The SC/water partition coefficients of acetamidophenol and pentyloxyphenol:* effect of delipidization

	Acetamidophenol		Pentyloxyphenol	
	A†	B‡	A†	B‡
Lipids removed§ (%)	25.6	16.4	25.6	16.4
PC (intact)	5.1 ± 0.3	4.3 ± 0.1	84 ± 14	100 ± 3.8
PC (delipidized)	6.2 ± 0.3	7.0 ± 0.0	80 ± 18	75 ± 1.4

* SC was separated by the 'heat treatment on metal' procedure described in the text. The equilibration time was 24 h. Values are means ± SD, $N = 5$.
† Thigh skin from a 27-year-old male.
‡ Abdominal skin from a 73-year-old female.
§ Percentage weight reduction in SC after delipidization treatment.

concomitant exposure of a potentially toxic chemical and, for example, industrial solvents is possible. However, one may question whether the delipidized PC data can be used to infer the chemical's preference for one region of the SC over another. It remains to be seen whether the delipidization process allows the chemical to have access to a domain within the SC from which it is excluded when the membrane is intact.

The different SC separation techniques employed did not influence the subsequently determined PC values of AC (Table 3). The isolation procedures were chosen for their relatively benign nature;[8] in particular, when elevated temperatures were employed, the level of heating did not take the SC through lipid phase transitions associated with enhanced permeability.[1,9] For PO, the PC was more sensitive to the separation procedure: the EDTA method gave a low and 'noisy' value; whereas 'sunburn' SC has a high and variable figure. Practically speaking, the 'heat treatment in water' was the most rapid and easy method. The use of EDTA was problematic because incomplete epidermal–dermal separation frequently occurred, reducing substantially the SC yield. One should also be cautious about the use of 'sunburn' SC, which is likely to have been treated with emollient creams and/or lotions prior to its removal. These caveats may explain, at least in part, the variable (EDTA and 'sunburn') results for PO.

Because human skin is not routinely available to all investigators, there has been considerable attention devoted to the identification of a suitable animal model for percutaneous penetration studies. For screening purposes, the animal model should be not only predictive of the human skin behaviour but also be readily available and relatively easy to manipulate. In the very few experiments summarized in Table 4, the SC/water PCs of AC and PO were compared for human, rhesus monkey and hairless guinea-pig membranes. These measurements were neither designed to be exhaustive nor suggestive of a 'lead' animal candidate; they were meant to illustrate the fact that the procedures described in this paper, and applied primarily to human SC, can also be used with tissue from animal models. The results themselves show a rather consistent outcome for the two phenols in the three different SC samples used. The ranking of PCs (rhesus monkey > guinea-pig > man) was identical for AC and PO. Technically the human SC was the easiest to isolate. The SC/epidermis sheets of monkey skin were extremely fragile, while those of the hairless guinea-pig were difficult to separate from the underlying dermis.

If the procedure is to be adopted as a component of the risk-assessment process, evaluation of inter- and intra-measurement variability must be undertaken and shown to be within acceptable limits. Using SC isolated from six 'donors' by two different techniques, results pertinent to this re-

Table 3 The SC/water partition coefficients of acetamidophenol and pentyloxyphenol:* effect of SC preparation technique.

Technique†	Acetamidophenol	Pentyloxyphenol
Heat treatment on metal‡	4.1 ± 0.6	105 ± 2.7
Heat treatment in water‡	4.7 ± 0.6	118 ± 6.3
EDTA‡	5.4 ± 0.4	76 ± 22
Sunburn§	4.7 ± 0.4	136 ± 15
Average	4.7 ± 0.5	109 ± 25

* The equilibrium time was 24 h. Values are means ± SD, $N = 5$.
† See text for details.
‡ SC from the thigh skin of a 47-year-old female Caucasian.
§ SC from the forehead of a 33-year-old male Caucasian.

Table 4 The SC/water partition coefficients (SC/W PC) of acetamidophenol and pentyloxyphenol:* species difference.

		SC/W PC	
Species	Source	Acetamidophenol	Pentyloxyphenol
Human	47/F/thigh†	3.8 ± 0.3	106 ± 3.0
Rhesus monkey	8/M/abdomen†	5.0 ± 0.3	153 ± 3.3
Hairless guinea-pig	300/F/back‡	4.5 ± 0.5	140 ± 9.5

* SC was separated by the 'heat treatment on metal' procedure described in the text. The equilibration time was 24 h. Values are means ± SD, $N = 5$.
† Age in years/sex (F, female; M, male)/anatomical site of skin used.
‡ Weight in grams/sex/anatomical site.

quirement have been obtained. In Table 5 repeat measurements on the same substrate indicate experiments conducted on different days (on each day, therefore, the chemical PC between SC and water was measured in quintuplicate). The data reveal that: for SC from a single donor, PC values are consistent from day to day; between 'donors' the variability in PC values is typically 10–20%, a reasonable range for a parameter associated with skin barrier function and permeability; and the method of isolation does not significantly affect the PC values of the AC and PO.

The manner in which chemical partitions into different layers of the skin may be important: when the SC is damaged and the compound has direct access to the lower cutaneous compartments; or in situations where systemic exposure has occurred and information relating to compound distribution and residence time within the body is required. We have also measured a number of apparent 'membrane'/water partition coefficients for AC and PO (Figure 2) to demonstrate the generality of our approaches for alternative partitioning phases. Detailed interpretation of the results shown in Figure 2 is probably unwarranted, but two aspects of physicochemical plausibility should be mentioned. First, for AC, a relatively hydrophilic chemical, the amount entering the 'membrane' phase is relatively independent of the latter's composition, indicating a generally low affinity of this phenol for any lipid phase. Second, for PO which, by contrast, is quite lipophilic, the PC values are significantly elevated when the SC forms a large part of the skin 'membrane'. In considering these results, it should be recalled that the PC is the equilibrium ratio of the amount of chemical per 1000 mg of 'membrane' to the amount of chemical per 1000 mg of water. It follows that 1000 mg of SC contains considerably more lipid, for example, than 1000 mg of full thickness skin.

Finally, in Table 6, the SC/water and SC/IPM partition coefficients of the four phenols, PCB and DDT are compared and presented together with the literature values of the PC of the chemicals between octanol and water, and between IPM and water.[11–13] PC[SC/water] and PC[SC/IPM] are inversely correlated as expected:

$$\log[K(SC/water)] = 2.12 - 1.08[\log K(SC/IPM)]; \ r = 0.96 \quad (1)$$

There are direct correlations between PC (SC/water) and both PC (octanol/water) [P] and PC (IPM/water):

Table 5 The SC/water partition coefficients (SC/W PC) of acetamidophenol and pentyloxyphenol: intra- and inter-stratum corneum variability.*

SC 'donor'†	SC preparation‡	Acetamidophenol	Pentyloxyphenol
57/M/C	Heat treatment on metal	5.0 ± 0.4	97 ± 7.1
57/M/C	Heat treatment on metal	5.8 ± 0.4	137 ± 12
57/M/C	Heat treatment on metal	6.1 ± 0.3	129 ± 17
24/M/C	Heat treatment on metal	5.0 ± 0.2	121 ± 4.0
46/M/B	Heat treatment on metal	4.8 ± 0.3	108 ± 5.8
47/F/C	Heat treatment on metal	4.1 ± 0.6	105 ± 2.7
47/F/C	Heat treatment on metal	3.8 ± 0.3	106 ± 3.1
Average		5.0 ± 0.8	116 ± 15
27/M/C	Heat treatment in water	4.8 ± 0.3	75 ± 6.0
27/M/C	Heat treatment in water	5.1 ± 0.3	84 ± 14
27/M/C	Heat treatment in water	4.6 ± 0.7	79 ± 14
47/F/C	Heat treatment in water	4.7 ± 0.2	118 ± 6.3
73/F/C	Heat treatment in water	4.3 ± 0.1	100 ± 3.8
73/F/C	Heat treatment in water	4.9 ± 0.5	97 ± 7.1
Average:		4.8 ± 0.2	92 ± 16
Overall average		4.9 ± 0.6	104 ± 19

* Equilibration time was 24 h. Values are means ± SD, $N = 5$.
† Age in years/sex (M, male; F, female)/race (C, Caucasian; B, black).
‡ See text for details.

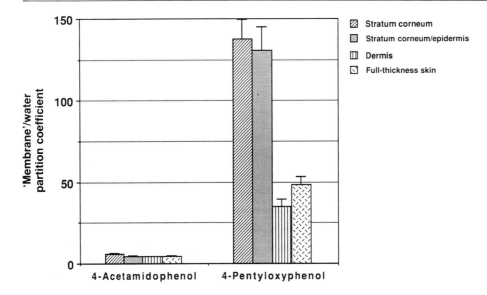

Figure 2

Partitioning of acetamidophenol and pentyloxyphenol into four skin 'membranes' from water (mean ± SD; $N = 5$). The equilibration time was 24 h.

Table 6 Partition coefficients of the chemicals studied.

Chemical	log [P]*	log K[IPM/water]†	log K[SC/water]‡	log K[SC/IPM]§
4-Acetamidophenol	0.3	−1.5	0.7	1.5
4-Cyanophenol	1.6	0.7	0.9	0.8
4-Iodophenol	2.9	1.9	1.8	0.3
4-Pentyloxyphenol	3.5	3.0	1.9	0.2
PCB	6.4	NA	2.3	−0.2
DDT	6.4	NA	2.5	−0.2

* Octanol/water partition coefficient from refs 12 and 13.
† Isopropylmyristate/water partition coefficient from ref. 11.
‡ SC/water partition coefficient.
§ SC/isopropylmyristate partition coefficient.
NA, Not available.

$$\log [K(SC/water)] = 0.69 - 0.28[\log P]; \quad r = 0.95 \quad (2)$$

$$\log [K(SC/water)] = 1.02 - 0.29[\log K(IPM/water)]; \quad r = 0.92 \quad (3)$$

Recently, we have made the corresponding comparison and correlations for atrazine and benz[a]pyrene and a total of 15 drugs (Surber and Maibach, unpublished data).[14] In Figure 3 the correlation of compound octanol/water PC (log [P]) with the compound SC/water PC [log PC (SC/water)] and the compound SC/IPM PC [log PC (SC/IPM)] is presented. Despite the wide spectrum of physicochemical and structural properties covered by the compounds included in the analysis, there is considerable overlap and consistency within the data. If these general patterns of behavior can be further substantiated with additional compounds, then one may ultimately be able to predict, for example, the SC/water PC from a suitable known (or readily obtained) oil/water PC. Of course, this objective has been sought in other studies with varying degrees of success. As PC

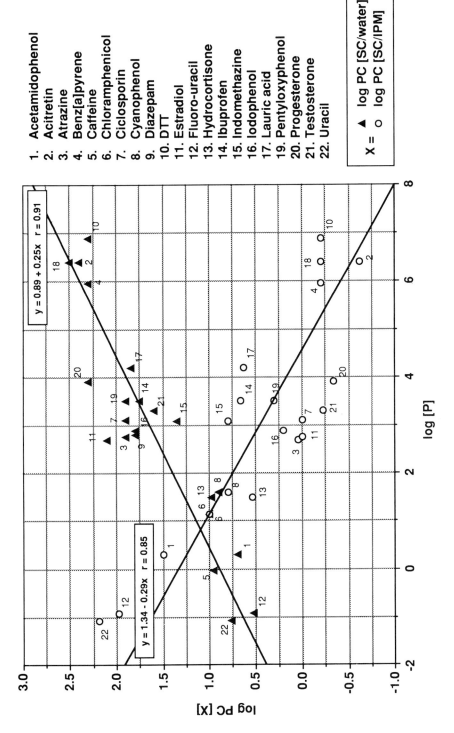

Figure 3
Correlation of compound octanol/water PC (log [P]) with the compound SC/water PC [log PC (SC/water)] and the compound SC/IPM PC [log PC(SC/IPM)].

values using human SC can be reproducibly evaluated, it should be possible to explore more rigorously the generality of the interrelationships between biological and 'physical/chemical' partitioning. These further experiments should investigate whether partitioning into SC from cadavers mirrors that into SC in vivo. Care should also be exercised in using PC values of compounds subject to significant skin metabolism to predict percutaneous permeability.

In conclusion, we have shown that simple and reproducible measurements of the partition coefficient of a chemical between the SC and a vehicle phase can be performed. The relevance of these parameters to the assessment of risk following dermal exposure has been discussed and illustrated. Furthermore, the relationship between SC/water PC and classic oil/water distribution coefficients has been suggested.

Acknowledgement

This work was supported by a Cooperative Agreement (CR-812474) from the US Environmental Protection Agency, the Swiss National Science Foundation and Deutsche Forschungsgemeinschaft.

References

1 Barry BW, *Dermatological formulations: percutaneous absorption*, Marcel Dekker: New York, 1983.
2 Kasting GB, Smith RL, Cooper ER, Effect of lipid solubility and molecular size on percutaneous absorption. In: Shroot B, Schaefer H, (eds). *Skin pharmacokinetics*, Karger: Basel, 1987, pp. 138–53.
3 Raykar PV, Fung M, Anderson BD, The role of protein and lipid domains in the uptake of solutes by human stratum corneum, *Pharm Res* (1988) **5**: 140–50.
4 Anderson BD, Higuchi WI, Raykar PV, Heterogeneity effects on permeability: partition coefficient relationships in human stratum corneum, *Pharm Res* (1988) **5**: 566–73.
5 Menczel E, Bucks DAW, Maibach HI et al, Malathion binding to sections of human skin: skin capacity and isotherm determinations, *Arch Dermatol Res* (1983) **275**: 403–6.
6 Saket MM, James KC, Kellaway IW, The partitioning of some 21-alkyl steroid esters between stratum corneum and water, *Int J Pharmacol* (1985) **27**: 287–98.
7 Wang JCT, Patel BG, Ehmann CW et al, The release and percutaneous permeation of anthralin products, using clinically involved and uninvolved psoriatic skin, *J Am Acad Dermatol* (1987) **16**: 812–21.
8 Bronaugh RL, Congdon ER, Percutaneous absorption of hair dyes: correlation with partition coefficients, *J Invest Dermatol* (1984) **83**: 124–7.
9 Potts RO, Physical characterization of the stratum corneum: the relationship of mechanical and barrier properties to lipid and protein structure. In: Hadgraft J, Guy RI, (eds). *Transdermal drug delivery: developmental issues and research initiatives*, Marcel Dekker: New York, 1989, pp. 23–57.
10 Southwell D, Barry BW, Woodford R, Variations in permeability of human skin within and between specimens, *Int J Pharmacol* (1984) **18**: 299–309.
11 Bucks DAW, Prediction of percutaneous absorption, Ph.D. thesis, University of California San Francisco, San Francisco, 1989.
12 Hansch C, Leo A, *Substituent constants for correlation analysis in chemistry and biology*, Wiley: New York, 1979.
13 Lyman WJ, Reehl WF, Rosenblatt DH, *Handbook of chemical property estimation methods*, McGraw-Hill: New York, 1982.
14 Surber C, Wilhelm K-P, Maibach HI et al, Optimization of topical therapy: partitioning of drugs into stratum corneum, *Pharm Res* (1990) **7**: 1320–5.

48
Skin surface pH after short exposure to model solutions

C. Surber, P. Itin and Th. Rufli
University of Basel, Department of Dermatology, CH-4031 Basel, Switzerland

Introduction

The acidic nature of the skin surface with gaps at intertrigineous sites is well documented.[1,2] Under normal conditions, skin-surface pH values are within a narrow range and pH 5 is generally considered as physiological.[2] Attempts have been made, with varying success, to investigate the relationship between alteration of skin surface pH and the development of skin irritation.[3] In a standardized experimental setting we investigated the ability of the skin to neutralize an artificially altered skin surface pH. The forearms of volunteers were exposed to various buffer solutions, to water from several sources (river Rhine, tap water, rain water, water polluted by a combustion engine) and to medical baths (Cremol and Balmandol). Skin surface pH was recorded before and at various time intervals after exposure.

Materials and methods

Test sites and exposure

Up to 16 test fields (1 × 1 cm) were outlined on the anterior aspect of the forearms. The forearms of the volunteers were submerged and exposed for 10 min at 23°C in the bathing solutions.

Bathing solutions

The following bathing solutions were used: glycine/HCl buffer (pH 2),[4] glycine/NaOH buffer (pH 10),[4] $NaHCO_3$ buffer (pH 8.4)[4] at two different concentrations (0.1 and 0.5 mol/l), water from several sources (river Rhine, tap water, rain water, and water polluted by a combustion engine) and two medical baths (Cremol and Balmandol).

pH determination

A flat surface glass electrode (Skin-pH-Meter, PH 900 PC, Courage + Khazaka, Köln, Germany) was used to measure the pH of the test sites. The pH meter was calibrated at pH 4 and 7 prior to each experiment. Distilled water (10 µl) was added to the test site and the flat head of the electrode was applied directly to the moist surface. Each measurement given is a mean value (delogarithmicated) of five consecutive measurements (pH is a logarithmic value. To calculate a mean value it is necessary to average the delogarithmicated values and to logarithmicate the mean value again to get the average pH.). The pH was determined first at test site 1, next at test sites 1 and 2, then at test sites 1, 2 and 3, and so on, at various time intervals (see Figures 1–4) yielding a pH value for a test site not previously used for measurement and various pH values for test sites previously used for measurement. Two types of pH values are shown in the figures: (A) the pH value for a test site not previously used; and (B) the pH value of test site 1 repeatedly used for measurement.

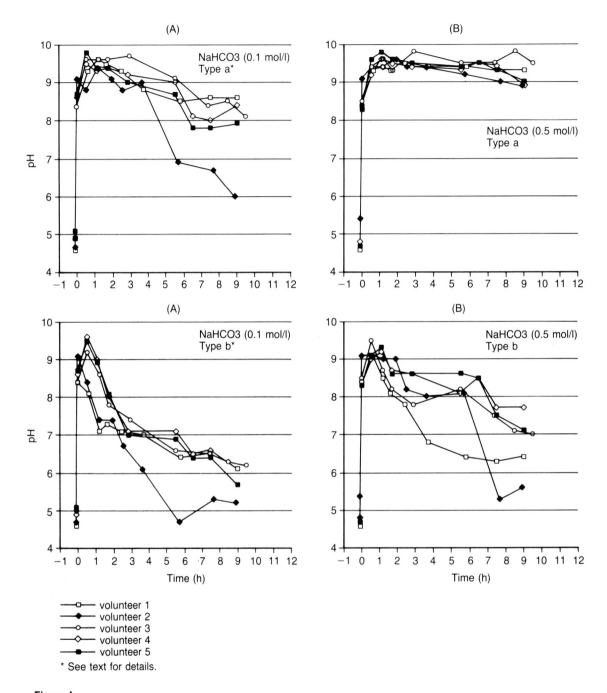

Figure 1

Skin surface pH after exposure to NaHCO₃ buffer in five volunteers. (A) pH 8.4, 0.1 mol/l; (B) pH 8.4, 0.5 mol/l.

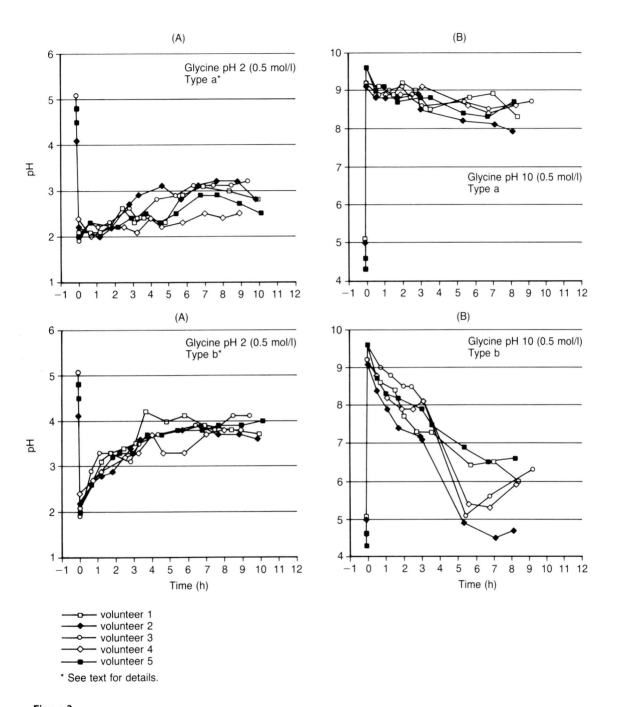

Figure 2

Skin surface pH after exposure to glycine buffers in five volunteers. (A) Glycine/HCl buffer pH 2, 0.5 mol/l; (B) glycine/NaOH buffer pH 10, 0.5 mol/l.

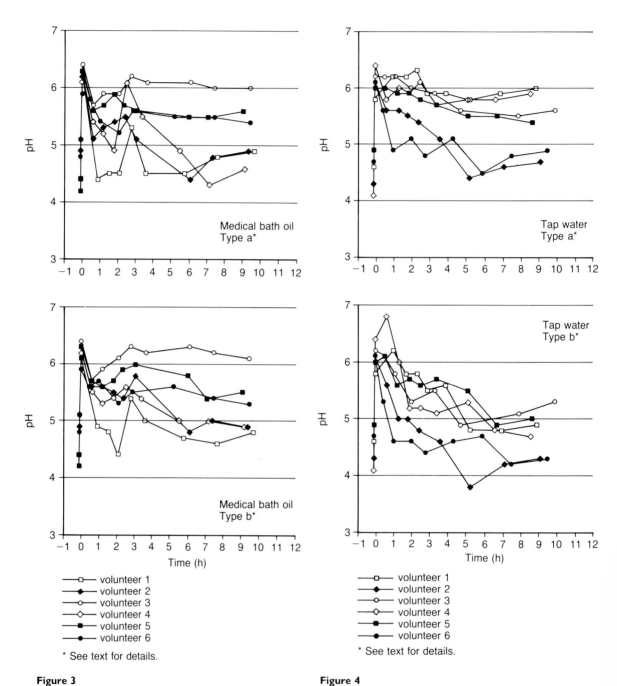

Figure 3

Skin surface pH after exposure to a medical bath oil (Cremol) in six volunteers.

Figure 4

Skin surface pH after exposure to tap water in six volunteers.

Results and discussion

NaHCO₃ buffers

The skin surface pH after exposure to NaHCO₃ buffer (pH 8.4) at two different concentrations (0.1 and 0.5 mol/l (oversaturated)) is shown in Figure 1. Note that the skin surface pH is initially about 1.5 pH units higher than the pH of the buffer solution itself due to changes in the carbonate buffer system, that repeated pH measurement results in a more rapid pH decline (type b), and that the skin surface pH tended to normalize more rapidly with the less concentrated buffer solution. Initial skin surface pH values were not reached by 10 h.

Glycine buffers

The skin surface pH after exposure to glycine/HCl buffer (pH 2, 0.5 mol/l) and glycine/NaOH buffer (pH 10, 0.5 mol/l) is shown in Figure 2. Note that repeated pH measurements (type b) resulted in a more rapid pH increase (glycine/HCl buffer, pH 2) or decrease (glycine/NaOH buffer, pH 10), and that this phenomenon is more distinct with the buffer solutions with the lower buffering capacity (0.1 mol/l) (date not shown).

Medical baths and water from several sources

The skin surface pH after exposure to a medical bath (Cremol) and tap water is shown in Figures 3 and 4. Note that, after exposure, skin surface pH was immediately elevated for a short period followed by a return to normal pH within 6 h, and that repeated pH measurement (type b) had no definite influence on skin surface pH. Observations made after exposure to the other solutions (Balamandol, river Rhine, rain water, and water polluted by a combustion engine) were similar to those made with Cremol and tap water.

It was demonstrated that repeated skin surface measurements in the same test field do influence pH when definite pH shifts are provoked. Return to normal pH was delayed when a new test field was chosen (type a) for each consecutive measurement. Because any reference to the pH of the tissue refers to the pH of the aqueous solution which bathes the cells of the tissue, it may be concluded that repeated measurements in the same test field influence the buffer system of the skin and/or dilutes the applied buffer system. The data show that exogenous influences can change the skin surface pH for an extended period of time. Attempts by different groups to study the relative irritancy of surfactants and model solutions as a function of skin surface pH have produced conflicting and often controversial results and the data reported have often been diametrically opposed when comparing, for example, synthetic detergent cleansers with classical alkaline soaps. Skin surface pH alterations caused by environmental factors, as simulated by the buffer solutions, the water from different sources and the medical baths, are probably of minor importance and have little or no influence on skin irritation. We believe that the skin surface pH and the alteration of the pH after short and prolonged exposure to detergents or model solutions are not parameters of high significance and are scarcely suitable for the study of environmentally induced skin damage. Furthermore it seems most doubtful whether it is possible to separate clearly the pH effects from the inherent irritancy of the xenobiotics themselves and other physicochemical parameters.[3,5]

References

1. Rothman S, *Physiology and biochemistry of the skin*, University of Chicago Press: Chicago, IL, 1954, pp. 221–32.
2. Braun-Falco O, Korting HC, *Hautreinigung mit syndets*, Springer-Verlag: Berlin, 1990, pp. 67–76.
3. Murahata RI, Toton-Quinn R, Finkey MB et al, Effect of pH on the production of irritation in chamber irritation test, *J Am Acad Dermatol* (1988) **18**: 62–6.
4. *Wissenschaftliche Tabellen Geigy*, Teilband Hämatologie und Humangenetik, 8. Auflage, Basel, 1979, pp. 60–2.
5. Surber C, Sucker H, Tissue tolerance of intramuscular injectables and plasma enzyme activities in rats, *Pharmacol Res* (1987) **4**: 490–4.

49
Surfactant damaged skin: which treatment?

Enzo Berardesca, Gian Piero Vignoli, Giovanni Borroni,* Christian Oresajo and Giacomo Rabbiosi

Department of Dermatology, University of Pavia, IRCCS Policlinico S. Matteo, 27100 Pavia, Italy, and *Elizabeth Arden Biosciences, Trumbull, CT, USA

Acute or chronic exposure to surfactants leads to the development of skin irritation.[1] Surfactants have several actions that contribute to their irritancy: they remove the stratum corneum lipids,[2,3] they extract aminoacids and proteins,[4] and they remove the natural moisturizing factors (NMF) from the stratum corneum.[5] Furthermore, these compounds have been shown in vitro to damage the skin barrier function increasing the permeability of the epidermis to water.[6] In vivo, the increased water evaporation from the skin surface can be detected using non-invasive techniques such as evaporimetry. This technique has been reported to be suitable for this purpose[7] and irritated 'dry' skin presents increased transepidermal water loss (TEWL) associated with reduced stratum corneum hydration and water-holding capacity.[8] The regulation of the stratum corneum barrier function is based on an heterogeneous two-compartment model which ascribes a special role to intercellular lipids.[9] Stratum corneum lipids consist mainly of cholesterol, free fatty acids and ceramides. The ceramides have given rise to great interest because they represent the major polar lipids of which the extracellular membranous structures of the stratum corneum are composed: the acylceramides contain a high proportion of esterified linoleic acid that have been postulated to play a predominant role in skin barrier formation.[10]

Moisturizers and emollients are commonly used in the treatment of rough dry skin, even though their role in the normalization of the damaged barrier is unclear.

In an experimental model of sodium lauryl sulphate (SLS) induced skin irritation, we compared the effects of two different treatments, based on NMF and ceramide I, in the recovery of barrier function and the normalization of TEWL to assess the usefulness of these treatments in these disorders.

Materials and methods

Ten healthy subjects of both sexes (age 26 ± 6 years) entered the study. Three different sites on the volar forearm were irritated by applying 1% sodium lauryl sulphate (SLS) in aqueous solution (Sigma Chemicals, St. Louis, USA) under 18 mm plastic chamber occlusion (Hill Top, Cincinnati, USA) for 24 h. At the removal of the occlusive devices, two sites were chosen at random for daily treatment with the moisturizing emulsion with NMF (NMF 4.5%, panthenol, allantoin, lactic acid, dimethicone and water) or the ceramide I (ceramide I 0.01%, cyclomethicone, squalene, dimethicone, neural lipid extract, epidermal lipid extract, retinyl palmitate, tocopheryl linoleate and evening primrose oil) lotion. The third irritated site served as a control.

Treatment was continued for 3 days; TEWL and skin conductance were measured daily to monitor skin barrier function and stratum corneum water content. TEWL was measured with an Evaporimeter EP 1 (ServoMed, Kinna, Sweden); skin conductance was measured using a Corneometer CM 820 PC (Courage and Khazaka, Cologne, Germany) at the end of the treatment. Baseline recordings were taken daily on non-irritated skin. Statistical analysis of the results was performed using ANOVA and the Scheffé test for multiple comparisons.

Results

The results obtained are shown in Tables 1 and 2 and in Figure 1. Lower mean TEWL values were recorded in baseline non-irritated skin. At the removal of occlusion, TEWL was significantly higher in the three irritated sites compared with the baseline value. In the irritated site that served as control (no treatment), TEWL reached a peak value after 48 h following irritation. In the ceramide treated site, no significant differences compared to baseline skin were recorded throughout the study; TEWL levels progressively decreased from day 1 to day 3, whereas in the site treated only with the moisturizer the TEWL was higher than the baseline value ($P < 0.05$) on days 2 and 3. At the end of treatment, the moisturizer treated site showed a significant increase in stratum corneum water content compared to the control site ($P < 0.01$) (Table 2).

Discussion

The stratum corneum is considered to form a uniform layer which constitutes the main skin barrier against water loss. Its structure is based on a model[11] consisting of an intracellular and an intercellular compartment. The former is constituted by corneocytes and is the largest regarding

Table 1 Mean TEWL values (g/m² h) ± standard deviation during the study

Group	Irritation	Day 1	Day 2	Day 3
Baseline	4.5 ± 1.1	5.5 ± 1.2	5.1 ± 1.4	5.1 ± 1.1
Control	8.4 ± 2.6	11.9 ± 8.7	8.9 ± 4.6	8.3 ± 2.5
Moisturizer	9.1 ± 3.3	9.3 ± 2.6	8.8 ± 1.4	8.1 ± 1.8
Ceramide	8.0 ± 2.3	9.2 ± 2.5*	7.6 ± 2.7*	7.0 ± 2.6*

* Values not significant compared to baseline.

Table 2 Water content of the stratum corneum (Corneometer units) after 3 days of treatment

Group	Count	Mean	SD	SE
Baseline	10	76.3	12.91	4.083
Control	10	71.1	13.56	4.288
Ceramide I	10	76.5	10.763	3.403
Moisturizer	10	82*	12.111	3.83

* Hydration is significantly ($P < 0.01$, ANOVA repeated measures test and Scheffé test) higher than the control value in the site treated with the moisturizing emulsion.

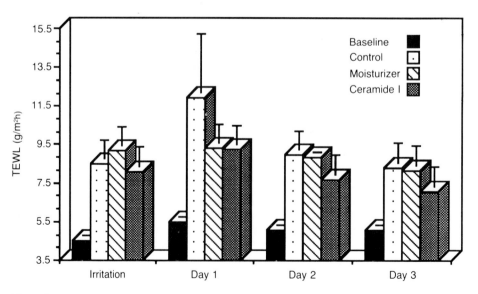

Figure 1

TEWL values during treatment of SLS irritated skin with ceramide I and a moisturizer containing NMF (see text for details).

volume; the latter is formed by intercellular lipids (neutral lipids, polar lipids and sphingolipids). Sphingolipids account for 18% of intercellular corneum lipids; among these, ceramides are predominant. In the cellular compartment, apart from keratin, the corneocytes contain a group of substances referred as 'natural moisturizing factors' (NMF) composed by pyrrolidonecarboxylic acid and other carbohydrate–protein complexes that are involved in maintaining the capacity of the corneum to hold and trap water.[12] In the lowest stratum corneum the cells are more tightly packed and represent the most efficient part of the barrier.[13]

Acute or chronic exposure to surfactants may cause irritant dermatitis leading to the development of dry or rough skin. From a biophysical point of view, this disorder is characterized by an increased TEWL[7] due to the defective water barrier and decreased stratum corneum water content.[14] Emollients and moisturizers are used to improve this condition, restoring normal water content levels and decreasing clinical symptoms of dry skin.

In the present study we compared the effects of a moisturizing emulsion containing NMF and a lotion containing ceramide I on the normalization of the water barrier after experimental exposure to SLS. The data obtained (Table I and Figure I) show a significant effect of the treatment with ceramide I on the barrier function as detected with TEWL measurements. Indeed, lower TEWL values compared to control and moisturizer treated sites were detected on days 2 and 3 ($P < 0.05$). Ceramide I is an acylceramide and plays a role in cementing the extracellular lipid sheets which constitute the barrier and prevents water loss from the skin. Its content is greater in lamellar bodies from which it is extruded into the intercellular compartment of the stratum corneum.[15]

At the end of the study, the stratum corneum water content was significantly increased in the site treated with NMF. Table 2 shows increased water content in the ceramide treated site compared to the control site; the values equal the baseline levels recorded in non-irritated skin. Higher values ($P < 0.01$) were recorded on the site treated with NMF compared to control.

The study shows that TEWL and skin hydration are not always strictly correlated; topical application of NMF increases skin hydration by trapping water in the corneocytes, but has little effect in restoring the intercellular compartment damaged by SLS. The use of moisturizers in the treatment of irritant contact dermatitis may be of value to improve the clinical signs of dermatitis, but should be used with other compounds capable of reducing water evaporation from the surface and improving skin barrier function.

Treatment with the ceramide containing preparation increases skin hydration (even though not so significantly as the NMF containing preparation) and leads to rapid restoration of the barrier function preventing prolonged water loss from the skin. This action may assist healing of the skin affected by irritant contact dermatitis.

References

1 Klauder JV, Actual causes of certain occupational dermatoses, *Arch Dermatol* (1962) **85**: 441–54.
2 Scheuplein R, Ross L, Effects of surfactants and solvents on the permeability of epidermis, *J Soc Cosm Chem* (1970) **21**: 853–73.
3 Kirk JF, Hand washing: quantitative studies on skin lipid removal by soaps and detergents based on 1500 experiments, *Acta Dermatol Venereol* (1966) **46** (suppl 57): 1–183.
4 Prottey C, Ferguson T, Factors which determine the skin irritation potential of soaps and detergents, *J Soc Cosm Chem* (1975) **26**: 29–46.
5 Imokawa G, Mishima Y, Cumulative effect of surfactants on cutaneous horny layers: absorption onto human keratin layers in vivo, *Contact Dermat* (1979) **5**: 357–66.
6 Smeenk G, The influence of detergents on the skin, *Arch Klin Exp Dermatol* (1969) **235**: 180–91.
7 Van der Valk PGM, Nater JP, Bleumink E, Skin irritancy of surfactants as assessed by water vapor loss measurements, *J Invest Dermatol* (1984) **82**: 291–3.
8 Tagami H, Kanamaru Y, Inoue K et al, Water sorption–desorption test of the skin in vivo for functional assessment of the stratum corneum, *J Invest Dermatol* (1982) **78**: 425–8.
9 Elias PM, Epidermal lipids, barrier function and desquamation, *J Invest Dermatol* (1983) **80** (suppl): 44–9.
10 Wertz PW, Downing DT, Ceramides of pig epidermis: structure determination, *J Lipid Res* (1983) **24**: 759–65.
11 Elias PM, Lipids and the epidermal permeability barrier, *Arch Dermatol Res* (1981) **270**: 95–117.
12 Middleton JD, The mechanism of water binding in the stratum corneum, *Br J Dermatol* (1968) **80**: 437–60.
13 Bowser PA, White RJ, Isolation, barrier properties and lipid analysis of the stratum compactum a discrete layer of the stratum corneum, *Br J Dermatol* (1985) **112**: 1–14.
14 Blank IH, Shapiro EB, The water content of the stratum corneum. III. Effect of previous contact with aqueous solutions of soaps and detergents, *J Invest Dermatol* (1955) **25**: 391–401.
15 Wertz PW, Downing DT, Freinkel RK et al, Sphingolipids of the stratum corneum and lamellar granules of fetal rat epidermis, *J Invest Dermatol* (1984) **83**: 193–5.

50
Three cases of urticaria caused by chronic exposure to pentachlorophenol

J. Lambert, L. Matthieu, Ph. Jorens,* P. Schepens* and P. Dockx
Departments of Dermatology and *Toxicology, University of Antwerp, B-2610 Antwerp (Wilrijk), Belgium

Introduction

Pentachlorophenol (PCP) is a commonly used wood preservative. It is used in industry to impregnate wood, leather, paper, paints and glues. PCP is also employed in homes and gardens as a fungicide, an algicide, an insecticide and a disinfectant. Its dose-dependent acute toxic effects on the phosphorylating process have been investigated in animals[1] and the symptoms of acute poisoning in man after massive exposure have also been described.[2]

Little is known about the effects of chronic exposure in man. Conjunctivitis, chronic sinusitis, upper respiratory complaints, recurring headache and neurological complaints have been reported.[3,4] In addition, some cases of aplastic anaemia and red cell aplasia have been related to repeated exposure to PCP.[5] Vaguely defined skin irritations and rashes, a susceptibility to skin infections,[3,4,6] chloracne[7] and contact urticaria[8] have been mentioned as skin disorders arising from PCP exposure.

Our personal experience with chronic PCP exposure causing dermatological lesions began in 1983.[9] We observed two cases of pemphigus vulgaris where PCP was a contributing factor: exacerbations of the disease were linked with elevated PCP levels in the serum. Since then we have been alert to the possible relationship of dermatological problems and chronic exposure to PCP, and have been able to pinpoint PCP as the cause of chronic urticaria in three patients.

Case reports

Case 1

A 35-year-old man had been suffering from urticaria for 4 months, with large weals scattered over the trunk and limbs. No obvious causes were noted. The dietary provocation tests were positive for salicylates and negative for penicillin, yeast extract, tartrazine and benzoates.

The treatment consisted of a salicylate free diet and different antihistamines including terfenadine, hydroxyzine and astemizole. However, the urticaria worsened. Two exacerbations with high fever, general malaise and arthralgia were observed. A new thorough clinical history revealed a possible PCP exposure when the patient was treating wooden windowframes shortly before the start of the urticaria and again just before the exacerbations. The serum PCP level was 58.7 µg/l. The serum PCP levels were measured following the analytical procedure described previously[10] with 30 µg/l as the highest dose acceptable as normal, being the mean of the PCP levels experienced in a population without any exposure. Other abnormal laboratory results were: C-reactive protein 9.9 mg/dl (normal <1.2 mg/dl); rheumatoid factor 57.4 IU/ml (normal <50 IU/ml); Rose Waaler 1/32. The circulating IgE immune complexes became positive at 3.03 TU/l (normal <2.74 TU/l). The titer for ANA was 1/40 with a mottled appearance and

1/120 up to 1/1200 for the anti-skin antibodies of the pemphigus vulgaris type.

Control investigations after 3 weeks still revealed a high PCP level of 143 µg/l. Because of the lack of any significant improvement the patient moved temporarily to another house in early September 1984. After 2 weeks the urticaria had decreased significantly. The serum PCP level declined to 50.9 µg/l and no further anti-skin antibodies were observed. A month later it decreased to 41.6 µg/l but increased to 96 µg/l when the patient returned home in January 1985. In the meantime all possible sources of PCP had been removed. Since then the patient has been free of urticaria and the last recorded value for his serum PCP level was 46 µg/l.

Case 2

A 30-year-old woman presented with a chronic urticaria, for the previous 10 months. In the same period she had moved to a new house where wood preservatives containing PCP had been used.

A first PCP level was markedly elevated (390 µg/l). All other blood results were normal except the circulating IgE immunocomplexes which were 2.94 TU/l (normal <2.74 TU/l).

A diet free of salicylates, penicillin, yeast extract, tartrazine and benzoates gave no improvement, not even in combination with dimenthidene maleate.

As soon as the patient had been informed about the high levels of PCP, all wood treated with PCP was coated with a specific protective layer to prevent further emanations. The urticaria gradually faded over several weeks. The PCP level was then 39 µg/l.

Case 3

A 36-year-old man presented with giant weals which had been present for several months. Other complaints included chronic fatigue, weight loss and non-specific upper respiratory problems. He too had treated a considerable amount of wood in his house with PCP and he, as much as the other patients, noted an improvement when leaving his house for holidays.

His PCP serum level was markedly elevated at 380 µg/l in December 1988. All other laboratory results were normal except a slight elevation of the cholesterol (274 mg/dl; normal 150–250 mg/dl).

The patient's symptoms were only partially relieved by antihistamine therapy and he decided then to remove much of the treated joists. The urticaria disappeared during the following month. The value for the serum PCP level was 48 µg/l in March 1989. Nevertheless, a problem of moderate itch persisted. Part of the wooden framework had not yet been removed and laboratory investigations confirmed that this had also been treated with PCP and the PCP levels remained elevated at 71 µg/l in June 1989, 55 µg/l in October 1989 and 55 µg/l in July 1990. Work to remove the PCP treated wood is underway at present. All other members of the family also had elevated PCP levels. Their values were also reduced after the first renovation and it is interesting to note that the patient's wife complained consistently of a slight itch and a chronic fatigue, which improved after the removal of the PCP treated joists.

Conclusion

We have presented three patients with chronic urticaria in whom we have been able to pinpoint PCP as the cause of the problem. The chronic intoxication was caused by emanation of PCP from wooden framework treated with a wood preservative containing PCP. The clinical course showed a striking parallel with the exposure to PCP. By taking the appropriate measures to remove all possible sources of PCP, the lesions of chronic urticaria subsided rapidly and serum levels of PCP declined significantly.

We hope that these observations will draw attention to the relationship between chronic PCP exposure and dermatological disorders and to possible new hazardous effects of PCP.

References

1 Williams PL, Pentachlorophenol, an assessment of the occupational hazard, *Am Ind Hyg Assoc J* (1982) **43**: 799–810.
2 Wood S, Rom WN, White GL Jr et al, Pentachlorophenol poisoning, *J Occup Med* (1983) **25**: 527–30.
3 Sterling TD, Stoffman LD, Sterling DA et al, Health effects of chlorophenol wood preservatives on sawmill workers, *Int J Hlth Serv* (1982) **12**: 559–71.
4 Klemmer HW, Wong L, Sato MM et al, Clinical findings in workers exposed to pentachlorophenol, *Arch Environ Contam Toxicol* (1980) **9**: 715–25.

5 Roberts HJ, Aplastic anemia and red cell aplasia due to pentachlorophenol, *South Med J* (1983) **76**: 45–8.
6 Sangster B, Wegman RCC, Hofstee AWN, Non-occupational exposure to pentachlorophenol: clinical findings and plasma PCP concentrations in three families, *Human Toxicol* (1982) **1**: 123–33.
7 O'Malley MA, Carpenter AV, Sweeney MH et al, Chloracne associated with employment in the production of pentachlorophenol, *Am J Ind Med* (1990) **17**: 411–21.
8 Kantor PM, Urticaria from contact with pentachlorophenate, *J Am Med Assoc* (1986) **256**: 3350 (letter).
9 Lambert J, Schepens P, Janssens J et al, Skin lesions as a sign of subacute pentachlorophenol intoxication, *Acta Dermatol Venereol (Stockh)* (1986) **66**: 170–2.
10 Janssens JJ, Schepens PJC, Chronic pentachlorophenol intoxication as a result of the usage of wood protectants, *Med Fac Landbouwwetensch Rijksunivers Gent* (1984) **49/3b**: 1175–84.

51
Non-melanoma skin cancer and therapeutic agents

J. H. Epstein
Department of Dermatology, University of California, San Francisco, CA 94143, USA

Non-melanoma skin cancers are by far the most common human malignancies that occur in the Caucasian population. They make up 30–40% of the cancers that occur in the USA. These lesions occur primarily through environmental influences. The most important of these influences are the rays of the sun. However, the sun is not the only carcinogen that we must deal with. Indeed our environment is full of carcinogenic substances such as those that are emitted from cars, chimneys and the like.

In this chapter we are concerned with a specific part of our environment which all of us are closely involved with, that is, or rather these are, topical medications. Obviously the vast majority of medications that dermatologists prescribe are not carcinogenic. However, there are a few commonly used and other not so commonly used agents which can or have produced cancers in humans, either by themselves or in conjunction with ultraviolet radiation (UVR).

The first topical medications that come to mind are coal tar and its derivatives which are commonly used in conjunction with UVB energy produced by fluorescent tubes or hot quartz units. Coal tar and its derivatives can produce cancer in at least seven ways. They contain complete carcinogens such as benz[a]pyrene and related polycyclic hydrocarbons, organ specific carcinogens such as β-naphthylamine, o-toluidine and quinoline which can produce bladder tumours, phenols and catechols which are tumour promoters, and naphthylenes which can produce lymphomas. Tar could also produce cancer through photoactivation by UVA rays, by additive effects of the full carcinogen and UVB photocarcinogenesis and promotion of UVB photocarcinogenesis by phenols and/or catechols.

All seven of these effects have been demonstrated in experimental animals. However, dermatologists are most interested in the presence of complete carcinogens such as the polycyclic hydrocarbon benz[a]pyrene, and the chemical promotion of chemcial carcinogenesis by phenols, catechols and the like. The possibility of a photosensitized carcinogenic effect with tar activated by UVA rays must also be considered. In general, most but probably not all of the tar molecules are removed before irradiation with primarily UVB rays. However, it is not likely that all of the tar is removed from all the cells of the epidermis and some UVA is included with the UVB exposures. Also, some physicians use a combination of UVA and UVB sources for their tar and UVR therapy. Experimental tar and UVA photocarcinogenesis has been definitively demonstrated.[1]

The additive carcinogenic effects of a chemical carcinogen such as the polycyclic hydrocarbon dimethylbenzanthracene (DMBA) which is similar to benz[a]pyrene and the physical carcinogen UVB energy have been demonstrated.[1] Hairless mice in one group received a single application of a subcarcinogenic amount of DMBA. Those in the second group received a single application of the diluent which was acetone. One month later tri-weekly exposures to UVB energy were initiated and carried out for the duration of the study. The cancers appeared significantly earlier in the mice which had received the DMBA application. In addition, the tumors grew more rapidly in the DMBA-treated group and all of these tumors were cancers. These are the three characteristic features of additive carcinogenesis rather than promotion.

Promotion of UVR initiated carcinogenesis by non-carcinogenic chemical promoters has also been confirmed experimentally with several agents.[1] The type of tumor that is seen in all these studies is squamous cell carcinoma. This of course is the type of tumor that is most dependent on sun exposure in human skin. It is quite feasible that the carcinogens in coal tar could act additively with the carcinogenic effects of UVB and the non-carcinogenic compounds such as the catechols and phenolic compounds in tar preparations could well function as promoters and might be responsible for the significant amount of industrial skin cancer that is induced by tar and tar products. In the USA 35% of all industrial cancers are considered to be produced by tar and tar derivatives.

This brings us to cancer and the Goekerman regimen. Despite multiple denials, retrospective studies and the like, Stern et al[2] have pointed out that, if you give enough UVB, that is over 300 UVB treatments, and/or enough tar (90 months) you would increase the cancer load at least to a small extent.[2] It is amazing that this cancer incidence is not much greater, especially if one considers that UVB is a much more effective carcinogen than PUVA, at least under experimental conditions. We found that UVB induced cancer in 60% of mice by 60 weeks with a total of 36 J/cm^2. It took 90 weeks and 1012 J of UVA plus psoralens (PUVA) to induce cancers in 60% of the mice.[3] Obviously, UVB is a much more efficient carcinogen experimentally than PUVA. We should also note that molecules from the tar are absorbed and there is an increased incidence of mutagens in the urine after crude-coal-tar applications.

Another group of medications, the alkylating agents, nitrogen mustard and the nitrosoureas carmustine (BCNU), methyl nitroso urea (MNU) and lomustine (CCNU), are not so commonly used but have been used therapeutically topically in mycosis fungoides (MF) and psoriasis with some success. Nitrogen mustard has also been used topically and intralesionally in various benign and malignant tumors ranging from keratoacanthomas to basal cell epitheliomas. Nitrogen mustard has also been used in vitiligo because of its pigment stimulating effects. We should note that the nitrosoureas also are potent pigmentation stimulators.

Nitrogen mustards are full carcinogens, perhaps through their effects on DNA. They cause strand breaks and cross-links in DNA molecules in cells. They also cause mutations and cancers experimentally. The nitrosoureas are also full carcinogens, most likely through their effects on DNA, but these effects are not clearly understood at present. Furthermore, carcinogenesis due to these nitrogen mustards and nitrosoureas may be due to direct alterations in DNA or through their immunosuppressive properties, as occurs in chemotherapeutic suppression for organ transplantation and the like.

Whatever the mechanism, these agents have proven to be carcinogenic in experimental animals.[1] As an example, 0.1 mg of nitrogen mustard in alcohol applied two times a week to the backs of hairless mice resulted in a significant production of cutaneous cancers. In addition the combined effects of chronic UVB exposures and nitrogen mustard markedly accelerated this cancer production as compared to UVB alone.

Topical methylnitrosourea (MNU) had an even more notable effect. By 6 months 50% of the mice had tumors larger than 100 mm^3, and by 10 months 96% had these large cancers. As with nitrogen mustard, the process was significantly accelerated when MNU was used in association with chronic UVB exposures. Almost 65% of the mice receiving both carcinogenic modalities had cancers at 6 months, and by 7 months 100% had such tumors.

In contrast, carmustine (BCNU) and lomustine (CCNU) are weak carcinogens in themselves but do markedly enhance UVR induced cancer formation. Topical applications of CCNU did not produce cancers in hairless mice. However, when chronic UVB exposures were added to the system there was indeed a definitive development of cutaneous cancers as compared to UVB alone. Similarly, topically applied BCNU was not carcinogenic to the hairless mice. However, topical application of BCNU plus UVB energy produced cancers much more rapidly than the UVR alone.

These experimental results indicate that nitrogen mustard and MNU are potentially potent carcinogens when applied topically. But perhaps the more important issue is that all these agents accelerate UVB induced cancer formation.[1]

Clinically, the induction of cutaneous cancers by topical nitrogen mustard therapy has taken the problem out of the laboratory and into the realm of the practice of medicine. Vonderheid et al[4] noted that 4% of their patients who had been treated for MF topically for up to 3 years developed premalignant and malignant cutaneous neoplasms, and 27% treated for more than 3 years developed such lesions. In addition, Kravitz and McDonald[5] reported two cases of squamous cell carcinoma (SCC) apparently related to nitrogen mustard therapy. One of these metastasized. Subsequently, Lee et al[6] reported that four patients with MF out of 29 treated with topical nitrogen mustard developed six skin cancers; two basal cell epithelioma (BCE) and four SCC on non-sun-exposed sites.

One more point with regard to nitrogen mustard is that it has been suggested that PUVA or UVB radiation, which are immunosuppressive, could be used to inhibit the common allergic reaction to nitrogen mustard in the treatment of psoriasis or MF. It should be pointed out that we found that nitrogen mustard can act as a promoter and cocarcinogen with UVB carcinogenesis. An interpretation of this finding is that it is the same concept as with PUVA. Thus, if experimental data can be related to human responses, it would seem that the combination of nitrogen mustard and UVB or PUVA should be avoided.

This brings us to a most important medication with a possible potential for promoting UV carcinogenesis, i.e. all-*trans* retinoic acid (Retin-A (RA)). It should be emphasized that RA has not been shown to be carcinogenic and, if it does stimulate cancer formation, it should be considered a promoter and not a full carcinogen.

A summary of the information available at this time concerning this problem is given below.[7] In the initial study, a 0.3% concentration of RA in a cream base was applied 3 times a week to albino hairless mice preceded by UVB irradiation from a hot quartz source. These RA applications did indeed accelerate the photocarcinogenic effects of the UVB. However, although these were the concentrations used by Bollag and Ott[8] in their early studies on the topical treatment of human actinic keratoses, they were quite irritating and toxic to the mice.

Because the concentration used in our study was so high, Forbes et al[9] examined lower, essentially non-irritating concentrations of the drug. They used 0.01 and 0.001% concentrations in methanol preceded by radiation from a solar simulator for 7 days a week. Under these circumstances the RA also accelerated UVR-induced carcinogenesis.

At the same time as Temple's[9] group was carrying out their studies, we were also looking at lower concentrations such as 0.05, 0.025 and 0.005% in a polyethyleneglycol alcohol base using thrice weekly applications and irradiation from a hot quartz source. The 0.025 and 0.005% applications had no significant detectable effect. However, in contrast to the previous studies, 0.05% RA significantly inhibited UVR-induced carcinogenesis.

Four subsequent studies have been reported. Davies[10] reported that using the true two-stage technique of irradiating for 6 weeks followed by topical applications of 0.01% RA for 14 weeks that the RA did indeed promote UVR initiated carcinogenesis. It should be noted that we have confirmed this promoting effect in our system.

In the next study the Kligmans[11] used FS-20 lamp radiation 3 times per week followed by topical 0.01 and 0.001% RA applications 5 times a week. These workers were unable to detect any difference between tumor formation in the irradiated control mice and those receiving the RA. Unfortunately all the mice had tumors by 30 weeks which clouded the issue.

Conner et al[12] reported a tendency to inhibition of tumor formation and size when 3.4 nm of RA were applied immediately after irradiation. This apparent inhibition was not statistically significant when the RA was applied only immediately after the UVB exposures (FS-40), but was when applied at 0, 1, 2, 3 and 4 h after irradiation ($P = 0.05$). The authors suggested that this inhibition might be due to inhibition of ornithine decarboxylase (ODC) activation by UVR, which they had reported earlier. It should be noted that Kligman[13] have reported that RA in a cream base did not inhibit UVR induced ODC activity and in fact increased it. High doses of RA in acetone also induced ODC activity.

The most recent review and evaluation of the relationship of retinoids to photocarcinogenesis is that by Davies and Forbes.[14] In this study non-irritating concentrations of RA (3.4 nm, 0.1 mg/ml) used in a concomitant study with UVR did indeed enhance photocarcinogenesis in two other less UVR sensitive rodents.

Thus from the experimental evidence it is clear that RA can both stimulate and inhibit photocarcinogenesis under different conditions. It should be noted that no evidence of a tumor promoting effect for RA has been reported in humans. In fact there is some evidence that RA may enhance the beneficial effects of 5FU on actinic keratoses. All the evidence for the promoting effects of RA in photocarcinogenesis has been gathered from experimental studies which, although not directly applicable to man, should alert us to the possibility of problems in the future.

The topical agent benzoyl peroxide (BPO) is even more frequently used than RA. Slaga et al[15] have published a study demonstrating that, although BPO was not carcinogenic it did promote tumor formation initiated by a subcarcinogenic application of DMBA. They used the tumor-susceptible Sencar mouse. The DMBA application was followed 1 week later by bi-weekly applications of benzoyl peroxide (BPO) in doses ranging from 1 to 40 mg for 52 weeks. Tumor promotion followed a dose–response pattern in general, although 20 mg was as effective as 40 mg. In a more recent report, these authors noted that lauroyl peroxide was as efficient a promoter as BPO and H_2O_2 was a weak promoter.[16] These agents are free-radical-generating compounds. O'Connell et al[17] and Athar et al[18] also noted enhanced malignant progression of chemically initiated and promoted papillomas by BPO. Athar et al also reported acceleration of malignant conversion of UVR-induced benign papillomas.

We examined the possible promoting effect of BPO on UVR-initiated carcinogenesis.[19] Used hairless mice were irradiated with 1.25 mJ/cm^2 of UVB energy 3 times a week for 8 weeks. Four weeks later BPO, BPO base, and croton oil and base were applied 5 times a week for 54 weeks. UVR produced a few tumors in the BPO and base treated mice. The croton oil promoted the UVR-initiated growths but BPO did not. Thus BPO did not promote UVR carcinogenesis, at least under the circumstances of the study. These findings were confirmed by Iversen.[20] A recent report by Hogan[21] on a large series noted no increased cancer risk in patients who had used BPO for acne.

The last treatment discussed here is not truly a topical medication but it does relate to local applications in part and that is PUVA therapy.

Unlike tar and UVB, the psoralens are not carcinogenic and, as far as is known, nor is UVA under clinical conditions. However, UVA can augment the carcinogenic effects of UVB energy and, in large amounts, can induce tumor formation in experimental animals.[1] The combination of the psoralens, 8-MOP and 5-MOP plus UVA radiation has proven to be both mutagenic and carcinogenic in experimental systems.[22,23] These effects appear to result from interactions with DNA. Both 8-MOP and 5-MOP produce monofunctional and bifunctional photoadducts with pyrimidine bases in DNA. The monofunctional adducts apparently are readily repaired whereas the bifunctional or cross-linking adducts are not and the latter are considered more mutagenic than the monoadducts. However, the angelicins which produce only monoadducts have been shown to be photocarcinogenic with UVA rays as well.[23] It should be noted that PUVA apparently can act as a promoter and an initiator of cutaneous carcinogenesis experimentally.

As far as the human experience is concerned there has been a concerted effort to reduce the amount of treatments for psoriasis as well as the total UVA used in order to avoid side effects which are primarily cutaneous cancer formation.

Stern and Lang[24] updated the original 2.5-year follow-up information on the 16 PUVA center statistics.[24] The 5-year findings confirmed and extended the initial data. There were three times as many cancers in the PUVA treated group as would be expected but, more notably, there were 8 times as many SCCs. The basal cell carcinoma (BCC)/SCC ratio was reversed and the distribution of the new cancers was on non-sun-exposed areas, emphasizing the fact that PUVA was responsible for these cancers.

Preceding therapy with ionizing radiation and tar and UVR, as well as having a light complexion predisposed to PUVA induced carcinogenesis. This plus the short incubation period and experimental evidence suggest that this early cancer response is due to tumor-promoting effects of PUVA. Since PUVA is also a carcinogen more cancers may occur. It was also clear from these studies that the more treatments, especially the more UVA joules used, the higher the cancer incidence.

As noted by Stern and Lang,[24] there is a dose-dependent increase in the risk of squamous cell carcinomas in all body sites exposed to the UVA radiation in patients with psoriasis treated with PUVA.[25] Patients who received more than 260 treatments had 11 times the risk as those who received 160 or fewer treatments. There was also a small dose-dependent increase in the risk of BCE formation.

Recently, Stern et al[25] have reported that PUVA induces a comparatively higher rate of squamous cell carcinoma on the male genitalia than elsewhere on the body.[25] Such cancers rarely occur in this anatomical location. However, in this 12.3 year prospective study of 892 men treated for psoriasis with PUVA, there was a 1.6% incidence of genital neoplasms. Patients with previous high levels of UVB therapy had a 4.6-fold increased risk of developing these cancers. These findings suggest that male genitalia are particularly susceptible to this carcinogenic stimulus. If this area is not involved it should be protected completely. If it is involved it should receive reduced dose.

In summary, tar is both carcinogenic and photocarcinogenic. It has been responsible for a significant number of industrial skin cancers. However, for practical purposes it is a safe, effective therapeutic modality. The nitrogen mustards and nitrosoureas are carcinogenic and have additive carcinogenic effects with UVB experimentally. Nitrogen mustard is proven to be carcinogenic in human skin under clinical circumstances. RA is proven to be a promoter and inhibitor of cutaneous carcinogenesis under experimental conditions. Clinically we have no evidence of this effect in humans. BPO has been shown to promote chemical- but not UVR-induced carcinogenesis in experimental animals. No clinical evidence is available for such an effect in human skin. PUVA has been shown to both initiate and promote cutaneous cancers in experimental animals. Clinically there has also been an increased incidence of human skin cancers. Most importantly the BCE/SCC ratio is reversed and the primary areas of involvement are the usually sun-protected areas. The rapid onset of such cancers suggests that this is a promoting or co-carcinogenic effect.

Acknowledgements

This study was supported by Grant No. CA15605 of the National Cancer Institute.

References

1 Epstein JH, Photocarcinogenesis, skin cancer and aging. In: AK Balin, AM Kligman (eds). *Aging and the Skin*, Raven Press: New York, 1988, pp. 307–29.
2 Stern RS, Zierler S, Parrish JA, Skin carcinoma in patients with psoriasis treated with topical tar and artificial ultraviolet radiation, *Lancet* (1980) i: 732–5.
3 Epstein JH, Cook WS, A comparison of PUVA and UVB photocarcinogenesis, *Photochem Photobiol* (1986) **43**: 17S.
4 Vonderheid EC, VanScott EJ, Johnson WC et al, Topical chemotherapy and immunotherapy of mycosis fungoides, *Arch Dermatol* (1977) **113**: 454–62.
5 Kravitz PH, McDonald CJ, Topical nitrogen mustard induced carcinogenesis, *Acta Dermatol Venereol (Stockh)* (1978) **58**: 421–5.
6 Lee LA, Fritz KA, Golitz L et al, Second cutaneous malignancies in patients with mycosis fungoides treated with topical nitrogen mustard, *J Am Acad Dermatol* (1982) **7**: 590–8.
7 Epstein JH, All-*trans* retinoic acid and cutaneous cancers, *J Am Acad Dermatol* (1986) **15**: 772–8.
8 Bollag W, Ott F, Vitamin A acid in benign and malignant tumors of the skin. *Acta Derm Venerol (Stockh)* (Suppl) (1975) **55**: 163–166.
9 Forbes PD, Urbach F, Davies RE, Enhancement of experimental photo carcinogenesis by topical retinoic acid. *Cancer Lett* (1979) **7**: 85–90.
10 Davies RE, Retinoic acid promotion of UVB initiated photocarcinogenesis presented. In ML Kripke, HN Glassman: *Retinoic Acid and Photocarcinogenesis Workshop. J Am Acad Dermatol* (1980) **2**: 439–42.
11 Kligman LH, Kligman AM, Lack of enhance of experimental photocarcinogenesis by topical retinoic acid. *Arch Dermatol Res* (1981) **270**: 453–62.
12 Conner MJ, Lowe NJ, Breeding JH, Chalet M, Inhibition of ultraviolet-B skin carcinogens by all-*trans*-retinoic acid regimens that inhibit ornithine decarboxylase induction, *Cancer Res* (1983) **43**: 171–4.
13 Kligman LH, Lack of inhibition of ultraviolet radiation-induced ornithine decarboxylase activity by retinoic acid. *Photochem Photobiol* (1986) **43**: 449–53.
14 Davies RE, Forbes PD, Retinoids and photocarcinogenesis: a review, *J Toxicol Cut Occular Toxicol* (1988) **7**: 241–53.
15 Slaga TJ, Klein-Szanto AJP, Triplett LL et al, Skin tumor-promoting activity of benzoyl peroxide, a widely used free radical-generating compound, *Science* (1981) **213**: 1023–5.
16 Klein-Szanto AJP, Slaga TJ, Effects of peroxides on rodent skin: epidermal hyperplasia and tumor promotion, *J Invest Dermatol* (1982) **79**: 30–4.
17 O'Connell JF, Klein-Szanto AJP, DiGovanni DM et al, Enhanced malignant progression of mouse skin tumors by free-radical generator benzoyl peroxide, *Cancer Res* (1986) **46**: 2863–5.
18 Athar M, Lloyd JR, Bickers DR et al, Malignant conversion of UV radiation and chemically induced mouse skin tumors by free radical generating compounds, *Carcinogenesis* (1989) **10**: 1841–5.
19 Epstein JH, Photocarcinogenesis promotion studies with benzoyl peroxide (BPO) and croton oil, *J Invest Dermatol* (1988) **91**: 114–6.
20 Iversen OH, Skin tumorigenesis and carcinogenesis studies with 7,12-dimethylbenz(a)anthracene, ultraviolet light, benzoyl peroxide (Panoxyl gel 5%) and ointment, *Carcinogenesis* (1988) **9**: 803–9.
21 Hogan DJ, Benzoyl peroxide: carcinogenicity and allergenicity. *Int J Dermatol* (1991) **30**: 467–479.
22 Grekin DA, Epstein JH, Psoralens, UVA (PUVA) and photocarcinogenesis; yearly review, *Photochem Photobiol* (1981) **33**: 957–60.
23 Mullen MP, Pathak MA, West JD et al, Carcinogenic effects of monofunctional and bifunctional furocoumarins, In: MA Pathak, JK Dunnick, (eds). *Photobiologic, Tociologic, and Pharmacologic Aspects of Psoralens*, NCI Monograph No. 66, National Cancer Institute, Bethesda, Maryland 1984, pp. 205–10.
24 Stern RS, Lang R, Nonmelanoma skin cancer occurring in patients treated with PUVA five to ten years after first treatment, *J Invest Dermatol* (1988) **91**: 120–4.
25 Stern RS, Members of the Photochemotherapy Follow-up Study, Genital tumors among men with psoriasis exposed to psoralens and ultraviolet A radiation (PUVA) and ultraviolet B radiation, *N Engl J Med* (1990) **322**: 1093–7.

52
Skin tumour promotion and the wound response: two sides of a coin

Friedrich Marks, Gerhard Fürstenberger and Michael Gschwendt
German Cancer Research Center, Institute of Biochemistry, D-6900 Heidelberg, Germany

Percivall Pott's famous work on skin cancer of chimney sweeps published in 1775 provided the first attempt to correlate a malignant skin disease with an environmental threat, i.e. the occupational contact with soot and tar. Moreover, the experimental induction of cancer by an environmental chemical agent (coal-tar) was shown for the first time using rabbit skin as a target tissue (Yamagiwa and Ichikawa, 1914). Later, it was found that skin carcinogenesis in experimental animals could result from a synergistic interaction of factors with different toxicological qualities (for a review of these historical aspects see Marks[1]). While the investigation of such factors, called initiators and promoters of carcinogenesis, has considerably increased our knowledge of the biological nature of tumour development, the threat exerted by them on human skin is still a matter of dispute.

Multistage carcinogenesis in animal skin

The multistage model of mouse skin carcinogenesis consists of a series of manipulations, i.e. initiation, conversion, promotion and malignant progression, which induce a sequence of events proceeding via hyperplastic and papilloma states to squamous carcinomas (see Figure 1; for reviews see Marks[1,2]).

Initiation, as brought about by any kind of carcinogen, results in a latent but irreversible neoplastic state, which is most probably due to irreversible genetic alterations such as point mutations of the Harvey-ras protooncogene.[3] Such alterations seem to be sufficient for a transformation into the papilloma state, whereas for malignant progression additional genetic effects appear to be necessary perhaps in analogy to the Vogelstein model of colorectal cancer.[4] In the mouse skin model malignant progression occurs spontaneously at a rate of 5–10%, most probably in a population of autonomous papillomas, but can also be enhanced by an additional carcinogen treatment.[5]

In contrast to initiation and malignant progressions, the stages of conversion and promotion are probably based on non-mutagenic mechanisms. The promotion of papilloma development from initiated epidermal cells requires an induction of sustained epidermal hyperplasia which can be brought about by chronic application of tumour promoting agents such as the phorbol esters and others.[6] In fact, all tumour promoters are also strong skin mitogens inducing hyperplastic transformation, i.e. a complex pattern of epidermal hyperplasia and inflammation.[7] However, because permanent stimulation of epidermal cell proliferation provides only a necessary but not a sufficient condition for tumour development, an additional stage (conversion) had to be introduced.[8] One distinguishes now between two classes of skin tumour promoters, i.e. converting ('complete') promoters, such as the phorbol ester 12-0-tetradecanoylphorbol-13-acetate (TPA), and non-converting ('incomplete') promoters such as the TPA derivatives retinoyl phorbol acetate (RPA) and $C_{14:4}PA$ (Ti8) or the plant poison mezerein (Figure 2). Both classes share the property of being highly hyperplasiogenic skin irritants. Since a short pretreatment with a converting tumour promoter, either prior to or after initiation, renders mouse skin susceptible to the papilloma-inducing effect of chronic mitogenic stimulation (as induced by a

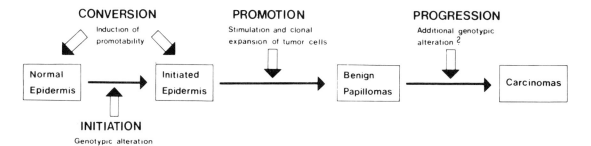

Figure 1

Schematic outline of the multistage approach to mouse skin carcinogenesis. Conversion, as defined as induction of promotability, can be induced within a certain time period either prior to or after initiation, indicating that it is not a component or 'stage' of tumour promotion proper. For other details see text. From Marks.[2]

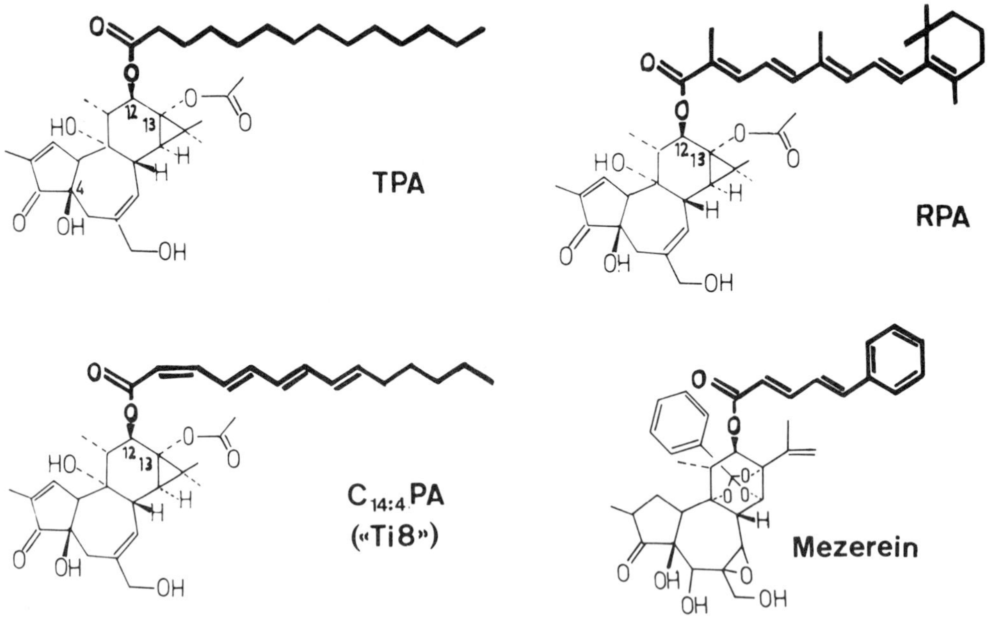

Figure 2

'Complete' and 'incomplete' tumour promoters. While the phorbol ester TPA is a converting (complete) tumour promoter, its unsaturated derivatives Ti8 and RPA (retinoyl phorbol acetate) are non-converting (incomplete) promoters in NMRI mouse skin, whereas mezerein exhibits incomplete promoting efficacy in SENCAR mouse skin.

non-converting promoter) conversion may be operationally defined as the induction of promotability.[8]

The mechanistic background of conversion is still unclear. Both an activation of initiated cells (whatever this means) and a stimulatory effect on stroma formation have been discussed.[8] The stroma hypothesis is based on a close relationship between conversion and tissue damage: (i) mechanical skin wounding provides a strong converting (and promoting!) stimulus;[8] (ii) conversion seems to be correlated with the induction of severe chromosomal damage in epidermis, which may be interpreted as a symptom of cell destruction resembling wounding;[8] and (iii) the 'wound hormones' TGFα and TGFβ exert a converting effect upon combined injection into initiated mouse skin[9] — in particular TGFβ has been shown to play a critical role in stroma formation.[10]

Exotic and abundant skin tumour promoters

Most skin tumour promoters used for experimental purposes are exotic compounds of rather remote origin (Figure 3; for a review see Fujiki et al[11]). Thus, they may not exert a significant environmental threat to the skin. On the other hand, agents which are in dermatological or cosmetic use such as anthralin and benzoylperoxide have been shown to possess tumour promoting efficacy in mouse skin.[12]

Finally, there are two abundant skin tumour-promoting agencies: ultraviolet radiation (UVR)[13] and mechanical wounding.[14] Both agencies exert a complete (converting) promoting stimulus. The tumour-promoting effect of UVR (especially of UVA[13]) and of wounding clearly demonstrates the critical role of endogenous factors in skin tumour development. These may be looked for among the large group of 'wound hormones' consisting of pro-inflammatory mediators, cytokines, growth factors, etc., which are released upon tissue damage (Figure 4).[14–17] As mentioned above, two of these hormones, i.e. TGFα and TGFβ, have indeed been found to exert converting efficacy in initiated mouse skin.[9] Moreover, locally released eicosanoids are essential mediators of both conversion and promotion (see below). Of course, a putative role for other 'wound hormones' in skin carcinogenesis still remains to be tested.

What then, are the relationships between such different tumour promoters as exotic poisons, sunlight and the scalpel? We postulate that the common denominator consists in their ability to evoke a wound response in skin.[14] A promoting agent may do this directly by damaging cell and tissue structures or indirectly by interacting with the signal-transducing pathways of wound hormones, thereby mimicking the effect of those factors. Benzoylperoxide and thapsigargin[18] may provide examples of directly acting promoters. Since the wound response seems to be controlled by a complex network of interactions consisting of paracrine and autocrine loops, a single stimulatory input at a critical point may well be sufficient to set in action the whole apparatus of wound healing (see Figure 8). A prominent example of such a mechanism seems to be provided by TPA-type tumour promoters which mimic the effect of the second messenger diacylglycerol in activating the enzymes of the protein kinase C (PKC) family. Actually, there is no other point of attack beside PKC known for these promoters, although the biological response they evoke largely resembles the wound response in all its complexity.

A key role for protein kinase C and eicosanoids

Protein kinase C is a component of signal-transducing pathways which are controlled by a wide variety of extracellular signals via second messengers such as diacylglycerol and probably arachidonic acid. PKC provides a family of at least seven closely related species, the expression of which depends on the tissue and the state of development.[19] The PKC enzymes can be grouped into two subfamilies depending on whether their activation requires Ca^{2+} ions (PKC of the α, β or γ type) or not (PKC of the δ, ε and ζ type). Epidermis has been shown to contain Ca^{2+} dependent αPKC and βPKC.[20] Recently, we have found that a Ca^{2+} insensitive δ-type PKC is the most abundant isoform in epidermis of both animal and human origin.[21,22] While αPKC and βPKC are cytosolic enzymes which upon activation are translocated to the inner side of the plasma membrane, δPKC is exclusively found in the particulate fraction probably being firmly associated with membranes and perhaps the cell nucleus (Figure 5).

Whilst the precise physiological roles of the different PKC isoforms in epidermis are far from understood, the fact that an over-stimulation of PKC by TPA-type tumour promoters gives rise to a complex and long-lasting response largely resembling the wound response indicates a key role

Anthralin, Dibenzoylperoxide, ICH₂–COOH Iodoacetic acid, TPA, Lyngbyatoxin A, Teleocidin B, Aplysiatoxin

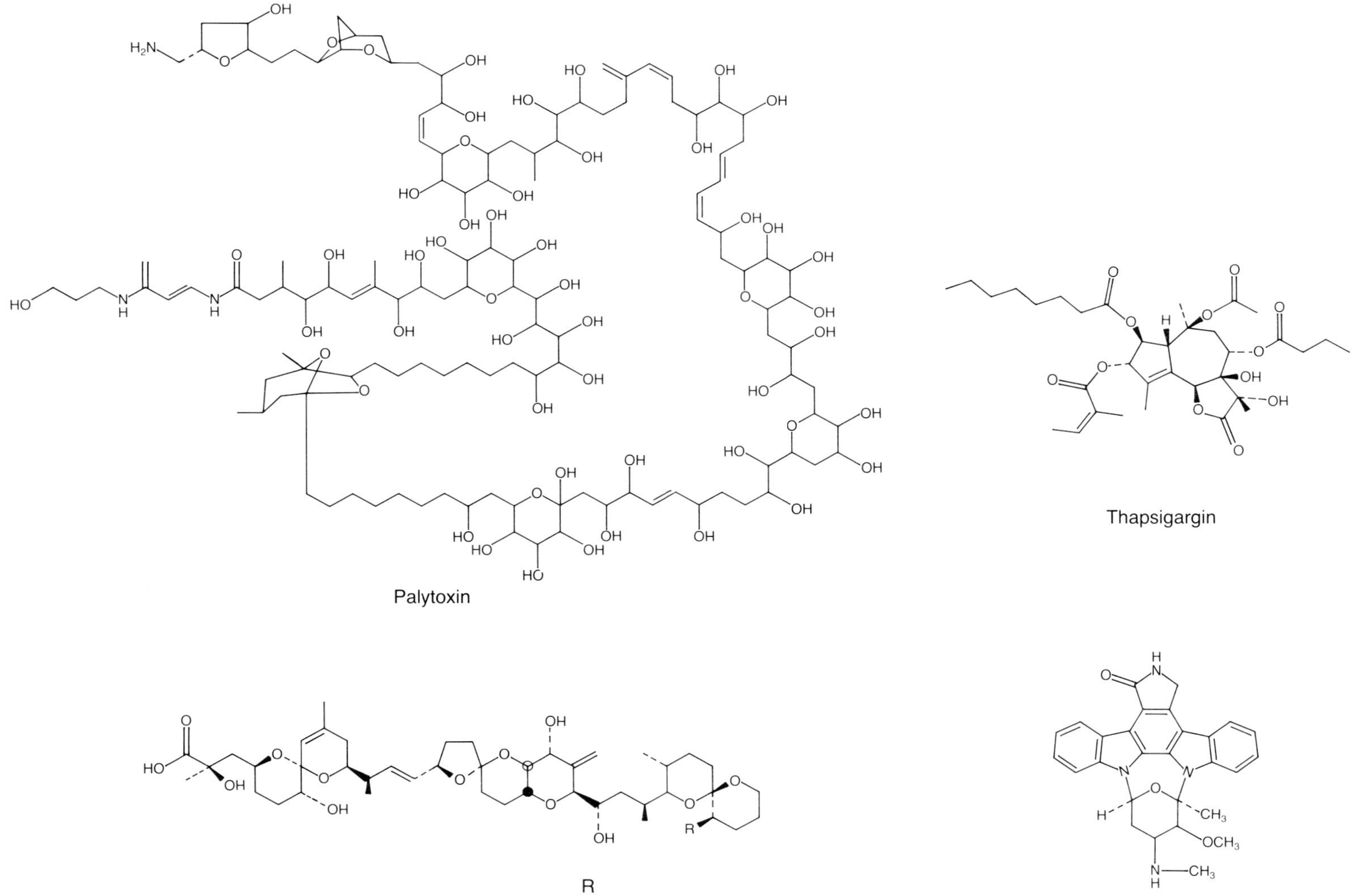

Palytoxin

Thapsigargin

	R
Okadaic acid	H
Dinophysistoxin – 1	CH_3

Staurosporine

Figure 3

Tumour-promoting agents used in experimental skin carcinogenesis. For details on the origin, isolation and properties of the compounds see Fujiki et al.[11]

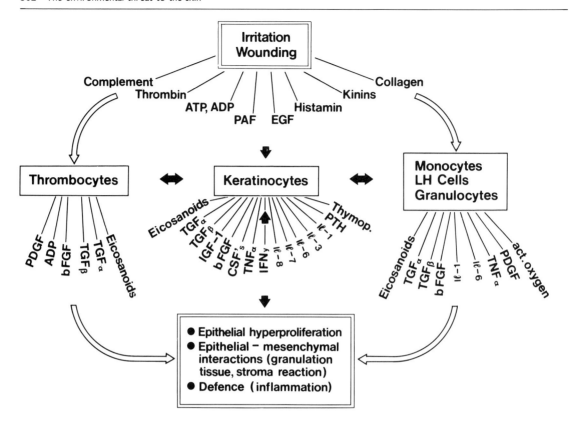

Figure 4

The 'wound hormone cascade' in skin. As shown, a series of primary wound factors released upon tissue damage or irritation stimulate cells involved in the early phases of the wound response to release a 'cocktail' of growth factors, cytokines, proinflammatory mediators, etc. These factors are thought to form a complex network of juxtacrine, autocrine and paracrine loops thus controlling the wound response which consists of epidermal hyperproliferation, formation of granulation tissue and activation of the immune system. The scheme is certainly far from being complete.

for these enzymes in tissue repair and defense reactions. It has indeed been proposed that PKC is involved in the control of certain genes such as c-fos, c-myc, ODC, TGFβ, etc., as well as of the eicosanoid cascade all of which have been found to be activated by TPA treatment. As shown by means of specific inhibitors, the eicosanoids released by both the cyclo-oxygenase and the lipoxygenase pathways have a crucial mediator function in the hyperplastic and inflammatory response as well as in conversion and tumour promotion (Figure 6, for a review see Fürstenberger and Marks[23]). Thus, the triggering of 'quiescent' (undisturbed) mouse epidermis into the hyperproliferative state depends on an early release of prostaglandin E_2 while tumour promotion by repeated hyperproliferative stimulation is crucially dependent on prostaglandin $F_{2\alpha}$ synthesis in epidermis. Conversion and the inflammatory response seem to be mediated by eicosanoids generated by the lipoxygenase pathways. The most dramatic effect on eicosanoid metabolism seen upon phorbol ester treatment of mouse skin is a strong de novo induction of the enzyme 8-lipoxygenase, which is almost undetectable in untreated skin.[24] The arachidonic acid metabolites generated by this pathway, i.e. 8-hydroperoxy-eicosatetraenoic acid (HPETE) and 8-hydroxy-eicosatetraenoic acid (HETE), but also

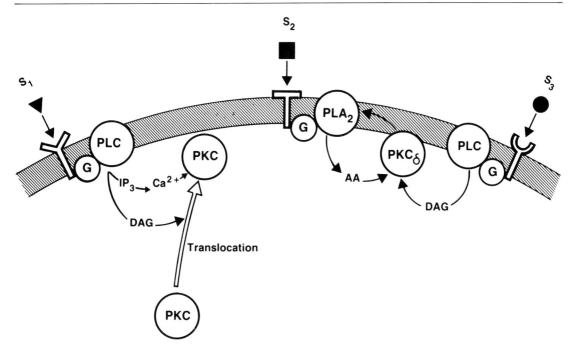

Figure 5

Putative role of different PKC species in intracellular signal transduction. (Left) The Ca^{2+} responsive PKC isoforms of the α, β and γ type are thought to be activated by the inositol-1,4,5-trisphosphate/1,2-diacylglycerol (IP_3/DAG) cascade. The two second messengers IP_3 and DAG are released from phosphatidylinositol bisphosphate by aspecific phospholipase C (PLC), which is activated by an external signal (S_1) via a receptor-controlled G protein. These cytoplasmic PKC isoforms are translocated to the inner side of the plasma membrane upon activation. (Right) A membrane-bound Ca^{2+} unresponsive PKC isoform of the δ type could be activated by DAG alone being released by a receptor–G protein controlled 'unspecific' phospholipase (PLC) upon stimulation by an external signal (S_3). Alternatively, δPKC might be activated by arachidonic acid (AA) which is released by phospholipase A_2 (PLA_2) stimulated by an external signal (S_2) via a receptor-controlled G protein. Conversely, δPKC may activate phospholipase A_2 thus generating a positive feedback loop. Due to its location in the membrane, δPKC may be assumed to interact particularly easily with other membrane proteins. 'Complete' and 'incomplete' tumour promoters of the phorbol ester type mimic the stimulatory effect of DAG in either case.

12-HETE produced by a constitutive epidermal 12-lipoxygenase, exert a clastogenic effect in keratinocytes and may, therefore, be considered as mediators of the chromosome-damaging effect of converting tumour promoters (see above). On the other hand, 8-lipoxygenase is also induced by a non-converting tumour promoter such as the phorbol ester RPA. It may be speculated that an incomplete tumour promoter stands in its own light by quenching the active clastogenic arachidonic acid metabolites perhaps due to an interaction with its unsaturated fatty acid side-chain. Eicosanoids may be also involved in the biological effects of several 'wound hormones' such as TGFα, bradykinin, TNFα, interleukin 1 and others which all have been shown to induce the eicosanoid cascade.

Eicosanoid formation is controlled by the availability of free arachidonic acid which is, for example, released from phospholipids by the enzyme phospholipase A_2 (PLA_2) upon cellular stimulation. PLA_2 occupies a central point in cellular regulation where several stimulatory pathways come together (Figure 7). There is evidence that this enzyme can be activated by phosphorylation catalysed either by a receptor–tyrosin kinase (such as the TGFα/EGF-receptor) or by protein kinase C.[25,26] Additional activating pathways involve an increase of cytoplasmic Ca^{2+} (as, for example, induced by the ionophore A23187 or the tumour promoter thapsigargin) or by a receptor-coupled G-protein as in the case of bradykinin.[26] While the essential involvement of eicosanoids in hyperplastic

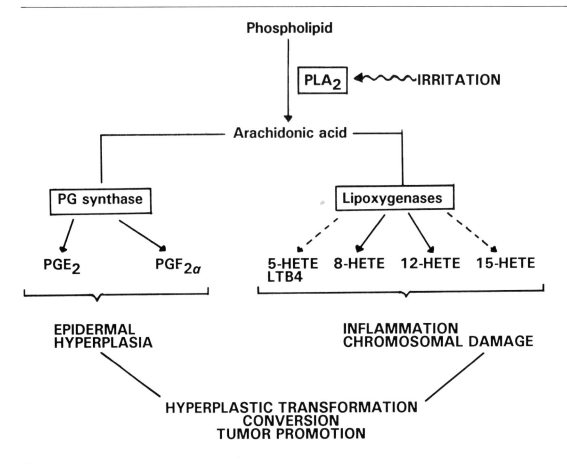

Figure 6

Putative physiological role of eicosanoids in the wound response and in tumour development in mouse skin upon irritation or injury. The prostaglandins E_2 and $F_{2\alpha}$ are essential mediators of the acute and chronic hyperplastic response of epidermis and of tumour promotion. Lipoxygenase derived arachidonic acid metabolites such as 8- and 12-HETE appear to be involved in the inflammatory response and in clastogenesis and conversion. In mouse epidermis 12-lipoxygenase activity is expressed constitutively, whereas 8-lipoxygenase activity is strongly induced only upon phorbol ester treatment. The 5- and 15-lipoxygenase activities are very low.

transformation and tumour promotion of skin has become evident,[7,23] the pathophysiological role as well as the precise mechanism of action of these factors in skin are not yet understood. Progress in this field will greatly improve our understanding of hyperplastic diseases, wound healing and tumour development.

While TPA-type tumour promoters seem to activate the eicosanoid cascade by PKC-mediated stimulation of phospholipase A_2 (as well as by induction of certain enzymes such as 8-lipoxygenase), tumour-promoting 'agents' such as wounding and UVR certainly open alternative pathways for the activation of both PKC and phospholipase A_2. As mentioned above, several 'wound hormones' which are released upon wounding or irradiation, do stimulate the eicosanoid cascade and PKC seems to be involved in intracellular signal transduction for many of these endogenous factors. As shown recently, UVR activates PKC and the arachidonic acid metabolism in skin as does the phorbol ester TPA.[13] This finding gave rise to the concept of UVB being an initiator and UVA a promoter of skin carcinogenesis.[13]

The putative relationship between the wound response and skin tumour promotion is summarized in Figure 8, emphasizing in particular the proposed key role of phospholipase A_2 and PKC.

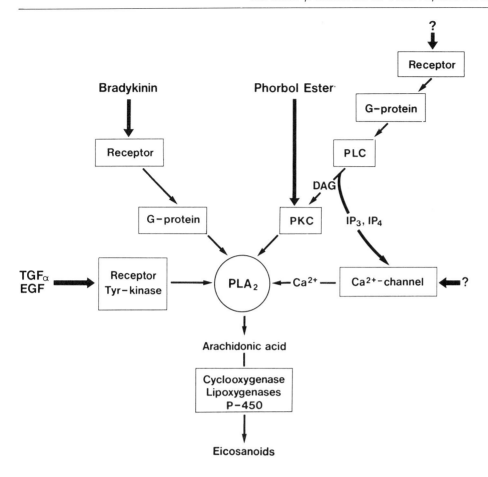

Figure 7

Multiple stimulation of phospholipase A_2 catalysed arachidonic acid release in mouse epidermis (for details see text). The multiplicity of stimulatory pathways easily explains the finding that arachidonic acid release and eicosanoid formation provide a general response to all kinds of irritating stimuli (TGFα, bradykinin, other 'wound hormones', phorbol ester, ionophore A23187, Ca^{2+} inducing thapsigargin, UVR, mechanical wounding, etc.). It is not clear whether receptor-tyr-kinases and PKC activate PLA_2 directly by phosphorylation or via additional enzymatic steps.

Conclusion

The rapid improvement in experimental technology has enabled us to dissect the complex pattern of tumour development in animal skin step by step. The picture which is emerging shows a very close relationship to the wound response. It appears as if Orth's classical statement of cancer being the result of 'immer wiederholter und gestörter Regeneration' (permanently repeated and disturbed tissue regeneration[27]) is not far from the truth. Any agent or manipulation which is able to evoke such a response must be considered a potential threat especially if, like UVR, it exhibits additional mutagenic potency, i.e. acts both as a tumour initiator and a complete tumour promoter in skin. An urgent need exists, therefore, for a reliable toxicological assay system for environmental tumour promoters possibly exerting a threat to human skin (and other organs). However, considering the extreme species variability in the skin's responsiveness to tumour promoting influences,[28] the animal models which are still employed for this purpose are not expected to fulfil this requirement.

Instead, an in vitro system based on our steadily increasing knowledge of molecular parameters may be more suitable. Such an in vitro test has yet to be introduced.

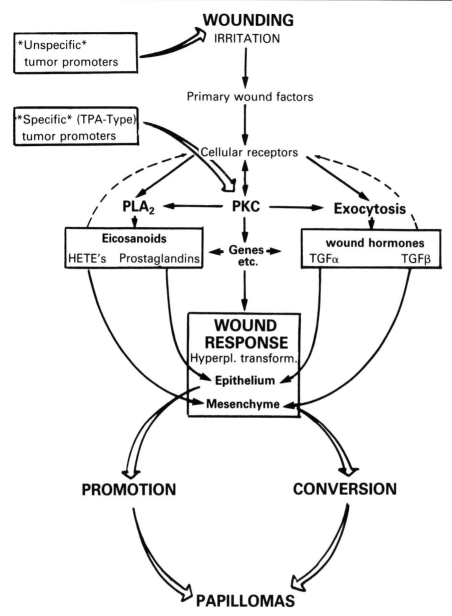

Figure 8

A speculative scheme illustrating the putative relationship between tumour promotion and the wound response. It is assumed that the interaction with cellular receptors of primary wound factors released upon tissue damage (see Figure 4) results in a series of molecular events. These include an activation of phospholipase A_2 (PLA_2) and subsequent eicosanoid formation (left) and of exocytotic processes resulting in a release of 'wound hormones' (such as TGFα, TGFβ and others, see Figure 4). Both eicosanoids and 'wound hormones' control the interaction of those cell types which are involved in wound healing thus giving rise to the wound response. Upon initiation, tumour development may be promoted in the course of this response via both epidermal hyperproliferation (promotion, probably controlled among others by prostaglandins and TGFα-type growth factors) and stroma function (conversion, probably controlled among others by HETEs and TGFβ). 'Unspecific' skin tumour promoters (wounding, UVR, organic peroxides, thapsigargin, etc.) are thought to induce the wound response by tissue damage, whereas 'specific' tumour promoters (phorbol ester type) may interact with components of intracellular signal transduction such as protein kinase C (PKC). PKC may occupy a central position in the response in that it not only transduces signals of wound hormones but may activate PLA_2, wound hormone release, de novo expression of eicosanoid forming enzymes (8-lipoxygenase!) and growth factors via effects on the corresponding genes and other molecular processes. By this a series of autocrine and paracrine feedback loops may develop which guarantee a rapid response of the damaged tissue.

References

1. Marks F, Skin cancer (excluding melanomas). In: Greaves MW, Schuster S, (eds). *Handbook of experimental pharmacology*, vol 87/II, *Pharmacology of the skin*, Springer: Berlin, 1989, p165.
2. Marks F, Fürstenberger G, From the normal cell to cancer: the multistep process of skin carcinogenesis. In: Maskens AP, Ebbesen P, Burny A, (eds). *Concepts and theories in carcinogenesis*, Excerpta Medica: Amsterdam, 1987, p169.
3. Balmain A, Brown L, Oncogene activation in chemical carcinogenesis, *Adv Cancer Res* (1988) **51**: 147–83.
4. Fearon ER, Vogelstein B, A genetic model for colorectal tumorigenesis, *Cell* (1990) **61**: 759–67.
5. Hennings H, Shores R, Wenk ML et al, Malignant conversion of mouse skin tumors is increased by tumor initiators and unaffected by tumor promoters, *Nature* (1983) **304**: 67–9.
6. Siskin EE, Gray T, Barrett JC, Correlation between sensitivity to tumor promotion and sustained epidermal hyperplasia of mice and rats treated with TPA, *Carcinogenesis* (1982) **3**: 403–8.
7. Marks F, Hyperplastic transformation: the response of the skin to irritation and injury. In: Galli CL, Hensby CN, Marinovich M, (eds). *Skin pharmacology and toxicology*, Plenum: New York, 1990, p121.
8. Marks F, Fürstenberger G, The conversion stage of skin carcinogenesis (commentary), *Carcinogenesis* (1990) **11**: 2085–92.
9. Fürstenberger G, Rogers M, Schnapke R et al, Stimulatory role of transforming growth factors in multistage skin carcinogenesis: possible explanation for the tumor-inducing effect of wounding in initiated NMRI-mouse skin, *Int J Cancer* (1989) **43**: 915–21.
10. *Ciba Foundation Symposium 157: Clinical applications of TGF-β*, Wiley: Chichester, 1991.
11. Fujiki H, Suganuma M, Significance of new environmental tumor promoters, *J Environ Hlth Sci (Environ Carcinogen Rev)* (1989) **C7(1)**: 1–51.
12. Fischer SM, Reiners JJ, Pence BC et al, Mechanisms of carcinogenesis using mouse skin: the multistage assay revisited. In: Langenbach R, Elmore E, Barrett JC, (eds). *Tumor promoters: biological approaches for mechanistic studies and assay systems*, Raven Press: New York, 1988, p11.
13. Matsui MS, Deleo VA, Longwave ultraviolet radiation and promotion of skin cancer, *Cancer Cells* (1991) **3**: 8–12.
14. Marks F, Neoplasia and the wound response: the lesson learned from the multistage approach of skin carcinogenesis. In: Paukovits WR, (ed). *Growth regulation and carcinogenesis*, vol 1. CRC Press: Boca Raton, FL, 1991, p53.
15. Kupper TS, Mechanisms of cutaneous inflammation, *Arch Dermatol* (1989) **125**: 1406–12.
16. Luger TA, Schwarz Th, Evidence for an epidermal cytokine network, *J Invest Dermatol* (1990) **95**: 100S–4S.
17. McKenzie RC, Sauder DN, The role of keratinocyte cytokines in inflammation and immunity, *J Invest Dermatol* (1990) **95**: 105S–7S.
18. Marks F, Hanke B, Thastrup O et al, Stimulatory effect of thapsigargin, a non-TPA-type promoter on arachidonic acid metabolism in the murine keratinocyte line HEL30 and on epidermal cell proliferation in vivo as compared to the effect of phorbol ester TPA, *Carcinogenesis* (1991) **12**: 1491–7.
19. Nishizuka Y, The molecular heterogeneity of protein kinase C and its implications for cellular regulation, *Nature* (1988) **334**: 661–5.
20. Fisher GJ, Tavakkol A, Griffiths CEM et al, Differential expression of protein kinase C isoenzymes in psoriatic lesions versus normal epidermis, *J Invest Dermatol* (1990) **94**: 524 (abstract).
21. Leibersperger H, Gschwendt M, Marks F, Purification and characterization of a calcium-unresponsive, phorbol ester/phospholipid-activated protein kinase from porcine spleen, *J Biol Chem* (1990) **265**: 16108–15.
22. Leibersperger H, Gschwendt M, Gernold M et al, Immunological demonstration of a calcium-unresponsive protein kinase C of the delta-type in different species and murine tissues. Predominance in epidermis, *J Biol Chem* (1991) **266**: 14278–84.
23. Fürstenberger G, Marks F, The role of eicosanoids in normal, hyperplastic, and neoplastic growth in mouse skin. In: Ruzicka Th, (ed.). *Eicosanoids and the skin*. CRC Press: Boca Raton, FL, 1990, p108.
24. Fürstenberger G, Hagedorn H, Jacobi T et al, Characterization of a novel 8-lipoxygenase activity induced by the phorbol ester tumor promoter TPA in mouse skin in vivo, *J Biol Chem* (1991) **266**: 15738–45.
25. Lin LL, Lin AY, Knopf JL, PDGF and EGF induce both the release of arachidonic acid and the phosphorylation of cPLA$_2$, *J Cell Biochem* (1991) 160 (abstract).
26. Kast R, Fürstenberger G, Marks F, Activation of keratinocyte phospholipase A$_2$ by bradykinin and phorbol ester TPA. Evidence for a receptor-G protein versus PKC-mediated mechanism, *Eur J Biochem* (1991) (in press).
27. Orth J, Präcarcinomatöse Krankheiten und künstliche Krebse, *Z Krebsforsch* (Precancerous diseases and artificial cancer) (1911) **10**: 42.
28. Fürstenberger G, Marks F, Mehrstufenmodelle zum Nachweis von tumorpromovierenden Substanzen: das In-Vivo-System Haut (Multistage models for the assay of tumour promoting substances: the skin in vivo system). In: Schlatterer B, (ed). *Chemische Krebsrisikofaktoren und Umwelt*. Veröffentlichungen des Fortbildungszentrums für Gesundheits- und Umweltschutz (Chemical carcinogenic risk factors and the environment), E Schmidt-Verlag: Berlin, 1991, p267.

53
The role of protein kinase C in epidermal differentiation and neoplasia

Andrzej A. Dlugosz, James E. Strickland, George R. Pettit* and Stuart H. Yuspa

*Laboratory of Cellular Carcinogenesis and Tumor Promotion, National Cancer Institute, Bethesda, MD 20892, USA, and *Arizona State University, Tempe, AZ 85287, USA*

Introduction

The epidermis provides a vital barrier separating host from environment. This specialized function is the result of a tightly regulated program of keratinocyte differentiation which begins in the first suprabasal layer of the epidermis. The movement of keratinocytes towards the surface of the skin is associated with the sequential induction of various proteins not expressed in basal cells. Keratins 1 and 10 (K1 and K10) are detected in the first suprabasal layer and higher, while filaggrin and loricrin are not expressed until cells are in the granular layer.[1,2] During the final stages of keratinocyte differentiation, activation of epidermal transglutaminase results in covalent cross-linking of various proteins into a rigid, detergent-insoluble cornified envelope characteristic of mature squames.[3] Although the mechanisms controlling keratinocyte differentiation have not been fully defined, extracellular Ca^{2+}, retinoids, and phorbol esters are potent modulators of this process.

Keratinocytes derived from newborn mouse skin provide a useful model for studying terminal differentiation in vitro. Cells cultured in medium with a reduced Ca^{2+} concentration (0.05 mM) exhibit a basal-cell-like morphology and do not express markers of terminal differentiation. Growth in medium with 0.12 mM Ca^{2+} for 24–48 h results in the sequential induction of K1, K10, loricrin, and filaggrin, as well as the activation of epidermal transglutaminase and formation of cornified envelopes.[4] These changes parallel those occurring as keratinocytes differentiate within the epidermis.

Protein kinase C (PKC) is an ubiquitous family of enzymes involved in various aspects of cell growth, differentiation, and neoplastic transformation.[5] Physiological activation of PKC occurs in response to a variety of extracellular stimuli, including hormones and growth factors. Ligand–receptor interaction results in activation of phospholipase C, which cleaves membrane phospholipids to the short-lived second messengers diacylglycerol and inositol trisphosphate. Inositol trisphosphate releases Ca^{2+} from intracellular stores, while diacylglycerol binds and activates PKC. PKC can be activated directly by phorbol ester tumor promoters such as 12-O-tetradecanoylphorbol-13-acetate (TPA), which bind to the same site as diacylglycerol.[6] Ultraviolet radiation (UVR), which is causally associated with the majority of human skin cancers, has also been reported to modulate PKC activity and to induce several biological responses in common with TPA.[7] Pharmacological activation of some PKC isoforms is associated with translocation from the cytoplasm to the particulate compartment followed by down-regulation. At the present time, seven genes encoding eight PKC isoforms have been described in mammalian cells: PKC α, β_I, β_{II}, γ, δ, ϵ, ζ, and η (PKC L in human cells).[5,8,9]

Several observations suggest that PKC is involved in keratinocyte differentiation. (1) The PKC activator TPA is a potent inducer of cornification in both mouse and human keratinocytes in vitro and mouse skin in vivo.[10,11] (2) A similar response occurs in cells exposed to exogenous phospholipase C, presumably as a result of increased production of the endogenous PKC activator diacylglycerol.[12] (3) A second set of phorbol ester binding sites appears during Ca^{2+} mediated keratinocyte differentiation, suggesting either an alteration of PKC or induction of a new species.[13] (4) Calcium (Ca^{2+}) mediated keratinocyte differentiation is associated with increased levels of diacylglycerol and inositol trisphosphates,[14–16] as well as an alteration in the subcellular distribution of PKC.[17] (5) Differentiation of keratinocytes in response to another stimulus, vitamin D_3, is associated with translocation of PKC from the cytosol to the particulate fraction, consistent with enzyme activation.[18] (6) Neoplastic keratinocytes lose the ability to differentiate in response to either Ca^{2+} or TPA,[19] which is consistent with the hypothesis that both inducers function through the PKC signal transduction pathway.

Ca^{2+}-mediated keratinocyte differentiation is blocked in cells depleted of PKC

To explore further the role of PKC in keratinocyte differentiation, we assessed the ability of cells deficient in PKC to respond to 0.12 mM Ca^{2+} medium. PKC was depleted by exposure of cultured keratinocytes to 60 nM bryostatin for 24 h. This treatment results in the rapid loss of immunoreactive PKCα and is associated with a block of PKC function based on the inability to elicit typical responses to TPA. Exposure of control cultures to 0.12 mM Ca^{2+} medium for 48 h results in induction of the differentiation markers K1, K10, loricrin, and filaggrin, based on immunoblot analysis. In contrast, in cells where PKC has been depleted by bryostatin pretreatment, induction of these markers in 0.12 mM Ca^{2+} medium does not occur or is markedly suppressed.[20] The block in marker expression is also detectable at the level of steady-state mRNA based on dot blot analysis using ^{32}P labelled probes identifying K1 and filaggrin transcripts. These findings suggest that PKC is necessary for induction of keratinocyte terminal differentiation by elevated extracellular Ca^{2+}. In vivo, TPA has been shown to cause prolonged down-regulation of PKC after the initial activation phase. TPA treatment of mouse skin rapidly reduced K1 mRNA levels,[21] suggesting that PKC is an important regulator of keratinocyte differentiation in vivo as well as in vitro.

Staurosporine induces terminal differentiation of normal and neoplastic mouse keratinocytes in vitro

The use of enzyme inhibitors provides another approach to studying the potential role of PKC in keratinocyte differentiation. Staurosporine is a potent inhibitor of PKC in in vitro assays using partially purified enzyme.[22] However, staurosporine was also found to inhibit several other classes of kinases at doses similar to those needed for PKC inhibition. Staurosporine blocks TPA-mediated responses in several cell types; however, in cultures of primary mouse keratinocytes, staurosporine not only fails to block TPA-mediated keratinocyte maturation,[23] but, paradoxically, also induces similar responses.[24] Exposure of primary mouse keratinocytes to staurosporine or TPA results in a 4- to 5-fold induction of epidermal transglutaminase activity and cornified envelopes, two markers of terminal differentiation. Because of the ability of staurosporine to induce cornification of primary keratinocytes, we examined its effects on two neoplastic keratinocyte cell lines: 308 and SP-1. Both cell lines contain an activating mutation of the c-ras^{Ha} gene, are resistant to the differentiating effects of Ca^{2+} or TPA in vitro, and produce papillomas when grafted onto the backs of nude mice.[25] Surprisingly, staurosporine is a potent inducer of maturation in both of these cell lines in vitro.[24] Exposure of SP-1 or 308 cells to staurosporine results in a 10-fold and 60-fold increase, respectively, in the number of cornified cells; epidermal transglutaminase assayed in SP-1 cells was also induced by staurosporine in a dose-dependent manner. In contrast, neither of these differentiation markers was induced by TPA.

Staurosporine inhibits tumor growth in vivo

The unique ability of staurosporine to induce terminal differentiation of neoplastic keratinocytes in vitro suggested that it may have similar effects in vivo. To address this question, tumors were produced by grafting 308 or SP-1 cells onto the backs of immune-deficient mice. Staurosporine or acetone was applied to the graft sites twice weekly beginning on the second week after grafting, and tumor volumes were determined weekly. Staurosporine markedly suppressed growth of tumors derived from either cell line in a dose-dependent manner.[26]

Staurosporine induces PKC agonist effects in cultured primary mouse keratinocytes

Because of the remarkable ability of staurosporine to restore the differentiated phenotype in neoplastic keratinocytes, we initiated a series of experiments to explore this drug's mechanism of action. Since many of the responses we observed in primary keratinocytes mimic those seen after TPA exposure, we evaluated the ability of staurosporine to act, paradoxically, as a functional PKC agonist in this cell type. Several responses characteristic of PKC activators were examined in primary keratinocytes exposed to staurosporine.[24] Like TPA, staurosporine causes a dose-dependent induction of ornithine decarboxylase activity. For this response, and several others, staurosporine exhibits a biphasic dose–response curve with a restricted effective dose range. These findings are consistent with the hypothesis that staurosporine selectively affects one of multiple targets within the cell. Both staurosporine and TPA also inhibit [^{125}I]EGF binding in a dose-dependent manner. In cells that were pretreated with bryostatin to down-regulate PKC, the effect on EGF binding is completely blocked in response to TPA, and partially blocked in response to staurosporine. These data indicate that PKC is involved in this response to both agents. Results of a similar experiment assessing the formation of cornified envelopes in bryostatin pretreated cells indicates that PKC is also involved in this response to staurosporine or TPA.

As an additional marker of PKC activation, expression of c-*fos* mRNA was examined by means of Northern blot hybridization. In primary keratinocytes, TPA is a potent inducer of *fos* transcripts which are detected within 30 min of exposure and remain elevated for at least 8 h. Staurosporine also induces *fos*, although to a lesser degree than TPA. In cultures exposed to both agents, higher levels of *fos* transcripts are detected than with either TPA or staurosporine alone. As with the other data presented thus far, these findings indicate that staurosporine induces PKC agonist effects in cultures of primary mouse keratinocytes. To study the ability of staurosporine to influence kinase activity directly, protein phosphorylation was studied in primary keratinocytes permeabilized with digitonin. Cells were incubated with [^{32}P]ATP, proteins from total cell lysates separated by polyacrylamide gel electrophoresis, and labeled phosphoproteins identified by autoradiography. In preliminary experiments, TPA enhanced the phosphorylation of a protein migrating at approximately 40 kDa. In contrast, staurosporine did not induce phosphorylation of this protein and blocked TPA-mediated phosphorylation, consistent with its reported activity as a PKC inhibitor. These results suggest that staurosporine behaves primarily as a functional PKC agonist in intact primary keratinocyte, but also possesses PKC inhibitory activity.

The biochemical basis for staurosporine's divergent effects on responses attributed to PKC activation may be the result of selective interaction with different targets within the cell, perhaps PKC isozymes. We have recently demonstrated expression of mRNA encoding PKC α, δ, ϵ, ζ, and η, but not PKC β or γ, in cultured primary mouse keratinocytes, making this a tenable hypothesis (A. A. Dlugosz, H. Mischak, F. Mushinski and S. H. Yuspa, unpublished observations).[27] An alternative explanation is that staurosporine functions primarily as a PKC agonist by selectively inhibiting another kinase which is normally a negative regulator of PKC activity. Indirect effects on PKC may be the result of staurosporine-mediated changes in the level of diacylglycerol or other endogenous modulators of PKC activity.

The remarkable ability of staurosporine to induce cornification of neoplastic keratinocytes in vitro, and suppress tumor growth in vivo, suggests that modulation of PKC may provide a novel approach for the treatment of epithelial neoplasms via the induction of terminal differentiation.

References

1. Roop DR, Nakazawa H, Mehrel T et al, Sequential changes in gene expression during epidermal differentiation. In: Rogers GE, Reis PJ, Ward KA et al, (eds). *The biology of wool and hair*, Chapman and Hall: London, 1988, pp311–24.
2. Fuchs E, Epidermal differentiation: the bare essentials, *J Cell Biol* (1990) 111: 2807–14.
3. Goldsmith LA, The epidermal cell periphery. In: Goldsmith LA, (ed.). *Biochemistry and physiology of the skin*, Oxford University Press: Oxford, 1983, pp184–96.
4. Yuspa SH, Kilkenny AE, Steinert PM et al, Expression of murine epidermal differentiation markers is tightly regu-

lated by restricted extracellular calcium concentrations in vitro, *J Cell Biol* (1989) **109**: 1207–17.
5. Nishizuka Y, The family of protein kinase C for signal transduction, *J Am Med Assoc* (1989) **262**: 1826–33.
6. Sharkey NA, Leach KL, Blumberg PM, Competitive inhibition by diacylglycerol of specific phorbol ester binding, *Proc Natl Acad Sci USA* (1984) **81**: 607–10.
7. Matsui MS, DeLeo VA, Induction of protein kinase C activity by ultraviolet radiation, *Carcinogenesis* (1990) **11**: 229–34.
8. Osada S, Mizuno K, Saido TC et al, A phorbol ester receptor/protein kinase, nPKCeta, a new member of the protein kinase C family predominantly expressed in lung and skin, *J Biol Chem* (1990) **265**: 22434–40.
9. Bacher N, Zisman Y, Berent E et al, Isolation and characterization of PKC-L, a new member of the protein kinase C-related gene family specifically expressed in lung, skin, and heart, *Mol Cell Biol* (1991) **11**: 126–33.
10. Yuspa SH, Ben T, Hennings H et al, Divergent responses in epidermal basal cells exposed to the tumor promoter 12-O-tetradecanoylphorbol-13-acetate, *Cancer Res* (1982) **42**: 2344–9.
11. Astrup EG, Iversen OH, Cell population kinetics in hairless mouse epidermis following a single topical application of 12-O-tetradecanoylphorbol-13-acetate II, *Virchows Arch [B]* (1983) **42**: 1–18.
12. Jeng AY, Lichti U, Strickland JE et al, Similar effects of phospholipase C and phorbol ester tumor promoters on primary mouse epidermal cells, *Cancer Res* (1985) **45**: 5714–21.
13. Dunn JA, Jeng AY, Yuspa SH et al, Heterogeneity of [3H]phorbol 12,13-dibutyrate binding in primary mouse keratinocytes at different stages of maturation, *Cancer Res* (1985) **45**: 5540–6.
14. Jaken S, Yuspa SH, Early signals for keratinocyte differentiation: role of Ca2+-mediated inositol lipid metabolism in normal and neoplastic epidermal cells, *Carcinogenesis* (1988) **9**: 1033–8.
15. Tang W, Ziboh VA, Isseroff RR et al, Turnover of inositol phopholipids in cultured murine keratinocytes: possible involvement of inositol trisphosphate in cellular differentiation, *J Invest Dermatol* (1988) **90**: 37–43.
16. Ziboh VA, Isseroff RR, Pandey R, Phospholipid metabolism in calcium-regulated differentiation in cultured murine keratinocytes, *Biochem Biophys Res Commun* (1984) **122**: 1234–40.
17. Isseroff RR, Stephens LE, Gross JL, Subcellular distribution of protein kinase C/phorbol ester receptors in differentiating mouse keratinocytes, *J Cell Physiol* (1989) **141**: 235–42.
18. Yada Y, Ozeki T, Meguro S et al, Signal transduction in the onset of terminal keratinocyte differentiation induced by 1 alpha, 25-dihydroxyvitamin D3: role of protein kinase C translocation, *Biochem Biophys Res Commun* (1989) **163**: 1517–22.
19. Hennings H, Michael D, Lichti U et al, Response of carcinogen-altered mouse epidermal cells to phorbol ester tumor promoters and calcium, *J Invest Dermatol* (1987) **88**: 60–5.
20. Dlugosz AA, Pettit GR, Yuspa SH, Involvement of protein kinase C in Ca2+-mediated differentiation of cultured primary mouse keratinocytes, *J Invest Dermatol* (1990) **94**: 519.
21. Toftgard R, Yuspa SH, Roop DR, Keratin gene expression in mouse skin tumors and in mouse skin treated with 12-O-tetradecanoylphorbol-13-acetate, *Cancer Res* (1985) **45**: 5845–50.
22. Tamaoki T, Nomoto H, Takahashi I et al, Staurosporine, a potent inhibitor of phospholipid/Ca^{++} dependent protein kinase, *Biochem Biophys Res Commun* (1986) **135**: 397–402.
23. Sako T, Tauber AI, Jeng AY et al, Contrasting actions of staurosporine, a protein kinase C inhibitor, on human neutrophils and primary mouse epidermal cells, *Cancer Res* (1988) **48**: 4646–50.
24. Dlugosz AA, Yuspa SH, Staurosporine induces protein kinase C agonist effects and maturation of normal and neoplastic mouse keratinocytes in vitro, *Cancer Res* (1991) **51**: 4677–84.
25. Strickland JE, Greenhalgh DA, Koceva-Chyla A et al, Development of murine epidermal cell lines which contain an activated rasHa oncogene and form papillomas in skin grafts on athymic nude mouse hosts, *Cancer Res* (1988) **48**: 165–9.
26. Strickland JE, Dlugosz A, Hennings H et al, Staurosporine inhibits tumor formation from grafted mouse papilloma cell lines, *Proc Am Assoc Cancer Res* (1991) **32**: 127.
27. Dlugosz AA, Knopf JL, Yuspa SH, mRNA encoding protein kinase C alpha, delta, epsilon, and zeta is expressed in normal and neoplastic mouse keratinocytes in vitro, *J Invest Dermatol* (1991) **96**: 566.

54
Effects of short-term surfactant exposure on stratum corneum capacitance and skin surface water loss

Klaus-P. Wilhelm,*† Anastasia B. Cua* and Howard I. Maibach*
*Department of Dermatology, School of Medicine, University of California San Francisco, California, USA and †Department of Dermatology, Medizinische Universität zu Lübeck, Ratzeburger Allee 160, D-2400 Lübeck, Germany

Introduction

Exposure of the skin to certain surfactants can result in denaturation of keratin proteins and removal of intercellular stratum corneum lipids. Both effects may result in a perturbation of stratum corneum barrier function and skin irritation, characterized by erythema, dry rough scaly skin and fissures. A relationship between surfactant induced irritation and the swelling of isolated stratum corneum by anionic and non-ionic surfactants has been demonstrated in vitro.[1,2] It has been suggested that the swelling of stratum corneum results from a reversible conformational change of keratin proteins exposing new water binding sites and thereby increasing the hydration of the membrane. The aim of the present study was to investigate the swelling effects of surfactant solutions on human stratum corneum in vivo.

Experimental methods

Chemicals

A homologous series of alkyl sulphates based on alkyl chain length (C_8 to C_{14}) was obtained from Research Plus (Bayonne, NJ, USA). Sodium lauryl-9-ethoxy sulphate was from Shell Development (Houston, TX, USA) and Tween 20 (polyoxyethylenesorbitan monolaurate) was from Sigma Chemicals (St Louis, MO, USA).

Study population

Healthy female Caucasians (aged 18–40 years) volunteered to participate after signing a consent form. Volunteers were deemed to be free of active skin disease and were instructed not to wash or treat their skin with any skin-care product for 24 h prior to the experiments. This study was approved by the University of California, San Francisco, Committee on Human Research.

Application

Surfactant solution (0.5 ml) was applied to the mid-volar forearm using occlusive polypropylene chambers (Hilltop Laboratory, Cincinnati, OH, USA). The patches were fixed with non-occlusive paper tape (Scanpore, Norgeplaster, Oslo, Norway). The application time was 5 min and the concentrations used were: 3, 10, 30 and 100 mmol/l. Phosphate buffered saline served as vehicle control. At the end of exposure, the skin was wiped with a soft paper towel (Kimwipes, Kimberly-Clark, Roswell, GA, USA) to remove remaining solution, rinsed with distilled water and gently dried with a soft paper towel.

Measurements

Before all measurements the subjects rested for 20–30 min at constant ambient room temperature

(20 ± 2°C) and relative humidity (40–65%). Skin surface water loss (SSWL), in the special case of occlusion or after application of water or of a solution to the skin, correlates positively with stratum corneum hydration, once the occlusive material (or the solution) is removed.[3] In essence, SSWL equal excess water evaporation plus baseline transepidermal water loss.[4] The SSWL was measured using an evaporimeter (EP1, Servo med, Stockholm, Sweden). This instrument uses the method of vapour pressure gradient calculation described in detail by Nilsson.[4] The probe was held in place for each measurement until a stable value had been established (approximately 30 s). Measurements were performed before and 1, 6 and 11 min after removal of the surfactant solutions. Skin temperature was measured using a thermistor (Tele-Thermometer, Yellow Springs Instruments, Yellow Springs, OH, USA). The SSWL values were corrected to a standard skin reference temperature of 30°C as described by Mathias et al.[5] Capacitance was determined as a measure of stratum corneum hydration in duplicate using a capacitance meter (Corneometer CM 820 PC, Courage & Khazaka, Cologne, Germany). The probe (7 × 7 mm) is applied to the skin surface with a constant pressure (3.5 N). The measuring principle is based on the distinctly different dielectric constants of water (approximately 81) and the other materials (<7).[6]

Results

The sodium lauryl sulphate (SLS) induced hydration of the stratum corneum was investigated in response to different concentrations over time. Immediately (1 min) after the 5-min application of the compound, the skin surface water loss (SSWL) was increased seven-fold over the control treatment (buffer) (Figure 1) and capacitance was increased by 150% as compared with pretreatment values (Figure 2). This increase was transient and only 5 min later baseline hydration values were regained. The increase in stratum corneum hydration was significantly increased by SLS in a dose-dependent manner as demonstrated by both the SSWL and the capacitance measurements. Again, baseline values were re-established 6 min after removal of the surfactant. Because of the rapid reversibility of the observed effect, only the hydration values obtained directly after the end of exposure are shown for the other surfactants tested. For the homologous series of alkyl sulphates a dose–response relationship was found for all four molecules (Figures 3 and 4). The SSWL increased with increasing alkyl chain length, the maximum values being obtained for the C_{12} homologue for all concentrations with a slight decrease for the C_{14} homologue. The data obtained are in agreement with in vitro experiments reported earlier[7] and reflect the irritation potential of these

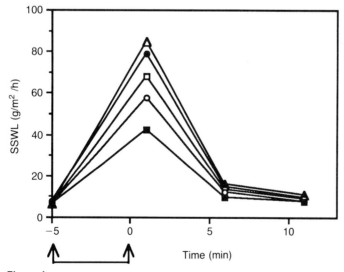

Figure 1

Mean skin surface water loss (SSWL) after a 5-min application (indicated by arrows) of sodium lauryl sulphate (SLS) at different concentrations (n = 10). △, 100 mmol; ●, 30 mmol; □, 10 mmol; ○, 3 mmol; ■, control.

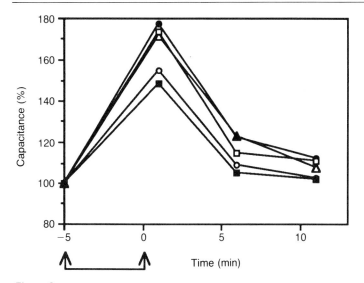

Figure 2

Mean stratum corneum hydration as evaluated by capacitance measurements after 5 min application (indicated by arrows) of sodium lauryl sulphate (SLS) at different concentrations ($n = 10$). (See Figure 1 for key.)

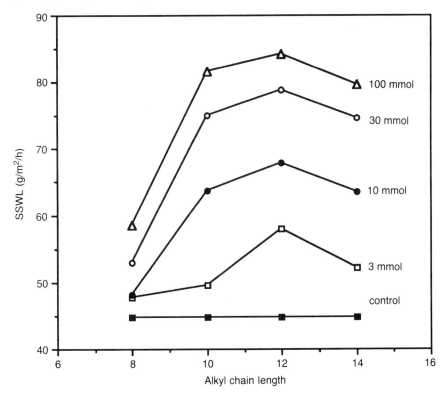

Figure 3

Mean skin surface water loss (SSWL) 1 min after a 5-min application of alkyl sulphates at different concentrations ($n = 10$).

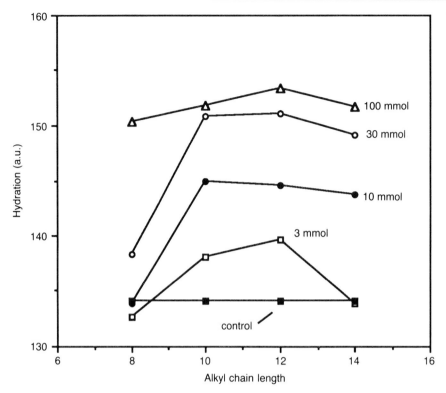

Figure 4

Mean stratum corneum hydration as evaluated by capacitance measurements 1 min after a 5-min application of alkyl sulphates at different concentrations ($n = 10$).

compounds.[8] Ethoxylation of SLS significantly reduced stratum corneum hydration in our model and the non-ionic surfactant Tween 20 had no significant effect (Figures 5 and 6). The mean SSWL values increased exponentially with increasing mean capacitance values (Figure 7). This explains why the SSWL data were more sensitive in detecting differences at high surfactant concentrations than were capacitance measurements.

Discussion

Using SSWL and capacitance measurements, surfactant-induced stratum corneum swelling could be conveniently measured. The swelling effect following application of surfactant solutions for quite a short period of time (5 min) was transient in nature and dependent on the surfactant concentration, although the effect appeared to flatten off for higher concentrations. The swelling mechanism is a two-step process: diffusion of the surfactant into the matrix is followed by expansion against the elastic forces of the membrane.[2] It has been suggested that the swelling results from a continuous disruption of the secondary and tertiary structures of keratin proteins exposing new water binding sites and, thereby, increasing the hydration of the membrane. Interactions with intercellular stratum corneum lipids may also occur, although it would be expected that the extraction of lipids would not be as readily reversible as observed in this study. The in vivo swelling response to the alkyl sulphates seems to parallel their irritation potential as reported by Kligman and Wooding.[7] Ethoxylation reduced the swelling effect, while the only non-ionic surfactant tested (Tween 20) had no significant effect. These observations are in agreement with the reported irritation potential of these compounds.[8] Future work will include other

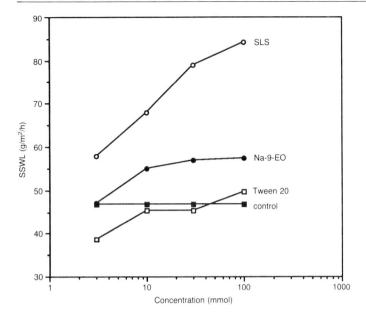

Figure 5

Mean skin surface water loss (SSWL) 1 min after a 5-min application of sodium lauryl sulphate (SLS), sodium lauryl-9-ethoxy sulphate (Na-9-EO), and Tween 20 at different concentrations ($n = 10$).

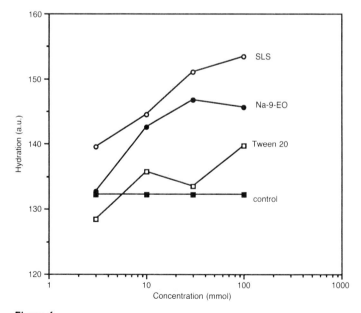

Figure 6

Mean stratum corneum hydration as evaluated by capacitance measurements 1 min after a 5-min application of sodium lauryl sulphate (SLS), sodium lauryl-9-ethoxy sulphate (Na-9-EO) and Tween 20 at different concentrations ($n = 10$).

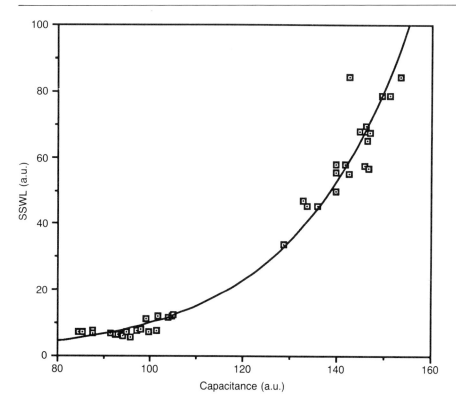

Figure 7

Plot of the mean skin surface water loss (SSWL) values versus capacitance.

substances with different structures in order to elucidate whether the simple in vivo functional assay described here, which results in no volunteer discomfort, can be used to predict the irritation potential of a broad range of molecules.

Acknowledgements

KPW was supported by a post-doctoral fellowship from the German Research Foundation (DFG, Bonn).

References

1 Putterman GJ, Wolejsza NF, Wolfram MA et al, The effect of detergents on swelling of stratum corneum, *J Soc Cosmet Chem* (1977) **28**: 521–32.

2 Rhein LD, Robbins CR, Ferne K et al, Surfactant structure effects on swelling of isolated human stratum corneum, *J Soc Cosmet Chem* (1986) **37**: 125–39.

3 Wilson D, Berardesca E, Maibach HI, In vivo transepidermal water loss and skin surface hydration in assessment of moisturization and soap effects, *Int J Cosmet Sci* (1988) **10**: 201–11.

4 Nilsson GE, Measurement of water exchange through skin, *Med Biol Eng Comput* (1977) **15**: 209–18.

5 Mathias CGT, Wilson DM, Maibach HI, Transepidermal water loss as a function of skin surface temperature, *J Invest Dermatol* (1981) **77**: 219–20.

6 Courage W, Khazaka G, Corneometer CM 820. Instrument manual, Cologne, Germany, 1990.

7 Kligman AM, Wooding WM, A method for the measurement and evaluation of irritants on human skin, *J Invest Dermatol* (1967) **49**: 78–94.

8 Tavss EA, Eigen E, Kligman AM, *J Soc Cosmet Chem* (1985) **36**: 251–4 (letter).

55
The influence of hyaluronic acid on wound healing controlled by a standardized model for humans

Katrin Winkler, Klaus Hoffmann*, Stefan el-Gammal, Barbara Karmann and Peter Altmeyer

Dermatology Department, University of Bochum, Gudrunstrasse 56, 4630 Bochum, Germany

Introduction

Hyaluronic acid

Hyaluronic acid (HA), a mucopolysaccharide synthesized by fibroblasts, is found in all connective tissue. It is the main component of connective tissue matrix. The long non-branching chains of up to 20,000 β-1,4-glycosidically bonded disaccharide units are characteristic of its structure. Each disaccharide (hyalobiuronic acid) unit consists of glucuronic acid and N-acetylglucosamine. The molecular weight of HA varies depending on the degree of polymerization; it can be more than 10^8 Da when obtained from natural substrate.[1] Despite their considerable length the polysaccharide chains are water soluble owing to the large number of dissociated carboxyl groups. The resulting solution is a highly viscous gel. It is this property that gives HA the ability to regulate the water content of tissues by slowing down water perfusion and thus increasing the moisture content. In addition, there is a controlled transport of proteins and metabolites in the interstitial spaces.[2] HA is depolymerized by the enzyme hyaluronidase, which is normally produced in tissues by hydrolytic splitting of the β-1,4 bonds. An extremely high rate of dissolution is found during the first few hours after injury in particular. Many bacteria produce the hyaluronidase which explains their ability to penetrate tissue.[3] The effect of HA on the progression of wound healing processes after skin injury has been evaluated using micro- and macroscopic techniques in both experimental[4,5] and clinical studies.[6-8]

More rapid onset of healing characterized by proliferation of granulation tissue in the filious replacement stage and in newly formed vessels in patients treated with HA compared to a control group, especially in those with poorly healing wounds, has been described. Furthermore, higher resistance to mechanical stress and increased activation of epithelial cell migration and cell differentiation has been observed.[9] Numerous in vitro investigations have shown that HA stimulates cellular processes involved in wound healing, including cell migration,[10] especially of fibroblasts,[11] macrophages,[12] polymorphonuclear leucocytes, lymphocytes and monocytes, fibroblast proliferation,[13] and phagocytosis by neutrophil leucocytes and monocytes.[14]

It has also been demonstrated that local accumulation of HA occurs around a wound during normal wound healing processes, which possibly stimulates healing, and continues until the wound is healed.[15]

Basal cell carcinoma

Basal cell carcinoma is an infiltrating destructive generally non-metastasizing epithelial tumour.[16] Basal cell carcinomas normally arise on clinically normal skin. Current investigations suggest that there is a correlation of the incidence of basal cell carcinoma with the degree of actinic elastosis. Histologically, basal cell carcinomas are characterized by proliferation of basaloid cells, a palisade-like arrangement of cells at the periphery of the

*Correspondence.

lobules. Various factors are important in the aetiopathogenesis, but particularly genetic and actinic factors. Excision including that by curettage and electrodesiccation, radiation treatment and cryosurgery are the methods of treatment for basal cell carcinoma.[17,18]

Cryosurgery

Cryosurgery is a popular method used for the treatment of basal cell carcinoma. Today, the cryogen used is liquid nitrogen which has largely superseded carbon dioxide. Control of the cold flux at the tumour base by means of a thermoneedle is indispensable in cryosurgery. This needle is placed below the tumour after local anaesthesia in order to measure the exact temperature in this area during freezing.

A distinction is made between two cryotechnical methods: the open spray method and the closed-contact method. In the open spray method, liquid nitrogen is sprayed directly onto the area to be frozen. The skin area to be treated is limited with a moulage of flexible rubber material. In the closed contact method, the nitrogen is pumped from the storage vessel into a cryopistol, as it is called, through a hose connector and into the stamp (Figure 1). A thermosensor continually records the cooling. The effect of the cold can be divided into two kinds of cell freezing: heterogenous and homogenous nucleation. In homogenous nucleation the extracellular water is frozen at a rate of $-10°C$/min, the intracellular water diffuses into the interstitium along the osmotic pressure gradient. Electrolytic displacements up to toxic concentrations cause cell death.

In heterogenous nucleation the toxic electrolyte concentrations are not reached homogenously throughout the whole freezing area so that cells can survive. Homogenous nucleation requires freezing rates of up to $-100°C$/min and a tissue freezing temperature of below $-20°C$ to obtain intra- and extra-cellular freezing. During the thawing phase the cells are destroyed as a result of the paradoxical growth of the ice cubes. Thus 100% cell necrosis is reached after one freezing cycle.

A moderate erythema persists after the tissue has thawed and an oedematous component then arises within a few hours. The epithelium becomes detached within 4 h and later the upper dermal layer becomes demarcated. This results in an ulcer, characterized by a fibrinous coat, the widening of which is defined exactly by the freezing temperature, the stamp size and the number of cryocycles. Some of the follicles and sweat glands remain intact in this type of cryosurgical procedure. A multicentred regeneration of the upper surface epithelium is therefore possible. If the tumour parenchyma proves more sensitive to freezing then the surrounding area is not destroyed. Cryosurgery can be used as a curative method for treating epithelial tumours. Cryosurgery provides excellent functional and cosmetic results. Owing to the ability to standardize, the procedure provides an excellent wound-healing model.

DAY	Cryo	0 x 1	2	3	4	7	10	14	21 ⟶
PHOTO		x x	x	x	x	x	x	x	x ⟶
SONO		x x	x	x	x	x	x	x	x ⟶
CRYOLESION				■━━ mm x mm ━━▶					
SMEAR					X				

Figure 1

Diagram of the study

Sonography

The recently available high-frequency digital 20-MHz B-scan ultrasound technique enables exact definition of tumour depth and the extent of the cryonecrosis. The healing processes can also be visualized by means of the technique. High-frequency 20-MHz sonography is thus a suitable tool for the in vivo measurement of wound healing.

Materials and methods (Figure 2)

A total of 66 patients (27 men, 39 women) were treated with HA cream (Jossalind) or unmedicated placebo cream base, in a randomized, double-blind study. Patient enrolment (33 active, 33 placebo) was done over a period of 1 year. After being informed of the nature and consequences of the study, all patients gave consent. The patients were selected according to previously defined criteria (Table 1). The basal cell carcinomas to be treated were on the head or neck areas only (Table 2). The basal cell carcinomas were not to exceed a pre-operative superficial area of 4.0 cm. A 2 mm punch biopsy was made pre-operatively to confirm the diagnosis after clinical evaluation of the type of the basal cell carcinoma (solid, sclerotic, superficial, or cystic) (Table 3).

Assessments were made *clinically*, by measuring the tumour area (diameter × diameter) and subsequent documentation by photography (polaroid and slide), and *sonographically* (lateral limitation and depth of invasion of the tumour).

Table 1 Primary criteria for exclusion.

(1)	Area of the BCC ≥ 4.0 cm or tumour invasion ≥ 2.5 cm
(2)	BCC in certain locations such as head/neck
(3)	Patients with other dermatological diseases surrounding the tumour
(4)	Age <50 or >85 years
(5)	Insulin-dependent diabetes mellitus or Hb A_1 > 10%
(6)	Severe systemic disease (i.e. kidney deficiency)
(7)	Hypertension with systolic values ≥180 mmHg
(8)	Poor compliance in following the study protocol
(9)	Known sensitivity to parabene
(10)	Relapsing tumour

BCC, basal cell carcinoma; Hb A_1, glycolised haemoglobin.

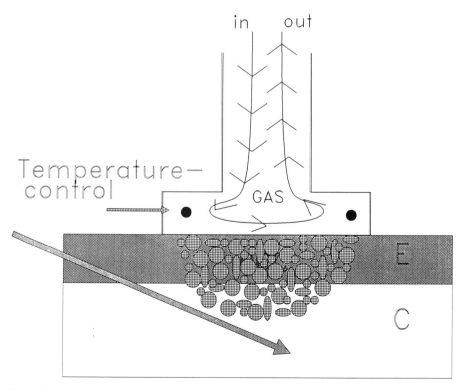

Figure 2

Design of the closed cryosurgery system. E, epidermis; C, corium.

Table 2 Location of basal cell carcinomas.

Upper third of the face	
Forehead/temple	23
Corner of the eye	5
Eyelid	1
Bridge of the nose	14
Side of the nose	14
Cheek	12
Lower third of the face	
Lips	1
Chin	1
Ear	6
Neck	3

Table 3 Histological classification of basal cell carcinomas.

Active-treatment group	
Solid	12
Sclerotic	12
Superficial	8
Cystic	1
Placebo group	
Solid	12
Sclerotic	11
Superficial	10
Cystic	0

The number of cryosurgical cycles used was selected according to the sonographically determined tumour depth of invasion. Prior to treatment any depth of invasion above the central dermis was excluded, since such depths of invasion would require at least two freezing cycles. Prior to cryosurgery, Scandicain (Mepivacain–HCL) without addition of adrenaline was used as a local anaesthetic in all patients and injected below the tumour parenchyma. Subsequently, a biopsy was taken. Exophytically growing tumours were removed with the aid of an electrocautery loop in order to guarantee better cold flux. In the closed-contact procedure, a stamp overlapping the tumour by 1–2 mm was chosen. In the open-spray procedure, the definitely healthy skin area was covered with a moulage and the cryogen was sprayed directly onto the affected skin areas. Size of stamp, the type of needles, the freezing temperature of the stamp and at the tumour base, quantity of freezing cycles and the expansion of the freezing area measured directly after cryosurgery were recorded. The freezing procedure was not permitted to last longer than 1 min, and the thawing phase was as long as possible (>5 min).

Hyaluronic acid or placebo was applied postoperatively three times daily in a thin layer so that the edge of the ulceration was overlapped by approximately 1 mm. The study medication was applied to the wound using an aseptic gauze pad.

Daily examination of the wound area was made and bacterial swabs were taken regularly.

On days 0, 1–4, 7, 10 and 14 ultrasound scans of the lesion were performed and, if the lesion was not completely healed, subsequent weekly sonographic investigations were performed until healing occurred. Table 4 shows the parameters obtained. On days 7 and 14 the efficacy of the study medication was rated by both examiners and patients using an ordinal scale level; the ratings were 'complete healing', 'significant healing', 'little healing' and 'no healing'. Moreover, the investigators rated the usefulness and the risk of the treatment. The tolerance and safety of the study medication were evaluated on days 7 and 14 on an ordinal scale. Unexpected and adverse experiences were recorded on forms specially designed for this purpose.

A 20-MHz digital ultrasound scanner (DUB 20, Taberna Pro Medicum Company, Lüneburg, Germany) was used. The transducer of the scanner, which generates ultrasound signals, operates at a frequency of 20 MHz. The system consists of an ultrasound pulse/receiver unit (Panametrics) and a digital oscilloscope (2430 Tectronics) with a GPIB interface and an 80286 computer (Tandon). Memory storage is done on a 5¼ in. floppy disk

Table 4 Sonographic parameters.

(1) Thickness of the skin (mm)
(2) Thickness of the entry echo/fibrinous coat (mm)
(3) Thickness (invasion) of the tumour/oedema (mm)
(4) Sonographic density of the entry echo/tumour/corium
(5) Granulation tissue measurable (yes/no)
    If yes: thickness (mm)
        density correlated to the surroundings
        re-epithelialization (yes/no)
        change of reflectivity (no, partial, complete)
    If reflectivity is changed:
        demarcation of the tumour/oedema at side (sharp/insufficient)
        demarcation of the tumour/oedema in depth (sharp/insufficient)
        tumour borders (regular/irregular)
        internal echos (normal, light reduced, decreased, increased reflections, echo distribution

and hard disk. The transducer is guided by stepping motor control across a skin area of 12.8 mm. After digitalization the received echo signals can be converted into a two-dimensional sectional view (B-scan image). While being moved linearly the transducer does not touch the skin. It is moved through a front water section over the skin area to be investigated. The tissue is presented to a depth of up to 7 mm entailing a presentation of entry echo, dermis, subcutis and, if applicable, muscle fascia. The resolution capacity is 80 μm axially and 200 μm laterally. In order to reproduce the signals in the form of a sectional view, the unit makes the received signals visible not only in the form of an amplitude but also in brightness values (grey shades). Since the human eye can discriminate colours better than grey shades, the usual grey shades are coded by 255 different colours (colour coding). The dark shades correspond to regions of low echo strength (black, no reflection; dark green, reflection poor). The bright shades correspond to strongly reflecting structures (blue, red, yellow and white indicate increasing echogenity). This has the advantage that even slight differences in the reflection behaviour can be evaluated by colour coding.

The sonogram is displayed true to scale on the screen with varying multiplication factors (8-fold for width and 24-fold for depth). The regions of interest (ROI) can be measured by the computer with the help of insertable measurement lines on the screen. Measurement of density was performed by computer control (image analysis) at the structures of interest (STOI).

A large-scale unit (Erbe, Mannheim, Germany) was used for cryosurgery. This unit operates with a built-in heat exchanger connected to the cryopistol via a hose. Nitrogen is pumped under pressure into the cryopistol through a highly insulated hose connector, thus guaranteeing a constant flow of the cryogen through the pistol. There are various kinds of cryostamps to be used with the pistol (as is also usual with small-scale units). Exact measurement of the temperature in the cryostamp is one of the most important advantages of the unit.

Results (see Figures 3, 4, 5, 6, 7 and 8)

Demographic data

A total of 33 patients (12 men, 21 women; average age 69.0 years, sd 8.3) were treated with the active material (HA) and 33 (15 men, 18 women; average age 66.4 years, sd 9.0) were treated with placebo (Table 5). The demographic data for both groups were comparable. In 26 patients in the active group and in 25 patients in the placebo group concomitant diseases were present which were judged not to affect wound healing.

Description of the basal cell carcinoma and cryosurgery

In the active-agent-treated group, the average diameter of the basal cell carcinomas was 16.1 mm, the tissue temperature was −29.4°C, the stamp temperature was −130.9°C and the duration of freezing was 55.1 s. One patient required two freezing cycles (Table 6). In the placebo-treated group, the average diameter of the stamp was 15.3 mm, the tissue temperature was −33.4°C, the stamp temperature was −124.9°C and the duration of freezing was 57.3 s (Table 6). The average size of the basal cell carcinomas of the active-agent-group patients (diameter × diameter) was 165.5 mm^2 and the average size of the set cryolesion was 364.2 mm^2; for the placebo-treated group these values were 99.8 and 319 mm^2, respectively.

Table 5 Demographic data for the 66 patients studied.

Parameter	Active-treatment group (n = 33)	Placebo group (n = 33)
Sex (M, F)	12, 21	15, 18
Age ±sd (years)	69.0 ± 8.3	66.4 ± 9.0
Weight ±sd (kg)	69.0 ± 10.4	73.4 ± 14.2
Height ±sd (cm)	165.9 ± 8.9	167.4 ± 9.7

Table 6 Description of basal cell carcinomas and cryosurgery (n = 66).

	Mean	sd
Duration of the BCC (months)	23.00	19.00
Area of BCC (mm^2)	132.12	152.20
Area of cryolesion (mm^2)	341.62	272.96
Size of the stamp (mm)	16.00	6.00
Skin temperature (°C)	31.42	9.07
Stamp temperature (°C)	127.89	39.78
Number of cycles (n)	1.00	0.00
Duration of cycles (s)	56.23	5.65

BCC, basal cell carcinoma.

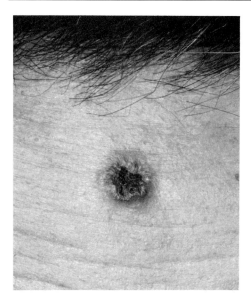

Figure 3

Ulcerated pigmented basal cell carcinoma (BCC) of a 65 year old female on the forehead before cryosurgery (6 × 9 mm).

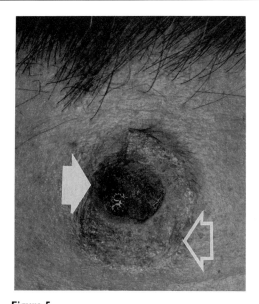

Figure 5

Cryolesion at day 3 after cryosurgery with remains of the (cryo-)blister (open arrow) and necrotic tumour masses (closed arrow) centrally.

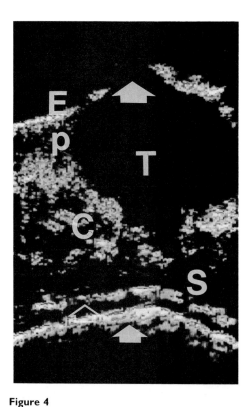

Figure 4

20–MHz sonogram of the BCC before cryosurgery. E, entry echo; P, echo-poor band; C, corium; T, tumour; S, subcutaneous fat; open arrow, muscle fascia; closed arrows, jump in impedance to the periosteum.

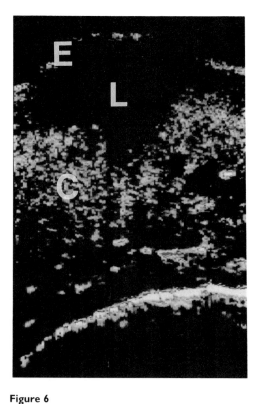

Figure 6

Sonogram of the cryolesion at day 3 after cryosurgery. E, entry echo; L, echolucent lesion; C, corium.

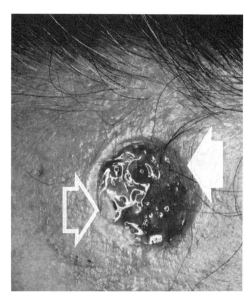

Figure 7

Cryolesion at day 14 after cryosurgery showing a sharply defined ulcer with lateral fibrinous islands corresponding to the granulation tissue (closed arrow).

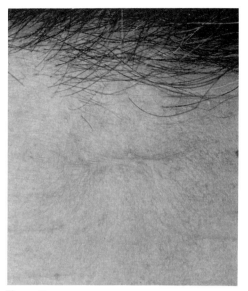

Figure 9

Cryolesion 3 months after cryosurgery showing a flat and slightly atrophic scar.

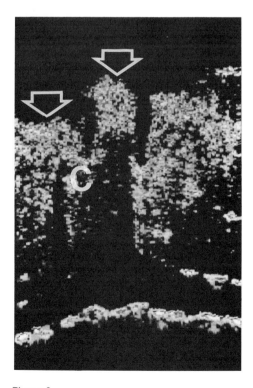

Figure 8

Sonogram of the cryolesion at day 14 after cryosurgery. C, corium; open arrows, granulation or collagen tissue showing as weak internal echos.

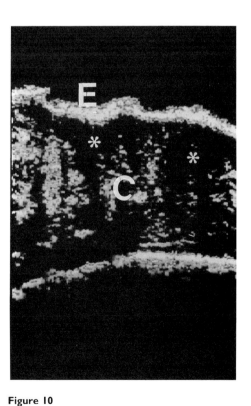

Figure 10

Sonogram of the cryolesion 3 months after cryosurgery. E, entry echo; C, corium; stars, irregular distributed bundles of newly formed connective tissue, the echo is therefore poor.

Eleven patients in the active-treatment group and three in the placebo group had an initial tumour volume of $\geqslant 100$ mm^3. The average tumour volume was 100.8 mm^3 (sd ± 130.6) in the active group and 50.4 mm^3 (sd ± 41.8) in the placebo group. The average tissue density (measured sonographically) was 3.5 (sd ± 3.9) in the active-agent group and 6.3 (sd ± 7.7) in the placebo group. On day 1 after cryosurgery, the lesion surface area and volume and the tissue density were similar in the groups. The efficacy parameters were stratified according to an initial tumour volume of <100 mm^3 ($n = 22 + 19$) and an initial tumour volume of $\geqslant 100$ mm^3 ($n = 11 + 3$) since size and, above all, the depth of the basal cell carcinoma influence the time taken for healing.

Time required for healing

Due to the non-uniform duration of the study, the duration of healing was divided into two groups: $\geqslant 14$ days and <14 days. In the active-agent group, the lesion healed in four of the 33 patients by day 14, and in 19 patients after day 14. In the placebo group, healing was complete in seven patients by day 14 and in 26 patients after day 14. The average healing time in the active-agent group was 17.5 days, and in the placebo group 21 days.

The difference between the treatment groups in the subjects with an initial tumour volume of <100 mm^3 was more marked. In this case, the lesion healed in 13 subjects (59.1%) in the active-agent group by day 14, and in nine patients (40.9%) after day 14 (Table 7). Seven patients (24.1%) in the placebo group required a healing time of <14 days and 22 patients (75.9%) required a time of >14 days.

Table 7 Duration of healing for patients with an initial tumour volume of <100 mm^3 active-treatment group, $n = 22$; placebo group, $n = 29$.

Duration of healing (days)	Active-treatment group		Placebo group	
	n	%	n	%
7	0	0.0	1	3.4
8–14	13	59.1	6	20.7
21	4	18.2	9	31.0
28	2	9.1	2	9.1
35	3	13.6	9	31.0
42	0	0.0	2	9.1
>42	0	0.0	0	0.0

The average time required for healing for patients showing complete healing of the wound was 14 days in the active group and 21 days in the placebo group. The number of placebo-treated patients having an initial tumour volume of $\geqslant 100$ mm^3 was too small to allow any conclusion to be drawn about the relative efficacy of the treatments. In the 11 patients of the active group, one patient was healed before day 14, five patients on day 21, one patient on day 28, and two patients on day 42. In two patients the time required for healing was longer than the duration of the study.

Surface area of the basal cell carcinoma
(see Figure 11a, c)

The average surface area of the lesion in the active-agent-treated group was 1.6 cm^2 (day 0) and 3.8 cm^2 (day 1). In the placebo group the average basal cell carcinoma area was 1.0 cm^2 and that of the cryolesion was 3.4 cm^2. The reduction in wound surface area began after 6 days in the active-agent group, and after 8 days in the placebo group. From treatment days 6 to 13, the wound surface area decreased at least 10% more quickly with HA treatment compared with placebo. There was similar progress in patients with a tumour volume of <100 mm^3, although in this case the wound surface decreased from days 6 to 10 roughly 20% more markedly with active treatment than with placebo. In the $\geqslant 100$ mm^3 group, the active-agent-treated patients, there was less increase in the surface area of lesion in the first few days after cryosurgery and a delayed wound healing, as compared with the active-agent group having an initial tumour volume of <100 mm^3.

Volume of basal cell carcinoma/cryolesion
(see Figure 11b, d)

The wound volume was calculated from clinical and sonographic parameters (diameter × diameter × sonographic depth). On day 1 the volume of the basal cell carcinoma was 100.8 mm^3 and that of cryolesion was 195.2 mm^3 in the active-agent-treated group, and 50.4 and 187.7 mm^3, respectively, in the placebo group. In the HA-treated group of patients the lesion was approximately twice and in the placebo-treated-group approximately three times as large as the original basal cell carcinoma. The wound reduced in size by 17.5% by day 7 in the active group, while in the placebo

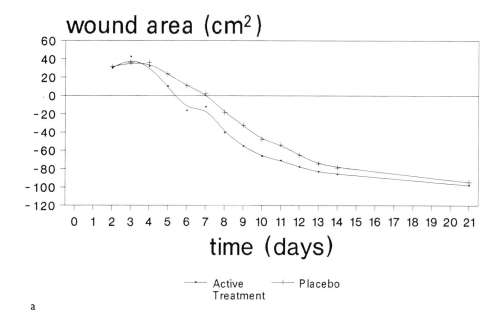

a

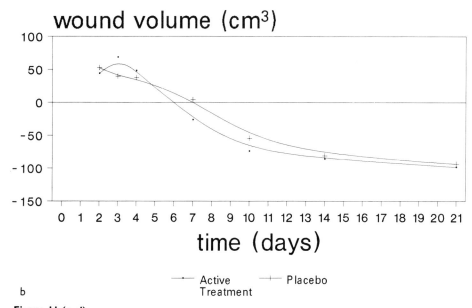

b

Figure 11 (a–d)

Follow up of the wound healing with the parameter "area of ulceration" and "volume of the ulceration"

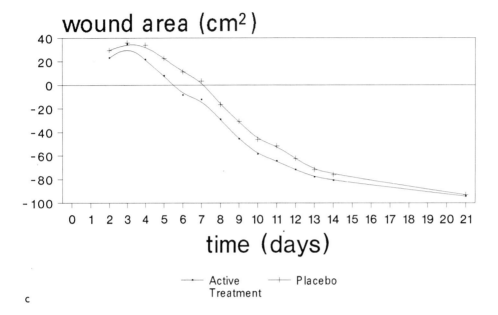

c

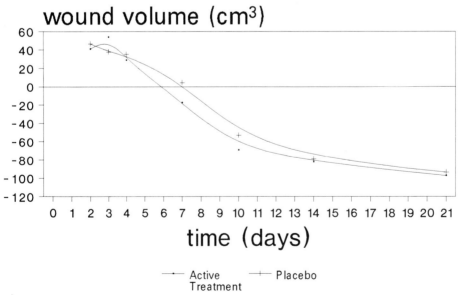

d

group a further slight increase in wound volume of 4.3% was observed. The reduction in volume by day 10 was 69.2% in the active group and 53.0% with placebo. The reduction was more than 90% in both groups by day 21. The pattern was similar in patients having an initial tumour volume of <100 mm³, although the differences between the active-agent and placebo groups were more marked (active-agent group: day 7, −26.3%; day 10, −74.0%. Placebo group: day 7, −4.1%; day 10, −54.5%).

Depth of basal cell carcinoma/cryolesion

The depth of the basal cell carcinoma was 1.8 mm in the active-agent group and 1.7 mm in the placebo group. The wound began to close after day 7 with both treatments. The percentage decrease in wound depth was greater in the active-agent group than in the placebo group.

Skin thickness

The average thickness of the skin at the edge of the wound in the active-agent group increased after the cryosurgery from 3.5 to 4.4 mm, and in the placebo group from 3.7 to 4.5 mm. The increase in skin thickness was caused by the post-operative oedema, which started to diminish from day 7. The average skin thickness in both groups on day 21 was 3.8 mm. At 3 months after the cryosurgery the skin thickness was similar to that before the surgery.

Granulation tissue

In the course of the study it proved very difficult to detect exactly the borders of the granulation tissue in the ultrasound picture. On day 4 after cryosurgery granulation tissue was distinguishable in seven patients in the active-agent-treated group and in eight patients in the placebo group; in both groups the average thickness of this tissue was 0.6 mm. The thickness of the granulation tissue on day 7 was 1.0 mm in 25 patients in the active-agent group and was 0.7 mm in 21 patients in the placebo group on day 21. In the following days, the number of patients in which borders of granulation could be recognized decreased continually.

Densitometry

The density (brightness) of the entry echo was reduced in more than half of patients by day 2 and had returned to normal in most patients by day 14. The density of the basal cell carcinoma was reduced or without reflection; the newly formed tissue began to normalize its density from day 21. In the same way, the density of the corium was slightly reduced after cryosurgery in about two-thirds of patients; it only became normal by day 21 in a few patients.

Discussion

Cryosurgery provides a wound-healing model by producing a well-controlled, almost painless defect in the epidermis and corium and is a suitable treatment for basal cell carcinoma.[19,20] With healing rates of 96% and a relapse frequency of 7.3%, cryosurgery is an alternative to conventional surgical methods.[17,18] The high incidence of basal cell carcinoma makes it possible, using strict inclusion criteria, to achieve a homogeneous patient group. The lesion caused by cryosurgery is, therefore, especially suitable for investigating the effect of the HA used in this study.

The reduced sonographic density of the corium after cryosurgery is caused by a reduction in the neighbouring interfaces of collagen bundles caused by dermal exudate and cellular infiltrate. It was shown in the present study that the observation of cellular repair processes is limited by the resolution of the 20-MHz scanner (80μm). Demarcation of the granulation tissue is only possible by comparing sonograms in temporal sequence. Internal echos in the lesion at the end of the healing phase can be interpreted as newly formed, fine fibrillar connective tissue, which forms reflective surfaces for the ultrasound signal because of its irregular cross-linking.

The exact determination of the depth of tumour invasion guarantees a safe choice of cryocycles, stamp size and freezing temperature, which are decisive factors in successful cryosurgery of a basal cell carcinoma.[17, 19, 28, 29]

Patients with a basal cell carcinoma often also suffer from actinic elastosis. This was frequently no longer detectable in the areas around the lesion after cryosurgery. Sonography offered the possibility of an improved comparison between the two treatment groups. Ulcer volumes, however, did not show any difference in reduction between the two groups, probably because the necrosis and inflammatory cell infiltrate made clear measurement difficult.

The sonographically determined thickness of entry echo scab correlated with the clinical parameters. Tumour volume and tumour surface area were different in the two groups. Both the tumour surface area and the tumour volume were larger in the actively treated group than in the placebo group. According to Altmeyer and Luther[17] the cryodamage is proportional to the mass of the tumour parenchyma since tumour parenchyma reacts more sensitively to the effect of cold than does the surrounding tissue and the tumour surface area (stamp size).[19] It was therefore logical to expect more cryodamage in the active group and this was observed clinically. After classifying the duration of healing as <14 days and ≥14 days there were differences in the rate of healing between the two groups. The more rapid healing started after about 1 week in the active-agent-treated group. Based on the above results it is concluded that treatment with HA significantly speeds up wound healing. The mode of action of this effect is not yet known.

One suggestion is that there is increased capillary perfusion after treatment with HA during the first few hours of healing. One possible explanation for this phenomenon is lower vessel permeability, and not an increase in angiogenesis as previously thought.[22] Other suggestions include vasodilatation and decreased vascular obstruction from cell debris and thiambi. Hyaluronic acid may also affect inflammatory cells, and increased granulocyte function has been reported. Moreover, there is an interdependence of HA synthesis and growth factors on the one hand, and some cytokines and hormones (insulin, prostaglandins and interleukins) on the other. This hypothesis is supported by the fact that the same factors causing a slowing down of HA synthesis also cause a slowing down of growth factor expression.[23,24]

Hyaluronic acid speeds up wound healing by promoting tissue formation rather than by early scar formation, as it supports cell migration and proliferation, which mainly take place during the initial phase of wound healing. In addition, there is a decrease in HA concentration in the tissue with increasing age of the wound. Therefore, it can be concluded that there is an increase in hyaluronidase concentration and an increased release of oxygen radicals from neutrophil leucocytes, which cause distintegration of the substance.[25,26] The treatment with HA possibly neutralizes this effect. It is interesting that HA is transformed into a smaller molecular substance which then promotes angiogenesis.[27] All in all, the extreme complexity of the suggested modes of action of HA should be emphasized. It would certainly be very useful to continue research in this field. According to our previous studies[28] we conclude that our model[29] is well suited to support this research.

References

1 Comper WD, Laurent TC, Physiological function of connective tissue polysaccharides, *Phys Rev* (1978) **58**: 255.
2 Lindahl, Hook M, Glycosaminoglycans and their binding to biological macromolecules, *Ann Rev* (1978) **47**: 385.
3 Siliprandi D, Siliprandi N, Mucopolysaccaridi. In: *Biochimica strutturale*, Libreria Cortina Padova, Chapter 1, p. 50.
4 Curri SB, Acido ialuronic e processi riparativi delle ferite, *Biochim Biol Sper* (1963) **2**: 235.
5 Abatangelo G, Martelli M, Vecchia P, Healing acid enriched wounds: histological observation, *J Surg Res* (1983) **35**: 410.
6 Passarini B, Tosti A, Fanti PA et al, Effetti dell'acido ialuronic sul processo riparativo delle ulcere trofiche *Stud Comp Giorn Dermatol Vener* (1982) **117**: 27.
7 Retanda G, Acido ialuronico nei processi di riparazione delle ulcere cutane, *Esp Clin Giorn Dermatol Vener* (1985) **120**: 71.
8 Sorrone A, Valci A, Nostra esperienza sull'uso dell'acido ialuronico *Riv Ital Chir Plast* (1986) **18**: 205.
9 Håkansson L, Hallgren R, Venge P, Regulation of granulocyte by hyaluronic acid, *J Clin Invest* (1980) **66**: 298.
10 Bernanke DH, Markwald R, Effects of glycosaminoglycans on seeding of cardiac cushion cells into a collagen-lattice culture system, *Anat Record* (1984) **210**: 25.
11 Abatangelo G, Cortivo R, Martelli M et al, Cell detachment mediated by hyaluronic acid, *Exp Cell Res* (1982) **137**: 73.
12 Shannon BT, Love SH, Myrvik GN, Participation of hyaluronic acid in the macrophage disappearance reaction, *Immunol Commun* (1980) **9**: 357.
13 Curri SB, Csermely E, Reperti morfohistochimici nell ulcere da varici infiltrate con acido ialuronico (Brevia n.3) *Biochim Biol Sper* (1963) **2**: 239.
14 Ahlgren T, Jarstrad C, Hyaluronic acid enhances phagocytosis of human monocytes in vitro, *J Clin Immunol* (1984) **4**: 246.
15 Shetlar MR, Shetlar CL, Kischer CW, Glycosaminoglycans in granulation tissue and hypertrophic scars, *Burns* (1981) **8**: 27.
16 Altmeyer P, Holzmann H, *Lexikon der Dermatologie*, Springer-Verlag: Berlin, 1986, pp64–8.
17 Altmeyer P, Luther H, Die dermatologische Kryochirurgie, *Akt Dermatol* (1989) **15**: 303–11.
18 Breuninger H, Schippert W, Black B et al, Untersuchungen zum Sicherheitsabstand und zur Exzisionstiefe in der operativen Behandlung von Basaliomen *Hautarzt* (1989) **40**: 693–700.

19 Zacarian SA, *Cryosurgery for skin cancers and cutaneous disorders*, C. V. Mosby Company: St Louis, 1985.
20 Luther H, Banas J, Darweke-Pickardt G et al, Die Kryochirurgie des Basalioms Ergebnisse einer retrospektiven Studie, Histologische Untersuchungen der Kryoläsion, *Zeit Hautkrank* (1989) **64**: 748–55.
21 Lawrence CM, Shuster S, Comparison of ultrasound and caliper measurement of normal and inflamed skin thickness, *Br J Dermatol* (1981) **112**: 195–200.
22 King SE, Hickerson WL, Kenneth GP et al, Beneficial actions of exogenous hyaluronic acid on woundhealing, *J Surg* (1991) **109**: 76–83.
23 Brecht M, Mayer U, Schlosser E et al, Increased hyaluronic synthesis is required for fibroblast detachment and mitosis, *Biochem J* (1986) **239**: 445–50.
24 Prehm P, Inhibition of hyaluronic synthesis, *Biochem J* (1985) **225**: 669–705.
25 Carlin G, Djursater R, Goldschmidt T et al, Degradation of hyaluronic acid and collagen by oxygen free radicals. In: Venge P, Lindbom A, (eds). *Inflammation: basic mechanism, tissue-injuring, principals and clinical models*, Alquist & Wiksell: Stockholm, 1985, pp297–301.
26 Greenwald RA, Moak SA, Degradation of hyaluronic acid by polymorphnuclear leukocytes, *Inflammation* (1986) **10**: 15.
27 West DC, Hampson IN, Arnold F et al, Angiogenesis induced by degradation of products of hyaluronic acid, *Science* (1985) **228**: 1324–6.
28 Hoffmann K, Winkler K, el Gammal S, A wound healing model under sonographic control. *Clin Exp Dermatol* (1991) in press.
29 Hoffmann K, Stücker M, el Gammal S, Digital 20 MHz sonography of basal cell carcinoma. *Hautarzt* (1990) **41**: 333–339.

56
Influence of short daily exposure to thermal water on the hydration state of the skin

P. Clarys, C. Eeckhout, J. Taeymans,* P. Gross* and A. O. Barel

*Algemene en Biologische Scheikunde, HILOK, Free University of Brussels, Brussels, Belgium, and *Kurzentrum, Lenk, Switzerland*

Introduction

The thermal Kurzentrum of Lenk (Switzerland) is one of the spas recognized by the Department of Health of Switzerland as a centre specialized in the treatment of rheumatic patients. Part of the typical 3-week cure in the centre consists of daily bathing in hot thermal water containing high concentrations of salts and sulphur (sulphates and hydrogen sulphide). According to recent data from balneotherapeutic treatments, the sulphur which penetrates the skin is oxidized and provokes various physiological responses in the skin: vasodilation in the microcirculation, an analgesic influence on the pain receptors and inhibition of the immune response.[1–3]

Patients undergoing the 3-week antirheumatic hydrotherapy in Lenk sometimes complain about modifications of the lipid film of the skin. Typically a drying of the skin and a reduction in the amount of skin-surface lipids are observed as side-effects.

The present study was concerned with an objective evaluation of the influence of the hot sulphur rich water on skin hydration and skin lipids. These physiological parameters of the skin surface were measured objectively using non-invasive biophysical methods. A Corneometer and Sebumeter (Courage-Khazaka, Germany) were used for the quantitative determination of skin hydration and skin lipids, respectively, before, during and after the thermal cure. The use of either a water/oil (W/O) or oil/water (O/W) emulsion containing urea as humectant was assessed objectively during exposure of the skin in order to minimize side-effects (dryness and diminution of skin lipids). A similar study was carried out in Brussels, Belgium, on a control group of volunteer subjects who were not exposed to the hot sulphur rich water treatment for a 3-week period.

Materials and methods

Subjects

Twenty four volunteers (males and females; mean age 59 years) with no skin disease took part in the experiments in the Kurzentrum of Lenk (Switzerland) during the 3-week thermal cure. All volunteers had relatively dry skin on the forearms and on the lower part of the legs as estimated visually and measured by means of capacitance values obtained with the skin Corneometer (arbitrary capacitance units (a.u.) of 63 on the forearms and 59 on the legs).

A control group comprising 12 volunteers (males and females; mean age 36 years) without skin disease was tested in our laboratory in Brussels. The control group was not exposed to the effect of the hot and sulphur rich thermal water. The members of the control group also had relatively dry skin on the forearms and legs (66 a.u. and 61 a.u., respectively) due to winter xerosis.

Test areas

Hydration and skin surface lipids were measured at two skin sites: the middle part of the volar side of both forearms and the middle part of the front side of the lower legs. Non-invasive biophysical measurements were always carried out before exposure of the skin to thermal water or bathing.

Hydration and lipid surface measurements were made on days 0, 4, 9, 14 and 18 or 19. Twelve volunteers were asked to apply once a day (in the evening) an O/W emulsion emollient (Excipial U Lotion®, Spirig Switzerland) containing 2% urea and 12 volunteers similarly applied a W/O emulsion emollient (Excipial U Lipolotion®, Spirig, Switzerland) product containing 4% urea. The volunteers applied the emollient on the left forearm and on the left lower leg during the 3-week thermal cure. The contralateral skin sites were not treated with moisturizers and were considered as control sites to evaluate the effect of daily exposure to thermal bathing.

The 12 volunteers of the control group were followed according to a similar protocol of exposure to normal tap water, measurements and daily application of an O/W emulsion emollient containing 2% urea.

Test solutions and products

Thermal water

Twenty four volunteers were exposed daily (20 min exposure) for three weeks to hot thermal water (34°C, pH 7.9) in the Kurzentrum of Lenk. The results of the chemical analysis of the spa water are given in Table 1. The 12 volunteers in Brussels were exposed to tap water.

Table 1 Chemical analysis of the thermal water at Kurzentrum Lenk, Switzerland.

Constituent	Concentration (mg/l)
Cations	
Sodium	9.5
Potassium	1.5
Magnesium	36
Calcium	594
Total	655
Anions	
Chloride	35
Nitrate	1
Bicarbonate	317
Sulphate	1350
Total	1671
Dissolved gas	
Hydrogen sulphide	44

Measurements

The hydration of the skin was evaluated using the Corneometer CM 820. The instrument measures the electrical capacity of the skin in arbitrary units. The electrical capacitance of the horny layer is proportional to the water content of this layer. The skin surface lipids were measured with the Sebumeter SM 820.

The method used is based on the increase in the transparency of a plastic strip after application of lipids from the skin surface. The increase in the transmission of light, which is measured by a photomultiplier, gives a measure of the quantity of lipids deposited on the plastic strip.

The Sebumeter gives lipid quantities (in arbitrary units) which are proportional to the quantity (in microgrammes) of lipids per square centimetre of skin surface.

Both measurements were carried out in a room where temperature and relative humidity (RH) were kept constant ($22 \pm 1°C$, $53 \pm 2\%$ RH). An acclimatization time of 30 min was allowed prior to carrying out measurements.

Statistics

Data were tested for normality using a Kolmogorov goodness-of-fit test.

The untreated areas were analysed with regard to time in order to detect possible changes in hydration state or changes in skin surface lipids due to daily bathing.

The efficiency of the applied emollients was tested by comparing the data from the treated and the untreated skin sites in each group.

Correlation tests were made between the two examined skin areas and between the two parameters (skin surface lipids and hydration state).

Results

The hydration state of the skin (forearms and lower legs) as a function of the duration of a 20-min daily exposure to sulphur rich thermal water is shown in Figure 1. The data in Figure 1 also include the results of the hydration of the same skin areas in the control group. After several days of exposure to thermal water a significant decrease of hydration was found at both skin sites ($p < 0.05$).

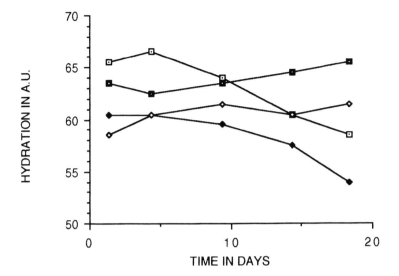

Figure 1

Effect of consecutive daily exposure of the skin to hot and sulphur rich thermal water. Hydration of the forearm (□) and of the lower leg (◆) as a function of duration of exposure to thermal water ($n = 24$). Hydration of the forearm (■) and the lower leg (◇) in the control group ($n = 12$). Hydration is expressed in arbitrary capacitance units (a.u.).

As expected the hydration of the corresponding skin areas in the control group remained constant.

Similarly, the amount of skin surface lipids showed a tendency to decrease after several days of exposure to the thermal water (Figure 2). The Sebumeter is not very sensitive in measuring the small amounts of skin surface lipid which are normally found on skin areas such as the forearm and the lower leg. Due to the large standard deviations, the decrease in the amount of surface lipids after daily exposure to sulphur rich thermal water was not statistically significant.

The moisturizing effect of 2% urea lotion on the forearm exposed to thermal water daily and on the non-exposed skin (control group) is shown in Figure 3. By comparing the hydration values for the two skin sites (forearm and lower leg) protected with the emollient with the values for the contralateral non-protected skin site a significant increase in hydration ($p < 0.05$) was observed for the thermal water exposed group ($n = 12$) and for the control group ($n = 12$). Similar significant results were obtained when assessing the moisturizing effects of 4% urea Lipolotion on the same skin areas exposed to daily sulphur rich thermal water ($n = 12$).

Figure 4 shows the increase in skin surface lipids on the forearms after treatment with the emollients. A significant increase in the amount of lipid occurred after 2 weeks of application of the emollient emulsions to the skin surface exposed to thermal water as well as the non-exposed sites ($p < 0.05$). Daily exposure of the skin to the sulphur rich hot water partially removed skin lipids and application of a moisturizing-emollient emulsion appears to restore the lipid film of the skin.

As previously reported,[4] a positive correlation was observed when comparing the mean hydration values on the untreated forearm and on the untreated lower leg ($r = 0.89$). When comparing the mean values of skin surface lipids of the untreated forearm with the mean values of lipids present on the untreated lower leg a positive correlation ($r = 0.72$) was obtained. In complete agreement with previous work,[5] no correlation could be detected between hydration values and the amount of skin surface lipid as measured at the two untreated skin sites.

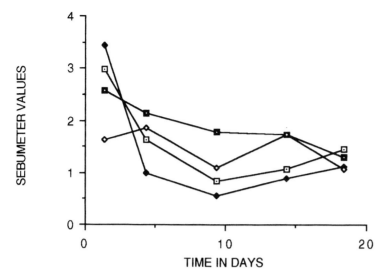

Figure 2

Effect of consecutive daily exposure of the skin to hot and sulphur rich thermal water. Amount of skin surface lipid on the forearm (□) and the lower leg (◆) as a function of duration of exposure to thermal water ($n = 24$). Amount of skin surface lipid on the forearm (■) and the lower leg (◇) in the control group ($n = 12$). Skin surface lipid is expressed in units proportional to microgrammes of lipid per square centimetre of skin.

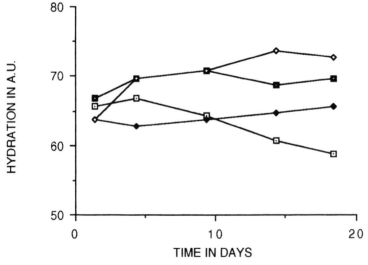

Figure 3

Moisturizing and protective effect of an emollient containing 2% urea on the hydration state of the skin (forearm). Hydration of the skin of the forearms exposed to thermal water ($n = 12$): protected skin site (■); unprotected skin site (□). Hydration of the skin of the forearms in the control group ($n = 12$): protected skin site (◇); and unprotected skin site (◆).

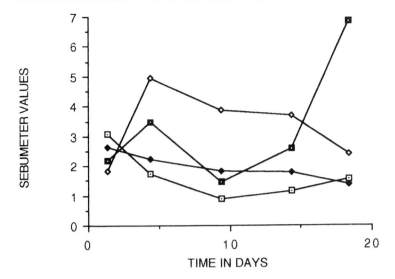

Figure 4

Recovery of the lipid content and protective effect of an emollient containing urea. Amount of skin surface lipid on the forearm exposed to thermal water (*n* = 12): skin site protected with an emollient containing 2% urea (■); unprotected skin site (□). Amount of skin surface lipid on the forearm in the control group (*n* = 12): skin site protected with an emollient containing 4% urea (◇); unprotected skin site (◆).

Conclusions

In agreement with the visual evaluations and with the more subjective perceptions of the 24 subjects themselves, daily exposure of the skin for approximately 19 days to hot sulphur rich water causes significant dehydration of the skin surface and a decrease in the skin surface lipids. Similar measurements carried out on a control group of 12 volunteers did not show any significant effect of normal bathing on the same skin parameters.

The decrease in hydration and skin lipids due to daily bathing in sulphur rich water can be easily avoided by the daily application of emollients containing urea as a humectant.

Finally, the use of non-invasive biophysical instruments demonstrates the advantage of objective quantitative measurements in evaluating the effect of environmental factors on the skin.

Acknowledgements

The authors are grateful to Mr Courage and Mr Khazaka, Courage+Khazaka electronics GmbH, Germany, for their valuable technical support in this study. The authors would like to acknowledge the support of Dr B. Gabard, Spirig, Switzerland.

References

1. Schmidt KL, Schwefelwässer (Sulphur water). In: Schmidt K, (ed). *Kompendium der Balneologie und Kurortmedizin* (Handbook of hydrotherapy and spa medicine), Steinkopff: Darmstadt, 1989, p. 195.
2. Pratzel HG, Zum Problem der chemischen Grenzwerte in der Balneologie (About the problem of chemical limitations in hydrotherapy). In: Schmidt K, (ed). *Kompendium der Balneologie und Kurortmedizin* (Handbook of hydrotherapy and spa medicine, Steinkopff: Darmstadt, 1989, p. 67.
3. Pratzel HG, Grundlagen des perkutanen Stofftransports in der Pharmako-Physicko-Therapie und Balneotherapie, Habilitationsschrift, (Principles of percutaneous transport in physicopharmaceutical therapy and hydrotherapy, Ph.D. thesis) Ludwig-Maximilians-Universität: Munich, 1985.
4. Tagami H, Impedance measurements for evaluation of the hydration state of the skin surface. In: Leveque J, (ed). *Investigation in health and disease*, Marcel Dekker: New York, 1989, p. 79.
5. Thune P, Nilsen T, Hanstad K et al, The water barrier function of the skin in relation to the water content of stratum corneum, pH and skin lipids, *Acta Dermat Venereol (Stockh)* (1988) **68**: 277–83.

57
Experimental modelling of percussive mechanical trauma to the skin and its monitoring in the workplace

C. J. Graves, C. Edwards and R. Marks
Department of Dermatology, University of Wales College of Medicine, Cardiff, UK

Introduction

It is likely that mechanical injury to the skin plays a significant contributory role in the development of industrial dermatitis. Simple clinical observation would suggest this, because industrial dermatitis often occurs at the sites of minor mechanical injury. However insufficient is known about the mechanical stimuli responsible and their effects on the skin.[1] Although our information is incomplete, data are available concerning the effects of challenge with a variety of substances on the range of clinical response,[2] the morphology of the tissue reaction[3] and the epidermal cell kinetic response.[4] Less information is available for the effects of chronic mechanical injury. There is limited evidence that such trauma does cause epidermal thickening and an increase in epidermopoiesis;[5-7] however, other data are lacking.

There are three main components of chronic mechanical trauma: abrasion, percussion and shearing. Preliminary work has been done by our group on the effects of abrasive trauma, using devices designed to deliver controlled and measured doses of abrasive trauma to the skin.[8,9] These studies have indicated that abrasive stimuli to the skin of the forearm produce an epidermal response that is similar, histomorphologically and from the cell kinetic viewpoint, to that of toxic chemical injury.

Our aim was to extend the work by modelling the percussive component of mechanical trauma through the development of a laboratory instrument for mimicking workplace percussive trauma. In addition to this we have developed a system for monitoring tasks undertaken in the workplace that involve percussive trauma to hands and other exposed areas of skin. The first part of this chapter deals with laboratory based work. The second part describes the workplace monitoring system and some results from its use in various industrial environments.

Experimental mechanical trauma

Methods

We have designed and constructed a device which supplies repetitive and measured percussive mechanical trauma to the skin (Figure 1). It was important that the device should model percussive rather than vibrational trauma. Vibrational trauma, although a problem, affects the whole limb involved rather than the skin. The vibrating object tends to remain in contact with the skin causing the whole limb to vibrate. In vibration white finger, for example, most of the energy of vibration is transmitted to the whole hand, arm and joints, eventually causing damage to the capillaries. With percussive trauma the energy is delivered to the skin rather than the whole limb, because the impinging object impacts at a speed where the hands and/or arms present themselves as a stiff system. The energy of impact produces sound, heat and compression of the skin, rather than significant movement of the limb.

The percussor device consists of an oscillating solenoid driven plunger. It is able to mimic percussive trauma by operating in the range 3–20 Hz and by lifting anything up to 10 mm off the skin. The impact head has an area of 2.5 cm^2. The instrument

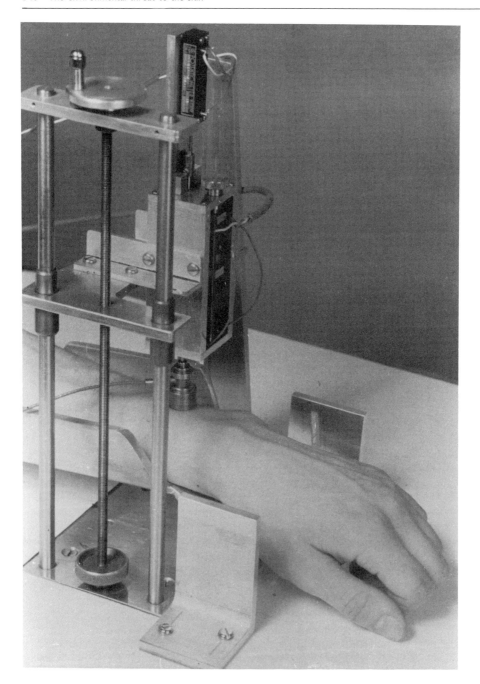

Figure 1

Device for delivering controlled repetitive and measured percussive mechanical trauma to the skin.

contains force and displacement transducers interfaced to a BBC microcomputer which monitors the dose delivered. It is the dose received by the skin rather than the power of the device which is monitored, because the force sensor is mounted directly behind the impact head. In this way we have been able to supply a dose of percussive trauma measured in joules (the internationally accepted unit of energy). This is a significant step towards the proper quantification of the effects of mechanical trauma.

Results

In trials carried out using the percussor device on the wrists of 8 volunteers, it was shown that there is a significant dose-related increase in transepidermal water loss (TEWL) after 5 day experimental schedules designed to mimic chronic percussive trauma. Doses of 2.5 mJ/cm^2/impact and 5 mJ/cm^2/impact were applied at a frequency of 7 Hz, in 10-min sessions three times a day, for 1 week (Figures 2 and 3). Measurements of TEWL, erythema[10] and skin thickness were made. Both regimens produced a statistically significant increase in water loss

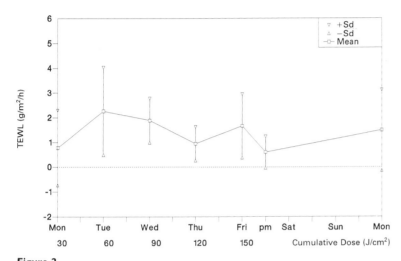

Figure 2

Difference in transepidermal water loss (TEWL) between percussively traumatized (2.5 mJ/cm^2/impact) and untraumatized sites.

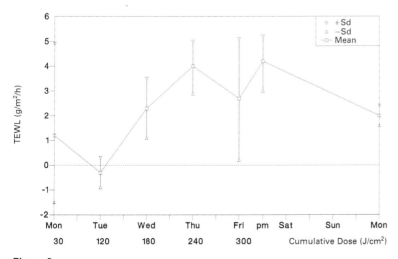

Figure 3

Difference in transepidermal water loss (TEWL) between percussively traumatized (5 mJ/cm^2/impact) and untraumatized sites.

(Mann–Whitney, $P>0.001$). Water loss measurements after trauma of 5 mJ/cm^2 were significantly greater than after trauma of 2.5 mJ/cm^2 (Mann–Whitney, $P>0.05$). There was a measurable increase in erythema after the chronic 5 mJ/cm^2 trauma regimen (Figure 4). There was, on average, an 8% change in whole skin thickness after application of the 5 mJ/cm^2 percussive trauma regimen (paired t-test, $P>0.05$).

Discussion

The TEWL results indicate that, for the volunteers used in our trials, a trauma threshold was reached after receiving a cumulative dose of greater than 150 J/cm^2. In line with this, an increase in erythema was only apparent after doses of greater than the threshold were given. These results show that chronic repetitive percussive trauma can reduce the barrier efficacy of the stratum corneum, and that the concept of a threshold is likely to be of value in further studies.

Workplace monitoring

System

The system we have developed to monitor percussive mechanical trauma to workers' hands in the workplace is based around piezo-electric polyvinylidene fluoride (PVDF) force sensors and an ambulatory data recorder. The requirements of monitoring such trauma in an industrial work environment placed tight constraints on our design and are worth mentioning.

In order to monitor unobtrusively in the workplace, the system had to be small, portable and battery powered. Percussive mechanical trauma, although often repetitive, is nevertheless intrinsically random in nature. Therefore long periods of monitoring are required in order to capture sufficient data of interest. This resulted in the decision to use an ambulatory tape recorder capable of recording for up to 2 h. It was deemed that four sensors would be the minimum number capable

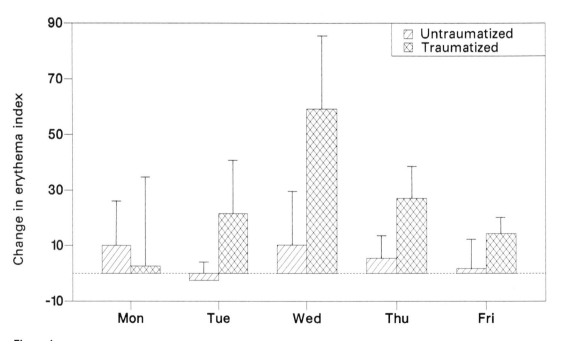

Figure 4

Erythema response to percussive trauma 1 min after dose (5 mJ/cm^2/impact).

of covering sufficiently an area of interest on the hands. The nature of percussive impacts is such that each channel requires a bandwidth of 1 kHz. This meant that we used analogue recording techniques in order to fit four channels onto the tape. In summary, the recording part of the system consisted of four piezoelectric PVDF force sensors interfaced to a four-channel amplitude-modulation unit. The modulated information was recorded on a Casio DA1 digital audio tape (DAT) recorder.

In order to recover the sensor signals, the recorded information was played back through a demodulator unit. The four channels were then input into an IBM PC/AT compatible microcomputer using a four-channel data-acquisition card. The data were analysed using signal-processing software. The software allows the form of the percussion signals to be examined and the type of impact detected to be assessed. It also allows measurement of the peak forces and the duration of an impact. The monitoring system is shown, being worn in Figure 5.

Calibration and validation

The system was calibrated using the percussor device (Figure 6). An output of 22 mV as measured by the computer is produced by an impact force of 1 N.

Validation of the system was accomplished using a pendulum. A simple dose–response experiment was set up to mimic a 'real life' percussion situation. We set up a pendulum with a large smooth weight. We placed the hand being monitored in a position so as to stop the weight at the lowest point of its swing. The weight was released to swing and impact with the hand from increasing heights. The sensors were mounted on the index finger, thumb, central palm and thenar eminence. The magnitudes of the impacts detected by each of the four sensors are plotted against the kinetic energy of the weight at impact in Figure 7. The graph shows that in this particular environment the index finger was always involved, the central palm was hardly involved at all. The thumb and thenar eminence were involved depending on the particular geometry of the impact.

This experiment demonstrates that the system is capable of identifying areas at greatest risk of damage from percussive trauma in the workplace.

Methods

The system was tested in various industrial environments. The worker being monitored was given a range of tasks to do, each lasting less than 5 min. There were two types of percussion involved in these tasks. The first type involved continuous contact between the hands and the object delivering the percussive trauma. In this category all the tasks involved using a hammer. The first two were onto a surface with low recoil, the third was onto a metal surface from which the hammer rebounded. The second type involved the separation and coming together of the hands and the object. In this category, all the tasks involved the handling of heavy objects. The results are shown in Figures 8–10.

Results and discussion

We can see clearly how with tasks involving hammering (Figure 8), the thenar received a consistently large dose of percussive trauma whereas the palm was hardly involved at all. The metal hammering produced larger vibrations in the handle and, as a consequence, the thumb and index finger received greater doses of trauma.

Turning to the second category (Figure 9) there was little difference between the tasks resembling hard and soft contacts. All monitored parts of the hand were involved. However, the percussive trauma brought about by operating a hand press (labelled 'open hand impact') affected the palm far more than in any other activity. Likewise, the index finger was involved the most whilst loading boxes. In this particular activity the worker was catching medium sized boxes containing heavy metal goods, in order to stack them away. It is not surprising that the index finger and thenar received large doses of percussive trauma as in this task it would be necessary for the thenar (as well as other peripheral parts of the palm) to take the weight of the box.

Figure 10 shows the distribution of forces over the four areas being monitored. It enables us to compare the two categories of tasks. It is clear that proportionately the thenar eminence receives a larger dose of percussive trauma from tasks involving hammering than from the 'make and break' category of tasks. Across the range of tasks of either type, the palm was minimally involved except in the operation of the hand press where the hand was required to be open.

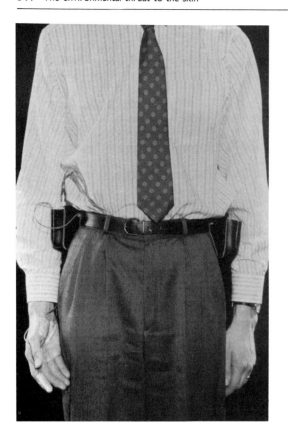
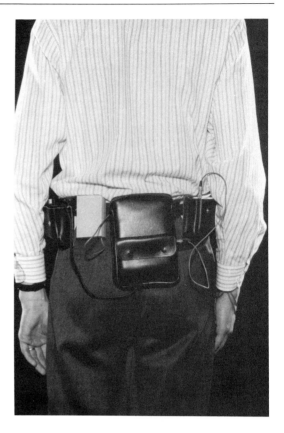
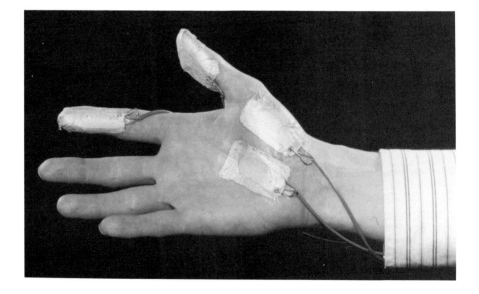

Figure 5

The monitoring system being worn.

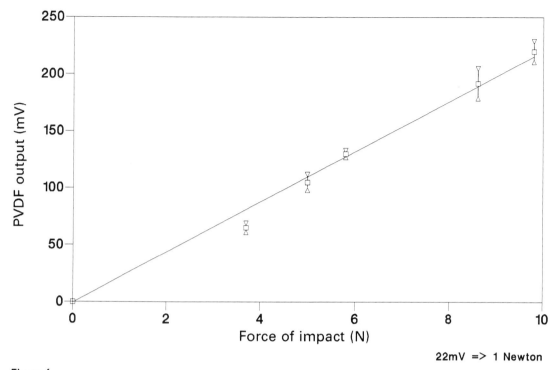

Figure 6

Percussion from percussor device as monitored by the PVDF sensor.

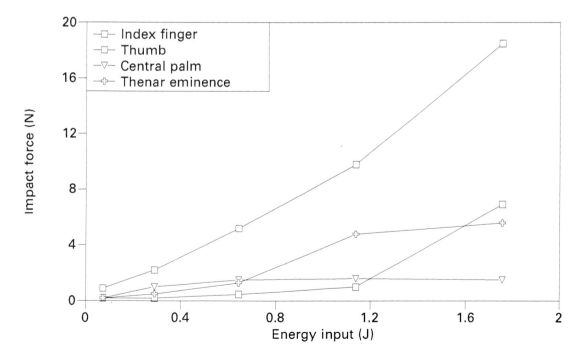

Figure 7

Impacts to the hand from a swinging pendulum as measured by the PVDF sensors.

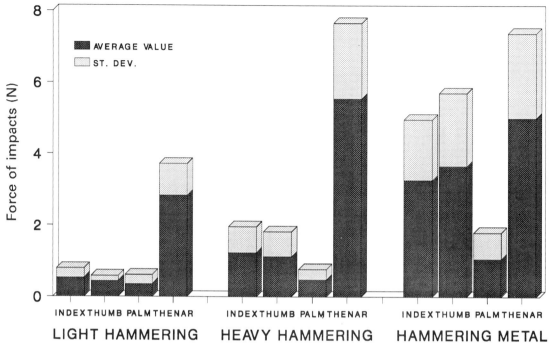

Figure 8

Percussive trauma in the workplace tasks involving hammering.

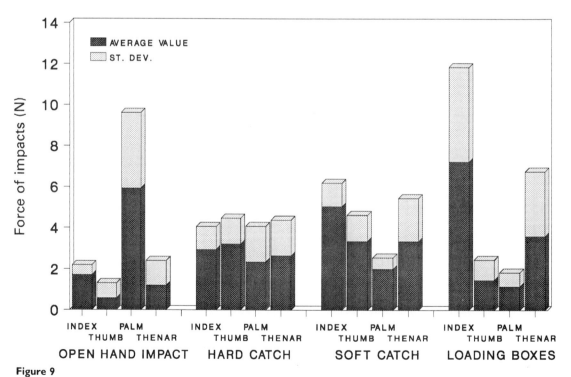

Figure 9

Percussive trauma in the workplace tasks involving handling objects.

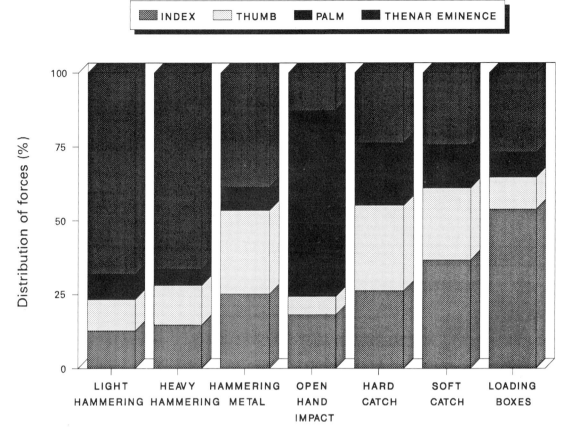

Figure 10

Percussive trauma in the workplace.

Conclusions

Experimental work investigating the effects of controlled repeated percussive injury has been carried out and the results indicate that the barrier property of skin is significantly impaired after cumulative doses of greater than 150 J/cm^2 are given using our trauma regimen.

We have designed and built a workplace monitoring system for the measurement of doses of mechanical trauma received by workers in industry. The system has been shown to monitor the detail of percussive trauma received by the hands, through the judicious placing of sensors on the areas of interest. For all the types of task investigated save one, the central palm receives minimal percussive trauma. In hammering tasks, the thenar eminence receives a larger proportion of percussive trauma than the index finger and thumb, and than it also receives from other types of activity involving percussive trauma.

This area of study is of prime importance if progress is to be made in correlating experimental laboratory based work with the real world of the industrial workplace.

Acknowledgements

This work was supported by a grant from the UK Health and Safety Executive.

References

1. Kligman AM, Klemme JC, Susten AS, (eds), The chronic effects of repeated mechanical trauma to the skin, *Am J. Ind Med* (1985) **8**: (4/5).
2. Kligman AM, Assessment of mild irritants. In: Frost P, Horowitz SN, (eds). *Principles of cosmetics for the dermatologist*, CV Mosby Co.: Missouri, 1982, pp. 265–73.
3. Lindberg M. Forslind B, Wahlberg JE, Reactions of epidermal keratinocytes in sensitized and nonsensitized guinea pigs after dichromate exposure: an electron microscope study, *Acta Derm Venerol (Stockh)* (1982) **62**: 389–94.
4. Marks R, Kingston T, Acute toxicity reactions in man. Tests and mechanisms, *Food Chem Toxicol* (1985) **23**: 155–63.
5. Mackenzie IC, The effects of frictional stimulation on mouse ear epidermis. I. Cell proliferation, *J Invest Dermatol* (1974) **62**: 80–5.
6. Mackenzie IC, The effects of frictional stimulation on mouse ear epidermis. II. Histologic appearance and cell counts, *J Invest Dermatol* (1974) **63**: 194–8.
7. Marks R, Hill S, Barton SP, The effects of an abrasive agent on normal skin and on photoaged skin in comparison with topical tretinoin, *Br J Dermatol* (1990) **123**: 457–66.
8. Marks R, Black D, Methodologies to produce and assess standardized trauma to the skin, *Am J Ind Med* (1985) **8**: 491–8.
9. Hamami I, Parameters and determinants of skin irritancy, Ph.D. Thesis, University of Wales, 1986.
10. Pearse AD, Edwards C, Marks R, The evaluation of sun protection factor (SPF) using a portable erythema meter, *J Invest Dermatol* (1988) **91**: 384.

Part III: The microbial threat

58
The effects of global warming on skin infections and infestations

David Taplin,* Alfred M. Allen,† Terri L. Meinking and Sherri L. Porcelain*
Departments of Dermatology & Cutaneous Surgery, and *Epidemiology & Public Health, University of Miami School of Medicine, Miami, FL, USA, and †Pierce County Public Health Department, Tacoma, WA, USA

> The earth was warmer in 1990 than in any other year since people began measuring the planet's surface temperature, separate groups of climatologists in the United States and Britain, said yesterday.
>
> *New York Times*, 10 January 1991

Introduction

Concern has been expressed in recent years over the effects on human health relating to the warming of our climate, commonly known as the 'greenhouse effect'. Largely as a result of increases in carbon dioxide (CO_2), methane, chlorofluorocarbons (CFCs) and nitrous oxide in the upper atmosphere, changes are taking place in the equilibrium between infra-red radiation lost into space, and that reflected back to the surface of the earth. The net result is predicted to be an increase in land mass and ocean surface temperatures, with potentially dramatic changes in climate and sea levels.

Opinions differ on how quickly, and to what extent these changes will occur, but there is a general consensus that many areas of the world are likely to become more tropical, particularly in the northern hemisphere. In addition to climatic changes, weather patterns may alter, so that some areas will become wetter, while some locations which now enjoy adequate rainfall may suffer drought conditions.

Considerable attention has been paid to the effects on the skin of increased ultraviolet B (UVB) radiation related to ozone depletion. Predictions have also been made concerning the expected increase in heat-related injury and death, which also involve the skin as our principal method of thermoregulation. Virtually no attention has been paid to other adverse effects on the skin which will result from these climate changes. In 1985, a US government state-of-the-art series on global warming devoted only five pages to the skin in over 1000 pages, and this concerned the effects of increased UVB radiation.

Among other diseases which may, with some confidence, be predicted to increase in incidence and severity are skin infections and infestations.

Since 1960, teams from the Departments of Dermatology, and Epidemiology and Public Health at the University of Miami, Florida, have studied environmental effects on the human skin.[1–4] From 1965 to 1972, working with colleagues from the Walter Reed Army Institute of Research in Washington, DC (WRAIR) and the Letterman Army Institute in San Francisco (LAIR), extensive studies were instituted to identify the incidence and causes of the devastating skin infections among US troops in Vietnam.[5–9] Subsequently, surveys were conducted in Panama,[10] Colombia,[11] Costa Rica[12] and Uganda[13] to define further the effects of warm moist climates on the skin, and to compare them with similar populations in cooler climates or higher altitudes. Space limitations preclude an exhaustive review of this work, but a few examples are presented here, prefaced by a brief and somewhat simplified description of the greenhouse effect.

What is the greenhouse effect?

Most of us know that the atmosphere of the earth is mainly composed of 78% nitrogen and 21% oxygen. If these were the only gases present, the average global surface temperatures would be around −18°C; far too low to support life as we know it. Fortunately, our surface temperature has been remarkably constant for many thousands of years at around 15°C global average. This is due to the fact that that the atmosphere also contains water vapour (0.2%) and carbon dioxide (0.03%). Together, these two naturally occurring gases form a warming protective blanket, which allows shorter wavelengths from the sun, including the invisible spectrum, to reach the surface of the earth, but blocks much of the longer wave infra-red energy from escaping into space.

Not all thermal energy from the earth is blocked (absorbed) by water vapour. It has a 'window' which is transparent to infra-red wavelengths between 8 and 18 μm. Carbon dioxide and other trace gases, some of which are man-made, exhibit strong absorption bands in this range, thus preventing escape of infra-red radiation. In effect, they dirty the window, trapping more infra-red radiation, throwing the natural flux off balance, and causing a warming of the lower atmosphere and surface of the earth. This has become known as the 'greenhouse effect'.

In addition to water vapour and carbon dioxide, other gases have the capability of trapping longer wavelengths. These include methane (CH_4), nitrous oxide (N_2O), and chlorofluorocarbons (CFCs).

Chlorofluorocarbons

The effects of CFCs on the depletion of the ozone layer in the stratosphere is dealt with elsewhere in this volume, and will not be discussed in detail. It should, however, be noted that CFCs, although present at much lower concentrations in the atmosphere than CO_2, are far more efficient in trapping outgoing infra-red radiation, so that they also directly contribute to the greenhouse effect. The depletion of the ozone layer, which is real, and increasing at a faster rate than originally predicted, may have consequences far beyond the cutaneous damage resulting from increased UVB. Ocean food chains, starved at the lower end by UVB damage to phytoplankton, could be severely affected, with disastrous results on a resource which supplies, for example, 40% of the protein in Asia.

Carbon dioxide

The level of CO_2 in the atmosphere is increasing by 0.5% per year. The life expectancy in the atmosphere is greater than 150 years. Prior to the mid-1800s, man's contribution to the CO_2 in the atmosphere was, for practical purposes, nil. Increases in world population demanded changes in farming practices, and large areas of forest were cleared by slash-and-burn techniques. This activity removes standing trees and foliage, which absorb CO_2. The subsequent processes of burning and decay of organic material absorb oxygen and release CO_2. In the last 120 years, as much CO_2 has been generated by deforestation as has been produced by the burning of fossil fuels, but that has changed dramatically since 1960. Today, fossil fuel consumption accounts for 3 to 5 times more CO_2 release than slash-and-burn deforestation.

Based on ice-core samples, tree-ring data, and marine-sediment analysis, the CO_2 content of the close earth atmosphere was around 260–280 ppm v/v (parts per million by volume) in 1800. It is now approximately 350 ppm v/v and rising. Measured as carbon, this is equivalent to 740 billion metric tonne (BMT), which exceeds the carbon reserves trapped in all of the world's forests put together. Since 1850, we have plumped over 150 BMT of carbon into our atmosphere!

Our ability to detect and measure this increase in CO_2 owes much to foresight of Roger Revelle and the persistence of Charles David Keeling of the Scripps Institution of Oceanography. In 1958 Keeling began continous measurements of atmospheric CO_2 at Mauna Loa in Hawaii. The tracing of his infra-red detector is reproduced in Figure 1. It will be noted that there is an oscillation of CO_2 levels each year. This reflects the spring awakening of foliage in the Northern hemisphere with the absorption of CO_2, and the autumn leaf drop and decay associated with release of CO_2. The consistency of the overall increase since 1960 is remarkable, and is largely due to the increased burning of fossil fuels.

Since 1974, air samples taken in Alaska, USA, Samoa, and the South Pole have confirmed this increase, with extremely consistent findings. Atmospheric CO_2 has risen by 20–25% since the start of the industrial revolution, but half of this increase has occurred since 1958.

Methane

The level of CH_4 in the atmosphere is increasing by 1% per year, and the life expectancy of this gas remains uncertain. Ice-core samples from Greenland have been used to measure CH_4/air ratios over a period of 600 years. There was a close correla-

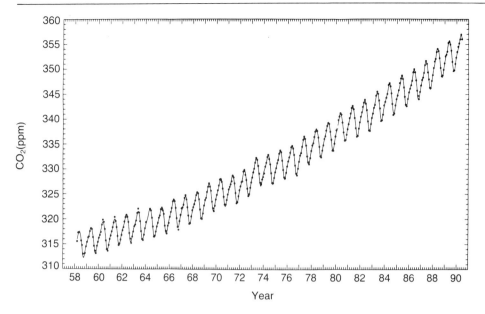

Figure 1
The annual atmospheric CO_2 concentrations measured at Mauna Loa Observatory, Hawaii. Oscillations reflect spring growth and autumn leaf drop in the northern hemisphere. (Reproduced with permission from Prof. Charles D. Keeling.)

tion between CH_4 concentration and population increase. From the 1300s to the 1800s, CH_4 was present at levels less than 0.8 ppm; the level is now around 2 ppm.

Methane (marsh gas) is produced naturally from decaying marshes and other biogenic sources. Increases in the last 50 years have been predominantly dictated by man's alteration of the ecosystem. Most of the increase is believed to come from the significant expansion of rice paddies. When rice plants are above water, they take up CO_2 and release oxygen in the same manner as other plants. For two-thirds of their growth cycle, however, the seedlings are underwater, where their metabolism is anaerobic, releasing methane. Another surprising, but significant, source is the expulsion of methane from belching ruminants, principally cattle. It is estimated that the 1.2 billion cows in the world release 90 million tons of methane per year.

Other sources include biomass burning (slash and burn), exploitation of natural gas resources, and coal mining. In 1980, the amount of CH_4 released by the actions of man had reached five times that calculated from natural biogenic sources. Methane is of concern in the greenhouse effect because it has strong absorption properties in the water vapour 'window' described above. Future man-made sources are unpredictable, and not all natural sources may have been identified.

Nitrous oxide

The level of N_2O in the atmosphere exhibits a slow but steady increase. The life expectancy of this gas is between 75 and 100 years. The primary source is microbial metabolism in soil and water. Increased use of fertilizers and higher crop yields, and increases in agricultural land use are the most likely origins of N_2O, which has increased by about 60% in the last 100 years. Some industrial sources, such as the production of nylon, also contribute to N_2O.

Skin conditions which are likely to increase in severity and incidence in warmer climates

Dermatophytosis

In countries where distinct differences between summer and winter temperatures occur, the increased incidence and severity of common dermatophyte infections is obvious in the summer months. In the USA, television commercials for athlete's foot (tinea pedis) remedies are notably absent in the winter months.

In the southern USA these conditions occur year round, but are more flamboyant in the more humid months of May to October. When persons are continuously exposed to hot humid conditions, particularly when wearing occlusive clothing, the results may be devastating. In Vietnam, it was a rare US soldier who escaped a ringworm infection. In some infantry units, up to 75% of the men suffered from severe, inflammatory infections, covering large areas of the body, precluding restful sleep, causing a significant effect on morale, and halving troop strength in forward combat units.[5,14]

We particularly noted the confluent lesions occurring under wet clothing worn by troops operating in flooded terrain. It was clear that whatever immunity they may have acquired from previous fungus infections during their 18 years or so growing up in the USA offered no protection from dermatophytosis when environmental conditions favoured the fungus, which in Vietnam was generally due to a local strain of zoophilic *Trichophyton mentagrophytes*.

We encountered a similar situation in soldiers operating in the lowland tropical areas of Colombia, except that the incidence and severity of their conditions were even worse. Eighty-five percent of infantry soliders had erosive, fissured, scaling and very painful feet due to dermatophytosis. Over half of them had inflammatory tinea corporis which extended over most of the trunk and buttocks. In this case, the offending dermatophytes were the strictly anthropophilic species, *Epidermophyton flocossum* and *Trichophyton rubrum*. It was evident that the species of fungus, state of nutrition, and immunological memory of the hosts played little role in susceptibility. The overriding factors controlling infections were climatic, coupled with the effects of occlusion, since we once again observed severe confluent lesions under damp clothing. The obvious role of occlusion led to practical remedial actions by military commanders. Allowing men to wear gym shorts and sandals when not on duty, and providing more time to dry underwear after laundering, made a significant impact on the severity of fungal infections, and had an enormous effect on morale. Table 1 illustrates the prevalence and 2-month incidence of dermatophytosis among Colombian infantry units conducting similar exercises, housed in the same type of accommodation, but exposed to different climates.

Following a series of elegant experiments by R. D. King and colleagues at the Letterman Army Institute of Research (LAIR), the occlusion phenomenon was finally explained in 1978.[15] Some CO_2 normally escapes from the skin surface, and diffuses into the air around us. Even more is released from damaged skin, such as may occur in dermatophytosis. The LAIR investigators showed that wet clothing traps CO_2, which may rise up to 200 times normal concentrations. Under increased CO_2 tension, the metabolism of dermatophyte fungi is substantially altered. They more readily digest stratum corneum, and exhibit morphological changes which we associate with invasive potential. The survey shown in Table 1 revealed clinical findings which supported the occlusion–CO_2 hypothesis. Note that 72% of the soldiers in the hot humid environment of El Centro developed extensive tinea corporis over a 2-month period. Only 9% of their counterparts, in the even hotter, but very dry desert of La Guajira had tinea corporis, reflecting the rapid evaporation of sweat from uniforms. Unlike damp or wet clothing, dry materials readily allow the escape of CO_2. A high prevalence of tinea pedis was found in all units where men were required to wear boots continuously during the day. The microclimate inside their boots was always tropical and probably main-

Table 1 Effects of climate on dermatophytosis among Colombian soldiers.*

Location (n)	Temperature (°C)	Relative humidity (%)	Point prevalence (%)		2-month incidence of tinea corporis (%)
			Tinea pedis	Tinea corporis	
El Centro (115)	28–38	80–90	85	55	72
Barranquilla (256)	24–32	60–70	64	38	50
La Guajira (75)	30–40	10–20	85	4‡	9
Santa Marta (348)	26–30	20–30	32†	17	20

* All men in the survey were exposed continuously to ambient conditions. Barracks were not air conditioned.
† The low prevalence of tinea pedis in this hot climate was related to the ability of this unit to conduct their 'boot training' barefoot on an ocean beach.
‡ In this hot dry climate, tinea corporis was uncommon, due to rapid evaporation of sweat from clothing.

tained high levels of CO_2. In Santa Marta, the opportunity to remove the boots for several hours every day reduced the prevalence of tinea pedis by 50%, and the severity of their infections was far less than in other units. Similar effects of CO_2 have been reported for *Candida albicans* and *Pityrosporum orbiculare*. The complex interactions between micro-organisms and the skin under occlusion deserve closer scrutiny. An understanding of these mechanisms should lead to novel ways of preventing and treating these conditions.[15]

Streptococcal pyoderma

The term streptococcal pyoderma is used here to describe any skin infection caused by β-haemolytic *Streptococcus pyogenes*. Since we believe the condition always requires some minor trauma or pre-existing lesion in order to become established, these infections may be initiated by a variety of cutaneous insults, including scabies, insect bites, pediculosis, or minor trauma. Thus, the prevalence varies according to the local conditions. There is no question, however, that streptococcal infections far exceed those caused by *Staphylococcus aureus* on a world-wide basis. Cultures of very early lesions indicate that *S. pyogenes* is the primary invader, but most cases become secondarily colonized by *S. aureus*. Moreover, in the tropics *S. aureus* can be cultured as readily from normal perineal skin as from purulent lesions. *S. pyogenes*, in contrast, is rarely recovered from normal skin except as an occasional transient contaminant in families where purulent children are crowded together.

Temperature, humidity, altitude, personal hygiene, age and overcrowded housing are the controlling factors of *S. pyogenes* infections. Figure 2 shows the relationship of climate (as measured by altitude) and level of hygiene, as observed by the investigators, with the prevalence of pyoderma. At all altitudes, poor living conditions, overcrowding and lack of running water increased the likelihood of streptococcal pyoderma. Conversely, higher altitudes, representing cooler conditions, particularly at night, decreased the incidence. Children living in overcrowded houses at sea level with limited bathing facilities showed a prevalence of culture positive streptococcal infections of over 30%. Very similar attack rates were found in lowland villages in Costa Rica, Uganda and Peru. The annual incidence under these conditions may exceed 100%. Not only is every child infected during a year, but some suffer from multiple episodes.

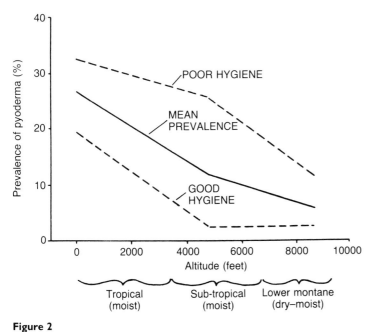

Figure 2

The relationship between climate, level of hygiene and prevalence of pyoderma. (From reference 11.)

Biting insects are a major cause of primary insults which precede streptococcal pyoderma. Depending on the local conditions, these may include mosquitoes (*Anopheles*, *Aedes* or *Culex*), sandflies (*Phlebotomus*), blackflies (*Simulium*) or biting midges (*Culicoides*). These pruritic bites when scratched can quickly become infected. There is no indication that any of these insects actually transmit the streptococci, although the hypothesis has not been investigated extensively.

Our observations of several hundred children over a period of months showed that the usual source of *S. pyogenes* infecting a new lesion is another purulent site on the same child. The next most likely origin is an infected sibling, particularly when they share the same bed or hammock. There is without question a role in transmission played by wound feeding flies (*Hippelates* eye gnats, *Musca domestica*, and other filth flies). Our studies indicate that these vectors ingest exudates containing *S. pyogenes* and *S. aureus*, and retain them in the gut for several days, later to regurgitate or defaecate them on open skin lesions. The higher incidence of streptococcal pyoderma in tropical climates is undoubtedly related to the greater abundance of biting insects and vector flies.

There is also evidence that *S. pyogenes* and *S. aureus* are more abundant in skin lesions in warmer climates.[11] In Bogota, Colombia (elevation 8700 feet) recovery of *S. pyogenes* from skin sores was only 67%, whilst *S. aureus* was cultured from 52%.

In Apartado, Colombia, a hot and humid sea level jungle town, 90% of lesions yielded both pathogens. It is tempting to suggest that if these organisms are more easily recovered on a swab in tropical conditions, they would also be more available to be transmitted by fingers and flies. We also noted that more colony-forming units (CFUs) of both organisms were recovered at the lower altitudes, although the cultures were all incubated at 35°C. It is probable that many factors combine to produce higher attack rates in the tropics, but they are all related to increased temperatures and humidity.

Scabies

Although thoughout history scabies has been recorded in all climates and among all races, it is, like fungal and bacterial infections, more prevalent, more severe and more often secondarily infected under tropical conditions. It is the frequent precursor of strepotoccal pyoderma.

In Panama, we have for many years studied crowded communities in which scabies had been endemic since 1973. In a recent survey, scabies was present in 78% of infants under 2 years old, 60% of children 2–6 years old and 54% of 6–10 year olds. Streptoccal pyoderma was reduced from 32% of all children under 10 years old to less than 2% by mass treatment of the scabies with permethrin cream without the use of antibacterial antibiotics.[16] Similar reductions of scalp pyoderma follows adequate treatment for head lice.

The presentation of scabies in the tropics differs in several respects from classic descriptions given by authors in temperate or cold climates. In addition to the high frequency of secondary bacterial infections, the tracts or burrows described in most textbooks are almost never found. We believe this represents the response of the female mite to environmental conditions, rather than the evolution of a 'tropical' strain of *Sarcoptes scabiei*. Our evidence for this is that subjects from a population at sea level with no scabies burrows often return from trips to the cooler mountains with burrows, which we can easily recognize. It has become dogma that scabies does not occur above the neck, but in warm, humid climates scabies is frequently found above the neck, in the scalp and behind the ears, particularly in children. In one study of children aged 2 months to 5 years, 41% had mite proven scabies of the scalp, and 18% had scabies of the face. Ninety percent had the condition on the buttocks.[17] Under occlusive clothing, in pregnant women and young infants, scabies lesions may cover the entire back or abdomen. Thus, the standard description of scabies confined to wrists, finger webs, elbows, male genitalia and female breasts is of little help in the tropics. Early lesions consist of 1–2 mm erythematous papules which may easily be mistaken for miliaria. In many populations in which we work, any cutaneous eruption, rash, pustule or papule is considered to be scabies until proven otherwise.

Discussion

The above samples illustrate the effects of warm climates on the initiation, exacerbation and transmission of skin infections and infestations. Other conditions which are more common and severe in the tropics include candidiasis, pitted keratolysis and tinea versicolor. We have not had the opportunity to evaluate the effect of climate on staphylococcal infections such as furunculosis and bullous impetigo, because these conditions were never present in more than 2% of the populations surveyed, regardless of climate.

Reports of skin conditions derived from clinic visits, hospital records, or chart reviews are a poor, and frequently erroneous method of determining community prevalence and incidence of infections, and should be viewed with suspicion.[18] For example, painful furuncles or disfiguring staphylococcal impetigo of the face may be sufficient reason to visit the local health post or clinic, because these conditions can be treated with antibiotics which are usually curative. The medical staff, therefore, perceive these conditions as the most prevalent type of skin infection. In reality, streptococcal pyoderma may be 50 times more common in the community, but treatment at the clinic offers only temporary relief, because the initiating factors, such as scabies, have not been eliminated, and the patients quickly become reinfected. The community may perceive these conditions to be inevitable and incurable, and avoid taking their children to the health post.[12, 18]

In evaluating the effects of environment on the skin, we know of no substitute for appropriately conducted surveys of the populations at risk. The data presented here were obtained by physical examination of all inhabitants of villages, military units, or schools, and represent true prevalence figures. They indicate that skin infections in warm climates among lower socio-economic groups constitute a significant proportion of the total health needs.

As summers become hotter and longer, and as the more tropical areas of the world expand north and south of the equator, we may expect substantial increases in the types of skin problems described above. The populations most at risk will be those most exposed to the environment; the millions without air-conditioning, or other means of escape from the heat and insects, large families in substandard housing with inadequate plumbing or lack of water, refugees from areas of drought, flood, and war and similar disadvantaged communities.

Even in more affluent societies, we expect a warming climate to affect adversely those with outdoor occupations. Examples include construction personnel, farm workers, road crews and aircraft mechanics. Particularly vulnerable will be the thousands of homeless who live on the streets of our cities. Exposed constantly to the elements, with little opportunity for personal hygiene, they suffer high attack rates of skin infections and infestations. The methods of reducing their disability are the same as those used in less developed tropical countries.

The drain on medical resources will fall on those agencies already overburdened with responsibilities to these populations, and eventually the costs will be borne by all of us. A recent Editorial in The Lancet, and our own experiences, indicate that prevention and early treatment of skin infections is a sound economic investment.[19]

The discipline of dermatology can and should play a vital role in this endeavour. Skin conditions are poorly understood and managed by those most likely to encounter them, particularly in rural areas of the tropics in the developing world. Conversely, trained dermatologists are rarely encountered in these locations. We can do much to alleviate suffering and disfigurement by disseminating what we already know where it is most needed, and to increase research on the mechanisms of the effects of climate on the skin. Finally, ministries of health and other government agencies need to recognize the enormous drain on their own resources caused by skin disability, and adjust their priorities accordingly.

References

1 Taplin D, Zaias N, Rebell G, Environmental influences on the microbiology of the skin, *Arch Environ Hlth* (1965) **11**: 546–50.
2 Taplin D, Zaias N, Tropical immersion foot syndrome, *Military Med* (1966) **131**: 814–18.
3 Taplin D, Zaias N, Rebell G, Skin infections in a military population, *Dev Ind Microbiol* (1967) **8**: 3–12.
4 Taplin D, Zaias N, Blank H, The role of temperature in tropical immersion foot syndrome, *J Am Med Assoc* (1967) **202**: 546–9.
5 Blank H, Taplin D, Zaias N, Cutaneous *Trichophyton mentagrophytes* infections in Vietnam, *Arch Dermatol* (1969) **99**: 135–44.
6 Allen AM, Taplin D, Twigg L, Cutaneous streptococcal infections in Vietnam, *Arch Dermatol* (1971) **104**: 271–80.
7 Allen AM, Taplin D, Lowy JA et al, Skin infections in Vietnam, *Military Med* (1972) **137**: 295–301.
8 Allen A, Taplin D, Epidemic *Trichophyton mentagrophytes* infections in servicemen, *J Am Med Assoc* (1973) **226**: 864–7.
9 Allen AM, Taplin D, Tropical immersion foot, *Lancet* (1973) **ii**: 1185–9.
10 Allen AM, Taplin D, Skin infection in Eastern Panama: survey of two representative communities, *Am J Trop Med Hyg* (1974) **23**: 950–6.

11 Taplin D, Lansdell L, Allen AM et al, Prevalence of streptococcal pyoderma in relation to climate and hygiene, *Lancet* (1973) **i**: 501–3.

12 Taplin D, Antibacterial soaps: chlorhexidine and skin infections. In: Maibach HI, Aly R, (eds). *Skin microbiology: relevance to clinical infections*, Springer-Verlag; New York, 1981, pp. 113–24.

13 Taplin D, Lansdell L, Value of desiccated swabs for streptococcal epidemiology in the field, *Appl Microbiol* (1973) **24**: 135–8.

14 Allen AM, *Internal medicine in Vietnam* Vol 1: *Skin diseases in Vietnam*, US Government Printing Office: Washington, DC, 1977.

15 Allen AM, King RD, Occlusion, carbon dioxide and fungal skin infections, *Lancet* (1976) **i**: 360–2.

16 Taplin D, Porcelain SL, Meinking TL et al, Community control of scabies: a model based on use of permethrin cream, *Lancet* (1991) **337**: 1016–18.

17 Taplin D, Meinking TL, Chen JA et al, Comparison of crotamiton 10% cream (Eurax) and permethrin 5% cream (Elimite) for the treatment of scabies in infants, *Pediatr Dermatol* (1990) **7**: 67–73.

18 Taplin D, Allen AM, Bacterial pyodemas, *Clin Pharmacol Ther* (1974) **5(2)**: 905–11.

19 Anon, Skin disease and public health medicine, *Lancet* (1991) **337**: 1008–9.

59
The effects of arthropods on the skin

D. A. Burns
Department of Dermatology, Leicester Royal Infirmary, Leicester LE1 5WW, UK

Arthropods are capable of damaging the skin by a variety of mechanisms, more than one of which may be implicated simultaneously.

Mechanical trauma from mouthparts

The trauma to the skin produced by penetration of arthropod mouthparts seldom causes severe disturbance to the host. The nature of the trauma inflicted depends upon the structure of the mouthparts and the method of feeding. There are basically two types of blood-feeding method: the 'vessel feeders' (solenophages) such as mosquitoes and sucking lice, whose delicate piercing mouthparts are inserted directly into capillaries; and 'pool feeders' (telmophages) such as tsetse flies and stable flies which lacerate the skin, damage blood vessels, and feed on the extravasated blood.

Reactions to retained mouthparts

Arthropod mouthparts retained in the skin may provoke a foreign-body reaction, and the response to retained Ixodid tick mouthparts is an example of this phenomenon. Ixodid ticks such as the common sheep tick *Ixodes ricinus* possess mouthparts designed to anchor them firmly to their hosts. The principal component of the mouthparts is a barbed hypostome. When attaching itself to the host the tick uses its toothed chelicerae to cut into the epidermis, the hypostome is then thrust through the opening, and gradually penetrates into the dermis. The tick salivary glands produce a protein cement material which forms a cone around the hypostome, interlocking with its barbs, and anchoring the hypostome in the dermis.[1] If the tick is suddenly wrenched from the host it is likely that fragments of the hypostome will remain in the skin to provoke a foreign-body reaction.

Invasion of the host's tissues

The larvae of certain Diptera (two-winged flies) cause myiasis, in which the host's tissues are invaded by the parasite.[2,3] Obligatory myiasis producers always pass their larval stage parasitically in the body of an animal, whereas the larvae of facultative myiasis producers usually develop on decaying flesh or vegetable matter, but may infest wounds. Obligate myiasis producers include *Dermatobia hominis* (the human bot fly), found in neotropical areas of the New World, and *Cordylobia anthropophaga* (the tumbu fly), which is widespread in tropical Africa south of the Sahara. The larvae of both these flies produce boil-like lesions on the skin (furuncular myiasis). The posterior end of the larva can be seen protruding from a punctum in the skin. *D. hominis* larvae have a bulbous anterior end equipped with rows of backward-pointing spines which help to anchor the larvae in the skin.

Other important obligate myiasis producers include species of *Chrysomya* (Old World screw worm) and *Cochliomyia* (New World screw worm), and some species of *Wohlfahrtia* and *Cuterebra*.[4]

Contact reactions

Contact with the secretions of certain arthropods, or with their living or dead bodies, may provoke reactions of an irritant or allergic contact nature.

Contact urticaria and dermatitis have been described in laboratory workers handling cockroaches[5] and locusts.[6]

Certain species of beetle release highly irritant, blister-provoking fluid when crushed.[7] Perhaps the best known of these is the Spanish fly, *Lytta vesicatoria*, which is a bright metallic green beetle found predominantly in the Mediterranean region. The pulverized beetles were once sold as an aphrodisiac, and have been used in the preparation of blistering plasters, in the treatment of warts, and as a component of hair-restorers. *Lytta vesicatoria*, a member of the Meloidae family of blister beetles, contains the vesicant cantharidin, which is highly toxic. Members of the family Staphylinidae (rove beetles) contain the vesicant pederin, which is chemically distinct from cantharidin. The other major family of vesicating species is the Oedemeridae.[8]

Also highly irritant to the skin are the defensive secretions of some tropical species of millipede.[9] Millipede chemical defences take the form of corrosive secretions containing aldehydes, cresols, benzoquinones and hydrogen cyanide, produced by repugnatorial glands distributed along the body segments. In the majority of species the secretions ooze out and form droplets around the foramina of the glands, but a few species, for example the giant Spirobolid millipedes of the tropics and subtropics, can squirt their secretions for some distance.

The hairs and spines of some caterpillars can produce urticarial papules on the skin by a combination of mechanical and pharmacological effects — the latter reaction being produced by venom present in the hairs and spines.[10,11] Hairs (setae), which are hollow, communicate with a poison gland cell. They are commonly barbed, and having penetrated human skin the barbs hold the setae in place. In some families of moths, caterpillars have clumps of much smaller hairs known as 'dart hairs'. These are pointed at both ends and carry fine barbs, and contact with the caterpillar may release huge numbers of these tiny darts. Dart hairs of this type are present on caterpillars of the brown-tail moth, *Euproctis crysorrhoea*, and the pine processionary caterpillar, *Thaumetopoea pityocampa*. Setae are also woven into cocoons and the webs of silk-spinning caterpillars.

Spines are an extension of the cuticle of the caterpillar, and contain venom. The spines either have a terminal plug of inspissated material at their open ends which is released by pressure, or a weak point at which the spine fractures, allowing the venom to escape when the skin is penetrated. Poisonous spines occur particularly on the caterpillars of the moth families Cochlididae, Saturniidae and Megalopygidae. The venom contained in the setae and spines of caterpillars contains histamine, histamine liberators, serotonin and proteases. In some moth species, for example moths of the genus *Hylesia*, irritating setae are carried by the adults. *Hylesia* moths are notorious for causing outbreaks of 'butterfly itch', 'moth dermatitis' or 'Caripito itch' in tropical South America.[12]

Injection of directly injurious substances

The venom injected by arthropods may contain pharmacologically active substances which produce local effects in the skin, and systemic effects if injected in sufficient quantity. Hymenoptera stings, for example, produce local pain, erythema and oedema, but the cumulative effect of a large number of stings may be fatal, particularly in children.

The clinical syndrome produced by the bite of a spider is known as arachnidism and, although most spiders are harmless to man because their chelicerae are not strong enough to penetrate human skin, there are some species which are well-known for the harmful effects of their bites.[13-15] The venom of the black-widow spider, *Latrodectus mactans*, is considered to be one of the most potent toxins, exceeding that of snake venoms. *Latrodectus hasselti*, the red-back spider, is a related species common in Australia. Black-widow spider bites (latrodectism) produce local erythema and oedema, accompanied by cramp-like or colicky abdominal pain, profuse sweating, paraesthesia, incoordination and paralysis, and without treatment the bite may be fatal in young children or in the elderly and frail.

The bites of species of spiders of the genus *Loxosceles* ('brown recluse', 'fiddleback', 'violin' spiders), which are found in North and South America, produce considerable local damage to skin and subcutaneous tissues (necrotic cutaneous loxoscelism), and occasionally severe systemic effects (viscerocutaneous loxoscelism). In viscerocutaneous loxoscelism the skin changes are accompanied by massive intravascular haemolysis, which may prove fatal.

The bites of the Australian funnel-web spiders *Atrax robustus* (the Sydney funnel-web) and *Atrax formidabilis* (the tree funnel-web) may be accompanied by severe systemic symptoms, and several fatalities following *Atrax* bites have been recorded. Other spiders with unpleasant bites include *Chiracanthium* species (Sac spiders), and *Tegenaria agrestis*, which has been reported as a probable cause of necrotic cutaneous arachnidism in northwestern USA.

There are a number of species of scorpion whose stings are dangerous, and may prove fatal, although many scorpions are quite harmless. Most of the dangerous species of scorpion belong to the family Buthidae. The local effects of scorpion stings are usually immediate severe local burning pain, hyperaesthesia and oedema.

The red and black imported fire ants, *Solenopsis invicta* and *Solenopsis richteri*, are troublesome pests in the southern states of the USA.[16,17] The fire ant uses its powerful mandibles to grip its victim, and then rotates about the point of attachment inflicting stings in a circular pattern. Skin lesions produced by fire ants typically occur in clusters, and initially take the form of weals, followed in a few hours by vesicles. The contents of the vesicles become cloudy, and after 8–10 h the typical lesion is an umbilicated pustule on an erythematous, oedematous base. Fire ant venom is composed of 90–95% piperidine alkaloids, which are responsible for the local reaction. In addition, four allergenic proteins have been isolated from the venom.

Injection of usually harmless substances into a previously sensitized host

The vast majority of reactions to arthropod bites or stings depend upon the presence of specific antibodies to antigenic substances in the arthropod saliva or venom. The type of reaction provoked by a bite or a sting in an individual patient depends to a large extent on previous exposure to the same or related species. A sequence of events demonstrated by Mellanby[18] with mosquito bites has been shown to occur with the bites of many other arthropods. When an individual is bitten for the first time by a species, if the salivary secretions do not contain pharmacologically active substances, there is commonly no reaction. After repeated bites, however, the individual begins to develop sensitivity, manifest initially by a delayed reaction (an itchy papule developing about 24 h after each bite, and persisting for several days). With further exposure to bites an immediate weal reaction occurs, followed by the delayed papular reaction. After a further period of exposure the delayed reaction no longer occurs, and eventually there is no reaction at all. The individual is then said to be immune.

The itching suffered by most patients with clothing louse infection is a manifestation of hypersensitivity to louse salivary antigens, and occasionally this mechanism is responsible for the development of a generalized pruritic papular eruption in patients with large numbers of head lice.

The local reaction to arthropod bites may result in bulla formation. Bullous reactions are common on the lower legs, but may occur in other sites, especially in children. The reaction to bed bug bites is frequently bullous.

The Blandford fly, *Simulium posticatum* (previously known as *Simulium austeni* Edwards), a small blackfly which is a pest in the Stour valley area of Dorset, is particularly notorious for the severity of the reaction to its bite. The female of this fly requires a blood meal prior to oviposition, and appears to have a preference for human blood, with a particular tendency to bite women's legs. Reactions to the bites vary from a small blister to large, haemorrhagic, indurated lesions.[19]

The venom of Hymenoptera (bees, wasps and ants), in addition to its pharmacologically active components, also contains a number of antigenic substances.[20] The three major allergens in vespid (wasp, yellow jackets and hornets) venoms are phospholipases, hyaluronidase and antigen 5. Honeybee venom contains three antigenic proteins (phospholipase A2, hyaluronidase and acid phosphatase) and the polypeptide melittin, which is also antigenic. Hypersensitivity to Hymenoptera venoms is mediated by IgE antibodies. The antigenic substances in the venom of many Hymenoptera are more liable to induce high degrees of immediate hypersensitivity than are the antigens of most other insects.

References

1. Arthur DR, *Ticks and disease*. Pergamon: Oxford, 1961.
2. Alexander JO'D, Cutaneous myiasis. In: *Arthropods and human skin*, Springer-Verlag: Berlin, 1984, pp. 87–113.
3. Lane RP, Lovell CR, Griffiths WAD et al, Human cutaneous myiasis — a review and report of three cases due to *Dermatobia hominis*, *Clin Exp Dermatol* (1987) **12**: 40–5.
4. Baird JK, Baird CR, Sabrosky CW, North American cuterebrid myiasis, *J Am Acad Dermatol* (1989) **21**: 763–72.
5. Zschunke E, Contact urticaria, dermatitis and asthma from cockroaches. *Contact Dermatitis* (1978) **4**: 313–4.
6. Monk BE, Contact urticaria to locusts, *Br J Dermatol* (1988) **118**: 707–8.
7. Theodorides J, The parasitological, medical and veterinary importance of Coleoptera, *Acta Trop* (1950) **7**: 48–60.
8. Nicholls DSH, Christmas TI, Greig DE, Oedemerid blister beetle dermatosis: a review, *J Am Acad Dermatol* (1990) **22**: 815–9.
9. Alexander JO'D, Centipede bites and millipede burns. In: *Arthropods and human skin*, Springer-Verlag: Berlin, 1984, pp. 383–9.
10. Alexander JO'D, Reactions to Lepidoptera. In: *Arthropods and human skin*, Springer-Verlag: Berlin, 1984, pp. 177–97.
11. Southcott RV, Lepidopterism in the Australian region, *Records Adelaide Children's Hospital* (1978) **2**: 87–173.
12. Dinehart SM, Archer ME, Wolf JE Jr, et al, Caripito itch. Dermatitis from contact with Hylesia moths, *J Am Acad Dermatol* (1985) **13**: 743–7.
13. Alexander JO'D, Spider bites. In: *Arthropods and human skin*, Springer-Verlag: Berlin, 1984, pp. 209–26.
14. Southcott RV, *Australian harmful arachnids and their allies*, Southcott RV: Mitcham, 1978.
15. Wong RC, Hughes SE, Voorhees JJ, Spider bites, *Arch Dermatol* (1987) **123**: 98–104.
16. Lofgren CS, Banks WA, Glancey BM, Biology and control of imported fire ants, *Ann Rev Entomol* (1975) **20**: 1–30.
17. de Shazo RD, Butcher BT, Banks WN, Reactions to stings of the imported fire ant, *N Engl J Med* (1990) **323**: 462–6.
18. Mellanby K, Man's reaction to mosquito bites, *Nature* (1946) **158**: 554.
19. Hansfield RG, Ladle M, The medical importance and behaviour of *Simulium austeni* Edwards (Diptera: Simuliidae) in England, *Bull Entomol Res* (1979) **69**: 33–41.
20. Reisman RE, Stinging insect allergy: progress and problems, *J Allergy Clin Immunol* (1985) **75**: 553–5.

60
Mediterranean sea and swimming pool dermatoses

Jean-Paul Ortonne, Michel Weiler, Philip el Baze* and Annick Genollier-Weiler
*Service de Dermatologie, Hôpital Pasteur BP No. 69, 06002 Nice Cedex, France and *Laboratoire de Bactériologie, Hôpital Pasteur BP No. 69, 06002 Nice Cedex, France*

The present vogue for vacations at the seaside and the popularization and diversity of sea sports indicate that many individuals are now exposed to a variety of aquatic-related skin disorders. For a large part of the year, several million divers, sea bathers, swimmers, water skiers and windsurfers live around the Mediterranean coast. Dermatologists who practise in coastal cities have to deal with more and more patients affected by water related dermatoses. In addition, there are large numbers of public and private swimming pools in these areas. Whereas skin disorders due to sun bathing have been extensively described, until recently water related diseases of the skin did not often appear in medical reports. It is only in the last few years that 'aquatic dermatology' has developed as a speciality in its own right.[1,2] In this paper, attention is focused on dermatoses related to contact with the Mediterranean sea and swimming pools.[3]

There are many dermatoses and mucosal changes related to contact with water or aquatic fauna. These include dermatoses due to marine animals and plants, dermatoses due to bacteria, dermatomycoses and viruses, skin lesions due to diving equipment, swimming-pool chemicals, etc., and aquatic-sport-related skin lesions. In addition, several cutaneous reactions due to contact with water such as water-induced pruritus and aquagenic urticaria[4,5] can be observed. These problems as well as dermatoses due to climate (sun, wind, etc.) are not discussed in this paper.

Dermatoses due to marine animals

These may be due to several different mechanisms: contact dermatitis resulting from irritation or allergy, primary or secondary infection, active (sting puncture or suction) or passive (abrasion or cuts) wounds, destructive and/or venomous bites.[1,2] Only the most common dermatoses found in the Mediterranean will be described. These are due to Coelenterates, Echinoderms or venomous spines of fish skin.

Coelenterate stings and wounds

Mode of contamination

Three major classes of coelenterates are included: Hydrozoa (hydroids, fire corals and the portuguese man of war), Scyphozoa (the jellyfishes) and Anthozoa (sea anemones and corals). These animals probably cause the most problems in swimmers.[1,2,6,7]

In the Mediterranean, *Physalia physalis* and *Pelagia nocticula* are most commonly the cause of dermatological problems. The sea anemone *Sagartia* induces a common skin condition which in some Mediterranean areas is called 'sponge fisherman's disease' or '*maladie des pêcheurs d'éponges nus*'.[2]

A dominant characteristic of the coelenterates is the presence of tentacles equipped with nematocysts or stinging organelles. The nematocysts discharge their contents through a thread-like tube of varying length, usually bearing a formidable array of spinules. The ability of a particular Coelenterate to sting the victim depends to a large extent on the ability of the thread tube to penetrate the skin. Our knowledge of the chemical and pharmacological properties of Coelenterate venoms is limited. It is likely that some clinical effects of Coelenterate stings are due to low-molecular-weight compounds present in nematocyst venoms, such as indole histamine, kinins, and prostaglandins, although some of these substances may be cytoplasmic contaminants. The venoms also contain many different peptides and proteins. Some venoms have also been found to possess enzymatic activity. The toxic effects of nematocyst venoms vary greatly from one Coelenterate species to another.[6,7]

The envenomation usually takes place by direct contact with tentacles. It must be noted that the sting of Physalia can penetrate a surgical glove and that the ejection force of a hydroid's nematocyst is approximately 40 000 g.[6,7] However, indirect contamination may occur in a variety of ways: detached tentacles with intact nematocysts; storage of intact nematocysts by another animal (such as the Mediterranean octopus); an aerosol of seaspray and tentacle fragments. The severity of a Coelenterate sting depends on a combination of many factors including the species of Coelenterate, the type of nematocyst it possesses, the penetrating power of the nematocyst needle, the surface of the exposed skin, the frequency and duration of exposure, the site of body injury, and the body weight and sensitivity of the victim to the venom. Usually there is a local reaction of a toxic nature.[6,7]

Clinical manifestations

The local reaction immediately after a sting is an acute local dermatitis.[6,7] Usually, a linear, urticarial, painful erythematous eruption follows the whiplike pattern of tentacular contact (Figure 1). The severity of the symptoms ranges from a mild stinging to a marked burning sensation, with pain and severe itching. In some cases, depending upon the age of the sting, the lesions may become vesicular, haemorrhagic, necrotizing or ulcerative.

Subacute and chronic changes include lichenification by persistent rubbing, localized hyperhydrosis, numbness or hyperaesthesia, lymphadenopathy, angioedema, urticaria and, rarely, vascular spasm and skin necrosis (Figure 2). Recurrent linear eruptions at original sting sites without repeated exposure to jellyfish envenomation have been described.[6,7]

The long-term sequelae of stings include keloids, scarring, hypo- and/or hyper-pigmentation, and fat atrophy (Figure 3). Systemic reactions rarely occur with Mediterranean species but occasionally a complex envenomation syndrome may occur. The most common manifestations are headache, malaise, weakness, increased perspiration and lacrimation. Less commonly, ataxia, paresthesiae, dizziness, muscle spasm and arthralgia may occur. Other reported manifestations are fever, chills, nausea and vomiting, diarrhoea, nervousness or extreme mental depression, throat constriction, respiratory depression, and cardiovascular impairment.[6,7] Fatal reactions have not been reported with Physalia physalis or Pelagia nocticula, the most common Mediterranean species.

Diagnosis and treatment

Clinical diagnosis is usually easy. Identification of the Coelenterate responsible for the skin manifestations, if possible, is very useful for management and treatment.

To decrease local reactions, further nematocyst discharge may be avoided by immobilizing the extremity. Toxin may be neutralized in different ways: diluted vinegar (3–10% acetic acid) soaks, sodium bicarbonate mixed with water, local heat (hot seawater 120°F for denaturalization of proteins), and proteolytic meat tenderizers. Never rub or use fresh water or alcohol as the change of tonicity will further activate nematocyst discharge. Tentacles should be removed carefully. In systemic reactions, depending on the severity and the symptomatology, systemic epinephrine or corticosteroid antihistaminics should be prescribed and the patient referred to the emergency department.[6,7]

Dermatitis caused by echinoderms

Mode of contamination

Sea urchins form part of the phylum echynodermata which also includes starfish and sea cucumbers. One of the echinoderm's principal means of defence is an array of sharp and/or toxic spines. Injuries from sea urchin spines are a familiar occupational hazard of fishermen in the Mediterranean area. In addition, the growing popularity of underwater activities among holidaymakers in these regions is presenting many dermatologists with a new diagnostic problem. Awareness of the hazard is the key to proper management.

Sea urchins are spherical organisms found on the rocky bottoms in salt water, although some species prefer to burrow in the sand. They are covered with numerous movable spines, the length of which varies with the species. Formed by the calcification of a cylindrical projection of subepidermal connective tissue, these spines are extremely brittle and may break off easily in the victim's skin. The spines of some species are venomous and may contain a neurotoxin.[2,8]

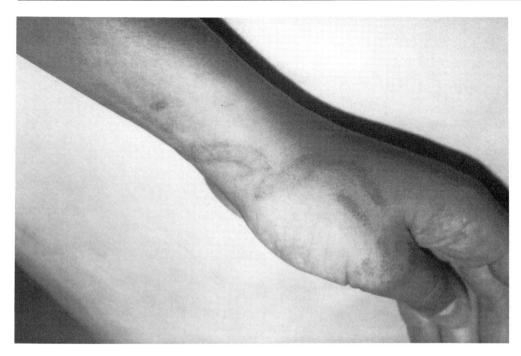

Figure 1

Jellyfish sting (*Pelagia noctiluca*). The immediate local reaction appears as a linear urticarial erythematous eruption following the whip-like pattern of tentacular contact. (Courtesy of Ph. Normand, M. D.)

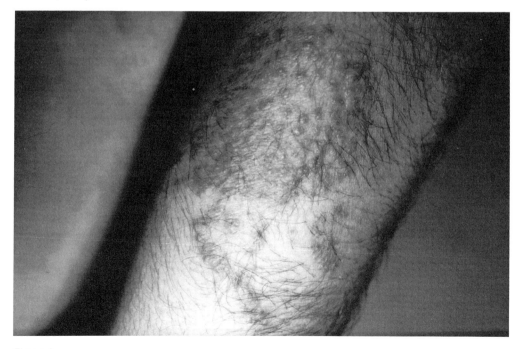

Figure 2

Jellyfish sting. Showing subacute local reaction with large erythematous plaque and multiple granulomas. (Courtesy of Ph. Normand, M. D.)

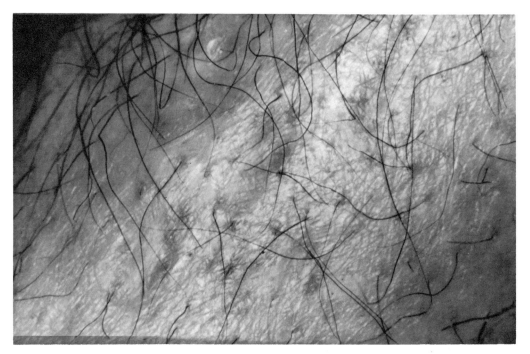

Figure 3

Jellyfish sting showing persistent long-term reaction with scarring and hypopigmentation.

Amongst the spines are pedicellariae (small pincer-like organs or fangs). These organs are attached to stalks that may be shorter or longer than the spines. Venom from the pedicellariae may be injected into the victim's skin via hook-like jaws or valves.[8]

Injury from sea urchins usually results from inadvertently coming into contact with the spines. The wound may occur on the hands as a result of picking the animal up, on the body or extremities by brushing against them or on the soles of the feet by walking in shallow water. Other methods of injury are losing one's balance and falling on them or being pushed by waves against a bed of sea urchins.

Clinical manifestations of injury: sea urchin dermatitis

Multiple puncture wounds occur, which initially produce little discomfort but, within several minutes, severe pain starts which lasts for up to 24 h. The victim instinctively pulls out the spines that are protruding from the skin and observes a black colour around the entrance wound in those species that are black.[8]

Many fragile broken spines may remain embedded in the skin, but the physician should be aware that some sea urchin spines contain a dye that may discolour the patient's skin and subcutaneous tissues, thereby giving the false impression that the spine is still embedded in the skin.[8]

A severe burning pain which may persist for several hours with or without oedema is the chief immediate symptom of sea urchin dermatitis. Some patients bleed profusely. Occasionally the spines may penetrate and remain intact. Although it is stated that the spines are readily reabsorbed, several observations suggest that many are extruded through the surface of the skin. Secondary infection may introduce further complications and may be severe when multiple lesions are present. Infected discharging wounds may be a means by which the tissues get rid of infected spines.

More severe reactions due to sea urchin spine injuries may occur.[8] Local reactions are papules or small nodules which may develop several months after the injury (Figure 4). These lesions may be nodular or diffuse. Lesions of both types are very persistent and, although spontaneous resolution may ultimately occur, it cannot be relied upon as a consistent eventuality. Small firm nodules which are

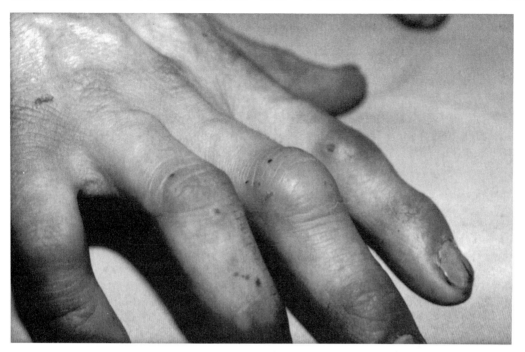

Figure 4

Sea urchin granulomas. The nodular lesions on the fingers of this patient occurred after an interval of two to three months after initial injury. (Courtesy of M. Weiller, M. D.)

granulomatous in nature are quite frequently seen. Some are flesh coloured, while others are violaceous or take on the colours of the dye in the spines. The granulomas that develop in some patients resemble sarcoid histologically. No organisms have been identified in most of these lesions. On rare occasions, examination by polarized light has revealed double refractile spine material. When the spines penetrate through the skin of the hands and feet or over joints a more severe reaction may ensue very soon after the injury, and the patient develops redness, swelling and pain typical of tenosynovitis. In other patients, the symptoms may develop much later with the appearance of subcutaneous nodules. X-Ray examination may reveal spines around the joints or in the tendon when done in the acute cases, while late developing nodules do not regularly show this. If the presence of spines is revealed upon X-ray examination, surgical removal is indicated.

Systemic reactions of sea urchin injuries are relatively uncommon but have been reported from contact with some poisonous species.[7] Symptoms may include nausea, fainting, paraesthesiae, ataxia, muscle weakness and respiratory distress. With subcutaneous injury, symptoms of malaise, fever and pain may be observed. These symptoms are presumably reactions to the inflammatory process.

Treatment

There is no specific treatment for the superficial type of injury other than support.[2,8] Analgesics may be indicated for the pain. If some spines are visible or protruding, one should always attempt to extract them. No attempt should be made to remove them in the way one usually removes a thorn since the spine is very fragile and readily fragments. Careful removal must be performed as soon as possible by a physician under local anaesthesia with specially designed forceps.

Regardless of treatment, superficially embedded lesions take several weeks or months to disappear. Spontaneous extrusion through the skin may be accelerated by white petroleum under occlusion or liquid nitrogen to create blisters. Deeply embedded spines, particularly when they have resulted in the formation of a granulomatous lesion, require excision.

These injuries may be quite severe and require extensive surgery to correct. One form of treatment that has been advocated in the past is crushing the spines by banging the entrance site with a stone. This supposedly fragments the spines into small pieces and allows them to be absorbed more rapidly. If the lithotriptor is easily available this may be used for the same purpose.

Injuries and eruptions caused by venomous fish stings

There are many venomous fish that are equipped with sharp, stout spines capable of easily penetrating human skin.[2,9] Some venomous fish can produce painful serious injuries and even death.

Injury is usually caused by venomous fish spines, but may also be due to poisoning by the fish's cutaneous glandular secretions, foams or slimes that usually produce an irritant contact dermatitis. Venomous marine fishes are present in large numbers in the Mediterranean Sea.

Most fish wounds are passive (the wader stepping on a stingray or a weaverfish) but active stabs also occur (jerky 'attack bounces' by some species such as the weaverfish).

Many injuries occur while fishermen handle their catch and even occur from dead, refrigerated fish in which the poison is still viable.

Stingrays

Stingrays probably constitute the most important group of venomous fish. The stingray can inflict painful and dangerous lacerations by means of dorsal or caudal spines equipped with complex venom glands.[2,9]

Most stingray wounds are acquired via contact with the smaller species which frequent shallow waters around rocky areas and burrow themselves in the sand. Stingrays are not aggressive. When startled, the ray will usually hasten away at great speed, leaving behind a muddy wake. But their habit of lying motionless in shallow water means they are easily stepped on by the unwary bather or wader.[2,9]

Stingray wounds are of either the laceration or puncture type. Penetration of the skin and underlying tissue is usually accomplished without serious damage to the surrounding structures but withdrawal of the sting may result in extensive tissue damage due to the barbed dentinal spines.

Pain is the predominant symptom and usually develops immediately or within 5 min of the attack. The pain has been described as sharp, shooting spasmodic and throbbing in character.[2,9]

More generalized symptoms of a fall in blood pressure, vomiting, diarrhoea, sweating, tachycardia, muscular paralysis and even death have been reported.[2,9]

Although stingray injuries occur most frequently around the ankle joint and foot as a result of stepping on the ray, instances have been reported in which the wounds were in the chest.

Weaverfish

Primarily dwellers of flat sandy or muddy marine bays, weavers are commonly seen burying themselves in the soft sand or mud with only their heads partially exposed. They are the most venomous fish found in the temperate zone. They are found all around the Mediterranean coast. The venom apparatus of weavers consists of the dorsal and opercular spines and associated glands.[2,9] Weavers may dart out rapidly and may strike an object with their opercular spines with unerring accuracy. When a weaver is provoked the dorsal fin is instantly erected and the gill covers expanded.

Weavers produce wounds that usually cause extremely intense pain, or a burning, stabbing or crushing sensation, initially confined to the immediate area of the wound and then spreading through the affected limb. The pain becomes progressively worse until it reaches an excruciating peak generally within 30 min. The severity is such that the victim may scream, thrash wildly about and lose consciousness. The pain commonly subsides within 24 h. Tingling followed by numbness develop around the wound.[2,9]

The skin around the wound is at first blanched, but soon becomes reddened, hot and swollen. The swelling may be quite extensive and continue for 10 days or longer (Figure 5). Oedema and erythema in the area of penetrated skin may simulate bacterial cellulitis. These wounds, notoriously slow in healing, often become infected.[2,9]

As with other venomous fish spines, the weaver sting produces rapid and severe systemic symptoms, including headache, fever, chills, nausea, vomiting, shock, abdominal pain, cyanosis, loss of speech, and tachycardia. Mental depression may be followed by convulsions, difficulty in breathing and even death. Gangrene has been known to develop as a complication.[2,9]

A swimmer stung by a weaver may die if not promptly rescued from drowning.

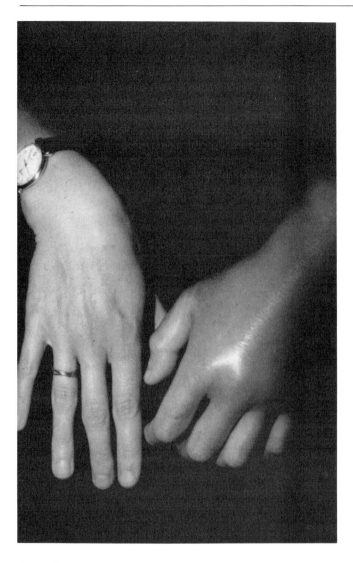

Figure 5

Weeverfish wound. The immediate reaction includes a quite extensive swelling as shown in this patient. (Courtesy of M. Weiller, M. D.)

Stargazers

These venomous fish spend a large part of their time buried in the mud or the sand. Wounds from the Mediterranean species *Uranoscopus scaber* may be fatal.[2]

Treatment

Efforts in treating venomous fish stings should be directed toward achieving three objectives: alleviating pain, combatting the effects of the venom, and preventing secondary infection.[2,9]

The pain results from the effects of the trauma produced by the fish spine and from the venom and the introduction of slimes and other irritating substances into the wound. In the case of stingray stings, the barbs of the spine may produce severe lacerations with considerable trauma to the soft tissues. Wounds of this type should be promptly irrigated or washed-out with salt water or sterile saline if such is available. Fish stings of the puncture wound variety are usually small and removal of the poison is more difficult. It may be necessary to debride the wound surgically in order to apply immediate migration and to remove as much of the venom as possible.[2,9]

Most physicians recommend soaking the injured member in hot water for 30 min to 1 h. The water should be maintained at as high a temperature (115–120°F or 50°C) as the patient can tolerate without injury, and the treatment should be instituted as soon as possible. If the wound is on the face or body, hot moist compresses can be employed.[2,9]

Another, easier way of producing local heat in order to destroy the thermolabile venom at the site of the wound is to hold a lighted cigarette as near as possible to the wound for 5–10 min. The local temperature obtained is about 50–55°C, which may alter the venom since heating readily destroys stringray venom in vitro.[2,9]

Intravenous calcium gluconate injections are sometimes helpful for muscle spasms. Infiltration of the wound area with 0.5–2% lidocaine has been used with good results. If local measures fail to prove satisfactory, narcotic analgesia (naloxone, reversible systemic opiates) are generally effective. Following the soaking procedure, debridement and further cleansing of the wound are mandatory. Wounds should be left open or closed loosely around packing or a small drain. The injured area should be covered with an antiseptic and sterile dressing.[2,9]

Prompt treatment usually eliminates the need for antibiotic therapy. If delay has resulted, the wound should be cultured prior to the administration of antibiotics. Tetanus prophylaxis is standard. Hypotension from the action of venomous fish spines on the cardiovascular system requires immediate and vigorous treatment. Treatment should be directed toward maintaining cardiovascular tone and the prevention of any further complications.[9]

The swimmer's itch and seabather's eruption

Swimmer's itch has also been called seabather's eruption, and clam digger itch, amongst other names.[10] This maculopapular eruption is caused by cercariae of infected animal schistosomes. The cercarial dermatitis may be acquired almost anywhere in the world, although it is more prevalent in fresh water, it may also be acquired in the sea. Cercariae that cause this dermatitis in man usually infect birds, rodents and ungulates. The dermatitis is caused by the destruction of invading cercaria in the human epidermis by a vigorous immune response.[10]

Swimmers do not feel the attacking cercariae. The penetration of skin by larvae causes itching which lasts about 1 h. This is followed within 10–20 h by the rapid development of urticarial wheals. Papules of 3–5 mm surrounded with erythema may coalesce and form large vesicles. They are associated with intense pruritus and may be complicated by excoriations. They disappear within 9–14 days if there is no secondary infection. There is no characteristic distribution of lesions but most patients are affected on skin exposed to water, particularly the surface of the water or where clothing was in contact with skin or in folds of skin.[10]

The diagnosis of cercarial dermatitis is by the characteristic clinical presentation and history. Searching for cercariae in biopsy specimens is futile, as they are already destroyed by the time the patient seeks aid.

Treatment is symptomatic: antihistaminics and antipruritic medications, rubbing with a towel to knock off the cercariae before they can penetrate and topical steroids.[10]

Another eruption called 'seabather's eruption' closely resembles cercarial dermatitis but apparently occurs only in sea water and affects mostly the covered areas (the buttocks and genital area for men, and the buttocks and breasts in women).[11] No obvious cause has been found and it is likely that it is not a specific disorder but caused by such agencies as algal toxins, enidarians, and pteropods as well as cercariae.[11]

Dermatoses due to marine plants

Cutaneous protothecosis or seaweed dermatitis is not observed in the Mediterranean.

Dermatoses due to bacteria and dermatomycoses and viruses

Infections due to bacteria

Most infections resulting from aquatic exposure are due to common micro-organisms (*Staphylococcus aureus*, Gram-negative bacteria) and otitis externa is probably the most common infection observed in bathers. However, the bacterial flora of sea water or fresh water may sometimes cause rapidly fatal infectious diseases. A careful recreational or occupational history may provide a clue to the aetiology. Bacteriologists should be alerted as to the possibility of aquatic bacteria because these organisms are unusual and sometimes difficult to identify.[12]

Bacteria acquired in the sea

Among marine bacteria responsible for distinct clinical disorders, Aeromonas hydrophila is the commonest and the uncommon Vibrio vulnificus is the species associated with the most serious infection.

Aeromonas hydrophyla Aeromonads are Gram-negative, non-sporulating, oxidase positive, facultative anaerobic rods. The primary reservoir of Aeromonas strains in nature is in stagnant or flowing fresh water, in salt water that interfaces with fresh water and in soil. Fishes may carry these organisms or may be infected by them. They have been found at temperatures between 4 and 45°C and are not considered halophilic since their sodium chloride tolerance ranges only from 0 to 4%. Human infections occur predominantly during the period between May and November. These microorganisms are considered opportunistic pathogens of low virulence. Serious infections develop mainly in immunocompromized patients with leukaemia, agranulocytosis or cirrhosis but Aeromonas can cause infections in healthy subjects.[13]

Aeromonas isolated from human sources are most often recovered from gastrointestinal and intra-abdominal sites. A. hydrophila seems to be responsible for a self-limiting cholera-like diarrhoea but it may be recovered in the stools of asymptomatic patients. Skin and soft tissue infections are directly associated with traumatic exposure to water or soil. The bacteria causes abscesses, cellulitis, necrotizing myositis or osteomyelitis. Gas gangrene associated with an A. hydrophila wound infection has been described in rare instances. Ecthyma gangrenosum has also been reported in immunocompromized patients.[14] Disseminated infections occur most often in immunosuppressed patients and may cause septicemia, endocarditis or meningitis. The diagnosis is quite easily made by cultures. However, in cutaneous infections, A. hydrophila is often mixed with other bacteria.

Infection of skin and soft tissues needs to be treated by incision, cleansing and drainage. A parenteral combination of two effective antibiotics is recommended. A. hydrophila is generally sensitive to aminoglycosides, trimethoprim-sulphamethoxazole, third-generation cephalosporins, imipenem and fluoroquinolones.

Vibrios Vibrios are Gram-negative rod-shaped usually curved micro-organisms with predominantly polar flagellae and are facultatively anaerobic. Their normal habitat is water sources. Halophilic Vibrios responsible for human diseases include V. parahaemolyticus, V. alginolyticus, V. vulnificus, V. metschnikowii and V. damsela. Their concentration in sea water is low and the survival of Vibrios depends on salinity, water temperature and associated microbial flora. Vibrios grow best at temperatures between 24 and 40°C and fail to grow at temperatures below 8–10°C. They are most often present in sea water during the warmer months and infections caused by these species are usually reported during this period. Vibrio species should be suspected in any acute infection associated with seafood ingestion or wound infections sustained in a marine environment.[15]

V. alginolyticus is the most frequently acquired Vibrio strain isolated in the Mediterranean. It may cause wound infections but otitis or conjunctivitis are more usual. V. vulnificus causes primary septicemia or severe wound infections. Soft tissue infections may rapidly progress to severe necrotizing cellulitis, myositis or fulminant bacteremia. Primary septicemia is a serious infection with a fatality rate of about 50%. It occurs most often in immunosuppressed patients and is frequently associated with petechiae, necrotic pustules, bullous lesions or ecthyma gangrenosum-like lesions. An infection caused by V. vulnificus was observed in an immunocompromised patient on the French coast of the Mediterranean (personal communication) but there are no other reports of human infection caused by the other species of marine Vibrios acquired in the Mediterranean. However, the possibility of such infections cannot be excluded. V. parahaemolyticus and V. metschnickowii cause vesticular or suppurative skin lesions which may be serious. V. parahaemolyticus is much more common in Japan where fish and other seafoods are eaten raw. V. damsela has also been reported to be responsible for wound infections but its causal role needs support.

Patients with wound infections frequently required surgical debridement and drainage. Serious wound infections should be treated with parenteral administration of two antibiotics. The organism is usually sensitive to tetracycline, trimethoprin-sulphamethoxazole, chloramphenicol, third-generation cephalosporins, imipenem and aminoglycosides. A combination of a tetracycline plus an aminoglycoside is generally recommended.

Erysipelothrix rhusiopathiae   *E. rhusiopathiae* is a Gram-positive facultatively aerobic rod found in fresh and salt water and in the flora of some aquatic animals. The bacterium is resistant, survives salting, drying, pickling and smoking and may be found alive after 12 days in sunlight. Fishermen, sea-food processors, sellers of fish, veterinarians, butchers and farmers represent groups at risk. This disease rarely seems to be acquired during bathing in the Mediterranean. This organism was in fact primarily a pathogen of swine and other animals, producing the disease referred to as swine erysipelas. In humans, the bacteria cause an erysipelas-like infection named erysipeloid, also known as fish-handler's disease and shrimp-picker's disease.[16]

The disease develops a few days after inoculation. It presents as a painful swelling usually localized to a finger, the back of the hand or wrist. The lesions are characterized by an elevated erythematous edge which spreads peripherally as discolouration of the central area fades. Fever and constitutional symptoms are usually mild or absent except when a more generalized infection occurs. Pitting and suppuration are absent. Regional lymph nodes may be inflamed. Disseminated infection may cause septicemia, endocarditis, arthritis, abscess and pulmonary involvement. Skin lesions are not always present in these cases. The diagnosis in the disseminated infection is made from blood culture or tissue samples. In a localized infection the organism may be obtained by a skin biopsy or by injecting saline into the edge of the lesion and then reaspirating without withdrawing the needle. However, skin cultures are often sterile and the diagnosis is usually made on the basis of an appropriate clinical picture with a compatible occupational history. Systemic ampicillin, trimethoprim-sulphamethoxazole or erythromycin are effective.

Mycobacterium marinum   *M. marinum* living in both salt and fresh water is described later.

Management of marine injuries   The role of various treatments for cutaneous injuries acquired in the sea is controversial. Some authors have shown that only mechanical cleansing of the wound is necessary and that antibiotics may be superfluous. One should bear in mind that bacteria recovered from marine injuries are usually similar to bacteria found in common cutaneous infections. However, in a patient at risk, the virulence of some strains of *Vibrios* and *A. hydrophila* may justify giving oral tetracycline or doxycycline for a wound acquired in sea water.[12] Severe *Vibrio* or *Aeromonas* wound infections are rare but should be suspected when tissue necrosis complicates a wound incurred in a marine environment. Antibiotics and surgical debridement are usually required in these cases. A suitable antitetanus immunization regimen should not be forgotten.[17,18]

Bacteria acquired in swimming pools

Infections acquired in swimming pools are rare and generally not severe. The risk of infection is higher in people who bathe in hot swimming pools, especially in whirlpools or spas.

Pseudomonas aeruginosa   *P. aeruginosa* is an aerobic Gram-negative rod recovered from soil, vegetation and water. This organism may proliferate in wet environments of low nutritional value such as swimming pools. It can ever grow in treated water when the free chlorine level falls below 0.5 mg/l or when the pH rises above 8. Despite its ubiquity in the environment, it rarely causes diseases in the competent host. However, outbreaks of a characteristic cutaneous infection due to *P. aeruginosa* may be acquired through bathing in inadequately treated pools. This problem is particularly associated with the use of whirlpools and spas. These devices have a filter arrangement, a heating system and a method of pulsating the water. The water is therefore warm (between 30 and 42°C) and oxygenated. These factors favour multiplication of *P. aeruginosa*.[19] Infections due to *Legionella pneumophila* and *Trichomonas vaginalis*[20] have also been reported in association with the use of spas.

The disease develops in persons who have shared the same bath within 2 days of exposure. The eruption may be follicular, maculopapular, vesicular, pustular or nodular.[21] The rash is distributed predominantly over the lateral aspects of the trunk, in the axillae and on the proximal extremities and buttocks. It does not occur on the palms or soles. This pruritic rash may also be associated with sore eyes, external otitis, mastitis, or axillary lymphadenopathy. Malaise, fever, nausea and urinary or respiratory tract infections have been reported. Clinical features heal spontaneously within

7 to 10 days. In immunocompromised hosts necrotic evolution or systemic involvement may occur leading to serious infection. The disease is generally diagnosed by means of the clinical features. Cutaneous cultures are often negative for P. aeruginosa except from larger pustules; however, the bacteria are easily found in the water of the pool. Most outbreaks of pseudomonal dermatitis have been associated with serotype 0:11, which is the one most commonly isolated from whirlpools. However, other serotypes have also been associated with this disease.[22]

In an immunocompetent patient, antibiotics are not necessary. Acetic acid soaks were proposed but do not appear to shorten the duration of the rash. Prophylactic measures are difficult because the ratio of bathers to water is generally high explaining why infections have occurred despite satisfactory maintenance. Moreover, the classical swimming pool bacteriological standards, of the absence of coliforms and a standard plate count limit of 200 bacteria per millilitre are unreliable guides to the control of P. aeruginosa infection risk in spas, especially when bromination is the mode of disinfection. Both bromination and chlorination are currently recommended for spa disinfection but it seems that chlorination is superior to bromination in reducing the risk of P. aeruginosa infection.[23] Continuous water filtration, maintenance of water with a free residual chlorine level of 1 ppm and a pH of 7.2–7.8 combined with the frequent changing of water reduce P. aeruginosa proliferation.

Mycobacterium marinum M. marinum is an atypical mycobacterium grouped with the photochromogens (Rumyon group I) living in an aquatic environment. It is found in fresh, brackish or salt water, in swimming pools, fish tanks, ocean beaches, rivers and lakes. Poikilothermic water animals such as salt water or freshwater fishes, shrimps, snails and water fleas have been reported as being vectors of human skin infection with M. marinum. Infection occurs as a result of contamination of trivial skin lesions and is frequently connected in some way with an aquatic environment.[24] In rare instances no history of exposure to water is elicited.

The incubation period of the disease is about 2 weeks in most cases and ranges from 1 week to 2 months. The lesions occur on the elbows, knees and feet in swimming-pool-related cases (swimming-pool granuloma) and on the hands and fingers of fish fanciers (fish-tank granuloma). After a few weeks the lesions are typically 1–2.5 cm in diameter. The lesions are described as non-tender inflammatory nodules, as ulcerated granulomata or as verrucous lesions (Figure 6). Occasionally subcutaneous nodules resembling sporotrichosis develop along lymph channels in the involved extremity. Synovial involvement also may occur following penetrating injury. Lymphadenopathy is usually absent. In immunocompromised patients, chronic skin ulcers may be observed. M. marinum is quite often isolated if a skin biopsy is processed at 33°C without removal of bacterial contamination. The bacteria grow optimally at 32°C in about 7–14 days. This psychrophilia may explain the rarity of internal dissemination. Histopathology reveals nonspecific inflammation or tuberculoid granuloma. Direct staining procedures have often failed to demonstrate acid-fast bacilli. Patients infected with M. marinum frequently have persistently positive tuberculin tests.

Excision of a small lesion by biopsy may be curative but adjunctive drug therapy is often needed. Tetracycline (usually 200 mg/day) is the drug of choice and should be continued for several weeks after clinical improvement. Some strains of M. marinum have been shown to be resistant to doxycycline.[25] Alternative therapies include rifampicin (often combined with ethambutol), sulphamethoxazole-trimethoprim or ciprofloxacin. The disease seems to be very unlikely to be transmitted via the water of swimming pools having residual chlorine levels of 2 mg/l or more.

Swimmer's ear Infection of the external ear canal causes more morbidity in those who engage in aquatic activities than any other infectious disease. Moisture retention is the main cause of this disorder as well as mechanical factors. *Pseudomonas* and *Staphylococcus* are the most common bacteria responsible for these infections but many other micro-organisms including fungi can be found. 'Swimmer's ear' develops in a few hours or days after exposure to water;[26] in contrast, symptoms of otitis media manifest themselves immediately. The signs of otitis externa include itching or pain in the ear canal and the feeling that the ear is 'wet' or 'full'. The definitive stage is characterized by suppuration and hearing may sometimes be impaired. Some complications may rarely occur including middle ear infection, cellulitis or the exceptional malignant otitis externa in a diabetic or immunocompromised patient.

Treatment is first directed at reducing the moisture in the ear canal. One of the most effective preparations for this purpose is a solution of 97% absolute alcohol and 3% glacial acetic acid. One

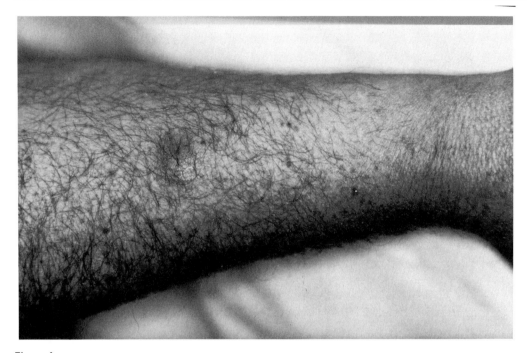

Figure 6

Cutaneous *Mycobacterium marinum* infection showing a typical erythematous nodular lesion.

should not use cotton-tipped applications which may worsen the disorder. If suppuration is present, antibiotic ear drops are given. Oral or intravenous antibiotics should be used if the infection does not resolve with these measures or if cellulitis is present. Prevention, especially for a person at risk, is accomplished by lessening the moisture in the external canal. Vigorously shaking the head or jumping with the head tilted to one side or using a hair dryer are the best means of preventing problems.[26]

Infections due to fungi

Hydration and maceration are well known to favour fungal infections but pityriasis versicolor and tinea pedis are the most frequent dermatomycoses associated with bathing.[27]

Pityriasis versicolor

Pityriasis versicolor is caused by the filamentous form of *Pityrosporum orbiculare*. The disease is most common in 10–30-year-olds with an increase in the hotter months. This may be a true increase or may be due to the hypopigmentation becoming more evident when tanning of the normal skin occurs. Sand abrasion of the skin and frequent application of oil may also favour this disease. Pityriasis versicolor is characterized by unobtrusive, scaly macules without marked inflammation, which may be hypo- or hyper-pigmented and which fluoresce yellow under Wood's light.

Tinea pedis

The presence of abrasive dust between the toes and the difficulty to getting toe webs adequately dry after bathing favour the development of tinea pedis, but occlusion by shoes is the most important factor.

Infections due to viruses

Plantar warts have frequently been associated with barefoot gymnastics or bathing. They are readily spread from person to person by contamination of the floor areas around the pool.

Swimming baths also seem to be an area of acquisition of molluscum contagiosum because outbreaks are occasionally seen in swimmers. It is believed that the structure of skin, which is changed by prolonged exposure to water, is of importance in determining the outcome of infection.[28]

Among other viruses the enteroviruses (Coxsackievirus and Echovirus) may theoretically be transmitted by swimming-pool water and outbreaks of conjunctivitis due to Adenovirus have also been reported after bathing.[29]

Contact dermatitis to swimming-pool disinfectants and diving equipment

Swimming-pool disinfectants

Chlorine is the most widely used swimming-pool disinfectant. Irritant and allergic reactions are very rare. A burning sensation at the tip of the penis, augmented by urination but without dermatitis has been reported in swimming pool users. Chlorinated swimming-pool water may also produce contact urticaria.[30]

Similar reactions have been described with sodium hypochloride, a swimming-pool disinfectant which is also present in many other products such as Dakin's solution and Eau de Javel.

Bromine is much less used as a swimming-pool disinfectant than chlorine and irritant dermatitis as well as allergic reactions are extremely unusual. Iodine has also been proposed for this use. It has been claimed that iodine offers several advantages over chlorine — including better disinfectant stability, with any irritation to bathers being of a very low order.[30]

It is sometimes necessary to use other products such as copper solutions or quaternary ammonium compounds to control algae. A very peculiar side-effect attributed to the use of copper algicides in swimming pools has been described. This is a green discoloration of the scalp hair in blond individuals. Regular shampooing decreases the tint and immersion of the hair in 3% peroxide solution will remove the green colour in a couple of hours.[30]

Diving equipment

Most diving equipment including underwater masks, mouth pieces, diving suits, swimming goggles, nose clips, ear plugs, fins and fin straps may produce allergic contact dermatitis occurring in rubber-sensitive patients.[30]

The skin reaction to the mask may vary from a reddish imprint on the face to a severe painful, sometimes disabling eruption characterized by vesiculation, weeping and crusting. Intra-oral irritation and inflammation accompanied by vesiculation of the oral mucosa gingiva and tongue may develop in patients who become sensitized to the mouthpiece.[30]

Contact dermatitis of the neck, trunk and extremities has been described in some divers whenever they wore their rubber diving suit.

A raccoon-like periorbital leukodermia has been described from contact with swim goggles. A toxic reaction has been postulated to have occurred from chemicals (a zinc bis(diethylcarbamothio) compound, a phenol methylene bis compound and a diethylthiourea) that leaked from the goggles and were eventually exhausted.[30]

In some cases, the chemicals in the equipment were the allergen responsible for these reactions. The causative chemical compounds identified by patch testing include the rubber antioxidant N-isopropyl-N-phenylparaphenylenediamine, N/N-diethylurea used to cement the nylon lining to the rubber diving suit, ethylbutylthiourea used as an accelerator, dibutylthiourea, and mercaptobenzothiazole. For patients who experience severe or frequent reactions, the use of 'hypoallergenic' diving equipment is mandatory.[30]

Windsurfing and boat equipment

Contact hand dermatitis may arise from rubber on wishbone handles. Contact with the back support may result in contact dermatitis on the abdomen.

Aquatic-sport-related dermatoses

Various traumas may occur during aquatic sports. Water-ski-cord strangulation around a wrist or an ankle may induce a wound, leaving a more or less deep scar. Corns and callosities of palms and soles are very common in windsurfers. In decompression sickness, the skin is also affected, showing erythema or pallor. Mottling is important as it can be a harbinger of the delayed onset of more serious problems. Nitrogen rash is seen in scuba divers when they stay beyond the time planned at a given depth. The transient rash consists of tender, pruritic erythematous lesions involving predominantly the elbows and the flanks.[31,32]

References

1. Mandojana RM, Letot B, Historical outlook of aquatic biotoxicology and balneology as related to dermatology: classification of aquatic dermatoses, *Clin Dermatol* (1987) **5**: 1–7.
2. Fisher AA, *Atlas of aquatic dermatology*, Academic Press: London, 1978, p. 113.
3. Genolier-Weiller A, Thesis, Marseille, 1987.
4. Steinman HK, Water-induced pruritus, *Clin Dermatol* (1987) **5**: 41–8.
5. Panconesi E, Lotti T, Aquagenic urticaria, *Clin Dermatol* (1987) **5**: 49–51.
6. Halstead BW, Coelenterate (Cnidarian) stings and wounds, *Clin Dermatol* (1987) **5**: 8–13.
7. Burnett JW, Calton GJ, Burnett HW et al, Local and systemic reactions from jellyfish stings, *Clin Dermatol* (1987) **5**: 14–28.
8. Baden HP, Injuries from sea urchins, *Clin Dermatol* (1987) **5**: 112–7.
9. Halstead BW, Vinci JM, Venomous fish stings (Ichthyoacanthotoxicoses), *Clin Dermatol* (1987) **5**: 29–35.
10. Baird JK, Wear DJ, Cercarial dermatitis: the swimmer's itch, *Clin Dermatol* (1987) **5**: 88–91.
11. Bernhardt MJ, Mandojana RM, 'Seabather's eruption', *Clin Dermatol* (1987) **5**: 101–2.
12. Auerbach PS, Natural microbiologic hazards of the aquatic environment, *Clin Dermatol* (1987) **5**: 52–61.
13. Dean HM, Post RM, Fatal infection with *Aeromonas hydrophila* in a patient with acute myelogenous leukemia, *Ann Intern Med* (1967) **66**: 1177.
14. Shackelford PG, Ratzan SA, Shearer WT, Ecthyma gangrenosum produced by *Aeromonas hydrophila*, *J Pediatr* (1973) **83**: 100–1.
15. Bonner JR, Coker AS, Berryman CR et al, Spectrum of *Vibrio* infections in a Gulf coast community, *Ann Intern Med* (1983) **99**: 464–9.
16. Klauder JV, Erysipeloid as an occupational disease, *J Am Med Assoc, Part III* (1938): 1345–8.
17. Pien FD, Ang KS, Nakashima NT et al, Bacterial flora of marine penetrating injuries, *Diagn Microbiol Infect Dis* (1983) **1**: 229–32.
18. Meislin HW, Lerner SA, Graves MH et al, Cutaneous abscess. Anaerobic and aerobic bacteriology and outpatient management, *Ann Intern Med* (1977) **87**: 145–9.
19. Jones F, Bartlett CLR, Infections associated with whirlpools and spas, *J Appl Bacteriol Symp* (1985) (suppl): 61S–6S.
20. Piekarski G, Saathoff M, *Trichomonas vaginalis* infections due to use of public swimming pools? *Immun Infect* (1973) **1**: 22–5.
21. Sausker WF, *Pseudomonas aeruginosa*. Folliculitis ('splash rash'), *Clin Dermatol* (1987) **5**: 62–7.
22. Gustafson TL, Band JD, Hutcheson RH Jr, et al, *Pseudomonas folliculitis*: an outbreak and review, *Rev Infect Dis* (1983) **5**: 1–8.
23. Shaw JH, A retrospective comparison of the effectiveness of bromination and chlorination in controlling *Pseudomonas aeruginosa* in spas (Whirlpools) in Alberta, *Can J Publ Hlth* (1984) **75**: 61–8.
24. Johnston JM, Izumi AK, Cutaneous mycobacterium marinum infection ('Swimming pool granuloma'), *Clin Dermatol* (1987) **5**: 68–75.
25. Lyungberg B, Christensson B, Grubb R, Failure of doxycycline treatment in aquarium-associated *Mycobacterium marinum* infections, *Scand J Infect Dis* (1987) **19**: 539–43.
26. Strauss MB, Dierker RL, Otitis extern associated with aquatic activities (swimmer's ear), *Clin Dermatol* (1987) **5**: 103–11.
27. Taplin D, Superficial mycoses, *J Invest Dermatol* (1976) **67**: 177–80.
28. Bader RE, Gehäuftes Vorkommen von Molluscum contagiosum in Bereich eines Schwimmbades, *Archiv Hygiene Bakteriol* (1967) **151**: 388–91.
29. Schmidt OW, Cooney MK, Foy HM, Adeno-associated virus in adenovirus type 3 conjunctivitis, *Infect Immun* (1975) **11**: 1362–70.
30. Fisher AA, Contact dermatitis to diving equipment, swimming pool chemicals, and other aquatic denizens, *Clin Dermatol* (1987) **5**: 36–40.
31. Mandojana RM, Sims JK, Miscellaneous dermatoses associated with the aquatic environment, *Clin Dermatol* (1987) **5**: 134–45.
32. Mandojana RM, Mini atlas of aquatic dermatologic lesions, *Clin Dermatol* (1987) **5**: 146–54.

61
The role of animals in the spread of fungal skin infections in humans

Christine M. Philpot
Mycology Unit, Department of Medical Microbiology, University Hospital of Wales, Heath Park, Cardiff, UK

As a general rule, the interaction of humans and animals in the transmission of fungal infections is not very great. As the fungi responsible are environmental organisms, humans and animals are exposed and acquire infection in a similar manner. For example, before the agent of blastomycosis was isolated from the soil, it was postulated that it must be present since dogs left out in the open in the endemic area acquired the disease. If the word 'animals' is taken to include other fauna, certain of the fungi causing systemic mycoses are found in association with birds, bats and rodents, e.g. *Histoplasma* and *Cryptococcus* are present in bird and bat faeces because of nitrogenous compounds present that enhance growth, and *Coccidioides* is present in rodent burrows where the fungus survives adverse weather conditions. However, the birds, bats and rodents do not transmit infection to man. One group of fungi, however, has a direct connection with both man and animals, causing infection in both, and some of these fungi are transmitted directly to man from animal hosts. This group is the dermatophytes or ringworm fungi. Dermatophyte fungi have the ability to break down keratin. Many soil fungi also possess keratinases, but are never pathogenic, presumably because they are unable to break down the keratins of humans and animals. Some of the ringworm fungi are similar. They live in the soil and are rarely pathogenic. The species most often isolated, *Microsporum gypseum*, produces low-grade infections, particularly in persons exposed to enriched soil, such as gardeners, or in animals.[1,2] Other species have become adapted to an existence on human keratin only.

A third group contains those species that have become adapted to life on animal keratin but which have the ability to attack human keratin as well, usually causing infection with much inflammation. Many of these species are host specific (Table 1), although they can and do infect other exposed animals. Not all these species have been recorded in the UK, or are found commonly here. Table 2 shows the range of species isolated in a veterinary practice over a 2.5-year period: six species are represented. It may be noted that *M. persicolor*, a fungus found on wild rodents, was isolated from dogs, *M. equinum* was isolated from farm dogs and cats, and *T. verrucosum* from a small herd of goats kept in a field in which cattle had been grazed earlier in the year.[3] These fungi can also be transmitted directly to humans. Acquisition may be by contact, the handling of an infected animal. For

Table 1 Animals as hosts for ringworm fungi.

Fungus	Main host
Microsporum spp.	
M. canis	Cat, dog
M. equinum	Horse
M. persicolor	Rodents
M. nanum	Pig
M. racemosum	Rat
Trichophyton spp.	
T. mentagrophytes	Rodents
T. erinacei	Hedgehog
T. equinum	Horse
T. verrucosum	Cattle
T. simii	Monkey
T. gallinae	Poultry, game birds

Table 2 Isolation of zoophilic ringworm fungi in veterinary practice.

	Dog	Cat	Goat	Horse
Microsporum canis	5	12		
M. equinum	1	1		8
M. persicolor	2			
Trichophyton mentagrophytes	1	3		
T. equinum				1
T. verrucosum*	1		3	

* T. verrucosum is under-reported since it is known to be present in the cattle in the area. It is usually diagnosed clinically without recourse to the laboratory.

example, ringworm of a very inflammatory, pustular type, was diagnosed in two women who had been caring for a hedgehog; they developed lesions on their hands, and the hedgehog was also infected. The same fungus, T. erinacei, was isolated from both human and animals cases.[4]

Cattle ringworm is endemic in the United Kingdom, as in most of the world, primarily in cattle (but other large ruminants may also have the fungus). Human infections with this fungus usually give a history of contact with these animals, such as in the case of a young girl who developed a lesion on her nose after being in contact with cows on holiday. Other cases seen in the Mycology Unit of the Department of Microbiology in the University Hospital of Wales (UHW) (Cardiff) are given in Tables 3 and 4 which also list infections due to M. canis, the cat ringworm fungus. Contact within a family with an infected cat, or kitten (often recently acquired), or with a dog, may give rise to a small cluster of cases, as illustrated in Table 4.

Table 3 *Trichophyton verrucosum* infections in the dermatology out-patient clinic of UHW Cardiff 1985–90.

Sex	Age (years)	Site	Clinical/epidemiological information
M	14	Arm	Lives on farm
M	28	Wrist	Farm worker
M	15	Thigh	Many animals
F	7	Arm	Very inflamed lesion. Exposure to cattle
F	11	Nose	Inflamed lesion tip of nose. Contact with animals including cows on holiday
M	1	Scalp	Lives on farm
F	4	Face	Eczema? Ringworm?

Acquisition of fungus from an animal may be indirect. For example, a patient developed a ring-like lesion on her back, which was followed 2 weeks later by the appearance of a second lesion on her shoulder. Her general practitioner diagnosed ringworm and advised her to take her cat to the veterinary practice. The cat also had an obvious infection, on its pinna with hair loss and scaling, and both the human and the animal case yielded M. canis. The girl, however, denied all direct contact with the cat, and thus she must have acquired her infection from picking up shed cat hairs and scales. Reports of the length of time for which fungus remains viable in such shed materials varies, but T. erinacei has been isolated from abandoned dry hedgehog nests after up to 1 year,[5] and, recently, T. verrucosum has been isolated from cattle hairs kept in a dry condition for over 1 year. It is probable that in dry conditions fungus will remain viable for a considerable period of time, but if the scales or hairs become wet overgrowth of bacteria and saprophytic moulds will prevent the growth of the ringworm fungus.[5] This indirect contact must be the way in which two cases of hedgehog ringworm recorded in the Mycology Unit were acquired: one case in a gardener who had no other relevant contact, and the other in a geologist who went out frequently into the field. Both patients had lesions on their hands. Contact with the original source of the fungus may be even more indirect; M. persicolor was isolated from the cheek of a child seen in the Dermatology Outpatient Clinic. The only relevant history was of contact with a cat that had 'bald patches'. If the cat was the source, it must have acquired its fungus from a wild rodent, and thus become an intermediary in transmission.

In all these cases, the clinical diagnosis was of ringworm, which was proven mycologically, and the relevant contact or source could be traced or indicated. If the clinical lesion is not diagnosed as ringworm, the connection with animals may be missed or delayed. This was the case in a patient who gave a history of the appearance of a single lesion, followed by the appearance of many lesions simultaneously. The preliminary diagnosis was of pityriasis rosea. However, the lesions were rather atypical, and scrapings were taken to exclude ringworm. Instead fungus was seen, and M. canis was isolated. On questioning, it was found that the patient owned a cat and a dog, and was in contact with neighbouring cats. Her own cat had bald patches from which M. canis was isolated. Both patient and animal were treated successfully with

Table 4 *Microsporum canis* infections in dermatology seen at the outpatient clinic of UHW Cardiff 1985–90.

Sex	Age (years)	Site	Clinical/epidemiological information
	Contact with cat and/or dog (animal not always infected)		
F	3	Scalp	Scalp scaling and hair loss. *Cat at home*
M	35	Body	Scaly rash? *Animal ringworm*
F	19	Abdomen	*Cat for 4 months, said to be healthy*
F	21	Arm	Contact with *cats* in the West Indies. Four lesions
M	10	Scalp	Two bald patches. Two other siblings affected. *Dog*
F	31	Face	Owns *cat*
M	8	Scalp	Scaly boggy patch on scalp. Mother lesions on leg, ankle. History of contact with *kitten with skin problems*. Other siblings not affected but patient had more contact. Mother's lesions developed after kitten removed from home
F	10	Chest	Clinical psoriasis, with scaly annular erythema. Had been on a *riding holiday*
M	7	Scalp	Mother and sister have lesions. *Cat with ringworm*
M	31	Back	Small inflamed scaly lesions over back and chest. Wife also has lesions. *Kitten recently acquired*
F	22	Forearm	Scaly patch. Owns *four cats*
M		Scalp	Three children with ringworm of scalp. Mother has lesion on body. *Two kittens with no lesions, one dog with lesion on the head*
F	24	Body	Atypical lesions over arms and back. *Contact with cat with lesions, also with dog*
F	7	Scalp	Typical bald scaly patch back of head. Sister lesion on upper shoulder. *Intermittent contact with cats. Dog in house, no obvious lesions*
F	1	Scalp	Typical bald patch side of head. *History of stray kitten*. Other family members also infected
	No contact with cats/dogs reported		
M	7	Scalp	Brother also has ringworm
M	6	Scalp	Scaly patchy alopecia
M	10	Face	Also on shoulder
M	5	Body	*Impetigo? Tinea?*
F	29	Arm	Scaly rash
F	33	Body	Multiple annular lesions on arms, neck and face. *Impetigo? Tinea?*
M	26	Body	Scaly rash, clinically ringworm
M	56	Thigh	*Impetigo? Tinea?*
F	21	Leg	Itchy rash. Recently in Greece. Fungus?
M	4	Scalp	*Clinically eczema*. Scalp scaling
F	18	Body	*Impetigo? Tinea?*
M	24	Body	Scattered patches. Other family members also
F	17	Face	Circular scaly patch. *Has eczema*
M	9	Scalp	*To exclude tinea capitis*

griseofulvin, and there has been no further outbreak of ringworm. Had the diagnosis of ringworm not been made, the patient would not have been cured, and the cat could have been a potential source of ringworm to other animal and human contacts.

The most serious aspect of the transmission of ringworm from animals to humans concerns the presence among the animal population of 'carriers', that is animals who carry fungus (often in considerable quantity) but show no signs of infection themselves. Cats, particularly long-haired cats, are often found by chance to harbour fungus. One survey found that up to 35% of long-haired cats attending a cat show yielded *M. canis* from brushings.[6] Often the first indication that a cat is carrying fungus is the development of lesions in another animal or in a human. For example, the presence of cat ringworm in a breeding cattery may not be suspected until a cat is sold and transmits its fungus to cat contacts or to its human owner; the cat itself shows no signs. Carrier states have also been reported in hedgehogs and rodents.[1]

It is possible to detect the presence of carriage in cats and other animals by using the Mackenzie hairbrush technique. A modification of this, using toothbrushes, has been used very successfully in the Mycology Unit at Cardiff to detect the presence of the carriage of *M. canis* in apparently normal cats, and to monitor the course of treatment of an infected cat. The toothbrush is brushed over the animal, and then pressed on to the surface of agar plates using an appropriate agar such as Dermatophyte Test Medium. This is a quick and efficient way of surveying a large number of animals.

Animals thus have a direct role in the transmission of ringworm to humans. Although the diagnosis may be obvious, and the relevant animal contact identified, this is not always the case. Animal derived ringworm is often very inflammatory and mimics acute infections such as bacterial impetigo. Such infections may be treated with antibacterial agents, and only later shown to be fungus; such cases have been seen in Dermatology Outpatient Clinics at the University Hospital of Wales, usually on an exposed site such as the face or leg. Appropriate laboratory investigations are most important in helping to elucidate such cases. The isolation of a species of ringworm fungus of the animal type should always be followed by the relevant epidemiological investigation, particularly in view of the presence of animal 'carriers'. Unless an animal contact is traced, it may remain a potential source of ringworm for other animals and humans. The use of the hairbrush technique may be most helpful in tracking down such carriers.

References

1 Philpot CM, Some aspects of the epidemiology of *Tinea*, *Mycopathologia* (1977) **62**: 3–13.
2 Philpot CM, Westcott G, Stewart JG, Microsporum gypseum ringworm, *Vet Rec* (1984) **114**: 22–3.
3 Philpot CM, Arbuckle JBR, *Trichophyton verrucosum* infection of goats, *Vet Rec* (1984) **114**: 550.
4 Philpot CM, Bowen RG, Hazards from hedgehogs. Two case reports with a survey of the epidemiology of hedgehog ringworm, *Clin Exp Dermatol* (in press).
5 English MG, Morris P, *Trichophyton mentagrophytes* var. *erinacei* in hedgehog nests, *Sabouraudia* (1969) **7**: 118–21.
6 Quaife RA, Womar SM, *Microsporum canis* isolations from show cats, *Vet Rec* (1982) **110**: 333–4.

62
Dermatophytes and human frequentation: a mycological environmental study

R. Mercantini, G. C. Fuga, D. Moretto and W. Marmo
S. Maria e S. Gallicano Dermatological Institute, Roma, Italy

Mammals shed hair and scale continuously and deposit these keratinous materials in their habitat. If this material is parasitized by keratinophilic fungi, it is logical to believe that humans and/or other mammals affected by dermatomycoses may spread fungal spores in proportion to the presence of the infected animal in that particular environment. In the study described here, we aimed to develop this hypothesis. Our first study was carried out in the National Park of Abruzzo (NPA), the only park of this kind in central Italy. The NPA was established in 1923 and to some extent has been protected from environmental alterations and human interference. Because of these characteristics, this park was chosen as the reference point for our study.[1]
The main characteristics of the NPA may be briefly summarized as follows. On an area of about 40 km^2 there are three small villages, each inhabited by a few thousand people. There are mountains covered by dense vegetation, a few valleys, a small river (The Sangro) and an artificial lake. The vegetation is mainly composed of beech tree (*Fagus silvatica*). The chamois (*Rupicapra rupicapra ornata*) represents the most common indigenous species of wildlife. A few dozen bears (*Ursus arctos marsicanus*) and a very few wolves (*Canis lupus italicus*) are also present. In the summer, the mountain prairies are visited by a few hikers and herds of sheep brought by the local shepherds according to old livestock traditions. Tourists increase the local population in the valley areas. Some parts of the park are completely inaccessible while others are strictly patrolled, being completely natural reserves.

Samples were taken from the surface layer of the soil in 161 different areas. To compare poorly populated areas like NPA with small areas that are more densely populated by similar animal species, we examined the soil of cages of wild animals as well as the enclosures of the zoo of NPA in Pescasseroli.[2] Using sterile procedures 20 samples were taken from the soil in enclosures and cages of wolves, foxes, roe, deer, bears, goshawks, kites, eagles, small birds and small mammals typical of the local fauna.

We also studied the microflora of public parks and gardens in various areas of Rome — areas that are much more frequented than the NPA. Samples were taken from the surface layer of the soil in 35 different areas.[3] As with the NPA, we also studied the zoological garden of Rome.[4] In particular, skin scrapings from different caged animals including birds, animals with both short and long hair, and with both thick and thin fur, were analysed. To obtain representative samples from closed areas we investigated some schools in Rome, and some airplanes, ferry boats and trains. We examined dust collected from the floors of 60 classrooms in different Roman schools: 20 kindergartens (children aged 2–5 years), 20 primary schools (aged 6–11 years) and 20 secondary schools (aged 11–14 years).[5,6]

In summary, we investigated various types of public transport (airplanes, ferry boats and trains) because these different forms of transport all carry many individuals who differ in age, race, origin and habits who share the same limited space while travelling. Moreover, the furnishings provide a microenvironment in which even very small particles, such as scales or hairs, can be found.

We studied the dust sucked from the floors of 20 Alitalia aircraft[7,8] on their arrival in Rome from various countries, of 10 ferry-boats of the Italian railways, arriving at Civitavecchia, the commercial harbour of Rome, from Olbia in Sardinia,[9] and of 11 trains of the Italian railway on their arrival in Rome from both Italian and other cities.[10]

It should be noted that not only did the NPA and the various vehicles studied differ in the degree of human frequentation, they also differed in the type of surfaces in the two habitats. Because the material collected differed so markedly, different microbiological techniques had to be employed. In NPA and the public gardens and parks of Rome we collected samples of the superficial layers of the soil. The samples were placed in sterile cellophane bags and sealed. Each sample was distributed to 10 sterilized Petri dishes of 10 cm diameter (30 g of soil per dish) and periodically moistened with sterilized water. Fragments of horse-hair previously sterilized in an autoclave at 120°C for 20 min were scattered onto the soil surface in the dishes. The dishes were incubated at 25°C for 180 days. Every other day, each dish was examined on alternate days at $25 \times$ magnification under a stereoscopic microscope. Mycelium growing on the horse-hair was periodically collected, deposited on dishes containing Mycosel agar (BBL), and incubated at 27°C. The colonies were then transferred to Sabouraud's dextrose agar (BBL) or to Phytone yeast extract, for the period necesssary for the growth of perfect forms and their identification.

In the zoos of NPA and Rome, samples were collected by brushing animals with sterilized brushes. The tips of the brush bristles were placed in Mycosel agar which was then poured into Petri dishes. The dishes were incubated at 27°C and observations were made from 24 h until 1 month after inoculation.

The dust taken from the floors and seats of the schools, aircraft, ferries and trains was weighed and placed in sterile flasks. An aqueous solution, containing gentamycin sulphate (2 mg/ml; Gentalyn, Essex), 1-chloramphenicol (20 mg/ml; Chemicetina Carlo Erba) and Nystatin (2000 IU/ml; Mycostatin Squibb) was added to the flasks. The total volume of the suspension was adjusted according to the amount of dust collected so that the concentration of the various antibiotics was kept constant. The flasks were placed on a rotary thermostat (New Brunswick Psycrotherm G-26) at 250 rpm with an eccentric rotation of 2 cm, at a temperature of 27°C for 24 h. The suspension was distributed uniformly onto the surface of the isolation medium (Mycosel agar BBL) in Petri dishes of 12 cm diameter (0.2/0.3 ml of suspension per dish). The dishes were incubated at 27°C and examined every 24–48 h over a period of 30 days. The fungal colonies which developed were isolated and transferred into tubes of Sabouraud's dextrose agar for identification.

Results

In the 161 samples from the NPA, no pathogenic fungi were found. In the soil from the cages and enclosures of the zoological garden of NPA, *Microsporum gypseum* was isolated from two samples: one from the deer enclosure and one from the bear enclosure.

In the samples taken from the parks of Rome, the most frequently found species was *Microsporum gypseum* (31 positive samples) A strain of *Microsporum canis* was isolated from a soil sample collected from the garden of the S. Gallicano hospital.

A total of 115 animals in the zoological garden of Rome were examined. Of these two leopards, one ox and one donkey were positive for *Microsporum gypseum* and one wild-boar was positive for *Microsporum nanum*.

Of the 60 samples taken from classrooms, one was positive for *Epidermophyton floccosum*, six for *Microsporum canis*, 10 for *Microsporum gypseum* and two for *Trichophyton mentagrophytes*. It is interesting to note that the sample positive for *Epidermophyton floccosum* was found in a secondary school.

From the dust from the seats and floors of 20 Alitalia aircraft we isolated three strains of *Epidermophyton floccosum*, two strains of *Microsporum canis* and one of *Microsporum gypseum*.

Of the ferry boat samples two were positive for *Epidermophyton floccosum*, three for *Microsporum canis*, four for *Microsporum gypseum*, and two for *Trichophyton mentagrophytes*.

Of the 11 train samples, eight were positive for *Epidermophyton floccosum*, 10 for *Microsporum canis*, and one for *Trichophyton tonsurans*.

Because unequal numbers of samples were taken from the various environments, it is only useful to discuss the percentage positivity. *Epidermophyton floccosum* was present in four environments (schools, aircraft, ferry boats and trains); the highest positive readings (72%) were found for trains. *Microsporum canis* was present in five different environments, with the highest frequency of recovery being from the trains (91%). *Microsporum gypseum* was the most widespread of the dermatophytes, with the greatest positivity being found for the samples from the public parks of Rome but with significant values for ferry boats and trains as well. *Microsporum nanum*, as already mentioned, was isolated from the hair of the wild-boar in the Rome zoo. *Trichophyton mentagrophytes* was present in three environments with high human frequentation, particularly trains which showed 73% positivity. *Trichophyton tonsurans* was only found on trains (9%).

We also examined keratinophilic fungi whose pathogenicity is uncertain. Among these were two strains of *Microsporum vanbreuseghem*: one from a school in Rome and the other from the soil of a small park in S. Andrea al Quirinale, Rome. *Trichophyton ajelloi*, *Microsporum cookei* and *Trichophyton terrestre* were isolated in all the environments studied. We also studied the genus *Chrysosporium* (of very low pathogenicity) which in certain cases was isolated in pure culture from nail diseases. The species *Keratinophilum* and *Tropicum* were also found in every environment. In particular 120 samples were positive for *Keratinophilum* and 61 for *Tropicum*. The species *Pannorum*, isolated from 102 samples, was present in every environment except the zoo in the NPA.

From these results it appears that the difference in the microflora from the different environments are in proportion to the degree of human frequentation which becomes an appreciable problem in closed environments. The NPA is a low human frequentation zone; not only were the number of the keratinophilic strains isolated significantly low but also there were no pathogenic species. In the open areas with moderate human or animal frequentation, of a total of 160 samples the percentage that were positive for dermatophytes was 22.96% with 0.6% being positive for *Microsporum canis*, 21.76% for *Microsporum gypseum* and 0.6% for *Microsporum nanum*. In much visited environments, such as schools, airplanes, trains and ferry boats (101 samples), the percentage positivity for dermatophytes was 67%, with 14% being positive for *Epidermophyton floccosum*, 21% for *Microsporum canis*, 19% for *Microsporum gypseum*, 12% for *Trichophyton mentagrophytes* and 1% for *Trichophyton tonsurans*. The results obtained are interesting, but need further in-depth investigation. Our present research is directed to this end.

Acknowledgements

This work has been accomplished thanks to Banco di Santo Spirito-Cassa di Risparmio di Roma and ACRAF Angelini.

The videotape 'Dermatophytes and human frequentation: a mycological environmental study' was awarded *cum laude* and with the special award for excellent scientific value by the jury of the Medikinale International Parma 91.

References

1 Marsella R, Mercantini R, Keratinophilic fungi isolated from soil of the Abruzzo National Park, *Mycopathologia* (1986) **97**: 97–107.
2 Mercantini R, Marsella R, Caprilli F, Isolation of keratinomicetes from the soil of wild animal cages and enclosures in the zoo of the National Park of Abruzzo, Italy, *Sabouraudia* (1978) **16**: 285–6.
3 Mercantini R, Marsella R, Caprilli F et al, Isolation of dermatophytes and correlated species from the soil of public gardens and parks in Rome, *Sabouraudia* (1980) **18**: 123–8.
4 Marsella R, Mercantini R, Spinelli P et al, Occurrence of keratinophilic fungi in animals of the zoological park of Rome, *Mycosen* (1985) **28**: 507–12.
5 Mercantini R, Marsella R, Lambiase L et al, Isolation of keratinophilic fungi from floors in riioman primary schools, *Mycopathologia* (1983) **82**: 115–20.
6 Mercantini R, Marsella R, Lambiase L et al, Isolation of keratinophilic fungi from floors in roman kindergarten and secondary schools, *Mycopathologia* (1986) **94**: 109–15.
7 Dal Fabbro G, Giammarruto R, Fuga GC et al, Primi risultati sull'isolamento di miceti cheratinofili dalla polvere di aerei di rotte intercontinentali Alitalia (First results on isolation of keratinophilic fungi from dust of intercontinental Alitalia aircraft), *Min Aerospaziale* (1985) **16**: 53–4.
8 Fuga GC, Mercantini R, Prignano G et al, Isolation of keratinophilic fungi from floors of intercontinental Alitalia aircrafts, *Proc Symp dermatophytes dermatophytoses in man and animals*, Izmir, 21–23 May 1986, pp. 211–13.
9 Marmo W, Serio A, Isolamento di funghi cheratinofili nella polvere di traghetti dell'Ente FS (Isolation of keratinophilic fungi from dust of Italian Railway ferries), *Atti Sez Stud CIRM Prem Med L. Guida* (1986): pp 4–8.
10 Fuga GC, Monti M, Mercantini R et al, Isolamento di funghi cheratinofili nella polvere dell carrozze viaggiatori di alcuni treni delle FS (Isolation of keratinophilic fungi from dust of passenger trains of Italian railways), *Atti IV Convegno del Collegio dei Medici dei Transporti*, Borca di Cadore, 1–5 October 1985, pp. 127–9.

63
The role of the cutaneous microflora in host defence and its response to the environment

J. H. Cove, E. A. Eady, J. L. Tipper and W. J. Cunliffe*

Department of Microbiology, University of Leeds, Leeds, UK, and *Department of Dermatology, The Leeds Foundation for Dermatological Research, The General Infirmary, Leeds, UK

Resident cutaneous micro-organisms

A combination of host and external environmental factors play a key role in the microbial colonization of mammalian skin. As may be expected, the resident microflora varies between different species and between different body sites. The microflora of man is believed to be unique in that it comprises three species of propionibacteria which do not generally colonize other mammals. These are *Propionibacterium acnes*, *Propionibacterium granulosum* and *Propionibacterium avidum*.[1] Other important components of the human cutaneous microflora include the *Micrococcaceae*, in particular *Staphylococcus epidermidis*, aerobic coryneforms (diphtheroids) and the yeast *Malassezia furfur*. Site-to-site variation in the distribution of these organisms is well documented and reflects differences in the cutaneous microenvironment.[1] For example, *P. acnes* predominate in sebum rich areas and colonize the pilosebaceous ducts of the face, chest and back, whereas aerobic coryneforms are more readily isolated from moist areas such as the axilla.[1] It should also be noted that, in adults, the resident microflora is remarkably stable both in composition and distribution, implying a considerable degree of resilience to environmental changes.

The relationship between the resident microflora and the human host is usually referred to as 'commensalism' indicating a one-sided association in which only the micro-organisms benefit, i.e. by gaining nutrients and a favourable physiochemical environment, but in which the host receives nothing in return. In reality a more appropriate description is 'mutualism' in which the association is beneficial to both man and microbes.[2] In this chapter we review the nature of the mutually beneficial association and then show how it may be perturbed by changes in either the host or the external environment. Perhaps the most important benefit conferred by the resident microflora is as an integral part of cutaneous host-defence systems.

Cutaneous host defence against microbial invasion

There are several mechanisms which protect the skin against colonization by pathogenic micro-organisms and their subsequent invasion into the epidermis or dermis. These have been described in detail elsewhere[1,2] but include: (i) the physical barrier provided by the epidermis, (ii) desquamation, (iii) the humidity of the skin, (iv) pH, (v) niche filling by the resident microflora, and (vi) the presence of inhibitory substances on the skin surface. The relative contribution of each of these mechanisms is unknown but will vary at different body sites and in different situations. For example, an intact upper epidermis is important for preventing infection by *Staphylococcus aureus*, e.g. in infected eczema, whereas for Gram-negative bacteria colonization is favoured by increased humidity and an altered resident flora. The intact epidermis with its multilayered structure and intercellular components presents a remarkably resilient physical barrier to invading micro-organisms. For example, keratin, the principal structural component of keratinocytes, is resistant to most, but not all, bacterial proteases. The epidermis is of course not a static environment. Desquamation continually removes both normal and resident micro-organisms together with chance contaminants. Only organisms capable of establishing growth at a rate equal to or greater than their rate of removal by desquamation would be expected to colonize the skin successfully. However, there are disease states of disordered desquamation, e.g. eczema, which are susceptible to infection.

The availability of water is probably the single most important factor which limits the size of the bacterial population at many body sites. Occlusion of the volar forearm and the concomitant increase in humidity at that site gives rise to a rapid increase in bacterial numbers, e.g. from 10^2 to 10^6 staphylococci per square centimetre of skin.[3] Indeed this has been widely used as the basis of a method for assessing the efficacy of antimicrobial products. The humidity of the skin differs in different parts of the body and this accounts to some extent for site-to-site variation in the composition of the microbial population. Desiccation also plays a major role in protecting normal skin from colonization by potentially pathogenic bacteria by, for example, S. aureus and Gram-negative bacteria.

The acidic nature of skin presents a hostile environment for would-be invasive micro-organisms. Measurements of the pH of normal skin show this to vary considerably (4.1–6.8), with a mean value of around 5.2.[4] Host factors, i.e. sweat production and microbial activity, contribute to the pH of the skin. The metabolic end-products of energy metabolism of propionibacteria include short-chain fatty acids such as acetic and propionic acids. Longer chain fatty acids are also released by the action of microbial lipases on sebum triglycerides.

A pre-existing and established population of cutaneous micro-organisms presents a formidable obstacle to colonization by other organisms.[2] The normal flora is well adapted to the physiochemical conditions of the skin and also to using the available nutrients. The ability of staphylococci and propionibacteria to adhere to each other and to keratinocytes and their production of exo-enzymes are examples of such adaptations. The skin flora can also reach high cell densities (often $\geq 10^6$ bacteria per square centimetre of skin), thereby removing all readily available nutrients. It is therefore possible to take the view that the resident flora fills all available ecological niches in the skin environment, thus protecting the host from less benign bacteria and fungi.

The cutaneous host-defence system comprises a variety of agents with varying complexity and specificities which not only serve to protect the host but also contribute to homeostasis within the resident microbial population. These agents are not only produced directly by the host but also include microbial products and compounds arising from the activities of microbial exo-enzymes. Important host derived factors include lysozyme, which is an enzyme in sweat capable of degrading bacterial cell walls, and lactoferrin and transferrin, found in the dermis and serum, respectively, which both chelate iron, an essential growth-limiting element. IgA is excreted in sweat and is known to have antimicrobial activity against certain bacteria.[5]

Short- and long-chain fatty acids produced by or as a result of microbial exo-enzyme activity (see above) not only contribute to the acidic pH of skin, but also possess non-specific antimicrobial activities. Clearly the relative susceptibilities of different micro-organisms to free fatty acids will shape the composition of the skin microflora and the ability of invading micro-organisms to compete. Non-resident bacteria are more susceptible to inhibition by acetate and propionate than the propionibacteria which produce them.[6] It should also be pointed out that there may well be significant interactions between different components of the cutaneous host-defence system. The antimicrobial properties of free fatty acids are well known, for example, to be highly dependent on pH.

The production of agents with more specific antimicrobial activity by the resident bacteria may be taken as evidence for the intense competition which exists between these organisms in their natural environment. Skin bacteria have been shown to produce both antibiotics and bacteriocins. Antibiotics in this context may be defined as relatively low molecular weight compounds of diverse chemical structure which exert either a narrow or broad spectrum of activity by inhibiting specific cellular targets. A well documented example of an antibiotic produced by cutaneous bacteria is epidermin, a polypeptide compound produced by S. epidermidis.[2,7] Bacteriocins are also produced by staphylococci and propionibacteria. These are high molecular weight proteins which are usually highly specific in their spectrum of antimicrobial activity.

Perturbations of the cutaneous host-defence system by environmental factors

The skin environment can be altered directly by changes in external conditions, by the physiology of the host (including the lesions of various dermatoses) or by interactions between the two. Within limits, which are not well defined, the cutaneous microflora possesses a remarkable capacity to regulate itself and can remain constant in healthy adults over a considerable period of time. The staphylococci and propionibacteria do, however, respond to changes in their environment, e.g. in pH, oxygen tension, and nutrients, as has been demonstrated in vitro by alterations in growth rate, growth yield and exo-enzyme production.[8-11] It would be expected, therefore, that similar, but not necessarily identical, responses would occur in vivo.

Generally, environmental changes which result in pronounced or lasting changes in the skin microflora and which are not part of normal development are associated with disease states, and vice versa. In addition, many therapies used to treat dermatological conditions may produce unexpected effects on the cutaneous host-defence system and on the micro-organisms involved.

External conditions, often related to climate or lifestyle, such as high humidity or dryness will exacerbate conditions such as athletes' foot or eczema, respectively. Cracking of the skin which represents a major alteration in the skin environment, i.e. in eczema and contact dermatitis, is also the principal factor which predisposes to colonization by *S. aureus*. Climatic variations may explain the distribution of certain skin diseases. For example, in temperate climates such as northern Europe impetigo is usually due to *S. aureus*, whereas in the tropics or subtropics the disease is often associated with a streptococcal infection.

Exposure to external agents which perturb the resident microflora is usually, but not always, due to therapeutic use. Even non-antimicrobial therapies may produce profound changes; for example, cytotoxic drugs and steroids affecting both immune function and cellular responses may facilitate invasion of the skin by pathogens and retinoids increase the risk of *S. aureus* infection by making the skin dry and cracked. However, the therapeutic use, and misuse, of antibiotics continues to have by far the most clinically significant and widespread impact on the skin microflora. This is manifest by the emergence of single and multiply antibiotic resistant bacteria which reside not only on the patients receiving the drugs, but have become widely disseminated among the untreated population.[12]

In order for an antibiotic to exert these effects it must reach the skin surface and retain its activity. This will of course depend on the route of administration, the antibiotic used and the type of skin lesions involved. The activity of an antibiotic at the skin surface depends on the physiochemical environment and the stability and solubility of the antibiotic. There are also more specific effects, it has been shown that sebaceous lipids reduce the effectiveness of bacterial cell wall synthesis inhibitors such as penicillin and bacitracin. Orally administered aminoglycoside antibiotics, e.g. gentamicin, do not reach the skin surface unless the epidermis is traumatized and broken. Other antibiotics, e.g. tetracyclines or erythromycin, used in acne therapy may be concentrated at sites of inflammation or within the pilosebaceous ducts, the density of which could determine the amount of antibiotic excreted at the skin surface. The concentration of active antibiotic at the skin surface is extremely difficult to quantify but it may be a key factor in the emergence of antibiotic resistant bacteria. Topically applied antibiotics will produce a range of drug concentrations at the skin surface, high concentrations being achieved at the site of application but lower, possibly subinhibitory levels being transferred to other body sites and, importantly, to non-treated individuals with whom the patient associates. The transfer of active drug to untreated individuals is obviously undesirable and likely to lead to the uncontrolled selection of antibiotic resistant bacteria. The emergence of widespread resistance to gentamicin in *S. aureus*, to mupirocin in coagulase-negative staphylococci and to macrolide–lincosamide–streptogramin B (MLS) antibiotics (including clindamycin and erythromycin) in cutaneous propionibacteria[13] were each preceded by the introduction of topical antibiotic preparations. However, a causal association has not yet been proven between topical antibiotic therapy and the emergence of resistance, as in each case resistance may have resulted from the increased general use of these antibiotics.

The microbial flora can maintain its stability of population size by regulating the density of its component subpopulations. This may reveal unexpected interactions or competition between different microbial types. If the numbers of propionibacteria are reduced by antibiotics, they are replaced by *Malassezia*.[14] A similar reciprocal relationship has been reported between staphylococci and corynebacteria.

Staphylococci and corynebacteria possess a large pool of antibiotic resistance genes so that their numbers are rarely decreased by most of the antibiotics used in dermatology. In addition they also possess resistance genes to a wide range of disinfectants, antiseptics and heavy metals (see Table 1). Coagulase-negative staphylococci are becoming an increasing problem in general medicine, for example, by causing infections in immunocompromised subjects, in continuous ambulatory peritoneal dialysis patients and in neonates. The emergence of multiply antibiotic resistant strains in these organisms should be viewed with concern, particularly as these resistances are genetically mobile and can be transferred between strains and species, including *S. aureus*, by conjugation, transposition and transduction.[15]

Until recently, propionibacteria have remained sensitive to a wide range of antibiotics, but strains resistant to erythromycin, clindamycin and tetracycline are now encountered increasingly frequently. This presents a clinical problem in the management of acne in which these organisms appear to have a pathogenic role.[16] Until 1975 acquired antibiotic resistance in *P. acnes* was rare, and was first reported in the USA in the late 1970s.[17] In the UK, 20% ($N = 49$) of patients with therapy-resistant (recalcitrant) acne, sampled during 1985–86, carried antibiotic resistant propionibacteria.[18] This group comprised approximately 8% of patients attending the clinic for treatment of their acne. Qualitative screening of similar patients ($N = 90$) in 1991 suggests that the incidence of propionibacterial antibiotic resistance is increasing, that resistance to trimethoprim is emerging and that multiply antibiotic resistant propionibacteria are becoming increasingly prevalent.

Propionibacterial antibiotic resistance is undoubtedly contributing to the increasing requirement for isotretinoin therapy originally reserved for very severe cases but now also required for the treatment of patients who no longer respond to antibiotic therapy.

The extensive dermatological use of oral and topical antibiotics has led to the selection of a predominantly resistant population of staphylococci and coryneforms. Even within the propionibacteria, multiply resistant strains are now being encountered. This trend is likely to continue at an increasing pace and will certainly adversely affect our ability to manage acne effectively. In the UK there are at least 54 alternative therapeutic combinations for treating patients with acne.[19] Some combinations of oral and topical antibiotics, e.g. oral tetracycline with topical erythromycin, are

Table 1 Acquired resistances in coagulase-negative staphylococci

Antibiotics	Heavy metals	Antiseptics/Disinfectants
Pencillins, including methicillin	Cadmium	Ethidium bromide
Tetracyclines	Mercury	Acriflavine
Macrolides, including erythromycin	Lead	Quaternary ammonium compounds including cetrimide and benzalkonium chloride
Lincosamides, including clindamycin	Arsenate/arsenite	
	Antimony	
	Bismuth	
Fusidic acid	Zinc	Diamidines
Chloramphenicol		Chlorhexidine
Trimethoprim		

highly inappropriate since they will select for multiply antibiotic resistant strains, and these are most likely to cause major problems in the future. There is now an urgent need for objective studies to identify the most effective therapeutic strategies for acne[20] which minimize the risk of further acquisition and dissemination of antibiotic resistance determinants.

Conclusions

A number of different mechanisms involving host factors and the skin microflora combine to prevent the establishment of pathogenic bacteria on human skin. Niche filling and the production of inhibitory substances by micro-organisms makes an important contribution to host defence. It is therefore important that the resident microflora has the ability to withstand perturbation by growth inhibitory environmental factors. At least four mechanisms can be identified which contribute to the stability of the resident cutaneous flora: (i) resistance to antimicrobials; (ii) the presence of protective factors on skin, e.g. lipids which reduce the activity of certain antibiotics; (iii) the inability of many orally administered antibiotics to reach the intact skin surface (exceptions being the anti-acne antibiotics); and (iv) the maintenance of a stable microbial population size through reciprocal interactions where one species takes the place of another when challenged by antimicrobials with selective action.

References

1 Noble WC, *Microbiology of human skin*, 2nd Edn, Lloyd-Luke: London, 1981.
2 Eady EA, Antimicrobiosis by members of the resident bacterial flora of normal and acne skin, Ph.D. Thesis, Department of Microbiology, University of Leeds, 1979.
3 Aly R, Shirley C, Cunico B et al, Effect of prolonged occlusion on the microbial flora, pH carbon dioxide and transepidermal water loss on human skin, *J Invest Dermatol* (1978) **71**: 378–81.
4 Holland DB, Cunliffe WJ, Skin surface and open comedone pH in acne patients, *Acta Dermatol Venereol* (1982) **63**: 155–8.
5 Gebhart W, Immunoglobulin A-mediated local immunity in the sebaceous follicle. In: Marks R, Plewig G, (eds). *Acne and related disorders*, Martin Dunitz: London, 1989, p. 23.
6 Ushijima T, Takahashi M, Ozaki Y, Acetic, propionic and oleic acid as the possible factors influencing the predominant residence of some species of *Propionibacterium* and coagulase negative *Staphylococcus* on human skin, *Can J Microbiol* (1984) **30**: 697–52.
7 Schnell N, Entian K-D, Schneider U et al, Prepeptide sequence of epidermin, a ribosomally synthesized antibiotic with four sulphide rings, *Nature* (1988) **333**: 276–8.
8 Cove JH, Holland KT, Cunliffe WJ, Growth yield, phosphatase and protease production by *Staphylococcus epidermidis* in batch and continuous culture, *Zentralbl Bacteriol* (1981) (suppl 10): 169–73.
9 Greenman J, Holland KT, Cunliffe WJ, Effects of glucose concentration on biomass, maximum specific growth rate and extracellular enzyme production by three species of cutaneous propionibacteria grown in continuous culture, *J Gen Microbiol* (1981) **127**: 371–6.
10 Greenman J, Holland KT, Cunliffe WJ, Effects of pH on biomass, maximum specific growth rate and extracellular enzyme production by three species of propionibacteria grown in continuous culture. *J Gen Microbiol* (1983) **129**: 1301–7.
11 Cove JH, Holland KT, Cunliffe WJ, Effects of oxygen concentration on biomass production, maximum specific growth rate and extra cellular enzyme production by three species of propionibacteria grown in continuous culture. *J Gen Microbiol* (1983) **129**: 3327–34.
12 Cove JH, Eady EA, Cunliffe WJ, Skin carriage of antibiotic-resistant coagulase-negative staphylococci in untreated subjects, *J Antimicrob Chemother* (1990) **25**: 459–67.
13 Eady EA, Ross JI, Cove JH et al, Macrolide-lincosamide-streptogramin B (MLS) resistance in cutaneous propionibacteria: definition of phenotypes, *J Antimicrob Chemother* (1989) **23**: 493–502.
14 Eady EA, Cove JH, Holland KT et al, Superior antibacterial action and reduced incidence of bacterial resistance in minocycline compared to tetracycline-treated acne patients, *Br J Dermatol* (1990) **122**: 233–44.
15 Lyon BR, Skurray R, Antimicrobial resistance of *Staphylococcus aureus*, *Microbiol Rev* (1987) **51**: 88–134.
16 Eady EA, Cove JH, Holland KT et al, Erythromycin resistant propionibacteria in antibiotic treated acne patients: association with therapeutic failure, *Br J Dermatol* (1989) **121**: 51–7.
17 Leyden JJ, McGinley KJ, Cavalieri S et al, *Propionibacterium acnes* resistance to antibiotics in acne patients, *J Am Acad Dermatol* (1983) **8**: 41–5.
18 Eady EA, Cove JH, Blake J et al, Recalcitrant *acne vulgaris*. Clinical, biochemical and microbiological investigation of patients not responding to antibiotic treatment, *Br J Dermatol* (1988) **118**: 415–23.
19 Cunliffe WJ, *Acne*, Martin Dunitz: London, 1989.
20 Eady EA, Cove JH, Joanes DN et al, Topical antibiotics for the treatment of *acne vulgaris*: a critical evaluation of the literature on their clinical benefit and comparative efficacy, *J Dermatol Treat* (1990) **1**: 215–26.

64
The host's immunological contribution to the ecological battle on the skin surface

Walter Gebhart and Astrid Kersten
IInd Department of Dermatology, University of Vienna, Alserstrasse 4, A-1090 Vienna, Austria

After birth, each individual enters a continuous phase of confrontation with numerous environmental impacts. To describe the successful management of such a complex battle, we use the simple word 'life'.

As with most mucous membranes, skin is colonized by enormous numbers of microbes. Resident bacteria and fungi are present in the follicles and on the skin surface of normal adults in such quantities that they outnumber normal human cells. Despite this numerical inferiority, highly organized multicellular systems can make use of foreign organisms by domesticating them in various ways.[1,2]

In and on human skin there is tough competition for nutritional sources such as protein-rich keratin, sebum and other tissue-derived sources of food. Most have a number of powerful weapons to fight off other micro-organisms. Therefore it appears wise for multicellular organisms to accept some of these microbes as symbionts in order to be protected by them from other, perhaps more harmful, invaders.

Antigenic material of any kind should be prevented from invading tissues as rapidly as possible, i.e. at the very surface. Therefore, cellular immune mechanisms are not appropriate tools for mediating surface immunity. Living and functionally immunocompetent cells will usually not be able to penetrate up to the outer body surface. However, mediators of specific humoral immunity can reach these areas via the typical cutaneous products of sebum and sweat. The following overview concentrates on immunoglobulin secretion as a mediator of skin surface protection.

Immunoglobulins in skin glands and their secretions

Cell-mediated immune reactions do not commonly occur on the healthy skin surface, which is inaccessible to living immunocompetent cells. Therefore, humoral secretory immune mechanisms must fulfil these functions. Little attention has been paid to immunobiological skin surface investigations in the past. Only small amounts of cutaneous secretions can be collected by conventional methods for biochemical investigation, resulting in a number of methodological difficulties.

In addition, low immunoglobulin concentrations in several secretions are another limiting factor. However, immunoglobulins in human sweat, cerumen and even in comedones, were demonstrated as long as 25 years ago. A number of theories concerning the control and even killing activity of these immunoglobulins on skin surface bacteria and fungi were suggested in early papers.[3-8]

During the past 5 years, our group has studied the question of cutaneous immunoglobulin secretion by various immunocytochemical techniques in order to analyse the production as well as the target sites of this humoral defense weapon. Immunoglobulins were demonstrated in glandular cells and in the secretions of human sebaceous and sweat glands by means of a post-embedding immunogold labelling technique. Finally, the secretory component was demonstrated in glandular cells and secretions using many antibodies.[9-12] Using these techniques it became clear, that immunoglobulin secretion is an active and purposeful contribution of the cutaneous glands and not just a passive diffusion into excretory body fluids. Furthermore, it was demonstrated that epithelial cells contribute an essential molecule to the active immunoglobulin dimer: the glycoprotein secretory component. At the same time epithelial cells can selectively bind immunoglobulins from the circulating pool, process them in their cytoplasm and excrete them to the outer surface.

Functional aspects of skin surface immunoglobulins

Despite considerable speculation over the function of immunoglobulin in cutaneous secretions, scientifically relevant studies have not been performed to determine their origin, binding sites or biological significance. Therefore, we designed the following experiments with the aim of obtaining a better understanding of humoral skin surface immunity.

Bacterial isolates and their reaction with sweat-derived immunoglobulins

Staphylococci were cultured from the skin surface of eight healthy volunteers and after two recultivation cycles investigated for surface immunoglobulins by using light microscopic immunoperoxidase techniques. As expected, these bacterial smear samples revealed no immunoglobulins on their cell walls.

However, preincubation of the isolates with the host's sweat before performing the immunostaining procedure resulted in a strongly positive surface coat on the bacteria. Immunoglublins A, G and M as well as a secretory component could be identified in various preparations. These findings point to a specific binding of sweat-derived immunoglobulins to surface receptors of resident skin surface staphylococci and yeasts.

In situ demonstration of secretory immunoglobulins on resident skin flora

Light- and electron microscopic immunostaining techniques were used to study the distribution and localization of secretory immunoglobulins on microbes of the skin surface and within pilosebaceous units. Immunoperoxidase and protein A gold techniques were applied to cytological preparations and paraffin or LR-White embedded sections.[9-12]

By analysing these preparations it was possible to demonstrate that numerous yeasts and bacteria of the normal skin flora are regularly coated in vivo by immunoglobulins. The secretory component was also present in the surface coats of the organisms (Figure 1).

Detailed ultrastructural studies revealed that the tracer particles were always bound to fimbrial or other adhesional structures in the glycocalyx and mucous capsule of microbes, respectively. Therefore, it seems that immunoglobulins are actively secreted by cutaneous glands in order to react and possibly interact with adhesional structures of fungal and bacterial skin surface symbionts.

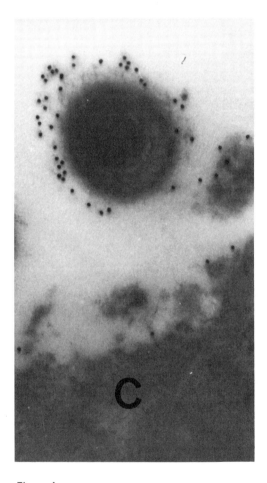

Figure 1

Immuno-electron-microscopic demonstration of the secretory component on the surface of a coccal organism adjacent to a corneocyte (C). Protein A gold labelled antibody is bound to surface coat structures of the bacterium. LR-White section, pre-embedding immunostaining technique, primary magnification ×10,000.

Interpretation of immunoglobulin-coating on cutaneous symbionts

Coating of viruses, bacteria or fungi with secretory antibodies is a basic biological principle, effective in preventing these microbes from penetrating the organism. It operates continuously in every healthy organism, regardless of whether the microbe is a harmless symbiont or an active pathogen.

The interaction between host and parasite is determined by the activity of adhesion molecules. These are important because adhesion is a major precondition for infectivity and thus microbial pathogenicity.[13,14] Whereas adhesion molecules of virulent microbes bind strongly to corresponding cellular receptors, the expression of these adhesins is low or blocked in non-pathogenic species by reaction with 'domesticating' factors of the host. Secretion of immunoglobulins obviously fulfils this 'domesticating' task, interacting specifically with the microbes living on the skin surface or in the pilosebaceous ducts. Invasion of these micro-organisms into the host is effectively blocked. Simultaneously, antigenic binding sites are occupied by secretory antibodies which do not activate the complement cascade. A further advantage of microbial coating with the host's proteins might be improved tolerance towards the parasite. This coating prevents recognition of non-self structures by the immune system. Continuous coating of micro-organisms with host molecules therefore seems to be a life-long 'domesticating' principle, enabling multicellular organisms to take advantage of other fauna by integrating it in a symbiontic way.

Final remarks

Numerous clinical observations, laboratory data and, in particular, certain diseases point to the significant role of immunoglobulins in skin physiology and pathology. The striking association of chronic and recurring infections of the skin in patients with congenital or acquired humoral immunodeficiency conditions is evidence for the clinical relevance of impaired potential for 'domestication'. Self-healing of acne was recently also interpreted as a consequence of adaptive immunization against the follicular microbial flora.[15] Thus, the phenomenon of inactivation of antigens in general can be partly explained on the basis of their interaction with secretory immunoglobulins.[16]

Further investigation of the interactions between cutaneous secretory immunomediators and their target structures should not only be restricted to microbes, but should also include allergens of any kind or 'foreign' molecules in general in order to reduce the gap between our present knowledge and the multiple and complex regulating factors influencing the ecosystems on the outer skin surface.

References

1. Davis BD, *Microbiology*, 3rd edn, Harper & Row: New York, 1980.
2. Kligman AM, Leyden J, McGinley K, Bacteriology, *J Invest Dermatol* (1976) **67**: 160–8.
3. Marghescu S, Immunoglobulingehalt der normalen Haut, *Arch Dermatol Res* (1972) **244**: 282–5.
4. Baart de la Faille-Kuyper EH, van der Meer JB, Baart de la Faille H, An Immunohistochemical study of the skin of healthy individuals, *Acta Dermatovenerol (Stockh)* (1974) **54**: 271–4.
5. Page CO, Remington JS, Immunologic studies in normal human sweat, *J Lab Clin Med* (1967) **69**: 634–50.
6. Petrakis NL, Doherly N, Lee RE et al, Demonstration and implications of lysozyme and immunoglobulins in human ear wax, *Nature* (1971) **229**: 119–20.
7. Corbel MJ (1974) Detection of antibodies to campylobacter fetus (vibrio fetus) in the preputial secretions of bulls with vibriosis, *Brit Vet J* (1974) **130**: 13–17.
8. Knop J, Ollefs K. Frosch PJ, Anti-P. Acnes antibody in comedonal extracts, *J Invest Dermatol* (1983) **80**: 9–12.
9. Gebhart W, Metze D, Jurecka W et al, Immunoglobulin A in sebaceous glands, *Wien Klin Wschr* (1986) **20**: 683–9.
10. Gebhart W, Metze D, Jurecka W et al, IgA in human skin appendages. In: Caputo R, (ed.). *Immunodermatology*, CIC Edizioni Internazionale: Rome, 1987, pp185–8.
11. Metze D, Jurecka W, Gebhart W et al, Immunohistochemical demonstration of immunoglobulin A in human sebaceous and sweat glands, *J Invest Dermatol* (1989) **92**: 13–17.
12. Gebhart W, Metze D, Mainitz M et al, Humorale Hautimmunität: Eine aktive sekretorische Leistung kutaner Strukturen (Humoral immunity: an active contribution of cutaneous glands), *Ellipse* (1989) **21**: 288–95.
13. Isenberg HD, Pathogenicity and virulence: another view, *Clin Microbiol Rev* (1988) **1**: 40–53.
14. Kilian M. Reinholdt J. Interference with IgA defence mechanisms by extracellular bacterial enzymes, *Med Microbiol* (1986) **5**: 173–208.
15. Gebhart W, IgA-mediated local immunity in the sebaceous follicle. In: Marks R, Plewig G, (eds). *Acne and related disorders*, Martin Dunitz: London, 1989, p23.
16. Metze D, Kersten A, Jurecka W et al, Immunoglobulins coat microorganisms of skin surface: a comparative study of cutaneous and oral microbial symbionts, *J Invest Dermatol* (1991) **96**: 439–45.

65
The aetiology and treatment of fungal nail infection

D. T. Roberts
Southern General Hospital, Glasgow, UK

Introduction

Nails may be infected by various fungi some of which are primary pathogens whilst others cause infection only when the nail apparatus is otherwise diseased or disturbed. Dermatophyte infection of nails is very common and is almost always a primary pathogen, although its occurrence is increased in some intercurrent conditions such as peripheral vascular disease. Dermatophyte fungi are keratolytic and initially attack the distal and lateral underside of the nail, gradually spreading proximally and eventually destroying the nail plate. Yeasts, mainly those of the *Candida* species are usually secondary pathogens and often cause a proximal nail dystrophy. They gain entry to the posterior nail fold when the cuticle becomes detached from the nail plate secondary to chronic immersion of the hands in water. Chronic inflammation of the posterior nail fold occurs, eventually disturbing the nail matrix which leads to a proximal dystrophy which spreads distally in contrast to dermatophyte infection. Other yeasts, notably *Scopulariopsis brevicaulis* are considered to be secondary pathogens of a previously traumatized nail. Some non-dermatophyte moulds commonly infect nails in tropical climates. The commonest of these is *Hendersonula toruloidea*, a soil saprophyte, which causes a characteristically black discoloration of the nail in affected patients.

It is important to differentiate between these various forms of infection because they do not all respond to the same antifungal drugs and accurate laboratory identification is essential prior to selecting therapy.

Dermatophytosis of nails

The remainder of this article concentrates on dermatophyte infection of nails as this is by far the commonest form of fungal nail infection and is the easiest to treat once an accurate diagnosis has been made. Dermatophytosis of nails is caused almost exclusively by anthropophilic dermatophytes which spread initially to the toenails from the feet and toeclefts. Thereafter, though not inevitably, spread to the hands and fingernails can occur. Three species of dermatophytes are notably involved, *Trichophyton rubrum*, *Trichophyton interdigitalae* and *Epidermophyton floccosum*. Because of its chronicity *T. rubrum* is by far the commonest pathogen of nails. These species of dermatophytes are endemic in communal bathing places such as swimming pools, sports clubs and industrial baths and infection is almost always picked up in such places because moisture and maceration of the toecleft skin are initially essential to the establishment of infection. Infection becomes established in patients who are repeatedly exposed to the fungus and the majority of infections are found in individuals using communal bathing facilities more than once per week.[1]

Prevalence of dermatophytosis of nails

Most of the data on the prevalence of nail disease are gathered by extrapolation from data of prevalence of toecleft and foot disease. Various studies have examined the incidence of dermatophyte infection of the feet in communal bathing places and the incidence varies from 8.5%[1] in a random sample of users to 80%[2] in coal miners who have a daily bath during the whole of their working lifetime. From these data plus a survey of London shopworkers it can be concluded that the incidence of dermatophyte infection of the feet in the overall population is of the order of 10–15%. Two studies have examined the incidence of nail infection in patients with known tinea pedis and this varies from 18%[3] to 33.5%.[4] It can thus be concluded that 2–5% of the population have a nail infection.

This is in agreement with a survey published in 1979 where a large population group was examined for evidence of skin disease by dermatologists in north-east USA. This survey concluded that the incidence of fungal nail infection was 2.18% which is in keeping with the previous assumption.

A recent and as yet unpublished questionnaire survey of a population sample of almost 10 000 using questions and photographs previously tested in known disease groups and found to be accurate, revealed an incidence of nail infection of 2.8% in men and 2.6% in women. In the 16–34 year old age group the incidence was 1.3%, increasing through 2.4% in the 35–54 year old age group up to 4.7% in patients of 55 years and over, thus indicating the chronicity of this infection and the length of time required for the infection to become established. Toenail infection was twice as common as fingernail infection in men and three times as common in women in this survey.

Environmental control measures

If no effort is made to reduce the reservoir of infection in the population then the incidence will gradually increase and there will be a larger innoculum of infection at new communal bathing establishments and the rate of spread of infection will also increase. However, such control measures are difficult to institute. It is obviously impossible to prevent entry of infected individuals, although a constant supply of plastic overshoes should be made available and their use encouraged at all times. In addition, a supply of antifungal foot powder, although of no value in the treatment of established infection, is useful prophylactically. Unfortunately it is likely that both of these measures will prove too costly to be used routinely.

It has been found impossible to kill the fungal innoculum effectively using disinfectants. Whilst many distinfectants will kill dermatophytes in vitro, the organism is enclosed in small pieces of keratin on the floors of communal bathing places and this tends to protect it from the effect of disinfectants. If the disinfectant used was powerful enough to destroy the keratin it would then of course become extremely irritant to the feet of users.

Washing floors in changing rooms and shower cubicles by hosing them down is effective but generally is not carried out often enough to prove completely beneficial. It is likely, therefore, that a reservoir of infection will remain in the population and effective treatment methods are required to reduce the incidence.

Treatment of fungal nail infections

Theoretically, nail infections can be treated topically, systemically or by surgical or chemical removal. The comparison given here of these methods of treatment concentrates on mycological cure rates as clinical improvement is an unreliable indicator of eradication of the organism.

Systemic treatment

Griseofulvin has, until very recently been the only available systemic drug useful for long-term treatment. It is a weakly fungistatic agent which affects the fungal cell nucleus. The drug must be given in nail infections until the whole of the nail has grown out. In the case of fingernail infection this amounts to a period of around 6 months and in toenails the period is 12–18 months. Griseofulvin is a disappointing drug, particularly in the treatment of toenail infections where mycological cure rates of only around 30% can be expected.[5] In addition, griseofulvin quite often causes troublesome side-effects such as nausea and headache and occasionally produces severe photosensitivity and can precipitate lupus erythematosus.

Ketoconazole is an imidazole available for systemic use. Like all imidazoles it acts by interference of fungal cell wall synthesis. It inhibits the cytochrome P450 system in the cell wall and blocks the conversion of lanosterol to ergosterol. The drug can thus also competitively inhibit other agents which act in the same way in human cellular systems. Ketoconazole is hepatotoxic and is not recommended for long-term treatment of nail infection. In any case it is no more effective than griseofulvin in eradicating the organism.[6]

Itraconazole is a new triazole which acts in the same way as ketoconazole but is rather more selective in inhibiting the fungal cytochrome P450 system. It is more effective in the treatment of nail infections than ketoconazole and is much less toxic. Cure rates of around 70%[7] have been achieved but the drug still requires to be given relatively long-term and it would also appear to be fungistatic rather than fungicidal, although this may be dose related.

The allylamines are a new group of antifungal agents which also affect fungal cell wall synthesis. The allylamines, however, inhibit the conversion of squalene to squalene epoxide by inhibiting the enzyme squalene epoxidase.[8] The build up of squalene within the cell is thought to be fungicidal rather than fungistatic. The allylamine terbinafine is available for systemic use and its minimum inhibitory concentration (MIC) against dermatophytes is the same as its minimum fungicidal concentration (MFC).[9] A study of this drug in moccasin tinea pedis over a 6 week treatment period revealed ongoing increasing cure rates long after the drug was stopped which contrasted with the high relapse rate using griseofulvin in the same condition. These results tend to support the contention that the drug is fungicidal.

A large multicentre study of terbinafine in the UK revealed 95% cure rates in fingernail infections after 6 months treatment and 86% cure rates in toenail infection after 12 months treatment.[10] Twelve months later the relapse rates in finger and toenail were 8% and 20%, respectively, which is remarkably low in this condition given the possibility of reinfection as well as relapse. The mean time to mycological cure was 29 weeks in the case of toenails and 14 weeks in the case of fingernails. This suggested that a shorter treatment period may be equally effective and an even more recent study using terbinafine for 3 months in nail infections resulted in cure rates of 80% in the case of toenails 48 weeks after the start of treatment, that is, 36 weeks after treatment ceased. It would appear, therefore, that this drug is far superior to griseofulvin in nail infections over a much shorter treatment period. This is likely to be because of its fungicidal mode of action. It has also been shown that the drug achieves reasonable concentrations in the distal nail 3–18 weeks (mean 7.8 weeks) after the start of treatment and thereafter a steady state is achieved.[11] No significant side-effects have been observed with this drug. These data suggest that terbinafine is likely to become the systemic treatment of choice in fungal nail infections in the near future.

Topical treatment does not compare with the cure rates obtained with terbinafine. Tioconazole nail lotion used over a 3 month treatment period produced only 22% mycological cure,[12] which is similar to the results obtained using a combination of 40% urea and bifonazole in a paste base.[13] This chemically removes the nail but is labour intensive to carry out and has not gained wide acceptance in the UK where the preparation is not commercially available. Combinations of topical treatment along with griseofulvin are likely to double the cure rates obtainable with griseofulvin alone over a prolonged treatment period,[14] but are still less good than those available with the newer systemic agents.

Conclusion

Fungal nail infection is likely to affect around 1.5 million of the population of the UK and is thus a relatively common disease. The incidence will probably increase with increasing use of communal bathing places as a leisure pursuit. It is not likely to be possible to eradicate the fungus from such communal bathing places and a reduction in the incidence of this infection is more likely to be achieved through more effective forms of treatment rather than by environmental protection methods. In this way the pool of infection in the population will become reduced, thus reducing the rate of spread of new infection.

References

1. Gentles JC, Evans EGV, Foot infection in swimming baths, *Br Med J* (1973) **3**: 260–2.
2. Götz H, Hantschke D, Einblicke in die Epidemiologie der Dermatomykosen in Kohlenbergbau (Examination of the epidemiology of dermatomycoses in coalmining), *Hautarzt* (1965) **16**: 543–8.
3. Alteras I, Cojocaru I, A short review on tinea pedis by dermatophytes, *Mykosen* (1973) **16**: 229.
4. Beare JM, Gentles JC, Mackenzie DWR, Mycology. In: *Textbook of dermatology*, vol 1. Blackwell: Oxford, 1972, p. 694.
5. Davies RR, Everall JD, Hamilton E, Mycological and clinical evaluation of griseofulvin in chronic onychomycosis, *Br Med J* (1967) **3**: 464.
6. Hay RJ, Clayton YM, Griffiths WAD et al, A comparitive study of ketoconazole and griseofulvin in dermatophytosis, *Br J Dermatol* (1985) **112**: 691–6.

7 Hay RJ, Clayton YM, Moore MK, An evaluation of itraconazole in the management of onychomycosis, *Br J Dermatol* (1988) **119**: 359–66.
8 Schuster I, Ryder NS, Allylamines — mode of action compared to azole antifungals and biological fate in mammalian organism, *J Dermatol Treat* (1990) **1** (suppl 2): 7–11.
9 Clayton YM, The in vitro activity of terbinafine, *Clin Exp Dermatol* (1989) **14**: 101–3.
10 Goodfield M, Clinical results with terbinafine in onychomycosis, *J Dermatol Treat* (1990) **1** (suppl 2): 55–7.
11 Finlay AY, Lever L, Thomas R et al, Nail matrix kinetics of oral terbinafine in onychomycosis and normal nails, *J Dermatol Treat* (1990) **1** (suppl 2): 51–3.
12 Hay RJ, Mackie RM, Clayton YM, Tioconazole nail solution — an open study of its efficacy in onychomycosis, *Clin Exp Dermatol* (1985) **10**: 111–15.
13 Hay RJ, Roberts DT, Doherty VR et al, The topical treatment of onychomycosis using a new combined urea/imidazole preparation, *Clin Exp Dermatol* (1988) **13**: 164–7.
14 Hay RJ, Clayton YM, Moore MIC, A comparison of tioconazole 28% nail solution versus base as an adjunct to griseofulvin in patients with onychomycosis, *Clin Exp Dermatol* (1987) **12**: 175–7.

66
Microbiological, environmental and industrial challenge to an industrially orientated hydrocolloid dressing

P. G. Bowler and H. Delargy
ConvaTec Wound Healing Research Institute, Clwyd, UK

Introduction

Protection of wounds or abrasions from environmental challenge leads to improved wound healing and skin quality.[1] Hydrocolloid dressings have been shown to have an interactive role in wound healing by providing a moist, occlusive environment,[2,3] by enhancing fibrinolysis,[4] angiogenesis (J. J. Pickworth, N. de Sousa and M. G. Rippon, unpublished observations) and by possessing growth factor stimulatory activity.[5] A hydrocolloid dressing (Granuflex Industrial, ConvaTec, Bristol-Myers Squibb) has been designed specifically for the industrial environment; it is adhesive and has a waterproof polymer film backing which affords a low vapour permeability. This product has been subjected to both chemical (industrial) and microbiological challenge. Chemical challenge involved subjecting the external backing polymer film to a variety of solid and liquid challenges for up to 1 h. Challenge materials included motor fuel (4 star), diesel fuel, mineral oil, brake/clutch fluid, grease, motor oil, industrial detergent, machine cooling oil (fresh and used), wet and dry cements, concentrated sulphuric and nitric acids and saturated sodium hydroxide solution. The microbial barrier function of the dressing was assessed using in vitro models in which the dressing was challenged with suspensions of *Pseudomonas aeruginosa* and *Staphylococcus aureus*.[6] (C. S. Clay and P. G. Bowler, unpublished observations).

Method

Chemical challenge

In vitro tests were set up to simulate conditions in which dressings may be subjected to solids and liquids commonly encountered in an industrial environment by both acute exposure (accidental spillage) and chronic exposure (complete immersion). The materials tested and the degree of exposure used are listed in Table 1.

Acute exposure

It was assumed that the challenge materials would be of a noxious or corrosive nature and would

Table 1 Solids and liquids used to test the dressings.

Materials	Exposure
Motor fuel (4 star)	Acute
Motor oil	Acute and chronic
Brake/clutch fluid	Acute
Industrial detergent	Acute and chronic
Machine cooling oil (used)	Acute and chronic
Machine cooling oil (neat)	Chronic
Diesel fuel	Acute
Wet and dry cement	Acute and chronic
Saturated sodium hydroxide	Acute
Nitric acid (concentrated)	Acute
Sulphuric acid (concentrated)	Acute

easily damage intact skin if not quickly removed. The apparatus consisted of a microporous filter holder into which the dressing was placed adhesive side down (Figure 1). The test substance, liquid or solid, was placed in the upper portion of the apparatus. A vacuum was applied to the lower limb for the 15 min test period. The sample was removed, the backing washed with water and then examined for any breakthrough.

Chronic exposure

In vitro tests were set up to assess the resistance of dressing samples to materials with which it may be in constant contact during a working day. The dressing sample was adhered to a polished stainless-steel plate and completely immersed in test substance for 1 h. The plate and dressing combined was then washed with water prior to removal of the dressing and examination for any breakthrough via the outer surface and edges of the matrix.

Microbiological challenge

Tryptone Soy Broth inoculated with *Pseudomonas aeruginosa* (NCTC 10332) or *Staphylococcus aureus* (NCTC 8532) was incubated overnight at 37°C to yield a growth of approximately 1×10^9 cfu/ml. Tryptone Soy Agar (TSA) was used for recovery of organisms in the event of penetration.

Dressing material was supported in an in vitro model as shown in Figures 2 and 3. Non-adherent gauze dressing (Johnson and Johnson) was used as a positive control. The inner adhesive dressing surface was challenged with approximately 250 ml of bacterial suspension and the apparatus was incubated at room temperature for up to 8 days. The outer dressing surface was kept dry and sampled daily by swabbing through each of the four ports. Recovery of the challenge organism on TSA was indicative of bacterial penetration. The bacterial suspension was tested for viability at the end of the study.

A supplementary dye penetration test was also performed to detect surface pin-holes in dressings. These can be observed by the application of a dye solution (0.15% methylene blue in alcohol) to the dry, outer dressing surface.

Results

Chemical challenge

None of the samples tested against acute or chronic challenge showed penetration via the back-

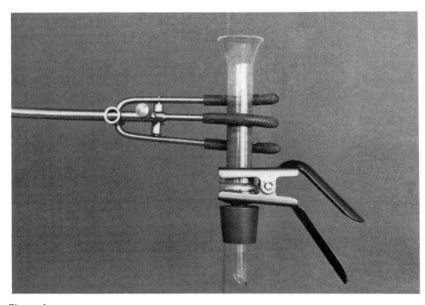

Figure 1

Acute exposure apparatus.

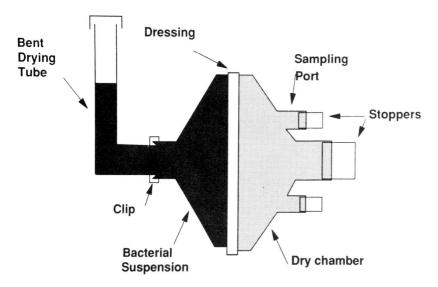

Figure 2

In vitro bacterial barrier model.

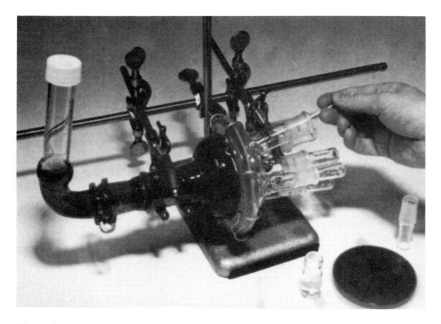

Figure 3

In vitro bacterial barrier apparatus.

ing or edges of the dressing into the matrix (Figures 4 to 10). Concentrated sulphuric acid reacted with the polyurethane film backing, but no breakthrough was observed. Motor fuel (4 star) deformed the backing film causing it to bubble, but no disruption of the matrix was detected.

Microbiological challenge

As shown in Table 2, penetration of challenge suspensions (P. aeruginosa and S. aureus) occurred rapidly (<24 h) through the control gauze dressing; in contrast, neither organism was seen to

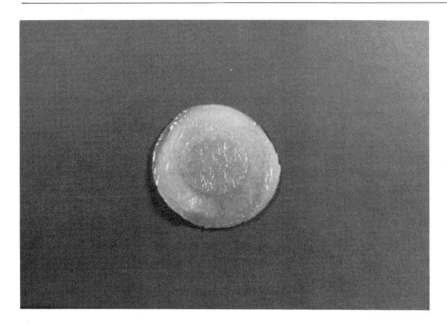

Figure 4

Acute exposure to concentrated nitric acid.

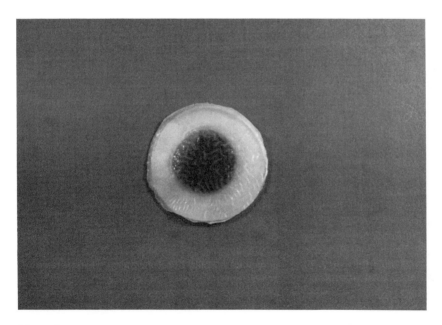

Figure 5

Acute exposure to concentrated sulphuric acid.

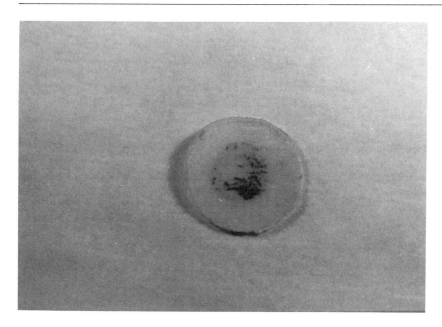

Figure 6
Acute exposure to wet cement.

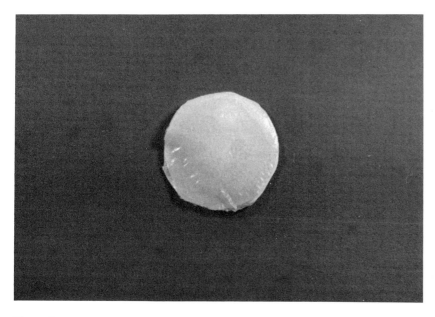

Figure 7
Acute exposure to motor fuel (4 star petrol).

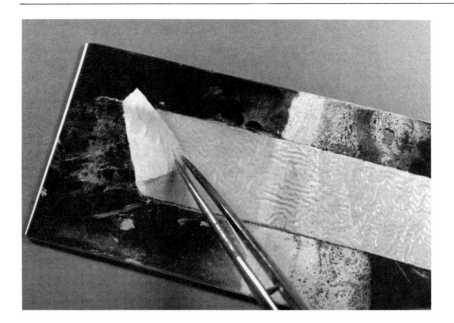

Figure 8
Chronic exposure to wet cement.

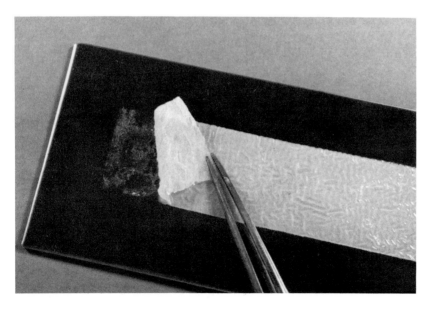

Figure 9
Chronic exposure to motor oil.

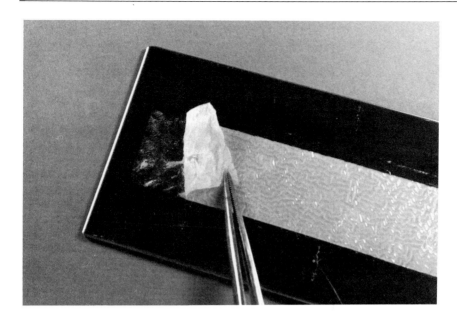

Figure 10
Chronic exposure to machine cooling oil.

Table 2 Microbial barrier properties of the Granuflex Industrial dressing.

Day	Granuflex Industrial dressing		Control dressing	
	P. aeruginosa	S. aureus	P. aeruginosa	S. aureus
1	−	−	+	+
2	−	−		
3	−	−		
4	−	−		
5	−	−		
6	−	−		
7	−	−		
8	−	−		

−, No organisms detected; +, organisms detected.

penetrate the Granuflex Industrial dressing over an 8-day period.

Conclusion

In vitro investigations have shown Granuflex Industrial dressing to be highly resistant to both chemical and microbiological challenge. As a consequence, the dressing may not only be of use in the clinical environment to protect health-care personnel in particular, from patients carrying infectious diseases, but its considerable chemical resistance may also favour the use of this dressing in the industrial environment for adequately protecting abrasions acquired by manual personnel.

References

1 Turner TD, Semi occlusive and occlusive dressings. An environment for healing — the role of occlusion. In: Ryan TJ, (ed). *Society of Medicine International Conference and Symposium Series 88*, The Royal Society of Medicine, London, 1985, pp. 5–14.
2 Cherry GW, Ryan TJ, McGibbon D, Trial of a new dressing in venous leg ulcers, *The Practitioner* (1984) **228**: 1175–8.
3 Cherry GW, Ryan TJ, Enhanced wound angiogenesis with a new hydrocolloid dressing. In: Ryan TJ, (ed). *An environment for wound healing: the role of occlusion*, ICSS No. 88, Royal Society for Medicine, London, 1985, pp. 61–8.
4 Lydon MJ, Hutchinson JJ, Rippon M et al, Dissolution of wound coagulum and promotion of granulation tissue under DuoDERM, *Wounds: Comp Clin Res Practice* (1989) **1**: 95–106.
5 Bolton L, Pirone L, et al, Dressings effects on wound healing, *Wounds: Comp Clin Res Practice* (1990) **2**(4): 126–34.
6 Dunn LJ, Wilson P, Evaluating the permeability of hydrocolloid dressings to multi-resistant *Staphylococcus aureus*, *Pharm J* (1990) **245**: 248–50.

Index (Page references in *italics* indicate figures)

acetaminophenol, partitioning study, 270–5
acidity, *see* pH of skin
   see also alkali irritancy test
acne, therapy resistance, 388–9
   see also chloracne, and tetrachlorodibenzo-*p*-dioxin
actinic elastosis, 83–4
   histology, 84
   ultrasonography, 84–90
actinic prurigo (AP), 68
   see also chronic actinic dermatitis (CAD)
adenovirus infection from bathing, 375
adhesion molecules
   expression, and UV irradiation, 125–7
   and pathogenicity of microorganisms, 393
Aeromonas hydrophilic, 371
age, and percutaneous absorption, 250
   see also photoaging
agriculture, and dermatitis, 177
alcohol intoxication, percutaneous, 255
algicides in swimming pools, 373
alkali irritancy test, 203
   and UV irradiation, 204–5
allergens
   arthropod secretions, 360
   in cosmetics, 175
   Euxyl K 400, 231–2
   transition metals, 216, 217
   see also irritants; photoallergens; xenobiotic skin penetration
allergy, photoimmunologic basis, 48–9
   see also contact dermatitis; cosmetic allergy; occupational problems; photoallergy
allylamines, for onychomycosis, 397
alopecia of fingers, and ionizing radiation, 122, 123
altitude, and sunlight exposure, 4
p-aminobenzoic acid (PABA), 131
   in toiletries, and photoallergy, 51
Aminoxide Ws 35, irritancy testing, 239–45
amiodarone
   metabolite phototoxicity, 63
   phototoxicity, 60

amyldimethylaminobenzoate, phototoxicity, 60
anaesthetics, topical, systemic toxicity, 255
ANAT3D, 105
angelicins, photocarcinogenicity, 294
animals
   in fungal transmission, 377–80
   in heavy metal immunotoxicity testing, 197–200
   for irritancy testing, 190–1, 240, 241
   for phototoxicity testing, 64
   see also marine animal dermatoses
ant stings, 361
Antarctica, ozone depletion over, 11
anthralin, *300*
   in carcinogenesis, 299
antibiotics
   for *Erysipelothrix rhusiopathiae*, 372
   from cutaneous bacteria, 386
   and skin microflora, 387–9
   topical, systemic effects, 250–1
   for *Vibrio* infection, 372
   see also antimicrobial agents, systemic effects
antigen-presenting cell function
   in photocarcinogenesis, 48
   and UV suppression of contact hypersensitivity, 47, 48
antihistamines
   for coelenterate stings, 364
   for solar urticaria, 70
   topical, systemic effects, 251
antimicrobial agents, systemic effects, 251–4
   see also antibiotics; disinfectants, swimming pool, and contact dermatitis
aplasia, bone marrow, after chloramphenicol, 250
aplysiatoxin, *300*
aquatic infections, 370–5
   bacterial, 370–4
   fungal, 374
   viral, 374–5
   see also marine animal dermatoses; swimming pools; water
aquatic sports

contact dermatitis from equipment, 375
   and dermatoses, 375
arachidonic acid, and eicosanoid formation, 303
arachnidisms, 360–1
arsenic toxicity, 253
arthropods, 359–62
   contact reactions, 360
   host invasion, 359–60
   injection of toxins, 360–1
   mouthpart penetration effects, 359
   see also insects
Atrax spider bites, 361
atrazine, 270
   skin vehicle partitioning, 274–5
Australia, skin cancer in
   basal cell carcinoma epidemiology, 19–21
   control programmes, 39–42
   factors in incidence, 39
avobenzene sunscreen, 133
azathioprine, for actinic dermatitis, 69

bacteria, cutaneous
   and antibiotics, 387–9
   antibiotics from, 386
   see also cutaneous microflora
   see also by species name
bacterial infections, aquatic, 370–4
   sea, 371–2
   swimming pools, 372–4
bacteriocins, 386
bacteriostats/bactericides
   toxicity, 251–4
   UVR as, 6
barrier function of epidermis
   and microbial invasion, 385–6
   and percutaneous absorption, 249
   stratum corneum regulation, 283
   see also immunoglobulins in skin protection; microorganisms, cutaneous defence; penetration of skin; percutaneous absorption, factors in; systemic effects of topical drugs; xenobiotic skin penetration

407

basal cell carcinoma (BCC), 319–20
  cryosurgery for, see wound healing, hyaluronic acid and
  epidemiology in Australia, 19–21
  and light exposure, 97–8
  and PUVA therapy, SCC ratio, 294, 295
basal cell naevus syndrome, 98
bath oil, and skin pH, 280, 281
bathing, see swimmer's ear; swimmer's itch; swimming, and sunlight exposure; swimming pools
bed bugs, 361
beetles, secretion reactions, 360
benoxaprofen
  photoproduct phototoxicity, 64
  phototoxicity, 60, 63
benzalkonium, epidermal response, 187
benz[a]pyrene, 270
  activation, 233–7
  carcinogenesis, 169–70, 291
  skin/vehicle partitioning, 274–5
benzathrone, phototoxicity, 60
benzocaine, topical, and methemoglobinemia, 255
benzoyl peroxide, and carcinogenesis, 293–4, 295, 299
black-widow spider venom, 360
Blandford fly, reaction to bite, 361
blastomycosis, 377
blister beetles, secretion reactions, 360
blistering, phototoxic, 61–2
Bloom's syndrome, 71
bone marrow aplasia after chloramphenicol, 250
boric acid toxicity, 251
bot fly myiasis, 359
bromination disinfection, 373
brown spots, facial, 91–6
  biopsy findings, 94, 95
  clinical appearance, 91–52, 92, 93
  diagnostic difficulties, 96
  histology, 92, 93, 94
  and malignant/premalignant skin disease, 95
  roughness, 92, 94
  and solar damage, 94–5
  study methods, 91
bupranolol, plasma levels, 182, 183

c-Ha ras oncogene, and UV irradiation, 33–7
c-myc oncogene, and UV irradiation, 33–7
calcium
  in keratinocyte differentiation, 310
  in water, adverse skin effects, 188, 190
camphor, 253–4
  toxicity, 254
cancer, see basal cell carcinoma (BCC); carcinogenesis, cytochrome P450 in; melanoma; non-melanocytic skin cancer; photocarcinogenesis, immune system in; promotion of skin cancer; proto-oncogene expression, and UV irradiation; skin equivalent culture; squamous cell carcinoma
Candida
  nail infection, 395
  in phototoxicity testing, 63
cantharidin, 360
capacitance of skin, and surfactant, 314–17

capillaroscopic studies
  in erythema quantification, 117–18, 119
  for ionizing radiation studies, 121–3
carbon dioxide, atmospheric increase, 352
  see also global warming
carcinogenesis, cytochrome P450 in, 169–70
  see also photocarcinogenesis, immune system in; promotion of skin cancer
carmustine
  carcinogenesis, 292
  topical, toxicity, 253
cashew nuts/oil sensitivity, 177
Castellani's solution, toxicity, 251, 253
caterpillars, toxic secretions, 360
cats, in ringworm transmission, 378–80
cattle ringworm, 378
'cemetery medals', see brown spots, facial
ceramides in epidermis, 283
  in repair, 185
  as treatment in surfactant study, 283–5
  UV modulation, 207–8
cercarial dermatitis, 370
chemical allergy, photoimmunologic basis, 48–9
chemical contamination, partitioning study, 269–76
  and animal species, 272
  compounds, 270
  and concentration, 270–1
  delipidization effect, 271–2
  and equilibration time, 270, 271
  'membrane'/water partitioning, 273
  partition coefficient determination, 270
  partition coefficients compared, 273–4
  skin preparation, 269–70
  and stratum corneum separation procedure, 272
  variability of measurements, 272–3
  see also irritants; percutaneous absorption, factors in; xenobiotic skin penetration
children, sun effect survey, 43–5
  see also schools
chloracne, and tetrachlorodibenzo-p-dioxin, 247–8
chloramphenicol, topical, systemic effects, 250
chlorine disinfection, 373
chlorofluorocarbons (CFCs)
  and global warming, 352
  and ozone depletion, 11–13
chlorpromazine
  metabolite phototoxicity, 63
  photoallergy, 62
  photosensitization mechanism, 59
  phototoxicity, 60, 61
CHROMA3D for skin colour analysis, 103, 105
chromium, and contact dermatitis, 215–17
chronic actinic dermatitis (CAD), 68–9
  see also actinic prurigo (AP)
chronic discoid lupus erythematosus (CDLE), and welding, 157
cinnamates as photoallergens, 51–2
classification of skin types, and UVB response, 112, 113
climate
  and dermatophytosis, 353–5

  and scabies, 356
  and skin diseases, 356–7, 387
  and streptococcal pyoderma, 355–6
clindamycin
  propionibacterial resistance, 388
  topical, systemic effects, 250
clothing for sun protection, 40
cloud cover, and sunlight exposure, 3–4
coal tar
  carcinogenicity, 169, 291–2, 294–5
  phototoxicity, 60
  systemic effects, 258
  see also dithranol, systemic effects
cobalt, and contact dermatitis, 215–17
Cockayne's syndrome, 71
colitis, pseudomembranous, and clindamycin, 250
collagen metabolism, and UVA, 77–81
colorimetry of skin, 100–3, 149–50
colour of skin, 99–115
  Chroma3D for analysis, 103, 105
  colorimetry, 100–3, 149–50
  and cumulative UVB dose, 113
  early studies, 99–100
  erythema quantification, 112, 117–19
  perception of, 99, 117, 149
  photoprovocation system for, 103, 104
  pigmentation and, 112–13
  reflectance photometric quantification, 150–4
  and skin type classification, 112, 113
  study subjects, 103, 105–6
  UVB dose responses, 106–12
  see also melanins; tanning
commensalism, microflora/human, 385
Compositae
  dermatitis, 52
  sensitization, 177
conjunctivitis from bathing, 375
contact dermatitis, 52
  to diving equipment, 375
  to p-phenylenediamine, 225–30
  to swimming pool disinfectants, 375
  to transition metals, 215–17
  see also allergens; allergy, photoimmunologic basis;cosmetic allergy; occupational problems
contact hypersensitivity, and UV suppression, 47–8
contact urticaria, from plants, 177
conversion, carcinogenic, 297–9
copper algicides, in swimming pools, 373
coproporphyria, hereditary, 70
corals, 363
Cordylobia anthropophaga myiasis, 359
corrosive substance testing
  predictive, 190–1
  in vitro, 192
corticosteroids, topical, systemic toxicity, 258
corynebacteria, antibiotic resistance, 388
cosmetic allergy
  allergens, 175
  products causing, 174–5
  frequency studies, 173–4
  photoallergic ingredients, 51
  transition metals, 216, 217
  see also Euxyl K 400 allergen
cosmetics, 173–6
  definition/purposes, 173

henna/p-phenylenediamine combination toxicity, 254
ingredient labelling, EC, 175–6
transition metals in, 216, 217
croton oil, epidermal response, 187
cryosurgery, 320
for basal cell carcinoma, see wound healing, hyaluronic acid and
sonographic evaluation, 321, 322–3
cutaneous microflora, 385–9, 391
and antibiotics, 387–9
and environmental factors, 387
in microbial invasion defence, 386
resident flora, 385
secretory immunoglobulin coating, 392–3
see also microorganisms, cutaneous defence; percutaneous absorption, factors in
cytochrome P450
cutaneous, 168–70
in xenobiotic metabolism, 167–8, 169–70

daffodil itch, 177
defence against microbial invasion, 385–6, 391
deforestation, and carbon dioxide release, 352
delayed hypersensitivity, and UVB radiation, 49
demethylchlortetracycline, phototoxicity, 61
dental amalgams, 195
dental resin polymerization, and UV exposure, 7
Dermatobia hominis myiasis, 359
dermatitis, see contact dermatitis
dermatophytes
animal hosts, 377
animals in transmission, 377–80
environmental distributions, 381–3
nail infection, 395–6
dermatophytosis incidence, and climate, 353–5
dermatoses from ionizing radiation, 122, 123
see also marine animal dermatoses; photodermatoses
detergents, and stratum corneum permeability, 211
see also sodium lauryl sulphate; surfactants
1,2–dibromo–2,4–dicyanobutan, in Euxyl K 400, 231
diethyltoluamide, toxicity, 254
3,4–dihydroxyphenylalanine(DOPA)– melanin, spectra, 112
dimethylbenzanthracene (DMBA), carcinogenesis
benzoyl peroxide promotion, 293–4
and UVB irradiation, 291–2
dimethylsulphoxide
irritancy test, 204, 205, 206
toxicity, 254
dinitrochlorobenzene (DNCB), 254–5
systemic effects, 255
dinophysistoxin, *301*
dioxin, see tetrachlorodibenzo-p-dioxin (TCDD)

diphenylpyraline hydrochloride, psychotic effects, 251
discotheques, UV exposure in, 8
disinfectants, swimming pool, and contact dermatitis, 375
see also antimicrobial agents, systemic effects
disodium aurothiomalate
immunopathological reactions, 195–6
immunotoxicity assays in mice, 198–9
Disperse Blue 35, phototoxicity, 60
dithranol, systemic effects, 258
see also coal tar
diving equipment, contact dermatitis to, 375
DNA probes, see RNA probes, for proto-oncogene study
dressings, see hydrocolloid dressing testing
drugs, see antibiotics; antihistamines; percutaneous absorption, factors in; photosensitization; photosensitizers; systemic effects of topical agents; topical medications, and non-melanocytic skin cancer; xenobiotic skin penetration
see also *by drug name*
dry skin study, and season, 159–64
dysplasia index, 30–31, *32*
see also photodysplasia

ear damage from neomycin, 251
see also otitis; ototoxicity of gentamicin
echinoderm dermatitis, 364, 366–8
clinical manifestations, 366–7
mode of contamination, 364, 366
treatment, 367–8
eczema, see contact dermatitis
eicosanoids
in carcinogenesis, 299
in tumour promotion, 302–4
in wound response, *306*
elastosis, see actinic elastosis; photoaging
ellagitannins, as cytochrome P450 inhibitors, 170
emollients, urea, 333–7
encephalopathy, toxic, diethyltoluamide-induced, 254
endothelial cell activation, and mast cell degranulation, 125–3
endothelial-leukocyte adhesion molecule–1 (ELAM–1) expression, 125–7
and UV irradiation, 126–7
enteroviruses in swimming pools, 375
enzymes, microbial exo-enzymes, 386
see also cytochrome P450
epicatechins, as cytochrome P450 inhibitors, 170
epidermin, 386
epidermis, response to irritants, 185–7
see also barrier function of epidermis; keratinocyte differentiation; stratum corneum; transepidermal water loss (TEWL)
Epidermophyton infections
and climate, 354
of nails, 395
epinephrine, for coelenterate stings, 364
Erysipelothrix rhusiopathiae, 372
erythema
curves, 99–100

and percussive mechanical trauma, 341–2
quantification, 112, 117–19
UVB provocation study, 103, 104, 106–12
see also sunburn, exaggerated, phototoxic
erythromycin, resistance in acne, 388–9
erythropoietic porphyrias, 70
estrogens, topical, systemic toxicity, 258
2–ethoxy-p-methoxycinnamate, photoallergy, 52
ethyl alcohol, percutaneous intoxication, 255
etretinate, phototoxicity, 63
European Community
on cosmetic labelling, 175–6
on irritant tests, 190–1
Euxyl K 400 allergen, 231–2

factories, UV exposure in, 8
fatty acids, from cutaneous microorganisms, 386
fenticlor, photocontact dermatitis, 53
filaggrin, 309
fire ants, 361
fire extinguishers, halon, and ozone depletion, 11, 12
fish stings, venomous, 368–70
fish involved, 368–9
treatment, 369–70
fish-handler's disease, 372
flaking skin study, and season, 159–64
flies
myiasis, 359
in bacterial infection transmission, 356
florists, occupational dermatitis in, 177
formaldehyde, irritancy testing, 239–45
fossil fuel consumption, 352
Fowler's solution, toxicity, 253
frusemide, phototoxicity, 62
fumaric acid monoethyl ester, percutaneous intoxication, 255
fungal infections, aquatic, 374
see also animals in fungal transmission; bacteria, cutaneous; bacterial infections; cutaneous microflora; dermatophytes; onychomycosis
funnel-web spider bites, 361
furocoumarins, photosensitization mechanism, 59

genital cancer, and PUVA therapy, 294
genophotodermatoses, 71
genotoxicity, skin equivalent model, 233–8
gentamicin
S. aureus resistance, 387
topical, ototoxicity, 250–1
germicidal lamps, 6
global warming
atmospheric gases in, 13, 352–3
environmental effects, 351
and ozone depletion, 13
reason for, 352
UVB skin effects, 351
see also climate
glycine buffer exposure, and skin pH, 279, 281
Goekerman regimen, cancer and, 292

gold
  clinical immunopathology, 195–6
  immunotoxicity assays in mice, 198–9
graft-versus-host disease phototherapy, 49
Granuflex dressing, see hydrocolloid dressing testing
greenhouse effect, see global warming
griseofulvin, for onychomycosis, 396, 397
gynecomastia, topical estrogen-induced, 258

haemolysis, see photohaemolysis
hairdressers, p-phenylenediamine contact dermatitis, 225–30
halons, and ozone depletion, 11, 12
health lamps, 4
heavy metal immunotoxicity, 195–201
  clinical immunopathology, 195, 196
  murine models, 197–200
  see also transition metals, and contact dermatitis; xenobiotics
hemeproteins, see cytochrome P450
Hendersonula toruloidea, nail infection, 395
henna/p-phenylenediamine combination, toxicity, 254
hepatic porphyrias, 70
herpes simplex infection, and UVB radiation, 49
hexachlorophene, 251–2
  toxicity, 252
hexachloroplatinates, immunogenicity assay, 199
histidine test for phototoxicity, 63
4–homosulfanilamide, toxicity, 252
horticulturalists, occupational dermatitis, 177
host defence against microorganisms, 385–6, 391
humidity
  atmospheric, and dry skin, 160, 162, 163
  of skin, and microbial invasion, 385–6
  see also climate; hydration of skin; water
hyaluronic acid, see wound healing, hyaluronic acid and
hybridization studies, for proto-oncogenes, 34
hydration of skin
  and surfactant exposure, 313–18
  and thermal water exposure, 333–7
  see also humidity; natural moisturizing factors (NMF); water
hydroa vacciniforme, 70
hydrochlorofluorocarbons (HCFCs), 13
hydrocolloid dressing testing, 399–405
  chemical challenge procedure, 399–400
  chemical challenge results, 400, *402–5*
  microbial challenge procedure, 399, 400, *401*
  microbial challenge results, 400, 405
hydrofluorocarbons (HFCs), 13
hydrotherapy, see thermal spa water exposure, and skin hydration
Hylesia moths, toxic secretions, 360
Hymenoptera
  antigens in venom, 361
  stings, 360

hypersensitivity
  to arthropod bites, 361
  contact, and UV suppression, 47–8
  delayed, and UVB irradiation, 49
hypochloride contact dermatitis, 373
hypotension, from fish venom, 370

immediate pigment darkening (IPD) in sunscreen evaluation, 133
immune system, UV radiation and, 47–50
  and contact hypersensitivity, 47–8
  and photodermatoses, 48–9
  and phototherapy, 49
  research needs, 49–50
  and skin cancer, 48
immunoglobulins, secretory, 391–3
  coating of cutaneous symbionts, 392–3
  skin surface secretion, 391–2
immunological photodermatoses, see photodermatoses
immunotoxicity, see heavy metal immunotoxicity
impetigo, and climate, 387
insecticides, topical, systemic effects, 256
insects
  and streptococcal pyoderma, 356
  UV traps, and UV exposure, 7–8
  see also arthropods
intercellular adhesion molecule–1 (ICAM–1) expression, 126
interleukin–4, in mercury immunopathology, 198
iodine, 252
  swimming pool disinfection, 373
ionizing radiation exposure, 121–3
irritant testing, 239–45
  in vitro, 191–2
  predictive, 190–1
  procedures, 203–4
irritants, 185–93
  adaptation to, 185
  arthropod secretions, 360
  cold dry wind, 188, *189*
  epidermal responses, 185–7
  factors affecting irritancy, 219
  hard water, 188, 190
  response, and application area, 219–23
  and UV irradiation, skin response study, 203–7, 208
  see also allergens; chemical contamination, partitioning study; detergents, and stratum corneum permeability; pentachlorophenol-induced urticaria; surfactant damage treatment study; xenobiotic skin penetration
isotretinoin for acne, and antibiotic resistance, 388
itraconazole for onychomycosis, 397
Ivy Shield efficacy study, 265–8
  see also Rhus dermatitis
Ixodes ricinus, reaction to mouthparts, 359

jellyfish, 363
  stings, *365*, *366*

Kathon CG, irritancy testing, 239–45

keratinocyte differentiation, 309
  protein kinase C in, 309–11
keratins, 309
keratoses, see photokeratosis in welders; solar keratoses
ketoconazole for onychomycosis, 396–7
ketoprofen phototoxicity, 63

labelling studies, for proto-oncogenes, 34
'Lab' system of colour representation, 103
laboratories, UV exposure in, 7
lactoferrin, 386
latitude (geographical), and sunlight exposure, 3
latrodectism, 360
legislation on photosensitizers, 63
Leishmania infection, and UVB radiation, 49
leukocytes
  in epidermal repair, 187
  migration, and endothelial cell activation, 125
leukopenia, silver sulfadiazine-induced, 253
lidocaine, topical, systemic effects, 255
lighting, general, and UV exposure, 8
lily rash, 177
lindane, topical, systemic toxicity, 256
lipids in stratum corneum, 283, 285
  delipidization, and chemical partitioning, 271–2
  and permeability, 211, 212, 214
  and thermal spa water exposure, 333–7
  UV modulation study, 204, 207–8
8–lipoxygenase in tumour promotion, 302–3
'liver spots', see brown spots, facial
lomustine (CCNU), carcinogenesis, 292
loricrin, 309
louse infection, hypersensitivity reaction, 361
loxoscelism, 360–1
lupus erythematosus, photoimmunologic basis, 49
  see also subacute cutaneous lupus erythematosus (SCLE), and occupational UV exposure
lyngbyatoxin, *300*
lysozyme, 386
Lytta vesicatoria, secretion reactions, 360

macrolide lincosamide streptogramin B (MLS), 387
macules, pigmented, see brown spots, facial
major histocompatibility complex (MHC), in mercury pathology, 198, 199
malathion, topical, 256
marine animal dermatoses, 363–70
  coelenterate stings/wounds, 363–4
  echinoderm dermatitis, 364, 366–8
  fish stings, venomous, 368–70
  swimmer's itch, 370
  see also aquatic infections; swimming pools; water
mast cell degranulation, 125–9
mechanical trauma, see percussive mechanical trauma; vibration trauma; wound healing, hyaluronic acid and; wound response

Mediterranean, *see* marine animal dermatoses
melanins
  colorimetric quantification, 149–50
  and erythema quantification, 112
  reflectance photometric meter, 150–4
  spectral characteristics, 112–13
  and UVR immune suppression, 49–50
  see also colour of skin; tanning
melanoma
  epidemiology, 15
  risk factors, 15–18
  see also brown spots, facial; non-melanocytic skin cancer NMSC); solar keratoses
mercury
  clinical immunopathology, 195, 196
  immunotoxicity assays, 197–8
  in topical medicines, systemic effects, 256
metals, *see* heavy metal immunotoxicity;transition metals, and allergic contact dermatitis
methane, atmospheric increase, 352–3
5–methoxypsoralen, government regulation, 63
8–methoxypsoralen, photosensitization skin cancer, 59
methoxypsoralens, carcinogenicity, 294
  see also psoralen, photosensitivity blistering reaction; PUVA therapy
methylnitrosurea (MNU), carcinogenesis, 292
N-methylpyrrolidone, skin penetration enhancer, 182
mezerein, carcinogenesis promoter, 297, *298*
microorganisms, cutaneous defence, 385–6, 391
  see also bacteria; barrier function of skin; cutaneous microflora; fungal infections; immunoglobulins in skin protection; penetration of skin
  see also by species name
Microsporum gypseum, 377
Microsporum spp
  animal hosts, 377
  animals in transmission, 377–80
  environmental distribution survey, 382–3
millipedes, defensive secretions, 360
modelling of xenobiotic skin penetration, 180–4
molluscum contagiosum, in swimmers, 374
monobenzone, topical, systemic effects, 256
monoclonal antibodies, in cytochrome 450 phenotyping, 168–9
Montreal Convention on CFC reduction, 11–12
mosquitoes
  feeding, 359
  sensitization to saliva, 361
moths, toxic secretions, 360
moulds, nail infection, 395
mouse tail test for phototoxicity, 64
mupirocin, resistance to, 387
Musca domestica, in infection transmission, 356

musk ambrette photoallergy, 51, 62
  new cases, 53
  presentation, 52
Mycobacterium marinum infection, 373, *374*
myiasis, 359

naevi, *see* brown spots, facial
nails, *see also* onychomycosis
nalidixic acid, phototoxicity, 62
2–naphthol, topical, 256
natural moisturizing factors (NMF), and surfactants, 283
  in surfactant damage study, 283–5
necrotic cutaneous loxoscelism, 360–1
neomycin, and ear damage, 251
nephrotic syndrome, topical mercury-induced, 256
neutrophils, in epidermal repair, 187
  see also leukocytes
nevi, *see* brown spots, facial
nickel, and contact dermatitis, 215–17
nitrogen mustards, carcinogenicity, 292–3, 295
nitrogen rash in divers, 375
nitrosureas, carcinogenicity, 292, 295
nitrous oxide, atmospheric increase, 353
non-melanocytic skin cancer (NMSC)
  epidemiology in Australia, 19–21
  and topical medications, 291–5
  see also melanoma
nonanoic acid, epidermal response, 187

oak, *see* Rhus dermatitis
occlusion
  by clothing, and dermatophytosis, 354–5
  of topical drugs, and absorption, 249
occupational problems
  plants, dermatitis from, 177–8
  platinum-related diseases, 196
  from UV exposure, 6–8, 155–8
  see also percussive mechanical trauma;visual display units, and facial rashes
ochronosis, phenol-induced, 252
oestrogens, topical, systemic toxicity, 258
offices, UV exposure in, 8
okadaic acid, *301*
oncogenes, *see* proto-oncogene expression, and UV irradiation
onychomycosis, 395–8
  dermatophyte environmental control, 396
  dermatophyte species, 395
  dermatophytosis prevalence, 395–6
  treatment, 396–7
  yeast/mould infections, 395
otitis, swimmer's ear, 373–4
ototoxicity of gentamicin, 250–1
ozone depletion, 11–12
  chlorofluorocarbons in, 352

palytoxin, *301*
partitioning, chemicals in skin, *see* chemical contamination, partitioning study
patch testing, *see* photopatch testing
pederin, 360
Pelagia nocticula, 363

penetration of skin
  by radiation, and wavelength, 105
  by sodium lauryl sulphate in vitro, 211–17
  see also barrier function of epidermis; microorganisms, cutaneous defence; percutaneous absorption, factors in; systemic effects of topical drugs; xenobiotic skin penetration
pentachlorophenol-induced urticaria, 287–9
pentyloxyphenol, skin vehicle partitioning study, 270–5
percussive mechanical trauma, 339–48
  experimental, 339–42
  workplace monitoring, 343–7
  see also wound healing, hyaluronic acid and; wound response
percutaneous absorption, factors in, 249–50
  see also barrier function of epidermis; penetration of skin; systemic effects of topical agents; xenobiotic skin penetration
pesticides
  experimentation problems, 179
  penetration modelling, 182, 183
pH of skin
  and microbial invasion, 386
  and model solution exposure, 277–81
phenol toxicity, 252
  in Castellani's solution, 251
phenols, partitioning study, 270–5
  and animal species, 272
  and concentration, 270–1
  and delipidization, 271–2
  and equilibration time, 270, *271*
  'membrane'/water partitioning, 273
  and stratum corneum separation procedure, 272
  variability of measurements, 272–3
2–phenoxyethanol
  in cosmetics, 232
  in Euxyl K 400, 231
p-phenylenediamine
  contact dermatitis, 225–30
  henna combination, toxicity, 254
phorbol ester, carcinogenesis promoter, 297, *298*
phospholipase A2 activation, and tumour promotion, 303–4
photoaging, 77
  see also actinic elastosis; brown spots, facial; collagen metabolism, and UVA
photoallergens, 51–5
  dermatitis diagnosis, 52–3
  exposure variation, temporal/geographical, 53
  photopatch testing for, 52–5
  in sunscreens, 51–2
  in toiletries, 51
photoallergy, 57, 59, 62
  mechanisms, 59
  photoimmunologic basis, 48–9
photocarcinogenesis, immune system in, 48
photodermatoses, 67–72
  actinic prurigo, 68

photodermatoses (cont'd)
  chronic actinic dermatitis, 68–9
  from photosensitizers, 71
  genophotodermatoses, 71
  hydroa vacciniforme, 70
  immune system in, 48–9
  listed, 67
  polymorphic light eruption, 67–68
  porphyrias, 70
  solar urticaria, 69–70
  UVR-exacerbated, 71
photodysplasia, 27–32
  quantification of, 28–31, 32
  therapeutic approaches, 31
  see also solar keratoses
photography, UV, and UV exposure, 7
photohaemolysis
  assay, in thiazide/UV study, 73–4
  in phototoxicity testing, 63
photoimmunology, see immune system, UV radiation and
photokeratosis in welders, 7
  see also solar keratoses
photopatch testing, 52–5
  procedure, 54
  results interpretation, 54–5
  standard light series, 53, 54
  UVA dose, 53–4
  UVA source, 54
photosensitivity diseases, 131
  see also hypersensitivity; photodermatoses
photosensitization, 57–59
  clinical reactions in, 71
  mechanisms, 57–9
  photoallergy, 48–9, 57, 59, 62
  see also phototoxicity; sensitization to arthropod bites
photosensitizers, 59–60, 131
  regulation, 63
  testing, 63–4
phototherapy, 5
  development, 100
  and immune function, 49
  and UV exposure of staff, 7
  see also PUVA therapy
phototoxicity, 60–2
  blistering, 61–2
  exaggerated sunburn, 61
  prickling/burning, 60–1
  skin fragility, 62
  sunscreen protection factors, 133
  testing, 63–4
  thiazide study, 73–6
Physalis physalis, 363
  sting, 364
phytophotodermatitis, 61–2
pigmentation, see brown spots, facial; colour of skin; melanins; tanning
pitch, phototoxicity, 60
Pityriasis versicolor infection, 374
plankton, and global warming, 13
plants
  Compositae, 52, 177
  occupational dermatitis from, 177–8
  phytophotodermatitis, 61–2
  see also animals; Rhus dermatitis
platinum
  clinical immunopathology, 196
  immunotoxicity assays, 199

podophyllum, toxicity, 256–7
poison oak/ivy, see Rhus dermatitis
  see also Ivy Shield efficacy study
polychlorinated biphenyls, 270
  skin/vehicle partitioning, 273–4
polymorphic light eruption (PLE), 67–68
popliteal lymph node (PLN) assay, 197, 199
  of gold, 198–9
  of platinum, 199
porphyrias, 70
  cutanea tarda, 62, 70
  turcica, 60
  see also 'pseudoporphyria', drug-induced
porphyrin metabolites, as photosensitizers, 60
portuguese man of war, 363
povidone iodine, 252
precocity, oestrogen-induced, 258
primula allergy, 177
profilometry, for macule study, 92, 94, 96
promethazine toxicity, 251
promotion of skin cancer, 297–307
  agents, 299, 300–1, 302
  eicosanoids in, 302–4
  multistage carcinogenesis model, 297–9
  protein kinase C in, 299, 302–304
  and wound response, 306
Propionibacteria cutaneous, 385
  antibiotic resistance, 387, 388
propylene glycol
  epidermal response, 187
  as skin penetration enhancer, 182
prostaglandins, in tumour promotion, 302
protein kinase C
  activation, 309
  in cancer promotion, 299, 302–304
  isoforms, 299, 309
  in keratinocyte differentiation, 309–11, 309–12
proto-oncogene expression, and UV irradiation, 33–8
pseudomembranous colitis after clindamycin therapy, 250
Pseudomonas aeruginosa
  in hydrocolloid dressing testing, 400, 405
  infection from swimming pools, 372–3
'pseudoporphyria', drug-induced, 62
psoralen photosensitivity, blistering reaction, 61–2
  see also 5–methoxypsoralen, government regulation; 8–methoxypsoralen, photosensitization skin cancer; methoxypsoralens, carcinogenicity; PUVA therapy
psychosis, and diphenylpyraline hydrochloride, 251
puberty, pseudoprecocious, oestrogen-induced, 258
public health programmes, skin cancer in Australia, 39–42
public transport, dermatophyte survey, 381–3
PUVA therapy, 5–6
  and carcinogenesis, 294, 295
  immunologic basis, 49
  and 8–methoxypsoralen

photosensitization, 59
  and nitrogen mustard carcinogenesis, 293
  for photodermatoses, 68, 69
pyoderma, streptococcal, and climate, 355–6

quaternary ammonium algicides, 373
quinozaline-n-dioxide, photoallergy, 62

rabbit irritation tests, 190–1
  splenocyte migration activity, 240, 241
resorcinol, toxicity, 252–3
Retin-A, and photocarcinogenesis, 293, 295
Rhus dermatitis, 177, 265
  barrier cream efficacy study, 265–8
ringworm fungi, see dermatophytes
RNA probes, for proto-oncogene study, 33
Rolipram, delivery system, 184
Rothmund-Thomson syndrome, 71
rove beetles, secretions, 360
rubber dermatitis, 375

Sagartia, 363
salicylanilides, halogenated
  photoallergy, 62
  photosensitivity, 51, 53
salicylic acid, toxicity, 257
scabies, and climate, 356
schools
  Australian, cancer control programmes, 40
  dermatophyte survey, 381–3
  see also children, sun effect survey
Scopulariopsis brevicaulis, nail infection, 395
scorpion stings, 361
screening programmes for skin cancer, 41–2
screw worms, myiasis, 359
sea, see marine animal dermatoses
sea anemone, 363
sea urchins, dermatitis
  clinical manifestations, 366–7
  mode of contamination, 364, 366
  treatment, 367–8
seabather's eruption, 370
season
  dry skin and, 159–64
  and sunlight exposure, 3
selenium sulfide toxicity, 257
sensitization, to arthropod bites, 361
  see also hypersensitivity; photosensitization
Seveso chemical accident, 247–8
sex hormones, topical, systemic toxicity, 258
shampoos, animal toxicity testing, 241, 244
shrimp-picker's disease, 372
silver nitrate, toxicity, 257
silver sulfadiazine, toxicity, 253
Simulium posticatum, reaction to bite, 361
skin equivalent culture
  as genotoxicity model, 233–8
  for irritant testing, 192
skin surface water loss (SSWL), and surfactant, 314–18
  see also transepidermal water loss (TEWL)

snow reflectance, 4
soaps, bacteriostats in, and photoallergy, 51, 53, 62
sodium bicarbonate buffer, and skin pH, 277, 278, 281
sodium hydroxide
    epidermal response, 187
    irritancy test, 203, 204–5
sodium lauryl sulphate
    epidermal response, 187
    in vitro penetration study, 211–17
    irritancy testing, 204, 205–7, 219–23, 239–45
    in stratum corneum hydration study, 313–17
    in surfactant damage treatment study, 283–5
solar keratoses
    transformation to SCC, in Australia, 20
    Welsh study, 23–6
    see also melanoma, malignant; photodysplasia; photokeratosis in welders
solar urticaria, 69–70
solaria, 4
Solenopsis richteri stings, 361
sonography, see ultrasonography
spa water
    and bacterial infections, 373
    disinfection, 373
    thermal, and skin hydration, 333–7
spectral characteristics of skin, 100
    melanins, 112–13
    and UVA exposure, 113
SPF factors of sunscreens, 40
    determination/testing, 132
sphingolipids in stratum corneum, 285
    see also ceramides
sphingosine, and epidermal proliferation, 185–6
spider bites, 360–1
splenocyte migration activity test, 240, 241
sponge fisherman's disease, 363
sports
    aquatic
        contact dermatitis from equipment, 375
        and dermatoses, 375
    and Australian cancer control programmes, 40
squamous cell carcinoma
    epidemiology in Australia, 19–21
    and PUVA therapy, 294, 295
staphylococci
    antibiotic resistance, 387, 388
    colonization, and skin cracking, 387
    cutaneous immunoglobulins on, 392
    in hydrocolloid dressing testing, 400, 405
    infection, and climate, 355, 356
stargazers (fish), 369
    wound treatment, 369–70
staurosporine, 301
    and keratinocyte differentiation, 310–11
STELLA, for penetration modelling, 182
sterilization (bacterial) by UVR, 6
steroids, topical, systemic toxicity, 258
stingray wounds, 368
    treatment, 369–70

stings
    of coelenterates, 363–4
    of fish, 368–70
    see also arthropods
stratum corneum
    barrier function regulation, 283
    integrity, and percutaneous absorption, 249
    structure, and permeability, 211
    and surfactants, 283–5, 313–18
    UV irradiation response study, 203–4, 207–8
    in xenobiotic penetration modelling, 180–3
    see also epidermis, response to irritants; keratinocyte differentiation; lipids in stratum corneum
streptococcal pyoderma, and climate, 355–6
stress, and rashes in VDU operators, 147–8
stroma formation in carcinogenesis, 299
subacute cutaneous lupus erythematosus (SCLE), and UV exposure, 155–8
sulphadiazine, silver, toxicity, 253
sulphamylon, toxicity, 252
sulphanilamide, photoallergy, 62
sulphonamide
    absorption, and silver sulfadiazine, 253
    toxicity, 252
sulphur water, see thermal water exposure, and skin hydration
sunbeds, and UV exposure of staff, 8
sunburn, exaggerated, phototoxic, 61
    see also erythema
sunlamps, 4
sunlight exposure, 3–4
    children's knowledge survey, 43–5
    and melanoma risk, 15–18
    prolonged, 27
    sunbathing, 4
    see also photodysplasia; solar keratoses; tanning
sunscreens, 131–5, 137
    adverse reactions, 51, 53, 62
    compounds used, 131–2, 134
    ideal, 135
    photoallergens in, 51–2
    phototoxic protection factor, 133
    recommendations, 40
    SPF factors, 40, 132
    titanium dioxide, microfine, 139–42
    titanium dioxide, pigmentary, 137–8
    transmission protection factors, 133
    usage study, Wales, 25
    UVA protection, 132–3
suntan, as cancer prevention target, 40–1
    see also tanning
suppressor T lymphocytes, in photocarcinogenesis, 48
surfactants
    damage treatment study, 283–5
    and stratum corneum hydration, 313–18
    see also detergents, and stratum corneum permeability
sweat, antimicrobial compounds in, 386
swimmer's ear, 373–4
swimmer's itch, 370
swimming, and sunlight exposure, 4
swimming pools
    bacterial infections, 372–4

disinfectants, and contact dermatitis, 375
and fungal infection of nails, 395, 396, 397
and viral infections, 374–5
see also marine animal dermatoses
systemic effects of topical agents, 250–8
    anaesthetics, 255
    antibiotics, 250–1
    antihistamines, 251
    antimicrobial agents, 251–4
    cosmetic agents, 254
    diethyltoluamide, 254
    dimethyl sulfoxide, 254
    dinitrochlorobenzene, 254–5
    ethyl alcohol, 255
    fumaric acid monoethyl ester, 255
    insecticides, 256
    mercurials, 256
    monobenzone, 256
    2-naphthol, 256
    podophyllum, 256–7
    salicylic acid, 257
    selenium sulfide, 257
    silver nitrate, 257
    steroids, 258
    tars, 258
    see also penetration of skin; percutaneous absorption, factors in; topical medications, and non-melanocytic skin cancer; xenobiotic skin penetration

T helper cells, in mercury immunopathology, 198, 199
    see also suppressor T lymphocytes, in photocarcinogenesis
tannic acid, as cytochrome P450 inhibitor, 170
tanning
    equipment, 4–5
    and erythema quantification, 112
    suntan, as cancer prevention target, 40–1
    see also melanins
tar, see coal tar
teleocidin B, 300
terbinafine, for onychomycosis, 397
tetrachlorodibenzo-p-dioxin (TCDD), cutaneous manifestations, 247–8
3,4',5',5-tetrachlorosalicylanilide (TCSA) photoallergy, 62
tetracyclines
    phototoxicity, 61
    resistance to, in acne, 388–9
    see also chlorpromazine
12-O-tetradecanoylphorbol-13-acetate
    carcinogenesis promoter, 297, 298, 300
    and keratinocyte differentiation, 310
    protein kinase C activation, 304, 309
thapsigargin, 301
    in carcinogenesis, 299
thermal spa water exposure, and skin hydration, 333–7
thiazide phototoxicity study, 73–6
ticks, reaction to mouthparts, 359
tinea infection, 374
    and climate, 353–5
tioconazole lotion, for onychomycosis, 397

titanium dioxide sunscreens, 137–42
  microfine, 139–42
  pigmentary, 137–8
TNF, see tumour necrosis factor-α (TNFα)
tobacco irritation/sensitization, 177
toothpastes, toxicity testing, 241, 245
topical medications, and non-melanocytic skin cancer, 291–5
  see also penetration of skin; percutaneous absorption; systemic effects of topical agents; xenobiotics; xenobiotic skin penetration
TPA, see 12-O-tetradecanoylphorbol-13-acetate
transepidermal water loss (TEWL)
  and percussive trauma, 341–2
  as repair stimulus, 185, 186
  in surfactant damage study, 283–5
  see also skin surface water loss (SSWL)
transferrin, 386
transforming growth factors in carcinogenesis, 299
transition metals, and contact dermatitis, 215–17
  see also heavy metal immunotoxicity
transport vehicles, dermatophyte survey, 381–3
trauma
  from arthropod mouthparts, 359
  vibration, 339
  see also percussive mechanical trauma; wound healing, hyaluronic acid and; wound response
1,1,1-trichloro-2,2-bis(p-chlorophenyl)ethane (DDT), 270
  skin/vehicle partitioning, 273–4
trichlorocarbanilide (TCC), percutaneous absorption, 253
Trichophyton infections
  and climate, 354
  of nails, 395
Trichophyton species, distribution survey, 382–3
Trichophyton verrucosum
  hosts, 377
  transmission, 378
triclocarban, percutaneous absorption, 253
tsetse flies, feeding, 359
tulip sensitization, 177
tumbu fly myiasis, 359
tumour necrosis factor-α (TNFα)

in collagen metabolism/UVA study, 77, 79, 81
  and mast cell degranulation, 126, 127
Tween 20, and stratum corneum hydration, 316, *317*

ultrasonography
  in elastosis, 84–90
  equipment, 83, 84, 322–3
  for wound healing, 321, 323
Umbilliferae phytophotodermatitis, 61–2
United Nations Environment Programme (UNEP), on ozone depletion, 11
urea emollients, and hydration/lipids, 333–7
urticaria
  contact, from plants, 177
  pentachlorophenol-induced, 287–9
  photoimmunologic basis, 48
  solar, 69–70

vaccination, UV exposure, 49
variegate porphyria, 70
vascular cell adhesion molecule-1 (VCAM-1) expression, 126
VDUs, see visual display units, and facial rashes
vehicles (for topical agents), and percutaneous absorption, 249–50
venom
  of arthropods, 360
  of coelenterates, 363–4
  of sea urchins, 364, 366
  of fish, 368–70
vesicating arthropods, 360
vibration trauma, 339
Vibrios, 371–2
Vienna Convention for the Protection of the Ozone Layer, 11
viral infections, aquatic, 374–5
viscerocutaneous loxoscelism, 361
visual analogue scale (VAS) scoring, for photodysplasia, 29–30, *32*
visual display units, and facial rashes
  prevalence study, 143–5
  psychophysiological study, 147–8
vitiligo, and monobenzone systemic effects, 256

warts, plantar, 374
water
  as irritant, hard water, 188, 190
  skin exposure, and pH, 280, 281
  UV transmission, 4

  see also aquatic infections; humidity; marine animal dermatoses; skin surface water loss (SSWL); swimming pools; thermal water exposure, and skin hydration; transepidermal water loss (TEWL)
weaverfish wounds, 368, *369*
  treatment, 369–70
welder's flash, 7
welding, and UV exposure, 6–7, 157
white finger, 339
Wilkinson's triangle, 51
wind, as irritant, 188, *189*
wood preservatives, pentachlorophenol, and urticaria, 287–9
Wood's lamp, 5, 7
wound healing, hyaluronic acid and, 319, 321–31
  BCC/cryolesion data, 323, 326, 329
  before/after illustrations, *324–5*
  healing time, 326, *327–8*
  mode of action, 330
  patients, 321, 323
  sonographic evaluation, 322–3
  treatment method, 322
  see also percussive mechanical trauma
wound response, 299, 302–4
  and tumour promotion, *306*
  wound hormone cascade, 302
  wound hormones, 299
wounds, of coelenterates, 363–4
  see also hydrocolloid dressing testing; trauma

X-rays, see ionizing radiation exposure
xenobiotic metabolism, cytochrome P450 in, 167–8
  cutaneous, 169–70
xenobiotic skin penetration, 179–84
  mathematical models, 180–4
  in vitro determination, 179–80, 184
  in vivo experimentation, 179, 184
  see also allergens; barrier function of epidermis; chemical contamination, partitioning study; cosmetic allergy; heavy metal immunotoxicity; irritants; percutaneous absorption, factors in; systemic effects of topical agents; topical medications, and non-melanocytic skin cancer
xeroderma pigmentosum, 71

yeast infection of nails, 395